Myocardial Viability:
A Clinical and Scientific Treatise

Edited by

Vasken Dilsizian, M.D.

Director of Nuclear Cardiology
National Institutes of Health, Bethesda, Maryland
Adjunct Professor of Medicine
Georgetown University School of Medicine and
The George Washington University School of Medicine
and Health Services, Washington, DC

Futura Publishing
Company, Inc.
Armonk, NY

Library of Congress Cataloging-in-Publication Data

Myocardial viability: a clinical and scientific treatise/edited by
  Vasken Dilsizian.
      p. cm.
    Includes bibliographical references and index.
    ISBN 0-87993-437-9 (alk. paper)
    1. Myocardium—Physiology. 2. Myocardium—Patho-
physiology.   3. Coronary heart disease—Pathophysiology.
4. Myocardial revascularization.   I. Dilsizian, Vasken.
    [DNLM: 1. Myocardium—pathology. 2. Heart Function
Tests. 3. Myocardial Diseases—physiopathology.
4. Myocardial Ischemia—physiopathology. 5. Ventricular
Function, Left—physiology.   WG 280 M99687 1999]
QP113.2.M95 1999
616.1′207 21—dc21

                                            99-039509

Copyright © 2000
Futura Publishing Company, Inc.

Published by
Futura Publishing Company, Inc.
135 Bedford Road
Armonk, NY 10504-1937

ISBN# 0-87993-437-9

Printed in the United States of America.
This book is printed on acid-free paper.

Dedication

This book is dedicated to my wife,
Madeline (Maddy) Erario, MD.
Her sustained love, devotion, and
encouragement made this endeavor possible.

Contents

Contributors vii

Preface ix

Part I. Introduction

Chapter 1. Perspectives on the Study of Human Myocardium: Viability
Vasken Dilsizian, MD 3

Part II. Basic Concepts and Mechanisms

Chapter 2. Modulation of Responses to Myocardial Ischemia: Metabolic
Features of Myocardial Stunning, Hibernation, and Ischemic
Preconditioning   Heinrich Taegtmeyer, MD, DPhil 25

Chapter 3. Reversible Myocardial Dysfunction: Stunning, Hibernation,
or What?   Francis J. Klocke, MD, Andrew J. Sherman, MD,
and Ada Jain, MD 37

Chapter 4. Preconditioning   James M. Downey, PhD and
Michael V. Cohen, MD 55

Part III. Vascular Biology and Cellular Physiology

Chapter 5. Experimental Models Useful in Evaluating Myocardial
Viability   James T. Willerson, MD and H. Vernon Anderson, MD 79

Chapter 6. Essential Fuels for the Heart and Mechanical Restitution
Heinrich Taegtmeyer, MD, DPhil and Raymond R. Russell III, MD, PhD 91

Chapter 7. Nitric Oxide and Energetics of the Heart: Physiology and
Pathophysiology   Joanne S. Ingwall, PhD 105

Chapter 8. Channels, Ischemia, and Stunning: Cellular Electrophysiology
and Intercellular Communication   Marc Ovadia, MD and
Peter R. Brink, PhD 115

Part IV. Advances in Functional Imaging

Chapter 9. New Methods for Measurement of Regional and Global
Ventricular Function   Stephen L. Bacharach, PhD 163

Chapter 10. Myocardial Contractile Reserve   Vera H. Rigolin, MD and
Robert O. Bonow, MD 181

Chapter 11. Morphological and Echocardiographic Features of Viable
and Nonviable Myocardium   Jamshid Shirani, MD, Madhulika Chandra, MD,
and Edmund H. Sonnenblick, MD 207

Chapter 12. Timing and Myocardial Salvage: Lessons Learned From the
Thrombolytic and Revascularization Multicenter Trials
Thomas J. Ryan, MD 233

Part V. Perfusion, Metabolism, and Cell Membrane Integrity

Chapter 13. Introduction to Tracer Kinetics
Stephen L. Bacharach, PhD. 251

Chapter 14. Thallium-201 Scintigraphy: Experience of Two Decades
Vasken Dilsizian, MD. 265

Chapter 15. Technetium-99m–Labeled Myocardial Perfusion Tracers:
Blood Flow or Viability Agents? Vasken Dilsizian, MD 315

Chapter 16. Myocardial Imaging of Lipid Metabolism with Labeled
Fatty Acids Ludwig E. Feinendegen, MD 349

Chapter 17. Positron Emission Tomography for the Assessment of
Myocardial Viability: Noninvasive Approach to Cardiac Pathophysiology
Heiko Schöder, MD and Heinrich R. Schelbert, MD, PhD 391

Chapter 18. Nuclear Magnetic Resonance and Myocardial Viability
William J. Thoma, PhD, Mark A. Lawson, MD, William T. Evanochko, PhD,
and Gerald M. Pohost, MD. 419

Index 437

Contributors

H. Vernon Anderson, MD   Professor of Medicine, University of Texas-Houston Medical School, Houston, Texas

Stephen L. Bacharach, PhD   Head, Imaging Science Group, Clinical Center, National Institutes of Health, Bethesda, Maryland

Robert O. Bonow, MD   Goldberg Distinguished Professor of Medicine, Chief, Division of Cardiology, Northwestern Medical School, Chicago, Illinois

Peter R. Brink, PhD   Department of Physiology & Biophysics, and the Institute for Molecular Cardiology, School of Medicine, State University of New York at Stonybrook, Stonybrook, New York

Madhulika Chandra, MD   Research Fellow, Division of Cardiology, Albert Einstein College of Medicine, Bronx, New York

Michael V. Cohen, MD   Professor of Medicine, Division of Cardiology, College of Medicine, University of South Alabama, Mobile, Alabama

Vasken Dilsizian, MD   Director of Nuclear Cardiology, National Institutes of Health, Bethesda, Maryland, Adjunct Professor of Medicine and Radiology, Georgetown University School of Medicine, Adjunct Professor of Medicine, The George Washington University School of Medicine and Health Sciences, Washington, DC

James M. Downey, PhD   Professor of Physiology, Department of Physiology, College of Medicine, University of South Alabama, Mobile, Alabama

William T. Evanochko, PhD   Associate Professor of Medicine, Division of Cardiovascular Disease, The University of Alabama at Birmingham, School of Medicine/Department of Medicine, Birmingham, Alabama

Ludwig E. Feinendegen, MD   Fogarty Scholar, Department of Nuclear Medicine, Clinical Center, National Institutes of Health, Bethesda, Maryland, Emeritus Professor of Nuclear Medicine, Heinrich-Heine University of Dusseldorf, Dusseldorf, Germany

Joanne S. Ingwall, PhD   Professor of Medicine (Physiology), NMR Laboratory for Physiological Chemistry, Cardiovascular Division, Brigham & Women's Hospital and Harvard Medical School, Boston, Massachusetts

Ada Jain, MD   Summer Research Fellow, Feinberg Cardiovascular Research Institute, Northwestern University Medical School, Chicago, Illinois

Francis J. Klocke, MD   Director, Feinberg Cardiovascular Research Institute, Division of Cardiology, Department of Medicine and Department of Surgery, Professor of Medicine, Northwestern University Medical School, Chicago, Illinois

Mark A. Lawson, MD   Fellow, Division of Cardiovascular Disease, The University of Alabama at Birmingham, School of Medicine/Department of Medicine, Birmingham, Alabama

Marc Ovadia, MD   Assistant Professor of Pediatrics (Cardiology), Cornell Medical College, Boas Marks Biomedical Research Facility, Manhasset, New York

Gerald M. Pohost, MD   Mary Gertrude Waters Chair in Cardiovascular Medicine, Professor of Medicine and Radiology, Division of Cardiovascular Disease, The University of Alabama at Birmingham, School of Medicine/Department of Medicine, Birmingham, Alabama

Vera H. Rigolin, MD   Assistant Professor of Medicine, Division of Cardiology, Northwestern University, Chicago, Illinois

Raymond R. Russell III, MD   Yale University School of Medicine, New Haven, Connecticut

Thomas J. Ryan, MD   Professor of Medicine, Department of Cardiology, Boston University School of Medicine, Boston, Massachusetts

Heinrich R. Schelbert, MD, PhD   Professor of Pharmacology and Radiological Sciences, Department of Molecular and Medical Pharmacology, UCLA School of Medicine, Los Angeles, California

Heiko Schöder, MD   Ahmanson Biological Imaging Clinic, Nuclear Medicine UCLA School of Medicine, CHS, Los Angeles, California

Andrew J. Sherman, MD   Research Fellow of the Thoracic Surgery Foundation for Research and Education, Feinberg Cardiovascular Research Institute, Northwestern University Medical School, Chicago, Illinois

Jamshid Shirani, MD   Associate Professor of Clinical Medicine and Pathology, Albert Einstein College of Medicine, Division of Cardiology, Bronx, New York

Edmund H. Sonnenblick, MD   Edmond J. Safra Professor of Medicine, Albert Einstein College of Medicine, Division of Cardiology, Bronx, New York

Heinrich Taegtmeyer, MD, DPhil   Professor of Medicine, Co-Director, Division of Cardiology, The University of Texas Houston Medical School, Houston, Texas

William J. Thoma, PhD   Instructor, Division of Cardiovascular Disease, The University of Alabama at Birmingham, School of Medicine/Department of Medicine, Birmingham, Alabama

James T. Willerson, MD   Medical Director; Director of Cardiology Research; Co-Director, Cullen Cardiovascular Research Laboratories, Texas Heart Institute, Houston, Texas

Preface

Myocardial viability is a major investigative area in contemporary cardiology with significant clinical and prognostic relevance. Despite remarkable advances in our understanding and clinical management of patients with impaired left ventricular function and heart failure, the prevalence of heart failure and the resultant death rates in the U.S. have almost tripled in the past three decades. Among patients with symptoms of heart failure, a significant majority have chronic ischemic heart disease as the cause of left ventricular dysfunction. The more severe the clinical failure and left ventricular dysfunction, the worse the prognosis.

Contrary to the conventional wisdom, impaired left ventricular function at rest in patients with coronary artery disease is not necessarily an irreversible process. New paradigms concerning the relationship between myocardial perfusion and left ventricular function have been described, such as stunning and hibernation. In these paradigms, myocardial function is depressed but myocytes remain viable, and therefore dysfunction may be completely reversible. The pathophysiology of these paradigms has been clarified, and novel diagnostic and therapeutic strategies have emerged. Myocardial reperfusion via revascularization ameliorates ischemic injury, recruits hibernating regions, and prevents future infarction. However, the success of myocardial reperfusion is critically dependent on the suitability of the coronary artery anatomy for revascularization. Among patients who are not candidates for conventional revascularization, novel therapeutic strategies such as percutaneous myocardial revascularization or treatment with pharmacological agents that cause angiogenesis may be considered. Because enhanced global left ventricular function after revascularization is associated with improved survival, early identification of viable myocardium in patients with coronary artery disease and left ventricular dysfunction has important prognostic implications.

Parallel advances have occurred in the noninvasive approaches used to study myocardial viability in patients with chronic ischemic heart disease. The importance and role of myocardial viability assessment is now widely appreciated, and great reliance is placed on such findings when patients are referred for coronary artery revascularization. New and sophisticated techniques have broadened the scope of the examination from anatomy and function alone to assessment of absolute myocardial blood flow, contractile reserve, cell membrane integrity, and metabolic substrate utilization. Advances in instrumentation have made it possible to introduce into clinical practice techniques that were once of purely academic interest. Imaging techniques that can identify patients with reversible left ventricular dysfunction, prospectively, before the transition to dilated phase of cardiomyopathy ensues, may result in more appropriate utilization of resources and enhanced efficiency of health care delivery.

The aim of this book is to bridge together basic cellular physiology and clinical decision making as it relates to myocardial viability. We were fortunate to have been able to gather some of the greatest minds in the field to assess the current state-of-the-art perspective of the field of myocardial viability and speculate areas of future research. All contributors have made sincere efforts to include the latest developments in their chapters and submit them in a timely manner.

In eighteen chapters, the monograph brings together into one volume various disciplines affecting myocardial viability in a manner that can be assimilated by the clinician, scholar, and students of physiology and metabolism. The chapters are organized into five sections that provide comprehensive review of cellular physiology as it relates to myocardial viability, clinical experience of recent years, and techniques which are most useful in clinical practice. In the introductory section (chapter 1) perspectives on the study of human myocardium are reviewed; cell death, histomorphologic and structural changes in ischemic cardiomyopathy, left ventricular remodeling, diagnostic techniques and treatment options. The second section (chapters 2–4) examines basic concepts and mechanisms of myocardial stunning, hibernation, and ischemic preconditioning. Modulation of responses to ischemia, the link between oxygen demand and supply in the coronary circulation, and their impact on contractile function are described. The third section (chapters 5–8) details fundamental cellular physiology and vascular biology as it pertains to myocardial viability. Essential fuels of the heart, complex regulation, and mechanical restitution are discussed. The role of nitric oxide in the heart, and experimental models useful in evaluating myocardial viability are presented. The function of various channels in regulating intracellular communication in normal, ischemic, and stunned myocardium is reviewed. The fourth section (chapters 9–12) addresses new methods for measurement of regional and global left ventricular function and contractile reserve. Morphologic and echocardiographic features of viable and nonviable myocardium and the impact of timing of reperfusion on myocardial salvage are presented. The fifth section (chapter 13–18) reviews principles of tracer kinetics and clinical application of SPECT, PET, and MRI technologies. Extensive review of the literature on myocardial blood flow, metabolism, and cell membrane integrity as it pertains to myocardial viability and recovery of function after revascularization is presented. In view of the comprehensive presentation of this topic, the monograph can serve as a reference source for those interested in the field of myocardial viability and improve communication between investigators from various disciplines.

Our knowledge of myocardial viability in normal and disease states stems from the work of many investigators and the continuing genesis of novel ideas. I have enormous admiration to the authors of this book for their outstanding contributions to the field. I feel privileged to have been part of this scientific endeavor as I learned much from the distinguished contributors. I offer profound gratitude to my mentors and the authors of each of the chapters. For it is their creative minds coupled with their magnanimity to share their expertise through lucid chapters that has made this book possible. My sincere appreciation to Steven Korn of the Futura Publishing, Inc., for providing me the opportunity to edit this monograph. But most of all, I would like to thank my patients who have served as my greatest teachers and whose clinical care in this area has been both challenging and enlightening.

Vasken Dilsizian, M.D.

Part I

Introduction

Perspectives on the Study of Human Myocardium: Viability

Vasken Dilsizian, MD

Introduction

The goal of myocardial viability assessment is to differentiate, prospectively, patients with potentially reversible from irreversible left ventricular dysfunction. Ideally, such information would be used to guide therapeutic decisions for revascularization. Therapeutic interventions that improve nonfunctioning but viable myocardial regions may improve significantly global left ventricular function[1-5] as well as impact left ventricular remodeling and patient prognosis.[6-10] Thus, among patients with preoperative left ventricular dysfunction in whom revascularization entails high perioperative morbidity and mortality, accurate assessment of myocardial viability may result in more appropriate utilization of resources and enhanced efficiency of health care delivery.

Left Ventricular Dysfunction and Heart Failure

Systolic left ventricular dysfunction is the final stage of most primary cardiovascular diseases that may manifest themselves clinically as heart failure. Heart failure is associated with poor morbidity and mortality; the more severe the clinical failure and left ventricular dysfunction, the worse the prognosis. Among patients with symptoms of heart failure, a significant majority may have underlying coronary artery disease as the cause of the chronic left ventricular dysfunction.[11,12] Because coronary artery disease is the most common cause of congestive heart failure in developed countries,[11-14] detection of myocardial viability within the subgroup of heart failure patients who may benefit from revascularization may significantly impact their survival.

Death rates (age adjusted per 100 000 population) for ischemic heart disease, stroke, and congestive heart failure from 1969 to 1995 are illustrated in Figure 1.[15] Despite the trend of decreasing death rates attributable to ischemic heart disease and stroke, the prevalence of heart failure and the resultant death rates in the United States have almost tripled between 1974 and 1994. It is estimated that 4.8 million Americans suffer from congestive heart failure. Of the 400 000 new heart failure patients diagnosed each year, it is estimated that 20% will be dead within 1 year and 50% within 5 years.[16,17] Although the

From Dilsizian V (ed). *Myocardial Viability: A Clinical and Scientific Treatise.* Armonk, NY: Futura Publishing Co., Inc.; © 2000.

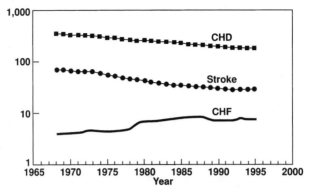

Figure 1. Death rates (age adjusted per 100 000 population) for ischemic heart disease, stroke, and congestive heart failure (CHF) in the United States from 1969 to 1995. Reproduced with permission from Reference 15.

incidence of heart failure is similar in men and women, the mortality rate is higher in men. In 1993, the death rate from heart failure was nearly 1.5 times higher in black men and women when compared with white men and women.

Contraction-Perfusion Mismatch (Stunning) and Match (Hibernation)

Over the past two decades, pathophysiological paradigms concerning the relationship between myocardial perfusion and left ventricular function have changed considerably with the introduction of stunned and hibernating myocardium.[18–20] These pathophysiological states have challenged the conventional wisdom that impaired left ventricular function at rest in patients with coronary artery disease and heart failure is an irreversible process. Substantial data now exist to indicate that under certain conditions, when viable myocytes are subjected to hypoperfusion and/or ischemia, prolonged alterations in regional and/or global left ventricular function may occur and that this dysfunction may be completely reversible.[1,2,21–28]

Stunned myocardium refers to the state of delayed recovery of regional dysfunction after a transient period of ischemia that has been followed by reperfusion.[18] Potential causes for the transient regional dysfunction may relate to myocardial injury caused by both ischemia and postischemic reperfusion.[29] Unlike stunning, hibernation is thought to be an adaptive rather than injurious response of the myocardium, in which viable but hypocontractile myocardium arises from prolonged myocardial hypoperfusion at rest in the absence of clinically evident ischemia.[20] The distinction between these two pathophysiological states may have important clinical implications. In the case of stunning, intervention aimed at reducing the number, severity, or duration of ischemic episodes would be expected to result in improvement in contractile function. In the case of hibernation, interventions that favorably alter the supply/demand relationship of the myocardium, either improvement in blood flow or reduction in demand, would result in functional improvement. However, in patients with coronary artery disease, it is more likely that injurious responses of stunning and adaptive responses of hibernation coexist. This may explain much of the controversy regarding definition of terms and variability among studies in patients.

If stunned and hibernating states indeed can be altered by therapeutic interventions, then the identification of such states prospectively in a particular patient may have signif-

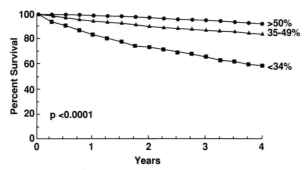

Figure 2. Cumulative 4-year survival of the medically treated Coronary Artery Surgery Study (CASS) registry patients on the basis of left ventricular ejection fraction (LVEF) at rest. Reproduced with permission from Reference 9.

icant clinical relevance, in part because left ventricular function is a major determinant of survival in coronary artery disease.[6–10,30–32] Although patients with normal (≥50%) or mildly reduced (35%–49%) left ventricular function have an excellent 4-year survival on medical therapy (92% and 83%, respectively), those with moderate to severely reduced (<35%) left ventricular function have a significantly lower 4-year survival (58%) when treated with medical therapy alone (Fig. 2).

In some patients with coronary artery disease and symptoms of heart failure, the severity of left ventricular dysfunction may be disproportionate to the extent of ischemic myocardial injury.[33,34] Thus, beyond the magnitude of necrotic injury, structure and performance of the remaining myocytes as well as the extracellular matrix of the nonmyocyte compartment may influence the left ventricular contractile function.

Myocardial Cell Death

Myocardial cell death in response to ischemic injury may occur via necrosis or apoptosis.

Necrosis

Until the early 1970s necrosis was the only clearly identified type of cell death. In necrosis, cell death is provoked by external (nonphysiological) injury (ie, ischemic, metabolic, or toxic) without active cellular participation or energy requirement. Ischemic injury first causes failure of the ionic pumps of the plasma membrane, which leads to full-blown necrosis 12–24 hours later. Cardinal features of necrosis secondary to ischemic injury include cellular swelling, disruption and lysis of the plasma membrane, release of the cytoplasmic and nuclear contents into the intercellular milieu, inflammation, and phagocytosis of necrotic cells. This uncontrolled process of cell death by necrosis usually involves patches of tissue rather than isolated cells.

Apoptosis

Apoptosis, also termed programmed cell death, is a form of suicide based on a genetic mechanism. This novel physiological process of cell death, first termed shrinkage necrosis and a year later apoptosis, was described by Kerr and colleagues in 1971.[35,36]

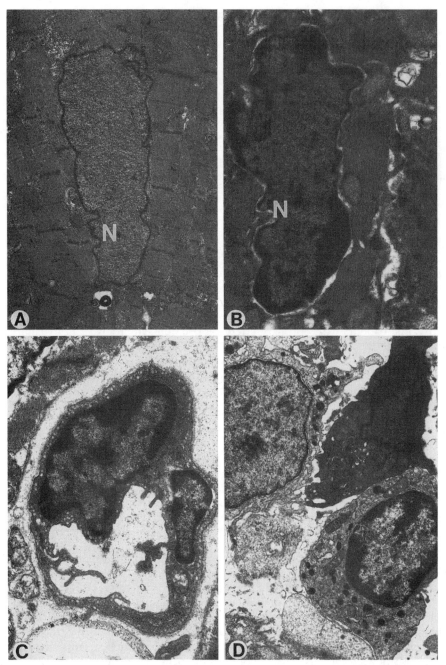

Figure 3. Cell death by apoptosis. Electron micrographs showing a normal myocyte (**A**) and apoptosis in a cardiac myocyte (**B**), an endothelial cell (**C**), and a large granular lymphocyte (**D**). **A.** The nucleus (N) of a normal myocyte shows a peripheral, narrow rim of heterochromatins and abundant euchromatins evenly distributed within the nuclear matrix. Cytoplasmic structures appear normal (magnification ×9000). **B.** Myocyte undergoing apoptosis shows sharply segregated, compact chromatin, convoled nuclear outline, and condensed cytoplasm (N, nucleus; magnification ×22 000). **C.** An apoptotic capillary endothelial cell is characterized by segregation of the chromatin into sharply circumscribed areas subjacent to the inner nuclear membrane (magnification ×15 000). **D.** A large granular lymphocyte undergoing apoptosis shows cell shrinkage, compact chromatin, and condensation of the cytoplasm. Compared with two other normal granular lymphocytes that have a large, round-shaped nucleus and electron-lucent cytoplasm (magnification ×11 000. Reproduced with permission from Reference 39.

Apoptosis is thought to be a fundamental part of normal human development (programmed cell death) but also can be triggered by extracellular agents such as hormones, cytokines, killer cells, and a variety of chemical, physical, and viral agents.[37,38] Unlike necrosis, apoptosis is an active, adenosine triphosphate (ATP)–dependent programmed cell death and usually involves single isolated cells (Fig. 3).[39] Cells undergoing apoptotic cell death usually shrink and exhibit dense chromatin condensation, nuclear fragmentation, cytoplasmic blebbing, and cellular fragmentation into small apoptotic bodies that are phagocytosed by neighboring cells or macrophages.[35,40,41] Because the plasma membrane is not lysed, no damaging inflammatory tissue reaction is elicited. Such histomorphological changes in apoptosis can be completed in less than an hour.

In a mature human, there is a fine balance between cell death and cell proliferation. The rates of apoptosis and proliferation vary widely from tissue to tissue and are critical during developmental stages as well as for regulation of tissue homeostasis. In cardiac tissue, myocytes are thought to be differentiated terminally and are unable to regenerate or proliferate.[42,43] In the disease state, such as acute ischemic injury, most myocytes die predominantly by cell necrosis. However, a number of normal or less badly damaged myocytes also may die prematurely by apoptosis. One therapeutic strategy, therefore, would be to develop apoptosis blockers to limit postischemic myocardial injury and subsequent left ventricular remodeling and cardiomyopathy.

Recently, several investigators have reported the extent of apoptosis and the level of molecular mediators of apoptosis in the failing human adult heart and in patients with arrhythmogenic right ventricular dysplasia.[44–46] Apoptotic nuclei were measured by specific labeling of fragmented DNA, an assay called terminal transferase-mediated deoxyuridine nucleotide end labeling (TUNEL)[47] and/or by observing the internucleosomal DNA laddering pattern characteristic of apoptosis when subjected to agarose gel electrophoresis.[48] These studies suggest that apoptosis may play a role in the progressive deterioration of left ventricular function observed in heart failure.

The identification of new genes and new effects of known genes that regulate or modify apoptosis raises fundamental questions about the pathophysiology of end-stage cardiomyopathy and heart failure. Because apoptosis can be modulated by growth factors and cytokines, the discovery of genes that regulate apoptosis may have important implications for the diagnosis and the development of new treatment strategies for patients with heart failure.[49–51] The balance between apoptosis-promoting and apoptosis-suppressing signals in normal, ischemic, and infarcted myocardium in relation to left ventricular remodeling and progressive cardiomyopathy remain uncharted.

Histomorphological and Structural Changes in Ischemic Cardiomyopathy

In the early 1980s, Flameng and coworkers described the structural component of long-term adaptive responses on the basis of biopsy specimens obtained during coronary artery bypass surgery from regions of reversibly dysfunctional myocardium.[28,51–53] These investigators and others[54] have shown an inverse relationship between functional improvement after revascularization and the extent and the severity of collagen replacement. In asynergic regions without prior myocardial infarction, myocardial cell degeneration without significant fibrosis was observed predominantly in the subendocardium.[28] This cell degeneration was characterized by progressive loss of contractile material secondary to ischemia with almost complete recovery of regional contractile function after revascularization. The authors attributed such improvement of regional function to regeneration of the contractile system within affected myocytes. In addition, morphologically normal-appearing myocytes in such regions often were structurally remodeled but metabolically active.[54]

The structural changes described in recent years[54,55] include (1) reductions in contractile filament material and sarcoplasmic reticulum, (2) accumulation and storage of glycogen, and (3) the appearance of numerous small mitochondria (Fig. 4). Because some of these structural changes of altered myocytes resemble those of embryonic cells, such changes have been attributed to a dedifferentiation process.[56,57] Furthermore, altered myocytes have been shown to reexpress contractile proteins that are specific to the fetal heart, such as the α-smooth muscle cell actin.[56] Whether these phenotypic changes are the result of prolonged hypoperfusion and/or ischemia or secondary to prolonged contractile unloading and are reversible after revascularization is unknown. Because these structural changes are chronic in nature and have developed over a prolonged period of time, this may explain why some regions viable by scintigraphic or echocardiographic techniques may be irreversible despite successful revascularization.[58]

Preliminary data indicate a time dependence of recovery of regional function after revascularization, with as much as 35% of the total improvement occurring 2–12 months after surgery.[59,60] Delayed recovery of function has been attributed to time-dependent recovery of energy stores and regeneration of cellular contractile material that were remodeled in consequence to chronic hypoperfusion. It is possible that long-term changes of functionally down-regulated myocytes might include the process of calcium flux and potassium pump activity[61] and alterations in gene expression that may lead to changes in contractile protein enzyme activity[62] and synthesis of new proteins,[63] which may take time to repair and recover after revascularization. Whether it is possible to distinguish such histomorphological and functional changes of reversibly dysfunctional from persistently dysfunctional myocardium, prospectively, by indirect imaging techniques is an area of intense investigation.

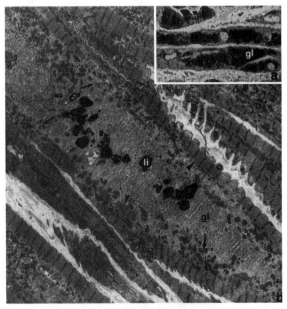

Figure 4. Light (a, top right) and electron micrograph (b) showing subcellular changes in cardiomyocytes of chronic hibernating myocardium: depletion of sarcomeres [present only at the cell periphery (arrowhead), accumulation of glycogen (gl), and the presence of numerous small mitochondria (arrows); li, lipofuscin; magnification: a ×350 and b ×3250. Reproduced with permission from Reference 56.

Left Ventricular Remodeling

After the initial ischemic injury, left ventricular dysfunction may continue to decompensate even in the absence of clinical signs and symptoms of heart failure. Pathophysiological processes involved in left ventricular remodeling and progressive systolic dysfunction may be related to the presence and extent of myocardial viability. For example, the left ventricular chamber can dilate on the basis of either direct loss of myocardial tissue (necrosis or apoptosis) or from altered hemodynamic processes (pressure overload or volume overload). Left ventricular dilatation and systolic dysfunction after an acute myocardial infarction have been shown to be predictors of survival.[64,65] Patients with dilated left ventricles and large end-diastolic[64] and end-systolic[65] volumes had significantly higher mortality when compared with those with small left ventricular volumes.

After an acute myocardial infarction, the myocardium is replaced by scarred tissue, which is susceptible to further thinning (replacement of myocardial cells by hydroxyproline) and elongation due to infarct expansion.[66-69] It has been demonstrated that this process of infarct expansion involves slippage of muscle bundles within the ischemic as well as nonischemic myocardial regions.[68-70] In addition to the infarct expansion, the process of left ventricular dilatation and remodeling ensues within days and months after the acute injury.[69-72] The morphological and geometric changes of the left ventricle as a result of remodeling affect regions of scarred as well as nonischemic, viable myocardium. The cardiac interstitium also may play a role in modulating muscle configuration after ischemic insults.[73]

The exact mechanism of left ventricular remodeling after myocardial infarction has not been established. Available data[74,75] suggest that in the setting of increased wall stress (due to neurohormonal changes), left ventricular cavity dilatation and hypertrophy of the remaining normal myocardium (to compensate for the loss function in the infarct territory) helps maintain stroke volume (Frank-Starling mechanism). However, if corrective measures are not taken, this leads to progressive morphological and geometric changes, which leads to further left ventricular dilatation.[75] The increased ventricular volume also leads to further increases in wall stress (Laplace's law), and the outcome of this vicious cycle is end-stage heart failure.

In left ventricular remodeling, cellular hypertrophy in normal myocardial regions may not necessarily translate to improved contraction. There may be reduced coronary flow reserve in regions with hypertrophy because of inadequate adaptation of the capillary vasculature.[76] In addition, changes in collagen replacement fibrosis[77] and connective tissue[78] also may contribute to progressive left ventricular dysfunction. Whether such deformations in left ventricular geometry and extracellular architecture are permanent or can be restored back to their original preischemic configuration remains uncertain.

Treatment Options of Heart Failure

Current treatment options for heart failure include (1) medical therapy, (2) revascularization, or (3) heart transplantation.

Medical Therapy

Despite improvement in heart failure symptoms with the addition of vasodilators,[13,14] angiotensin-converting enzyme inhibitors,[11,12,14,79-81] and/or β-adrenergic blocking agents[82-84] to standard medical treatment of heart failure, the resultant improvement in survival has been modest. In the era of prevasodilator and angiotensin-

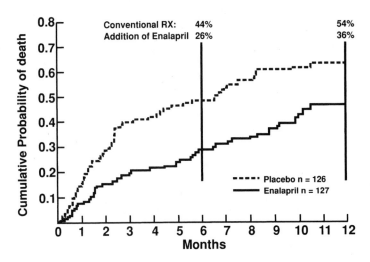

Figure 5. Cumulative probability of death in the placebo and enalapril groups from the Cooperative North Scandinavian Enalapril Survival Study (Consensus I Trial) of Class IV patients with severe CHF. Reproduced with permission from Reference 79.

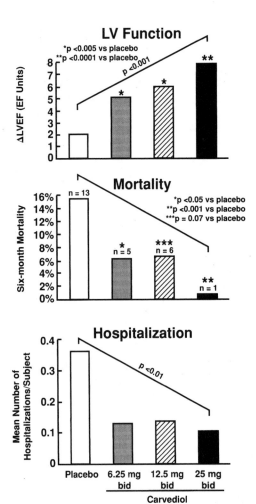

Figure 6. Carvedilol protocol 220 [Multicenter Oral Carvedilol Heart Failure Assessment (MOCHA)] data for mild to moderate CHF. **Top panel,** LVEF data at the end of a 6-month maintenance period as change from baseline values; **middle panel,** 6-month crude mortality as deaths per randomized patients ×100; **lower panel,** cardiovascular hospitalizations: mean number of hospitalizations per subject during maintenance period of 2–6 months. Reproduced with permission from Reference 82.

converting enzyme inhibitor therapy, the 1-year mortality among patients with severe chronic heart failure was approximately 50% when treated with conventional therapy.[85] In the Cooperative North Scandinavian Enalapril Survival Study (CONSENSUS I Trial), in which patients with severe heart failure (New York Heart Association functional class IV) were randomized to receive placebo (in addition to digitalis and diuretics) or enalapril (an angiotensin-converting enzyme inhibitor), the 6-month and 12-month mortality rates of enalapril-treated patients were 26% and 36% in contrast to 44% and 54% in the placebo-treated patients, respectively (Fig. 5).[79] However, despite the improvement in survival, the long-term survival on medical therapy remains discouraging.[11–14,80,81] The addition of cardioselective or third-generation β-adrenergic blocking agents to angiotensin-converting enzyme inhibitors in patients with mild symptoms of heart failure can increase left ventricular ejection fraction (LVEF) and retard progression of heart failure (Fig. 6).[82–84] Whether β-adrenergic blocking agents will produce improvement in symptoms and survival in patients with severe clinical heart failure remains uncertain. Therefore, any therapeutic intervention that has the potential to improve left ventricular function and symptoms of heart failure should be received favorably.

Revascularization

There is still some controversy regarding the selection of patients with ischemic left ventricular dysfunction and heart failure for coronary artery bypass surgery. Myocardial reperfusion via revascularization ameliorates ischemic injury, recruits hibernating regions, and prevents future infarction. Prior clinical trials have shown that patients with multivessel coronary artery disease and reduced left ventricular function benefit most from revascularization in terms of survival.[86–90] However, the operative risk of coronary artery bypass surgery is increased in this patient population explaining the reluctance of cardiac surgeons to operate on them.[91,92] With increased surgical expertise, aggressive use of intravenous medications in the operating room, combined with improved intraoperative myocardial preservation techniques, surgical mortality rates have decreased substantially over the last two decades.

Among patients with severely impaired left ventricular function undergoing coronary artery bypass surgery, the in-hospital mortality rates have declined to approximately 8% in

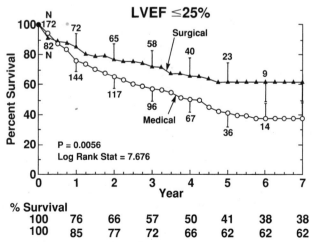

Figure 7. Life table cumulative survival for medically treated and surgically treated patients with severely reduced LVEF at rest. Reproduced with permission from Reference 7.

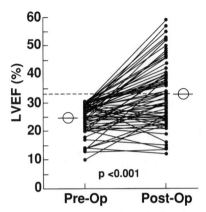

Figure 8. Change in LVEF at rest before (pre-op) and after (post-op) coronary artery bypass surgery. Reproduced with permission from Reference 4.

recent studies.[4,7,93] In the Coronary Artery Surgery Study (CASS), the overall surgical mortality rate was 6.9% in patients with LVEF of ≤35% compared with 1.55% for patients with LVEF of >35%.[7] Short- and long-term surgical survival benefits were shown to be greatest in patients with the most severe left ventricular dysfunction.[4,7,90,94] Among patients with LVEF of ≤25%, the 5-year survival rate was 62% with surgical treatment and 41% with medical treatment.[7] The 1- and 2-year survival of medically treated patients were 76% and 66%, in contrast to 85% and 77%, in the surgically treated patients, respectively (Fig. 7).[7]

Beyond survival, successful revascularization in patients with severely impaired LVEF has resulted in improved left ventricular function in up to one-third of patients, as well as improved anginal and heart failure symptoms.[3-5] The severity of the left ventricular dysfunction at rest did not predict the results of revascularization (Fig. 8). Such improvement in survival and left ventricular function was observed even in patients who had minimal or absent anginal symptoms. Although there have been some concerns regarding the use of the internal mammary artery conduit as well as maintaining saphenous vein graft patency among patients with severely impaired left ventricular function, recent data indicate no particular problems with the use of either conduits.[4]

The acceptable risk of revascularization along with the improvement in global left ventricular function, heart failure symptoms, and survival argue for serious consideration of bypass surgery in selected patients with suitable coronary anatomy. Among those who are not candidates for surgical revascularization, percutaneous myocardial revascularization or treatment with pharmaceutical agents that cause angiogenesis or improve blood flow and/or oxygen delivery to collaterally dependent viable myocardium should be considered.

Heart Transplantation

Since its introduction into clinical practice in 1967, cardiac transplantation has become an effective and accepted therapeutic alternative for patients with end-stage severe congestive heart failure. However, the great discrepancy between heart donors and candidates for transplantation renders the treatment ineffective in epidemiological terms. It is estimated that more than 150 patients with end-stage heart failure are added to the cardiac transplant list each month and the length of time required to identify a suitable donor organ exceeds 7 months or more. Approximately one-third of patients with end-stage heart failure die while waiting for a donor heart. This has propelled the development of left ventricular assist devices to serve as a bridge to cardiac transplantation until a donor organ becomes available.

Nearly 45% of all adult patients who require heart transplantation have ischemic cardiomyopathy as the underlying etiology. For the subset of patients who are fortunate enough to receive a heart transplant, their actuarial survival rate is 79% at 1 year with a constant mortality rate of approximately 4% per year over the next 13 years.[86] However, these survival rates should be viewed from the perspective that transplant recipients are, on the average, approximately 20 years younger than the average age of all patients with heart failure. Time to 50% survival after heart transplantation (patient half-life) is 8.7 years.[86] The majority of deaths are caused by nonspecific allograft failure (early 0–30 days after transplantation), acute rejection and infection (1–12 months after transplantation), cardiac allograft vasculopathy, and malignancy and acute rejection (>1 year after transplantation). Repeat heart transplantation is necessary in 2.1% of the total patient population.[86] Thus, despite being efficacious treatment for end-stage heart failure, cardiac transplantation is not a realistic solution for the majority of patients with congestive heart failure, especially for the elderly, because of the limited donor resource.

Diagnostic Techniques for Assessing Viability

Currently, there are a number of diagnostic techniques for assessing myocardial viability, prospectively, in patients with coronary artery disease.[95–99] Among them, eval-

THALLIUM-201

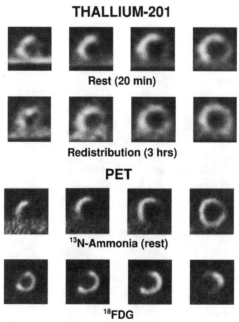

Rest (20 min)

Redistribution (3 hrs)

PET

^{13}N-Ammonia (rest)

^{18}FDG

Figure 9. Concordance between thallium single photon emission tomography (SPECT) and positron emission tomography (PET) is demonstrated in this patient example. Rest redistribution short-axis thallium tomograms (top two rows) and ^{13}N-ammonia and ^{18}F-fluorodeoxyglucose (FDG) PET images (lower two rows) are displayed from a patient with coronary artery disease. There are extensive thallium abnormalities in the lateral and inferior regions on the initial rest images that are partially reversible on 3 to 4-hour redistribution images, suggestive of viable myocardium. The corresponding ^{13}N-ammonia and FDG PET images (acquired after an overnight fast) show severely reduced ^{13}N-ammonia uptake in the lateral and inferior regions at rest (similar to the initial thallium images) with enhanced FDG uptake (mismatch pattern), suggestive of viable myocardium.

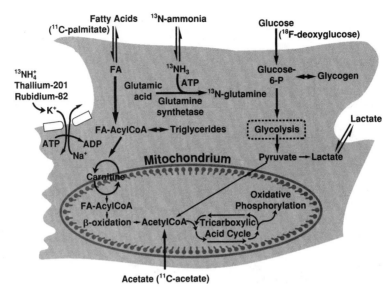

Figure 10. Schematic representation of a myocyte with its major metabolic pathways and regulatory steps.

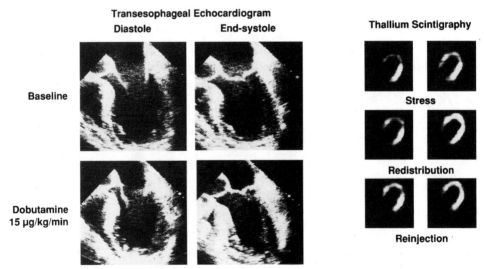

Figure 11. Example of concordance between thallium scintigraphy with reinjection and low-dose transesophageal echocardiography. Left panels show echocardiographic images obtained from the four-chamber view in diastole (**left**) and at end systole (**right**), at baseline (**top**), and during low-dose dobutamine infusion (**bottom**). Right panels show two consecutive transaxial thallium tomograms obtained immediately after stress (**top**), after 3- to 4-hour redistribution (**middle**), and after reinjection (**bottom**). Echocardiographic images show severe hypokinesis of the basal septum with akinesis of the apical region. With dobutamine, systolic thickening of the septal and apical regions significantly improves. This correlates with ischemic and viable myocardium in the corresponding areas by thallium scintigraphy. Reprinted with permission from Reference 96.

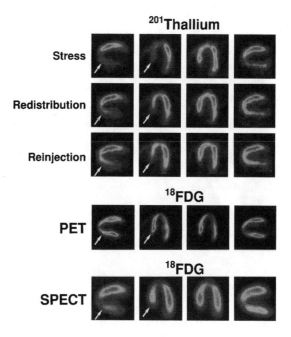

Figure 12. Concordance between stress-redistribution-reinjection thallium SPECT, FDG PET, and FDG SPECT is demonstrated in this patient example. Four radial long-axis tomograms are displayed for thallium stress, redistribution, and reinjection with corresponding tomograms of FDG PET and FDG SPECT. On the thallium images, reversible defects are seen in the apical and inferoseptal regions (shown by the arrowhead), suggestive of ischemic but viable myocardium. As in the findings on thallium, FDG PET and FDG SPECT studies show preserved metabolic activity in the apical and inferoseptal regions (viable by FDG).

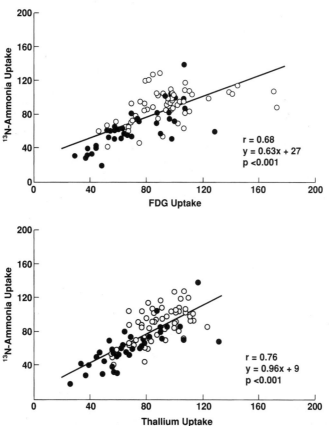

Figure 13. Relation between percent late ^{13}N-ammonia uptake and FDG uptake (**top**) and thallium uptake on redistribution imaging (**bottom**) in reversible (open circles) and irreversible (closed circles) asynergic regions after revascularization. There is a linear relationship between late ^{13}N-ammonia uptake, FDG uptake, and thallium uptake in all asynergic regions. Reprinted with permission from Reference 98.

uation of myocardial cell membrane integrity (see Chapters 14 and 15; Fig. 9) and metabolism (see Chapters 16 and 17; Fig. 10) using nuclear techniques, as well as contractile reserve with low-dose dobutamine echocardiography (see Chapters 10 and 11; Fig. 11), have gained considerable interest for differentiating viable from nonviable myocardium in asynergic regions. Although more conventional approaches of identifying scarred and necrotic myocardium, including determining the presence of occluded coronary arteries, regional contractile dysfunction and electrocardiographic Q-waves, these approaches have been shown to be less accurate. New modalities on the horizon include the use of metabolic tracers with single photon emission tomography (SPECT) (see Chapters 14 and 16; Fig. 12), more precise quantitative metabolic evaluations with positron emission tomography (PET) (see Chapter 17; Fig. 13), echocardiographic assessment of perfusion with contrast agents (Chapters 10 and 11), and the use of magnetic resonance imaging (Chapter 18).

Definition of Myocardial Viability

A number of important clinical questions still remain, relating to how the extent of viability may correlate to improvement in function, the degree to which hibernation and stunning are operative clinically, and the standardization of approaches to viability assessment. However, the most important questions relate to the definition of myocardial viability itself and to the clinical end points that are used to confirm or refute the presence of viable myocardium.

To date, the most common definition of myocardial viability has been the temporal improvement in contractile function of an asynergic region after restoration of blood flow. This end point has served as a gold standard for determining the accuracy of a particular tracer or technique for assessing myocardial viability (Fig. 14). However, recovery of global and/or regional left ventricular dysfunction after revascularization may not be the most appropriate definition of myocardial viability because it may underestimate the potential benefits of revascularization and thus the significance of the delineation of viable myocardium. Recovery of global and/or regional left ventricular function may be influenced by the duration and extent of hypoperfusion (hibernation and repetitive ischemia), suitability and completeness of revascularization, and long-term patency of revascularized coronary arteries, as well as other local and extrinsic conditions.[100] The restoration of blood flow to an epicardial rim of viable myocardium in the setting of nontransmural infarction, for example, may not result in significant improvement in regional function, but may result in stabilization of the electrical milieu and prevention of extensive ventricular remodeling in nontransmural infarct zones. These important effects of reperfusion of viable myocardium on left ventricular geometry, remodeling, and arrhythmias may result in long-term survival benefit even in the absence of changes in regional and global function.

There is a body of retrospective clinical data to support the hypothesis that a patent infarct-related artery improves clinical outcome independent of left ventricular function.[101–104] A prospective study in patients with acute myocardial infarction and moderately reduced LVEF confirmed that after adjustment for differences in baseline characteristics and left ventricular function, the patency of infarct-related arteries remained an independent predictor of mortality from all causes and of cardiovascular mortality.[105] Potential mechanisms for the improved survival among patients with patent infarct-related artery have not been elucidated fully. However, the auxiliary potential benefits of revascularization (independent of regional contraction) raise additional, as yet unanswered, questions, with regard to how and why we assess myocardial viability in coronary artery disease patients.

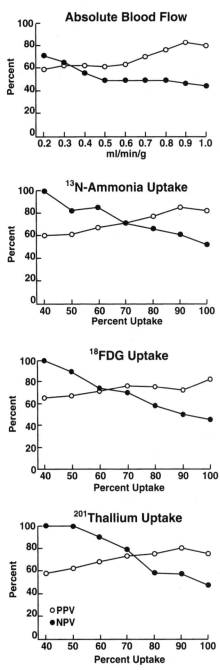

Figure 14. Positive and negative predictive values in predicting recovery of asynergic regions after revascularization are shown in relation to the magnitude of absolute blood flow, late ^{13}N-ammonia uptake, FDG uptake, and thallium uptake (maximum on either redistribution or reinjection). When ^{13}N-ammonia uptake and FDG metabolic data were combined, none of the asynergic regions demonstrating uptake of <50% on both ^{13}N-ammonia and FDG images showed improvement in systolic wall thickening after revascularization (negative predictive accuracy of 100%). Reprinted with permission from Reference 98.

In the future, it seems prudent to design large clinical trials to evaluate not only the benefit of revascularization on left ventricular function, but also on left ventricular cavity size, heart failure symptoms, arrhythmias, recurrent ischemic events, and long-term survival. To reduce the risk of heart failure and associated high mortality among patients with ischemic cardiomyopathy, attenuation of myocardial ischemia (revascularization/angiogenesis) and prevention of left ventricular remodeling (medical therapy) may be the optimum goals for managing such patients clinically.

References

1. Rozanski A, Berman DS, Gray R, et al. Use of thallium-201 redistribution scintigraphy in the preoperative differentiation of reversible and nonreversible myocardial asynergy. *Circulation* 1981;64:936–944.
2. Brundage BH, Massie BM, Botvinick EH. Improved regional ventricular function after successful surgical revascularization. *J Am Coll Cardiol* 1984;3:902–908.
3. Bonow RO, Dilsizian V. Thallium-201 for assessment of myocardial viability. *Sem Nucl Med* 1991;21:230–241.
4. Elefteriades JA, Tolis G Jr, Levi E, et al. Coronary artery bypass grafting in severe left ventricular dysfunction: Excellent survival with improved ejection fraction and functional state. *J Am Coll Cardiol* 1993;22:1411–1417.
5. Christian TF, Miller TD, Hodge DO, et al. An estimate of the prevalence of reversible left ventricular dysfunction in patients referred for coronary artery bypass surgery. *J Nucl Cardiol* 1997;4:140–146.
6. Nesto RW, Cohn LH, Collins JJ Jr, et al. Inotropic contractile reserve: A useful predictor of increased 5-year survival and improved postoperative left ventricular function in patients with coronary artery disease and reduced ejection fraction. *Am J Cardiol* 1982;50:39–44.
7. Alderman EL, Fisher LD, Litwin P, et al. Results of coronary artery surgery in patients with poor left ventricular function (CASS). *Circulation* 1983;68:785–795.
8. Pigott JD, Kouchoukos NT, Oberman A, et al. Late results of surgical and medical therapy for patients with coronary artery disease and depressed left ventricular function. *J Am Coll Cardiol* 1985;5:1036–1045.
9. Mock MB, Ringqvist I, Fisher LD, et al. Survival of medically treated patients in the Coronary Artery Surgery Study (CASS) registry. *Circulation* 1982;66:562–568.
10. Sheehan FH, Doerr R, Schmidt WG, et al. Early recovery of left ventricular function after thrombolytic therapy for acute myocardial infarction: An important determinant of survival. *J Am Coll Cardiol* 1988;40:633–644.
11. The SOLVD Investigators. Effects of enalapril on survival in patients with reduced left ventricular ejection fractions and congestive heart failure. *N Engl J Med* 1991;325:293–302.
12. The SOLVD Investigators. Effect of enalapril on mortality and the development of heart failure in asymptomatic patients with reduced left ventricular ejection fractions. *N Engl J Med* 1992;327:685–691.
13. Cohn JN, Archibald DG, Ziesche S, et al. Effect of vasodilator therapy on mortality in chornic congestive heart failure: Results of a Veterans Administrative Cooperative Study. *N Engl J Med* 1986;314:1547–1552.
14. Cohn JN, Johnson G, Ziesche S, et al. A comparison of enalapril with hydralazine-isosorbide dinitrate in the treatment of chronic congestive heart failure. *N Engl J Med* 1991;325:303–310.
15. National Heart, Lung, and Blood Institute. *Morbidity, and Mortality. Chartbook on Cardiovascular, Lung, and Blood Diseases.* Bethesda, Md: National Institutes of Health; 1998.
16. Yusuf S, Thom T, Abbott RD. Changes in hypertension treatment and in congestive heart failure mortality in the United States. *Hypertension* 1989;13(suppl 5):I74–I79.
17. Senni M, Tribouilloy CM, Rodeheffer RJ, et al. Congestive heart failure in the community: A study of all incident cases in Olmsted County, Minnesota, in 1991. *Circulation* 1989;98:2282–2289.
18. Braunwald E, Kloner RA. The stunned myocardium: Prolonged, postischemic ventricular dysfunction. *Circulation* 1982;66:1146–1149.

19. Diamond GA, Forrester JS, DeLuz PL, et al. Post-extrasystolic potentiation of ischemic myocardium by atrial stimulation. *Am Heart J* 1978;95:204–209.
20. Rahimtoola SH. A perspective on the three large multicenter randomized clinical trials of coronary bypass surgery for chronic stable angina. *Circulation* 1985;72(suppl V):V123–V135.
21. Rees G, Bristow JD, Kremkau EL, et al. Influence of aortocoronary bypass surgery on left ventricular performance. *N Engl J Med* 1971;284:1116–1125.
22. Chatterjee K, Swan HJC, Parmley WW, et al. Influence of direct myocardial revascularization on left ventricular asynergy and function in patients with coronary heart disease. *Circulation* 1973;47:276–286.
23. Dilsizian V, Bonow RO, Cannon RO, et al. The effect of coronary artery bypass grafting on left ventricular systolic function at rest: Evidence for preoperative subclinical myocardial ischemia. *Am J Cardiol* 1988;61:1248–1254.
24. Rahimtoola SH. Coronary bypass surgery for chronic angina-1981: A perspective. *Circulation* 1982;65:225–241.
25. Topol EJ, Weiss JL, Guzman PA, et al. Immediate improvement of dysfunctional myocardial segments after coronary revascularization: Detection by intraoperative transesophageal echocardiography. *J Am Coll Cardiol* 1984;4:1123–1134.
26. Braunwald E, Rutherford JD. Reversible ischemic left ventricular dysfunction: Evidence for the "hibernating myocardium." *J Am Coll Cardiol* 1986;8:1467–1470.
27. Ross J Jr. Myocardial perfusion-contraction matching: Implications for coronary heart disease and hibernation. *Circulation* 1991;83:1076–1082.
28. Flameng W, Suy R, Schwartz F, et al. Ultrastructural correlates of left ventricular contraction abnormalities in patients with chronic ischemic heart disease: Determinants of reversible segmental asynergy postrevascularization surgery. *Am Heart J* 1981;102:846–857.
29. Bolli R. Myocardial "stunning" in man. *Circulation* 1992;86:1671–1691.
30. Bruschke AVG, Proudfit WL, Sones FM. Progress study of 590 consecutive nonsurgical cases of coronary artery disease followed 5–9 years. II. Ventriculographic and other correlations. *Circulation* 1973;47:1154–1163.
31. Hammermeister KE, DeRouen TA, Dodge HT. Variables predictive of survival in patients with coronary disease: Selection by univariate and multivariate analysis from the clinical, electrocardiographic, exercise, ateriographic, and quantitative angiographic evaluations. *Circulation* 1979;59:421–430.
32. Harris PJ, Harrel FE, Lee KL, et al. Survival in medically treated coronary artery disease. *Circulation* 1979;60:1259–1269.
33. Burch GE, Giles TD, Cololough HL. Ischemic cardiomyopathy. *Am Heart J* 1970;79:291–292.
34. Schuster EH, Bulkley BH. Ischemic cardiomyopathy: A clinicopathologic study of fourteen patients. *Am Heart J* 1980;100:506–512.
35. Kerr JFR. Shrinkage necrosis: A distinct mode of cellular death. *J Pathol* 1971;105:13–20.
36. Kerr JFR, Willie AH, Currie AR. Apoptosis: A basic biological phenomenon with wide-ranging implications in tissue kinetics. *Br J Cancer* 1972;26:239–257.
37. Kerr JFR, Winterford WM, Harmon BV. Apoptosis: Its significance in cancer and cancer therapy. *Cancer* 1994;73:2013–2026.
38. Wyllie AH. Death gets a brake. *Nature* 1994;369:272–273.
39. Zhang J, Andrade ZA, Yu ZX, et al. Apoptosis in a canine model of acute chagasic myocarditis. *J Mol Cell Cardiol* 1999;31:581–596.
40. Clarke PGH. Developmental cell death: Morphological diversity and multiple mechanisms. *Anat Embryol* 1990;181:195–213.
41. Majno G, Joris I. Apopstosis, oncosis, and necrosis: An overview of cell death. *Am J Pathol* 1995;146:3–15.
42. Li F, Wang X, Capasso JM, et al. Rapid transition of cardiac myocytes from hyperplasia to hypertrophy during postnatal development. *J Mol Cell Cardiol* 1996;28:1737–1746.
43. Soonpaa MH, Field LJ. Survey of studies examining mammalian cardiomyocyte DNA synthesis. *Circ Res* 1998;84:15–26.
44. Narula J, Haider N, Virmani R, et al. Apoptosis is myocytes in end-stage heart failure. *N Engl J Med* 1996;335:1182–1189.

45. Olivetti G, Abbi R, Quaini F, et al. Apoptosis in the failing human heart. *N Engl J Med* 1997;336:1131–1141.
46. Mallat A, Tedgui A, Fontaliran F, et al. Evidence of apoptosis in arrhythmiogenic right ventricular dysplasia. *N Engl J Med* 1996;335:1190–1196.
47. Gavrieli Y, Sherman Y, Ben-Sasson SA. Identification of programmed cell death in situ via specific labeling of nuclear DNA fragmentation. *J Cell Biol* 1992;119:493–501.
48. Wyllie AH, Morris RG, Smith AL, et al. Chromatin cleavage in apoptosis: Association with condensed chromatin morphology and dependence on macromolecular synthesis. *J Pathol* 1984;142:67–77.
49. Yonish-Rouach E, Resintzky D, Lotem J, et al. Wild-type p53 induces apoptosis of myeloid leukemic cells that is inhibited by interleukin-6. *Nature* 1991;352:345–347.
50. Her E, Frazer J, Austen KF, et al. Eosinophil hematopoietins antagonize the programmed cell death of eosinophils: Cytokine and glucocorticoid effects on eosinophils maintained by endothelial cell-conditioned medium. *J Clin Invest* 1991;88:1982–1987.
51. Williams GT, Smith CA, Spooncer E, et al. Haemopoietic colony stimulating factors promote cell survival by suppressing apoptosis. *Nature* 1990;343:76–79.
52. Flameng W, Wouters L, Sergeant P, et al. Multivariate analysis of angiogaphic, histologic and electrocardiographic data in patients with coronary artery disease. *Circulation* 1984;70:7–17.
53. Maes A, Flameng W, Nuyts J, et al. Histological alterations in chronically hypoperfused myocardium: Correlation with PET findings. *Circulation* 1994;90:735–745.
54. Depre C, Vanoverschelde JJ, Melin JA, et al. Structural and metabolic correlates of the reversibility of chronic left ventricular ischemic dysfunction in humans. *Am J Physiol* 1995;268:H1265–H1275.
55. Vanoverschelde JL, Woijns W, Borgers M, et al. Chronic myocardial hibernation in humans: From bedside to bench. *Circulation* 1997;95:1961–1971.
56. Borgers M, Ausma J. Structural aspects of the chronic hibernating myocardium in man. *Basic Res Cardiol* 1995;90:44–46.
57. Borgers M, Thone F, Wouters L, et al. Structural correlates of regional myocardial dysfunction in patients with critical coronary artery stenosis: Chronic hibernation? *Cardiovasc Pathol* 1993;2:237–245.
58. Schwarz ER, Schaper J, vom Dahl J, et al. Myocyte degeneration and cell death in hibernating human myocardium. *J Am Coll Cardiol* 1996;27:1577–1585.
59. Mintz LJ, Ingels WB, Daughters GT, et al. Sequential studies of left ventricular function and wall motion after coronary artery bypass surgery. *Am J Cardiol* 1980;45:210–216.
60. Vanoverschelde JJ, Melin JA, Depre C, et al. Time-course of functional recovery of hibernating myocardium after coronary revascularization. *Circulation* 1994;90:I-378. Abstract.
61. Steenbergen C, Fralix TA, Murphy E. Role of increased cytosolic free calcium concentration in myocardial ischemic injury. *Basic Res Cardiol* 1993;88:456–470.
62. Capasso JM, Malhotra A, Li P, et al. Chronic nonocclusive coronary artery constriction impairs ventricular function, myocardial structure, and cardiac contractile protein activity in rats. *Circ Res* 1992;70:148–162.
63. Nomura K, Teraoka H, Arita H, et al. Disorganization of microfilaments is accompanied by downregulation of alpha-smooth muscle actin isoform mRNA level in cultured vascular smooth muscle cells. *J Biochem (Tokyo)* 1992;112:102–106.
64. Hammermeister KE, DeRouen TA, Dodge HT. Variables predictive of survival in patients with coronary disease. *Circulation* 1979;59:421–430.
65. White MD, Norris RM, Brown MA, et al. Left ventricular end-systolic volume as the major determinant of suvival after recovery from myocardial infarction. *Circulation* 1987;76:44–51.
66. Eaton LW, Weiss JL, Bulkley BH, et al. Regional cardiac dilatation after acute myocardial infarction: Recognition by two-dimensional echocardiography. *N Engl J Med* 1979;300:57–62.
67. Pirolo JS, Hutchins GM, Moore GW. Infarct expansion: Pathologic analysis of 204 patients with a single myocardial infarct. *J Am Coll Cardiol* 1986;7:349–354.
68. Hutchins GM, Bulkley BH. Infarct expansion versus extension: Two different complications of acute myocardial infarction. *Am J Cardiol* 1978;41:1127–1132.
69. Weisman HF, Bush DE, Mannisis JA, et al. Cellular mechanisms of myocardial infarct expansion. *Circulation* 1988;78:186–201.

70. Olivetti G, Capasso JM, Sonnenblick EH, et al. Side-to-side slippage of myocytes participates in ventricular wall remodeling acutely after myocardial infarction in rats. *Circ Res* 1990;67: 23–34.
71. Pfeffer JM, Pfeffer MA, Braunwald E. Influence of chronic captopril therapy in the infarcted left ventricle of the rat. *Circ Res* 1985;57:84–95.
72. Pfeffer MA, Braunwald E. Ventricular remodeling after myocardial infarction. *Circulation* 1990;81:1161–1172.
73. Eng C, Zhao M, Factor SM, et al. Post-ischaemic cardiac dilatation and remodelling: Reperfusion injury of the interstitium. *Eur Heart J* 1993;14:27A–32A.
74. Francis GS, Benedict C, Johnstone DE, et al. Comparison of neuroendocrine activation in patients with left ventricular dysfunction with and without congestive heart failure: A substudy of the Studies Of Left Ventricular Dysfunction (SOLVD). *Circulation* 1990;82:1724–1729.
75. Francis GS, McDonald KM, Cohn JN. Neurohormonal activation in preclinical heart failure: Remodeling and the potential for intervention. *Circulation* 1993;87:IV90–IV96.
76. Karam R, Healy BP, Wicker P. Coronary reserve is depressed in postmyocardial infarction reactive cardiac hypertrophy. *Circulation* 1990;81:238–246.
77. Shirani J, Lee J, Ohler L, et al. Impact of the severity of coronary artery stenosis on pathologic remodeling of viable myocardium in chronic ischemic cardiomyopathy. *Circulation* 1998;98: I-769.
78. Weber KT. Cardiac interstitium in health and disease: Remodeling of the fibrillar collagen matrix. *J Am Coll Cardiol* 1989;13:1637–1652.
79. The Consensus Trial Study Group. Effects of enalapril on mortality in severe congestive heart failure: Results of the Cooperative North Scandinavian Enalapril Survival Study (CONSENSUS). *N Engl J Med* 1987;316:1429–1435.
80. Swedberg K, Held P, Kjekshus J, et al. Effects of the early administration of enalapril on mortality in patients with acute myocardial infarction: Results of the Cooperative New Scandinavian Enalapril Survival Study II (CONSENSUS II). *N Engl J Med* 1992;327:678–684.
81. Pfeffer MA, Braunwald E, Move LA, et al. Effect of captopril on mortality and morbidity in patients with left ventricular dysfunction after myocardial infarction: Results of the Survival and Ventricular Enlargement Trial. *N Engl J Med* 1992;327:669–677.
82. Bristow MR, Gilbert EM, Abraham WT, et al for the MOCHA Investigators. Carvedilol produces dose-related improvements in left ventricular function and survival in subjects with chronic heart failure. *Circulation* 1996;94:2807–2816.
83. Packer M, Colucci WS, Sackner-Bernstein JD, et al for the PRECISE Study Group. Double-blind, placebo-controlled study of the effects of carvedilol in patients with moderate to severe heart failure: The PRECISE Trial. *Circulation* 1996;94:2793–2799.
84. Colucci WS, Packer M, Bristow MR, et al for the US Carvedilol Heart Failure Study Group. Carvedilol inhibits clinical progression in patients with mild symptoms of heart failure. *Circulation* 1996;94:2800–2806.
85. Smith WM. Epidemiology of congestive heart failure. *Am J Cardiol* 1985;55(suppl):3A–8A.
86. Hosenpud JD, Bennett LE, Keck BM, et al. The Registry of the International Society for Heart and Lung Transplantation: Fifteenth official report—1998. *J Heart Lung Transplant* 1998;17:656–668.
87. Alderman EL, Bourassa MG, Cohen LS, et al. Ten-year follow-up of survival and myocardial infarction in the randomized Coronary Artery Surgery Study. *Circulation* 1990;82:1629–1646.
88. Varnauskas E. Twelve-year follow-up of survival in the randomized European Coronary Surgery Study. *N Engl J Med* 1988;319:332–337.
89. Veterans Administration Coronary Artery Bypass Surgery Cooperative Study Group. Eleven-year survival in the Veterans Administration randomized trial of coronary bypass surgery for stable angina. *N Engl J Med* 1984;311:1333–1339.
90. Bounous EP, Mark DB, Pollock BG, et al. Surgical survival benefits for coronary disease patients with left ventricular dysfunction. *Circulation* 1988;78:I151–I157.
91. Cohn PF, Gorlin R, Cohn LH, et al. Left ventricular ejection fraction as a prognostic guide in surgical treatment of coronary and valvular heart disease. *Am J Cardiol* 1974;34:136–141.

92. Kennedy JW, Kaiser GC, Fisher LD, et al. Clinical and angiographic predictors of operative mortality from the collaborative study in Coronary Artery Surgery (CASS). *Circulation* 1981; 63:793–802.

93. Zubiate P, Kay JH, Dunne EF. Myocardial revascularization for patients with an ejection fraction of 0.2 or less; 12 years' results. *West J Med* 1984;140:745–749.

94. Kirklin JW, Blackstone EH, Rogers WJ. The plights of the invasive treatment of ischemic heart disease. *J Am Coll Cardiol* 1985;5:158–167.

95. Dilsizian V, and Bonow RO. Current diagnostic techniques of assessing myocardial viability in hibernating and stunned myocardium. *Circulation* 1993;87:1–20.

96. Panza JA, Dilsizian V, Laurienzo JM, et al. Relation between thallium uptake and contractile response to dobutamine: Implications regarding myocardial viability in patients with chronic coronary artery disease and left ventricular dysfunction. *Circulation* 1995;91:990–998.

97. Srinivasan G, Kitsiou AN, Bacharach SL, et al. ^{18}F-fluorodeoxyglucose single photon emission computed tomography: Can it replace PET and thallium SPECT for the assessment of myocardial viability? *Circulation* 1998;97:843–850.

98. Kitsiou AN, Bacharach SL, Bartlett ML, et al. ^{13}N-Ammonia myocardial blood flow and uptake: Relation to functional outcome of asynergic regions after revascularization. *J Am Coll Cardiol* 1999;33:678–686.

99. Kitsiou AN, Srinivasan G, Quyyumi AA, et al. Stress-induced reversible and mild-to-moderate irreversible thallium defects: Are they equally accurate for predicting recovery of regional left ventricular function after revascularization? *Circulation* 1998;98:501–508.

100. Ross J Jr. Mechanisms of regional ischemia and antianginal drug action during exercise. *Prog Cardiovasc Dis* 1989;31:455–466.

101. Cigarroa RG, Lange RA, Hillis LD. Prognosis after acute myocardial infarction in patients with and without residual anterograde coronary blood flow. *Am J Cardiol* 1989;64:155–160.

102. Schroder R, Neuhaus KL, Linderer T, et al. Impact of late coronary artery reperfusion on left ventricular function one month after acute myocardial infarction: Results from the ISAM study. *Am J Cardiol* 1989;64:878–884.

103. Galvani M, Ottani F, Ferrini D, et al. Patency of the infarct-related artery and left ventricular function as the major determinants of survival after Q-wave acute myocardial infarction. *Am J Cardiol* 1993;71:1–7.

104. Braunwald E. Myocardial reperfusion, limitation of infarct size, reduction of left ventricular dysfunction, and improved survival: Should the paradigm be expanded? *Circulation* 1989; 79:441–444.

105. Lamas GA, Flaker GC, Mitchell G, et al. Effect of infarct artery patency on prognosis after acute myocardial infarction. *Circulation* 1995;92:1101–1109.

Part II

Basic Concepts and Mechanisms

Modulation of Responses to Myocardial Ischemia: Metabolic Features of Myocardial Stunning, Hibernation, and Ischemic Preconditioning

Heinrich Taegtmeyer, MD, DPhil

Introduction

Myocardial stunning, hibernation, and ischemic preconditioning are terms used to describe modulated responses to myocardial ischemia. Like the term ischemia, the three terms are descriptive and in many ways their definitions also are arbitrary. At the outset it seems therefore useful to consider the origin of the terminology.

In the middle of the 19th century, Virchow performed experiments under a microscope and observed "focal anemia in blood vessels" from the web of a frog's foot after the application of vasoconstrictive stimuli. He called the phenomenon ischemia.[1] In this century, Braunwald and Kloner examined the literature and drew attention to reversible mechanical dysfunction that persists after ischemia following the return of normal perfusion. They called the phenomenon myocardial stunning.[2] Stunning is of clinical importance in the context of reperfusion after acute coronary occlusion. At about the same time, Rahimtoola also examined the literature and drew attention to reversible contractile dysfunction of ischemic heart muscle when regional wall motion improved with inotropic stimulation and/or coronary revascularization. He called the phenomenon myocardial hibernation.[3] Hibernation has long been of clinical importance in the context of myocardial revascularization.[4] Last, Murry, working in the laboratory of Jennings and Reimer, performed experiments in the dog lab and observed that canine myocardium subjected to four brief episodes of ischemia and reperfusion would tolerate a more prolonged episode of ischemia better than heart muscle not subjected previously to ischemia. The authors called the phenomenon ischemic preconditioning.[5]

This research was funded by National Heart, Lung, and Blood Institute Grant RO1 HL-43133.

Programmed Cell Survival

A common feature of these phenomena is the response of the heart to an altered physiological environment created by a temporary or sustained reduction in coronary flow. The myocardial response to ischemia is determined by both the severity and the duration of ischemia.[4,6–8] It also is determined by environmental factors including workload of the heart, hormonal stimulation, temperature, and release of autocrine and paracrine factors.[8–10] It is very difficult to understand the relative contributions of each of these components without first considering the function of the heart as a whole.

Heart muscle is both a consumer and a provider of energy, and energy transfer occurs through a series of highly conserved cyclic processes. The control of energy transfer in the heart is discussed elsewhere in this book. Since the discovery that the mammalian heart receives its nutrients through the coronary circulation[11,12] (Fig. 1) the tight coupling of coronary flow, myocardial oxygen consumption, and contractile performance (Fig. 2) is one of the fundamental principles of cardiovascular physiology.[13,14] The cellular responses to a decrease in coronary flow are both immediate and sustained. Immediate responses are those affecting the transfer of energy from substrates to adenosine triphosphate (ATP) and entail the activation of inactivation of highly regulated enzymes. Signaling pathways are those of metabolic regulation and are well delineated. Sustained responses involve adaptive changes in gene expression, the mechanisms of which are not so well understood.

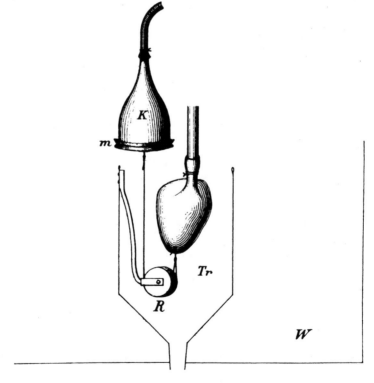

Figure 1. By showing that the isolated cat heart continued to beat when perfused through an aortic cammula, Langendorff demonstrated that the heart receives its nutrients through the coronary circulation. The figure is taken from his original publication and shows the heart mounted by tying the aorta to a steel cammula. Mechanical activity is recorded by displacement of a membrane (m) on a transducer (K).

Coronary Flow

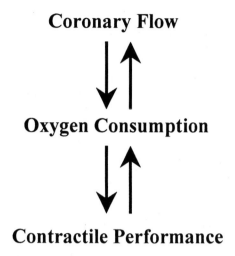

Oxygen Consumption

Contractile Performance

Figure 2. The coupling between coronary flow, oxygen consumption, and contractile performance is a cornerstone of cardiac physiology.

A reasonable working hypothesis links energy substrate metabolism with gene expression and enzyme regulation on the one hand and contractile function on the other hand (Fig. 3). In this scheme, there is a clear interdependence of metabolism, contractile function, and gene expression. Many of the signals, sensors, transducers, and effectors in this system have been identified only recently and continue to be the subject of intense investigation. Although there seems to be a dichotomy between the myocardial responses to acute and chronic changes in coronary flow, there also are certain commonalties. With respect to ischemia and the immediate or eventual return of contractile function, all adaptive processes ultimately are processes of "programmed cell survival." Although the molecular mechanisms of stunning, hibernation, and ischemic preconditioning may differ, a common feature of programmed cell survival is an intact, functioning nucleus of the cardiac myocyte. This term contrasts the well-known phenomenon of programmed cell death, or apoptosis, in the cardiovascular system.[15,16]

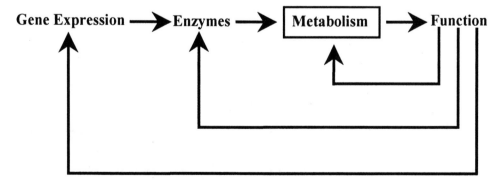

Figure 3. Metabolism and the activation of enzymes link function and gene expression in the heart.

Principal Observations: Aerobic versus Anaerobic Energy Production

Energy reserves in heart muscle are insufficient to sustain contractile function in the absence of a continuous flux of energy from oxidizable substrates. For this reason heart muscle is so richly endowed with mitochondria.[17] The principle of limited energy reserve is illustrated by a simple calculation. At an ATP content of approximately 20 μmol/g dry weight,[18] and at a myocardial O_2 consumption rate of 5 mmol/h per gram dry weight,[19] the heart turns over its entire ATP pool every 4–5 seconds. Although phosphocreatine (approximately 30 μmol/g dry weight) through the creatine kinase reaction and adenosine diphosphate (ADP) through the adenylate kinase reaction buffer ATP, the energy reserve in the absence of oxidizable substrates is still very limited. The heart therefore requires a continuous supply of energy providing substrates. Under aerobic conditions heart muscle prefers fatty acids to glucose as fuel for respiration. Under anaerobic conditions energy production relies on the mobilization of glycogen and anaerobic glycolysis, which amounts to approximately 5% of the energy derived from oxidative metabolism of glucose. Fatty acid oxidation ceases altogether. The combined effects of ATP hydrolysis and lactate production result in intracellular acidosis, accumulation of protons, inorganic phosphate, sodium, and calcium (Fig. 4). Note that the main source of protons is ATP hydrolysis[20,21] and also that adenosine is released, which results in an irreversible loss of purine nucleotides. The production of adenosine and the depletion of glycogen are both thought to be mediators of improved ischemia tolerance by ischemic preconditioning. As will be discussed below, the evidence is equivocal and the signal transduction pathways in

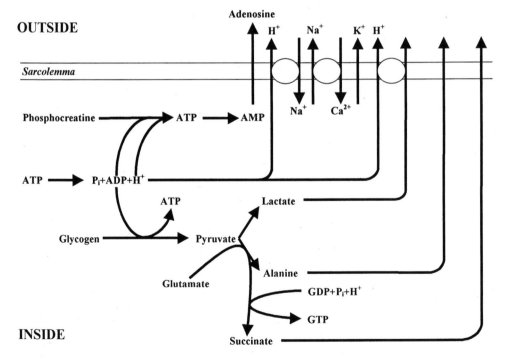

Figure 4. Salient metabolic responses to ischemia include glycogen breakdown, hydrolysis of adenosine triphosphate (ATP), proton production, cellular loss of potassium, and overloading of Ca^{2+}. Outside, extracellular space; inside, intracellular space. See text for details. Modified with permission from Reference 8.

ischemic preconditioning are complex. The accumulation of inorganic phosphate and of protons has been implicated as a causal link to decreased contractile performance,[22,23] while the accumulation of calcium in mitochondria and cytosol has been implicated as a causal link to irreversible cell damage.[24,25] Energy derived from glycolysis may be essential for the support of ion pumps and maintenance of cellular integrity as may be energy derived from the catabolism of glutamate (see review by Taegtmeyer et al.[8]). Indeed, physiological modulators of stress responses including glycogen may improve ischemia tolerance in vitro.[26–28] However, sustained, severe ischemia inevitably leads to cell death and necrosis.

Graded Ischemia and Graded Metabolic Responses

The myocardial response to ischemia is regulated[7] perhaps to preserve sufficient energy to protect the structural and functional integrity of the cardiac myocyte.[29] Ischemia tampers myocardial energy metabolism by slowing aerobic metabolism and by accelerating anaerobic metabolism—a reversal of the well-known Pasteur effect.[30] Just as there is a continuum of the relative restriction of oxygen delivery, one might expect that there is a continuum of metabolic responses to ischemia.[6,31,32] As coronary flow decreases in vivo, there is an increase in the uptake of glucose and, paradoxically, also of fatty acids.[33] Enhanced myocardial glucose uptake and metabolism are controlled further by the transmembrane glucose gradient, the rates of glucose phosphorylation, and glycogen turnover[34] and at the reactions of the glycolytic pathway. With sustained low-flow ischemia in vivo the up-regulation of glucose metabolism is limited to the cytosolic pathway (increased glycolysis and glycogen synthesis), while fatty acids continue to be the major source of oxidative substrate.[35] With acute low-flow ischemia in vitro glucose uptake is either unchanged[31] or increased.[32] Only with severe ischemia does the uptake of fatty acids cease, and glucose uptake dominates. The increase in glucose uptake relative to coronary flow is termed "metabolism/perfusion mismatch."[31,36] Metabolism/perfusion mismatch can be the result of either preserved metabolic activity with decreased flow or increased metabolic activity with preserved flow. Its long-term consequences are no longer metabolic but cellular: chronic or repetitive ischemia results in the dedifferentiation of cardiac myocytes to a fetal phenotype[37] with enhanced glycogen deposition, which corresponds to preserved metabolic activity[38] and correlates linearly with the retention of [^{18}F]2-fluoro-2-deoxy-D-glucose.[39] Reactivation of fetal genes is the hallmark of adaptation to changes in workload by the overloaded and by the unloaded heart.[40]

Although the mechanisms for stunning, hibernation, and ischemic preconditioning are still not defined very precisely,[41] the three phenomena have one feature in common: they are tissue responses related to ischemia and reperfusion. In principle they may occur in any tissue, with the brain showing the closest similarity to the heart. Understanding ischemia and understanding reperfusion is the clue to understanding stunning, hibernation, and ischemic preconditioning. The problem is quite simple: ischemia, or the response of cells to decreased blood flow, as we know it today, is more than a simple imbalance between supply and demand. The hibernating myocardium has adapted successfully to a decrease in supply without evidence of a switch to anaerobic metabolism. This switch occurs at a metabolic/enzymatic as well as at a genetic level. Some investigators tried to do justice to the diversity of the tissue response to reduced blood flow by defining two specific forms of ischemia: biochemical ischemia and physiological ischemia. These two definitions conveniently leave out any consideration of stunning or ischemic preconditioning. The stunned myocardium enjoys a normal blood supply although contraction is reduced while the myocyte repairs itself. In other words, while myocardial ischemia is associated with contractile dysfunction, contractile dysfunction can be present in the absence of ischemia and in the midst of plenty with respect to substrate supply and oxygen.

Reperfusion Injury: The Work of Oxygen-Derived Free Radicals?

Before we consider stunning or ischemic preconditioning it is necessary to address briefly the cellular events of reperfusion. Ischemia results in structural and functional damages of contractile proteins and cell membranes, including mitochondria, where the cells generate energy aerobically by reducing molecular oxygen to water. The metabolic events during reperfusion are complex[42] and dominated by the generation of oxygen-derived free radicals.[43–45] The cytochrome C oxidase reaction involves the transfer of four electrons to oxygen. Partial reduction of oxygen leads to multiple reactive oxygen species through superoxide anion radical. Superoxide dismutates to hydrogen peroxide (H_2O_2) + O_2. Further addition of electrons requires cleavage of the bond between oxygen atoms (Fenton reaction) to form the highly reactive hydroxyl radical (OH). In addition, NO forms nitrogen dioxide radicals, and myeloperoxidase forms hypochlorous acid.

Reactive oxygen species, particularly the hydroxyl free radical, can react with all biological macromolecules (lipids, proteins, etc.). The initial reaction generates a second radical, which reacts with a second macromolecule and generates a chain reaction. Proteins are modified in structure and function by radical reactions. Mammalian cells possess elaborate defense mechanisms to detoxify (metabolic) radicals. These include superoxide dismutase (SOD) and catalase,[46,47] inhibitors of free radical formation, radical scavengers, and the glutathione system.[48] Energy substrate metabolism during reperfusion of reversibly ischemic myocardium is characterized by a rapid return of long-chain fatty acid oxidation, which is uncoupled from contractile function[49] and associated with impaired glucose oxidation.[50] Postischemic recovery of function requires glucose.[51–53] Enhanced glucose uptake by reperfused myocardium in vivo may not manifest itself through enhanced retention of FDG because of a profound change in the tracer/tracee relationship under these conditions.[54] Postischemic recovery also is enhanced by pyruvate[55] or lactate,[56] most likely as a result of the anaplerotic requirement of the energy-depleted heart muscle.[9] Consistent with this hypothesis is the recent observation that mitochondrial metabolism of pyruvate is required for its enhancement of cardiac function and energetics.[57] In addition, pyruvate is an effective scavenger of oxygen-derived free radicals.[58]

Stunning, Hibernation, and Ischemic Preconditioning in Context

The hallmark of stunning is reperfusion without injury, either because ischemia was only mild (collaterals) or brief (thrombolysis) or controlled (reperfusion after cardiopulmonary bypass). Reversible contractile dysfunction with stunning has already been observed several years before the term "stunning" was introduced by Braunwald and Kloner in 1982.[59,60] Today, there is growing evidence, that decreased calcium sensitivity of the myofilaments is a hallmark of stunned myocardium.[61,62] Consistent with this concept is the inotropic stimulation of stunned myocardium by catecholamines, which entrances calcium sensitivity.[63,64] There also is growing evidence that stunning is a time of myocyte repair, including the degradation of damaged proteins and resynthesis of normal cell constituents.[65] Recently, we have observed that mechanical unloading may accelerate this process.[40] Whichever the mechanism may be, it is clear that stunning is not caused by adenine nucleotide depletion or to impairment in energy production but rather by a primary reduction in energy production.[66]

In contrast, the adaptive processes observed with reduced flow in hibernating myocardium are characterized by down-regulation of metabolic processes and reactivation of a fetal phenotype. This process is best described as "altered perfusion with long-term metabolic memory." This long-term memory is reflected in reexpression of fetal gene products. Fetal myocardium is characterized by reduced contractile function of the left ventricle, reliance on glucose for energy production, and an abundance of glycogen.[67] Adrenergic stimulation of adult myocardium results in preferential oxidation of glycogen for energy production.[68] It is reasonable to assume that the same occurs when hibernating or fetal myocardium are stimulated with epinephrine. More importantly, the salient feature of hibernating (or "viable") myocardium is the enhanced uptake of glucose and its tracer analog FDG and of glutamate,[69] which is metabolized to succinate and alanine.[70] Hibernating myocardium salvaged by reperfusion has a prolonged and gradual recovery of function analogous to the phenomenon of postischemic stunning seen experimentally.[71]

Hibernating myocardium should not be confused with low-flow ischemia. Recently, we examined contractile performance and glucose metabolism in response to a transient (60-minute) reduction in coronary flow.[31,32] In this model a fall in coronary flow was paralleled by a fall in cardiac output. The metabolic fate of glucose was assessed by employing three different tracers and measuring ^3H_2O production from [2-^3H] glucose for glucose transport and phosphorylation, [5-^3H] glucose for glycolysis, and [6-^3H] glucose for glucose oxidation. In the acute experiment reduction in coronary flow results in no change of glucose uptake but in a redirection of glucose oxidation to lactate production.

The term ischemic preconditioning now can be introduced as a form of short-term metabolic memory. The phenomenon, first observed in Dr. Jennings' laboratory in the mid-1980s,[5] is based on the observation that a brief period of ischemia, followed by reperfusion, lessens the effects of a subsequent, long period of ischemia. It was first seen (and is still most readily assessed) by a reduction in infarct size. Ischemic preconditioning also is readily observed in isolated perfused hearts[28,72] and even in isolated papillary muscles.[73] However, there is no question that ischemic preconditioning also is a clinically observed phenomenon in patients with unstable angina[74] or in patients undergoing percutaneous transluminal coronary angioplasty (PTCA).[75–77]

No other phenomenon in cardiovascular physiology has generated more interest in a search for the underlying mechanism. There are those who suggest that ischemic preconditioning depletes glycogen, lessens lactate accumulation, and reduces intracellular acidosis.[78–80] There are others, including this author, who suggest the opposite that glycogen actually lessens ischemic damage to the heart.[27,28] Preischemic glycogen levels do not determine the extent of acidosis during prolonged ischemia[81] and the recovery of function.[82] Studies using ^{31}P nuclear magnetic resonance (NMR) spectroscopy have shown that improved functional recovery in preconditioning is not caused by a higher level of high-energy phosphates or less acidosis during reperfusion.[83]

Perhaps most importantly, the search for a mechanism of ischemic preconditioning has initiated an unprecedented interest in receptor activation and signal transduction among cardiovascular physiologists. In short succession, it was discovered that activation of the adenosine A_1 receptor, of the α-adrenergic receptor, of the sarcolemmal and mitochondrial K_{ATP} channel and of the mitochondrial ATPase all mimic the phenomenon, and that activation of phospholipase C and translocation of protein kinase C isoforms also are involved.[84] Presently, known targets of protein kinase C include Ca^{2+}-ATPase, troponin T and I, myosin light-chain kinase, phosphofructokinase, and guanylate cyclase. Because each of these molecules is a potential participant in the metabolic effects of preconditioning,[85] these molecules may be targets for pharmacologic interventions mimicking the protective effects of ischemic preconditioning.[86]

Summing Up

An overview of the phenomena of myocardial stunning, hibernation, and ischemic preconditioning shows that the phenomena are part of the spectrum of myocardial ischemia and reperfusion (Fig. 5). By different mechanisms of acute and chronic adaptation to ischemia the different phenomena all result in a spectrum of programmed cell survival. To recapitulate:

- Stunning refers to reperfusion without injury.
- Hibernation refers to perfusion with long-term metabolic memory.
- Preconditioning refers to reperfusion with short-term metabolic memory.

Those who studied medicine in the 1960s may remember a spectrum displaying the different forms of endocarditis. It is not to be presumed that the model shown in Figure 5 answers all questions. Myocardial stunning, hibernation, and ischemic preconditioning trigger programmed cell survival most likely by different mechanisms. By drawing attention to programmed cell survival the model seems best suited to identify commonalties

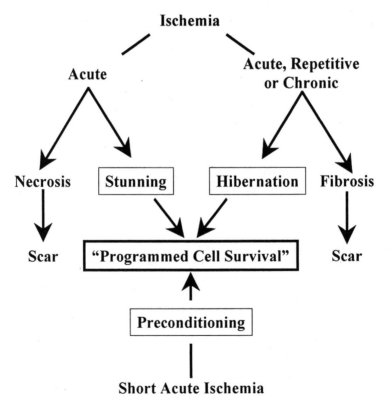

Figure 5. Myocardial stunning, hibernation, and ischemic preconditioning trigger programmed cell survival, most likely by different mechanisms. Common to all three phenomena is an intact, functioning nucleus of the cardiac myocyte. See text for further discussion.

rather than mechanistic detail. The issues undoubtedly are complex, but a better, more unifying concept undoubtedly will emerge in the age of cardiovascular molecular biology.

Acknowledgments: I thank Rachel Ralston for help with the preparation of this chapter.

References

1. Virchow R. *Die Zellularpathologie und ihre Begründung auf physiologische und pathologische Gewebelehre* [in German]. Berlin, Germany: Hirschwald; 1858.
2. Braunwald E, Kloner RA. The stunned myocardium: Prolonged, postischemic ventricular dysfunction. *Circulation* 1982;66:1146–1149.
3. Rahimtoola SH. A perspective on the three large multicenter randomized clinical trials of coronary bypass surgery for chronic stable angina. *Circulation* 1985;72:V123–V135.
4. Gorlin R. *Coronary Artery Disease.* Philadelphia, Pa: W B Saunders; 1976:316.
5. Murry CE, Jennings RB, Reimer KA. Preconditioning with ischemia: A delay of lethal cell injury in ischemic myocardium. *Circulation* 1986;74:1124–1136.
6. De Boer L, Rude R, Kloner R, et al. A flow- and time-dependent index of ischemic injury after coronary occlusion and reperfusion. *Proc Natl Acad Sci U S A* 1983;80:5784–5788.
7. Ross JJ. Myocardial perfusion-contraction matching. Implications for coronary heart disease and hibernation. *Circulation* 1991;83:1076–1083.
8. Taegtmeyer H, King L, Jones B. Energy substrate metabolism, myocardial ischemia, and targets for pharmacotherapy. *Am J Cardiol* 1998;82:54K–60K.
9. Taegtmeyer H, Goodwin GW, Doenst T, et al. Substrate metabolism as a determinant for postischemic functional recovery of the heart. *Am J Cardiol* 1997;80:3A–10A.
10. Taegtmeyer H, Peterson MB, Ragavan VV, et al. De novo alanine synthesis in isolated oxygen-deprived rabbit myocardium. *J Biol Chem* 1977;252:5010–5018.
11. Taegtmeyer H. One hundred years ago: Oscar Langendorff and the birth of cardiac metabolism. *Can J Cardiol* 1995;11:1030–1035.
12. Langendorff O. Untersuchungen am uberlebenden Saugethierherzen. *Arch Ges Physiol Menschen Ture* 1895;61:291–332.
13. Langendorff O. Zur kenntniss des blutlaufs in den kranzgefassen des herzens. *Arch Ges Physiol Menschen Ture* 1898;78:423–440.
14. Taegtmeyer H. Energy metabolism of the heart: From basic concepts to clinical applications. *Curr Prob Cardiol* 1994;19:57–116.
15. MacLellan W, Schneider M. Death by design. Programmed cell death in cardiovascular biology and disease. *Circ Res* 1997;81:137–144.
16. Haunstetter A, Izumo S. Apoptosis: Basic mechanism and impliation for cardiovascular disease. *Circ Res* 1998;82:1111–1129.
17. McNutt N, Fawcett D. *Myocardial ultrastructure.* New York: John Wiley & Sons; 1973:1–50.
18. Taegtmeyer H, Roberts AFC, Rayne AEG. Energy metabolism in reperfused rat heart: Return of function before normalization of ATP content. *J Am Coll Cardiol* 1985;6:864–870.
19. Taegtmeyer H, Hems R, Krebs HA. Utilization of energy providing substrates in the isolated working rat heart. *Biochem J* 1980;186:701–711.
20. Dennis S, Gevers W, Opie L. Protons in ischemia: Where do they come from, where do they go to? *J Mol Cell Cardiol* 1991;23:1077–1086.
21. Gevers W. Generation of protons by metabolic processes in heart cells. *J Mol Cell Cardiol* 1977;9:867–864.
22. Katz AM, Hecht HH. The early "pump" failure of the ischemic heart. *Am J Med* 1969;47:497–502.
23. Jennings R, Hawkins H, Lowe J, et al. Relation between high energy phosphate and lethal injury in myocardial ischemia. *Am J Pathol* 1978;92:187.
24. Fleckenstein A, Janke J, Doring H, et al. Myocardial fiber necrosis due to intracellular Ca^{2+} overload: A new principle in cardiac pathophysiology. *Rec Adv Stud Card Struct Met* 1974;4:563–580.
25. Katz A, Reuter H. Cellular calcium and cell death. *Am J Cardiol* 1979;44:188.
26. McElroy DD, Walker WE, Taegtmeyer H. Glycogen loading improves left ventricular function of the rabbit heart after hypothermic ischemic arrest. *J Appl Cardiol* 1989;4:455–465.

27. Schneider CA, Taegtmeyer H. Fasting in vivo delays myocardial cell damage after brief periods of ischemia in the isolated working rat heart. *Circ Res* 1991;68:1045–1050.

28. Doenst T, Guthrie P, Chemnitius J-M, et al. Fasting, lactate, and insulin improve ischemia tolerance: A comparison with ischemic preconditioning. *Am J Physiol* 1996;270:H1607–H1615.

29. Bristow JD, Arai AE, Anselone CG, et al. Response to myocardial ischemia as a regulated process. *Circulation* 1991;84:2580–2587.

30. Krebs H. The Pasteur effect and the relation between respiration and fermentation. *Essays Biochem* 1972;8:1–34.

31. Bolukoglu H, Goodwin GW, Guthrie PH, et al. Metabolic fate of glucose in reversible low-flow ischemia of the isolated working rat heart. *Am J Physiol* 1996;270:H817–H826.

32. Chen TM, Goodwin GW, Guthrie PH, et al. Effects of insulin on glucose uptake by rat hearts during and after coronary flow reduction. *Am J Physiol* 1997;273:H2170–H2177.

33. Young LH, Renfu Y, Russell R, et al. Low-flow ischemia leads to translocation of canine heart GLUT-4 and GLUT-1 glucose transporters to the sarcolemma in vivo. *Circulation* 1997;95:415–422.

34. Russell R, Cline G, Guthrie P, et al. Regulation of exogenous and endogenous glucose metabolism by insulin and acetoacetate in isolated working rat heart: A three-tracer study of glycolysis, glycogen metabolism and glucose oxidation. *J Clin Invest* 1997;100:2892–2899.

35. McNulty PH, Sinusas AJ, Shi CQX, et al. Glucose metabolism distal to a critical coronary stenosis canine model of low-flow myocardial ischemia. *J Clin Invest* 1996;98:62–69.

36. Tillisch J, Brunken R, Marshall R, et al. Prediction of reversibility of cardiac wall motion abnormalities predicted by positron tomography, [18]fluoro-deoxyglucose, and [13]NH$_3$. *N Engl J Med* 1986;314:884–888.

37. Borgers M, Thoné F, Wouters L, et al. Structural correlates of regional myocardial dysfunction in patients with critical coronary artery stenosis. *Cardiovasc Pathol* 1993;2:237–245.

38. Maes A, Flameng W, Nuyts J, et al. Histological alterations in chronically hypo-perfused myocardium. Correlation with PET findings. *Circulation* 1994;90:735–745.

39. Depre C, Vanoverschelde JL, Gerber B, et al. Correlation of functional recovery with myocardial blood flow, glucose uptake, and morphologic features in patients with chronic left ventricular ischemic dysfunction undergoing coronary artery bypass grafting. *J Thorac Cardiovasc Surg* 1997;113:82–87.

40. Depre C, Shipley G, Chen W, et al. Unloaded heart in vivo replicates fetal gene expression of cardiac hypertrophy. *Nat Med* 1998;4:1269–1275.

41. Kloner RA, Bolli R, Marban E, et al. Medical and cellular implications of stunning, hibernation, and preconditioning. An NHLBI workshop. *Circulation* 1998;97:1848–1867.

42. Becker L, Ambrosio G. Myocardial consequences of reperfusion. *Prog Cardiovasc Dis* 1987;30:23.

43. Ferrari R, Ceconi C, Curello S, et al. Oxygen-mediated myocardial damage during ischemia and reperfusion. Role of cellular defences against oxygen toxicity. *J Mol Cell Cardiol* 1985;17:937–943.

44. Zweier J, Flaherty J, Weisfeldt M. Direct measurement of free radical generation following reperfusion of ischemic myocardium. *Proc Natl Acad Sci U S A* 1987;84:1404–1407.

45. Bolli R, Patel B, Jeroudi M, et al. Demonstration of free radical generation in a "stunned" myocardium of intact dogs with the use of spin trap alpha-phenyl N-Tertbutyl nitrone. *J Clin Invest* 1988;82:476–485.

46. Ambrosio G, Weisfeld M, Jacobus W, et al. Evidence for a reversible, oxygen radical-mediated component of reperfusion damage: Reduction by recombinant human superoxide dismutase administered at the time of reflow. *Circulation* 1987;75:282–291.

47. Gross G, Farber N, Haroman H, et al. Beneficial actins of superoxide dismutase and catalase in stunned myocardium of dogs. *Am J Physiol* 1986;250:H372–H377.

48. Bolli R. Oxygen-derived free radicals and myocardial reperfusion injury: An overview. *Cardiovasc Drugs Ther* 1991;5:249–268.

49. Liedtke AJ, Renstrom B, Hacker TA, et al. Effects of moderate repetitive ischemia on myocardial substrate utilization. *Am J Physiol* 1995;269:H246–H253.

50. Liu B, Clanachan AS, Schulz R, et al. Cardiac efficiency is improved after ischemia by altering both the source and fate of protons. *Circ Res* 1996;79:940–948.

51. Mallet RT, Hartman DA, Bünger R. Glucose requirement for postischemic recovery of perfused working heart. *Eur J Biochem* 1990;188:481–493.
52. Fralix TA, Steenbergen C, London RE, et al. Metabolic substrates can alter postischemic recovery in preconditioned ischemic heart. *Am J Physiol* 1992;263:C17–C23.
53. Jeremy RW, Ambrosio G, Pike MM, et al. The functional recovery of post-ischemic myocardium requires glycolysis during early reperfusion. *J Mol Cell Cardiol* 1993;25:261–276.
54. Doenst T, Taegtmeyer H. Profound underestimation of glucose uptake by [18F]2-deoxy-2-fluoroglucose in reperfused rat heart muscle. *Circulation* 1998;97:2454–2462.
55. Bunger R, Mallet RT, Hartman DA. Pyruvate-enhanced phosphorylation potential and inotropism in normoxic and postischemic isolated working heart. Near-complete prevention of reperfusion contractile failure. *Eur J Biochem* 1989;180:221–233.
56. Goodwin GW, Taegtmeyer H. Metabolic recovery of the isolated working rat heart after brief global ischemia. *Am J Physiol* 1994;267:H462–H470.
57. Mallet R, Sun J. Mitochondrial metabolism of pyruvate is required for its enhancement of cardiac function and energetics. *Cardiovasc Res* 1998. 42:149–161.
58. De Boer L, Bekx P, Han L, et al. Pyruvate enhances recovery of rat hearts after ischemia and reperfusion by preventing free radical generation. *Am J Physiol* 1993;265:H1571–H1576.
59. Weiner JM, Apstein CS, Arthur JH, et al. Persistence of myocardial injury following brief periods of coronary occlusion. *Cardiovasc Res* 1976;10:678–686.
60. Heyndrickx G, Baig H, Nellens P, et al. Depression of regional blood flow and wall thickness after brief coronary occlusions. *Am J Physiol* 1978;234:H653–H659.
61. Carrozza J, Bentivegna L, Williams C, et al. Decreased myofilament responsiveness in myocardial stunning follows transient calcium overload during ischaemia and reperfusion. *Circ Res* 1992;71:1334–1340.
62. Marban E. Myocardial stunning and hibernation. The physiology behind the colloquialisms. *Circulation* 1991;83:681–688.
63. Becker L, Levine JD, Paula A, et al. Reversal of dysfunction in post-ischemic stunned myocardium by eprinephrine and postextrasystolic potentiation. *J Am Coll Cardiol* 1986;7:580–589.
64. Bolli R, Zhu X, Myers M, et al. Beta-adrenergic stimulation reverses postischemic myocardial dysfunction without producing subsequent functional deterioration. *Am J Cardiol* 1985;56:964–968.
65. Schaper W. Stunned myocardium, an opinionated review. *Basic Res Cardiol* 1995;90:273–275.
66. Zucchi R, Yu G, Ronca-Testoni S, et al. Energy metabolism in myocardial stunning. *J Mol Cell Cardiol* 1992;24:1237–1252.
67. Shelley H. Cardiac glycogen in different species before and after birth. *Brit Med Bull* 1961;17:137–156.
68. Goodwin G, Ahmad F, Taegtmeyer H. Preferential oxidation of glycogen in isolated working rat heart. *J Clin Invest* 1996;97:1409–1416.
69. Zimmermann R, Tillmanns H, Knopp W. Regional myocardial ^{13}N-glutamate uptake in patients with coronary artery disease. *J Am Coll Cardiol* 1988;11:549–556.
70. Taegtmeyer H. Metabolic responses to cardiac hypoxia: Increased production of succinate by rabbit papillary muscles. *Circ Res* 1978;43:808–815.
71. Patel B, Kloner R, Przyklenk K, et al. Postishemic myocardial "stunning": A clinically relevant phenomenon. *Ann Int Med* 1988;108:626–628.
72. Cave A. Preconditioning induced protection against post-ischaemic contractile dysfunction: Characteristics and mechanisms. *J Mol Cell Cardiol* 1995;27:969–979.
73. Walker D, Marber M, Walker J, et al. Preconditioning in isolated superfused rabbit papillary muscles. *Am J Physiol* 1994;266:H1534–H1540.
74. Kloner R, Yellon D. Does ischemic preconditioning occur in patients? *J Am Coll Cardiol* 1994;24:1133–1142.
75. Deutsch E, Berger M, Kussmaul W, et al. Adaptation to ischemia during percutaneous transluminal coronary angioplasty: Clinical, hemodynamic, and metabolic features. *Circulation* 1990;82:2044–2051.
76. Heibig J, Bolli R, Harris S. Initial coronary occlusion improves tolerance to subsequent prolonged balloon inflations. *Cathet Cardiovasc Diagn* 1989;16:99–104.
77. Yellon D, Alkhulaife A, Pugsley W. Preconditioning the human myocardium. *Lancet* 1993;342:276–271.

78. Asimakis GK, Inners-McBride K, Medellin G, et al. Ischemic preconditioning attenuates acidosis and postischemic dysfunction in isolated rat hearts. *Am J Physiol* 1992;263:H887–H894.
79. Wolfe CL, Sievers RE, Visseren FLJ, et al. Loss of myocardial protection after preconditioning correlates with the time course of glycogen recovery within the preconditioned segment. *Circulation* 1993;87:881–892.
80. Weiss R, De Albuquerque C, Vandergaer K, et al. Alternated glycogenolysis reduces glycolytic catabolic accumulation during ischemia in precondioned rat hearts. *Circ Res* 1996;79:435–446.
81. Soares P, De Albuquerque C, Chacko U, et al. Role of preischemic glycogen depletion in the improvement of postischemic metabolic and contractile recovery of ischemic-preconditioned rat hearts. *Circulation* 1997;96:975–983.
82. Doenst T, Guthrie PH, Taegtmeyer H. Ischemic preconditioning in rat heart: No correlation between glycogen content and return of function. *Mol Cell Biochem* 1998. 180:153–161.
83. Schjott J, Bakoy D, Jones R, et al. Preconditioning by brief ischaemic episodes in the isolated rat heart assessed by ^{31}P NMR spectroscopy: Dissociation between metabolic and functional recovery? *Scand J Clin Lab Invest* 1995;55:67–78.
84. Cohen M, Downey J. Myocardial preconditioning promises to be a novel approach to the treatment of ischemic heart disease. *Annu Rev Med* 1996;47:21–29.
85. Parratt JR. Protection of the heart by ischaemic preconditioning: Mechanisms and possibilities for pharmacological exploitation. *Trends Pharmacol Sci* 1994;15:19–25.
86. Cohen M, Downey J. Ischaemic preconditioning: Can the protection be bottled? *Lancet* 1993;342:6.

Reversible Myocardial Dysfunction: Stunning, Hibernation, or What?

Francis J. Klocke, MD,
Andrew J. Sherman, MD, and Ada Jain, MD

Introduction

Viable, reversibly hypocontractile myocardium in ischemic heart disease usually is characterized as either "stunned" or "hibernating." In recent years it has become apparent that reductions in flow can induce protective as well as injurious responses in the heart's contractile processes and that some of these beneficial adaptations develop quickly. This chapter will review studies pertinent to these adaptations and will attempt to clarify issues that complicate the characterization of hypocontractile myocardium as simply hibernating or stunned.

Stunning Versus Hibernation—Usual Definitions

In ischemic heart disease, the judgment as to whether viable, reversibly hypocontractile myocardium is stunned or hibernating traditionally has been made on the basis of whether coronary blood flow measured under resting conditions is normal or reduced.

Stunning refers to a delayed recovery of contractile function following a period of ischemia. Although myocardial function is depressed, coronary flow has returned to a normal (or "near-normal") resting level. The apparent imbalance between flow and function is characterized as a flow-function "mismatch."[1] Because coronary flow is taken as a surrogate for myocardial O_2 consumption, the implication is that a similar mismatch occurs for O_2 consumption and function. Stunning represents a transient reversible injury; potential causes relate to effects of both ischemia and postischemic reperfusion.[2]

Interest in stunning was stimulated by several studies in experimental animals in the mid-1970s. In 1975 Heyndrickx, Vatner, and colleagues demonstrated that reductions in regional mechanical function following coronary occlusions that produced severe ischemia without myocardial infarction could persist for hours.[3] Following a plethora of experimental studies, the concept of stunning has been extended to a variety of clinical situations associated with recent ischemia and reduced contractile function.[2]

From Dilsizian V (ed). *Myocardial Viability: A Clinical and Scientific Treatise.* Armonk, NY: Futura Publishing Co., Inc.; © 2000.

Hibernation is thought of as an adaptive rather than injurious response, in which myocardial contractile performance and O_2 consumption are reduced proportionately in the setting of a limited blood supply. Because the reductions in energy utilization and contraction are proportionate, a normal "match" between flow (or O_2 consumption) and function is maintained. Originally, it was proposed that the reduced energy utilization was related directly to the reduction in flow, that is, that local flow reserve was exhausted under resting conditions. Because this is not always the case,[4-8] it has alternatively been proposed that the adaptation represents a primary down-regulation of O_2 demand to accommodate a limited flow reserve, thereby reducing the likelihood of demand-induced ischemia. In either case, myocardial O_2 demand and supply remain in balance, favoring myocardial viability.

Interest in myocardial hibernation arose from clinical rather than experimental observations. The term hibernation initially was used by Diamond in the late 1970s[9] and Rahimtoola in the early 1980s.[10] It became apparent that regionally hypocontractile areas of the left ventricle in patients with ischemic heart disease sometimes showed substantial improvements in function following bypass graft surgery. Using positron emission tomography (PET), Tillisch, Schelbert, and colleagues demonstrated in 1986 that measurements of flow and glucose uptake could identify prospectively hypocontractile segments that benefited from revascularization.[11] Because reductions in perfusion and function and increases in glucose uptake were demonstrated when ischemia was not evident, this form of reversibly reduced function appeared to represent a chronic adaptation rather than an acute response to recent ischemia.

More recently, on the basis of studies during sustained partial reductions in coronary flow in experimental animals, it has been demonstrated that some beneficial adaptive responses to flow limitation can develop quickly, that is, within an hour or two.[12] The term "short-term" hibernation has been used to describe these findings, which will be reviewed later in this chapter.

There is now agreement that stunning and hibernation can occur in the same area, that is, a hibernating area can experience superimposed stunning following a period of ischemia. Some investigators have come to feel that reversibly hypocontractile myocardium usually is caused by repeated episodes of stunning (often clinically inapparent) and have even questioned whether hibernation is a clinically important entity. Conversely, others invoke the hibernation response to explain the persistence of viable but hypocontractile myocardium in the absence of clinically evident ischemia. Still others use the term "chronic" hibernation to include all chronic reversibly hypocontractile myocardium caused by coronary artery disease.[13] As discussed subsequently, these differences in viewpoint relate in part to methodological limitations in determining whether coronary flow is normal or reduced under resting conditions.

Issues in Design of Experimental Studies

When considering experimental studies of stunning or hibernation, several points need to be kept in mind.

1. Many animal studies intended to investigate these entities have been complicated by use of an ischemic stimulus that was severe enough to produce irreversible myocardial injury. In both acute and chronic preparations, it is difficult to separate effects of infarcted tissue on flow and function from effects of stunning or hibernation. When irreversible injury occurs, chronic studies can be complicated further by remodeling and hypertrophy. To avoid irreversible injury when a coronary artery is occluded completely, the duration of occlusion cannot exceed 15–20 minutes in intact animals such as the dog and pig. Durations of occlusion that

avoid irreversible injury are less well defined in smaller animals (particularly those with rapid resting heart rates) and in isolated heart preparations. Irreversible injury is especially difficult to exclude in isolated hearts in which diastolic pressure rises above baseline levels and developed pressure is reduced when perfusion is restored.

2. For a given degree and duration of ischemia, the severity of myocardial stunning is substantially less in conscious chronically instrumented animals than in acute open-chest or isolated heart preparations.[14,15]

3. Measurements of coronary flow usually are interpreted as reflecting myocardial O_2 consumption; that is, coronary arteriovenous O_2 differences are assumed to remain constant. This assumption is especially hazardous in anesthetized, open-chest and isolated heart preparations, in which there often is a progressive loss of normal autoregulation of coronary flow. When autoregulation is compromised, coronary flow increases and arteriovenous O_2 differences narrow; that is, coronary venous O_2 levels increase. Changes in O_2 consumption therefore can be accomplished through changes in O_2 extraction as well as flow, and the usual close correspondence between flow and O_2 consumption may not be present. In conscious, normally autoregulating preparations, oxygen extraction is near maximal under resting conditions, with coronary venous O_2 saturations of 20%–25% and P_{O_2}s of 15–20 mm Hg. However, changes in O_2 extraction can occur even in these preparations,[16] and measurements of O_2 consumption are again preferable.

4. Periods of ischemia frequently are followed by a transient increase in myocardial function when perfusion is restored. Although this phenomenon was noted in studies of myocardial stunning as early as 1978,[17] it remains incompletely understood. Pagani et al felt that it was dependent on the reactive hyperemia associated with reperfusion and were unable to abolish it with propanolol, reserpine, verapamil, or general anesthesia.[17] In addition to this phenomenon, effects of factors such as catecholamine release during a coronary occlusion may require significant time to abate. Thus, postischemic reductions in myocardial function may not be apparent or may not reach their nadir for 15–60 minutes after the onset of reperfusion.

5. Moderate degrees of flow reduction apparently can be sustained for at least a few hours without irreversible injury to the affected myocardium. In 1983, Matsuzaki et al maintained a partial coronary constriction sufficient to reduce regional systolic wall thickening (WT) by ~40% (and regional flow by a similar amount) for 5 hours in chronically instrumented dogs.[18] Function remained depressed when the flow restriction was removed but returned to the control level over the ensuing week. In 1986 Neill et al reported that alterations in adenosine triphosphate (ATP) metabolism stabilized during sustained 30%–80% reductions in coronary flow also lasting as long as 5 hours.[19]

Coronary Flow and Myocardial Oxygen Consumption in the Early Postischemic Period

As previously noted, stunning and hibernation usually have been distinguished on the basis of whether coronary flow is normal or reduced in the hypocontractile area. Experimentally, most studies of stunned myocardium have used total occlusions of sufficient duration to produce postreperfusion dysfunction ranging from near akinesia to dyskinesia. As illustrated in Figure 1, corresponding values of coronary flow and myocardial O_2 consumption have been more variable than often appreciated.

In one of the earliest studies of postischemic dysfunction, Heyndrickx et al reported subnormal levels of transmural flow and endocardial/epicardial flow ratio for up to 1 hour

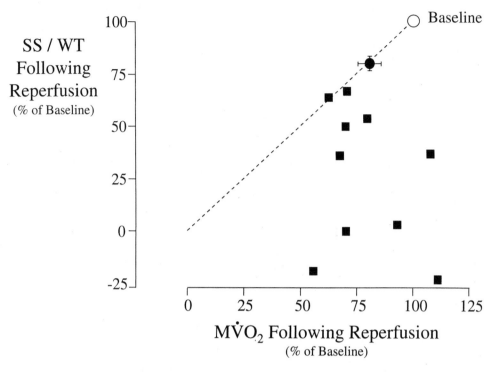

Figure 1. Values of regional function [as measured by segment shortening (SS) or wall thickening (WT)] and myocardial O_2 consumption after reperfusion. Values are taken with permission from Reference 16 and published reports are presumed to represent stunned myocardium. The open circle represents the baseline situation for all studies, with both regional function and myocardial O_2 consumption normalized to a value of 100%. The solid circle represents the average findings ±1 SEM found in Reference 16 after the restoration of unrestricted inflow. The solid squares represent average values of regional function and myocardial O_2 consumption after reperfusion in other studies. Reprinted with permission from Reference 16.

after the onset of reperfusion in conscious dogs subjected to a 15-minute coronary occlusion.[20] Conversely, while also studying conscious dogs, Laxson, Bache, and colleagues found flow and O_2 consumption to be unchanged 1 hour after three 10-minute coronary occlusions; regional function remained depressed to 37% of its original value.[21]

Variable results also have been obtained in open-chest preparations.[22–28] Stahl et al[22] and Dean et al[23] found coronary flow and myocardial O_2 consumption to be unchanged essentially in the setting of akinesia or dyskinesia following reperfusion in dogs, while Vinten-Johansen et al[24] reported that O_2 consumption was decreased by ~45% in the setting of dyskinesia. Schaper reported decreases in O_2 consumption and regional shortening averaging 30% and 50%, respectively, in open-chest dogs.[25] When open-chest pigs were studied in the same laboratory, reductions in O_2 consumption were less clear and decreases in regional function more pronounced, causing the authors to suggest a species variation.[25] While also studying open-chest pigs, McFalls et al observed reductions of ~30% in O_2 consumption and ~60% in segment shortening (SS) after two 10-minute coronary occlusions,[27] but found more concordant reductions of ~40% in regional O_2 consumption and function after one to three 5-minute partial occlusions.[28]

A limited number of additional measurements have been reported during open-chest studies directed at other issues. While investigating responses to isoproterenol, Smith found that control (preisoproterenol) values of flow and O_2 consumption were 20% less following a 10-minute coronary occlusion.[29] While studying effects of nicorandil and nifedipine on postischemic function, Lamping and Gross noted that subendocardial flow was lower in postischemic areas than in nonischemic areas for 5 hours after a 15-minute occlusion; flows were not measured prior to occlusion, however.[30] During a study of three sequential coronary occlusions Lange et al reported that flows in ischemic zones tended to be reduced following reperfusion for 15 minutes, but not 5-minute occlusions.[31]

In addition to these direct measurements of flow and O_2 consumption, Buxton et al[32] and Heyndrickx et al[33] have calculated values of myocardial O_2 consumption from the early myocardial clearance of ^{11}C-acetate administered intravenously and quantified by PET in chronically instrumented dogs. The Heyndrickx study[33] reports a 1- to 2-week reduction in calculated O_2 consumption despite the restoration of normal flow following a 1-hour reduction in flow sufficient to produce akinesis. Buxton et al[32] report similar decreases in acetate-derived O_2 consumption lasting up to a month in reversibly injured portions of canine myocardium following a 3-hour coronary occlusion.

Difficulties in Distinguishing Between Proportionate and Disproportionate Reductions in Flow and Function In Vivo

The variability of the findings just reviewed complicates any attempt to generalize them as representing simply stunning or hibernation. In several cases, the degree of postischemic dysfunction was severe and clearly "mismatched" with segmental flow and/or O_2 consumption. The high level of O_2 utilization in such studies has been referred to as the O_2 consumption "paradox" of stunned myocardium.[23] Although the basis for near-baseline O_2 consumption remains unclear, some workers have suggested that it relates to passive systolic stretch, that is, to energy expended to counteract the distending effect of overall ventricular contraction. In 1989 Gayheart et al reported that O_2 consumption in a pharmacologically arrested myocardial segment undergoing systolic bulging was paradoxically high (70% of that in normally contracting segments) when the heart was beating but decreased markedly when the heart was placed on cardiopulmonary bypass and vented.[34] Subsequent studies support the concept that reperfused stunned myocardium performs more total work in vivo than appreciated from measurements of systolic shortening or WT alone. After four 12-minute coronary occlusions in open-chest pigs, Vinten-Johansen et al found that changes in myocardial O_2 consumption (44% decrease from baseline) were more proportional to decreases in regional work calculated from pressure-segment length loops (67%) than to decreases in systolic SS (119%).[24] Also using pressure-segment length loop areas as a measure of regional work, McFalls et al likewise found that the total energy expended during mechanical contraction in stunned myocardium is higher than expected from changes in systolic segment length.[27] Chiu et al have suggested that asynchrony between regional force development and SS decreases systolic work to a greater degree than total positive work and that the latter exerts the dominant effect on regional O_2 consumption.[35] Other possibilities suggested to explain a mismatch between function and flow (and presumably O_2 consumption) include an increased use of energy for noncontractile activities, inefficient transfer of energy into myocyte contraction, and shunting of energy supplies toward cellular repair.[36]

Although these studies have all been performed in experimental animals, distinctions between "proportionate" and "disproportionate" reductions in flow and function are even more difficult in clinical situations. In situations in which coronary flow and myocardial O_2 demand may be more appropriately balanced than can be appreciated from conventional measurements of function, attempts to distinguish stunning from hibernation on the basis of the resting level of flow become problematic (Fig. 2).

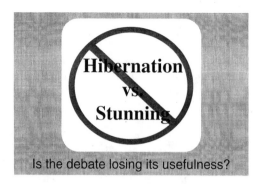

Figure 2. During the past few years limitations of the traditional definitions of hibernation and stunning and the dichotomous characterization of viable hypocontractile myocardium as hibernating or stunned have become increasingly apparent. Most individual situations probably represent a combination of beneficial adaptive responses, transient postischemic injury, and ultrastructural changes.

Early Adaptive Responses to Ischemia and/or Flow Reduction—Short-Term Hibernation

Studies from several laboratories indicate that apparently beneficial responses to flow reduction and ischemia can develop quite quickly, that is, within an hour or two. These responses usually have been identified in open-chest or isolated heart preparations, using sustained partial reductions in coronary flow.

1. In 1988 Fedele, Gewirtz, and colleagues followed metabolic responses to a 50% reduction in subendocardial flow over 3 hours in closed-chest pigs.[37] Lactate production developed during the first 5 minutes of flow reduction and was accompanied by a decrease in pH and increase in P_{CO_2} in regional venous blood. However, these abnormalities cleared during the subsequent hour and did not recur during the remaining 2 hours of flow reduction. Regional myocardial O_2 consumption decreased by ~20% when the flow reduction was initiated and remained at this lower level throughout the 3-hour period. The authors suggested that myocardial O_2 demand decreased to a level more appropriate to the reduced O_2 supply in response to the flow limitation.

2. In a study of isolated rabbit hearts also reported in 1988, Marshall found that developed pressure and myocardial O_2 consumption decreased progressively with flow reduction, while tissue lactate and high-energy phosphate levels remained normal until flow was reduced by >50%.[38] He too suggested that contractile performance can be coupled to oxidative energy production to maintain energy balance during partial flow restriction. A recent study of interstitial purine and lactate levels during graded ischemia by Delyani and Van Wylen[39] supports this conclusion.

3. In 1989 Kitakaze and Marban[40] reported that moderate reductions in perfusion pressure (and therefore flow) in ferret hearts cause reductions in developed pressure and the intracellular calcium transient without a decrease in intracellular pH or an increase in tissue lactate or inorganic phosphorus concentration.

4. The concept of early beneficial responses received further support in a series of studies of moderate flow reduction in open-chest pigs by Pantely et al in the early 1990s.[41] Subendocardial phosphocreatine levels fell by 50% in the first 5 minutes

of a 50% reduction in subendocardial flow but returned to normal as the flow reduction was continued for an hour.[42] In a subsequent similar study, subendocardial lactate accumulation initially rose to 300% of control levels and was accompanied by net arteriovenous lactate production; by the end of an hour tissue lactate levels were near normal and arteriovenous lactate extraction had returned.[43] When a period of rapid atrial pacing was superimposed on the continuing flow reduction at the end of the hour, lactate production and phosphocreatine depletion recurred, indicating that the heart was capable of utilizing the phosphocreatine it was accumulating during the continuing flow reduction prior to pacing. Schulz et al also demonstrated inotropic reserve at the completion of a 1-hour period of moderate flow reduction in pigs.[44] Regional myocardial WT and regional myocardial O_2 consumption were decreased proportionately to the degree of flow reduction throughout the studies of Pantely et al. Thus, function appeared to stabilize at a level consistent with but not exceeding O_2 supply. More recently, both this group[45] and Ito[46] have demonstrated similar findings using reductions in flow that were sufficiently gradual to result in minimal metabolic evidence of ischemia. The observation that the down-regulation of metabolic requirements can "almost keep pace" with the gradual decline in coronary flow raises the possibility that the down-regulatory process relates more directly to the level of flow than to ischemia per se.

5. ^{31}P nuclear magnetic resonance (NMR) spectroscopy studies of Keller and Cannon[47] in isolated rat hearts also indicate that modest reductions in coronary flow produce proportionate reductions in myocardial O_2 consumption and contractile performance with only slight reductions in creatine phosphate and insignificant lactate production.

6. Partial restoration of myocardial creatine phosphate levels during sustained reductions in coronary flow has been suggested to reflect a down-regulation of oxidative metabolism.[42,43] Alternatively, Kroll et al have presented an "open-system kinetics" hypothesis in which adenosine monophosphate (AMP) hydrolysis to adenosine and membrane adenosine efflux cause a decrease in the cytosolic concentration of adenosine diphosphate (ADP) linked to the myokinase reaction.[48] Schaefer et al have further defined changes in high-energy phosphates and lactate release during moderate flow reductions.[49] They propose that glycolytic production of ATP (as opposed to ATP production by mitochondrial oxidative phosphorylation) is needed for phosphocreatine normalization during such reductions.[50]

These situations are now frequently referred to as short-term hibernation, that is, a circumstance in which sustained reductions in coronary flow are associated with (1) reductions in systolic function of similar magnitude, (2) progressive restoration of initially depressed levels of myocardial creatine phosphate, and (3) persistence of inotropic reserve.[12] The reductions in coronary flow are presumed to trigger an acute down-regulation of myocardial O_2 demand during the period of flow reduction.

Whether such a response can persist after the restoration of unrestricted coronary inflow has been unclear. To address this point, our laboratory has evaluated O_2 consumption and function following sustained 2-hour reductions in coronary flow of ~50%, and repeated 2-minute total coronary occlusions, in chronically instrumented dogs.[16] Both flow restriction protocols were followed by proportionate reversible reductions in regional systolic function and myocardial O_2 consumption lasting up to 24 hours. A similar response has been observed by Berman et al following demand-induced ischemia in lightly anesthetized closed-chest swine.[51] Thus, perfusion-contraction matching can occur in the postischemic period in some experimental settings.

The characterization of reversibly hypocontractile myocardium as hibernating or stunned in studies such as these remains problematic. The proportionate reductions in function and O_2 consumption fit the usual definition of hibernation. They are consistent with the concept that the heart has an inherent but limited ability to down-regulate metabolic activity beneficially in response to flow restriction, and that stunning results when more severe degrees of flow reduction exceed this limit and cause transient myocardial injury. This scenario could explain much of the variability in the studies summarized in Figure 1 and earlier portions of this review. Findings in individual studies would represent the net result of beneficial hibernation responses and injurious stunning responses, with reductions in function becoming disproportionate to changes in O_2 consumption when the degree of flow reduction is severe enough to overcome beneficial adaptive processes.

An alternate possibility is that proportionate reductions in myocardial function and O_2 consumption represent an O_2-sparing effect of reversible ischemic injury to the contractile process that is milder than in previous studies of stunning. In this scenario, even though the mismatch of O_2 utilization and function that is accepted as the defining criterion for stunning is not present, the response underlying the proportionate reductions could be similar but less pronounced than when flow restriction is more marked. Recently, our laboratory has observed reductions in myofibrillar creatine kinase activity in myocardium meeting the criteria of short-term hibernation as well as in myocardium, which all would consider stunned.[52]

Models of Chronic Hibernation

Chronic adaptations have been difficult to study because of the lack of an animal model that is agreed to represent the hibernating state. Chronic studies of flow and function, that is, those lasting days or weeks, require the use of large animals that can be studied repeatedly, for example, dogs and pigs. Attempts to produce an anatomically and functionally stable partial stenosis of a major coronary artery are notoriously difficult. This situation has led to the frequent use of ameroid constrictors to produce a total coronary occlusion sufficiently gradually to allow the development of a collateral-dependent bed with negligible myocardial fibrosis and a limited flow reserve. The collateral-dependent bed is presumed to simulate the situation that would be imposed by a chronic stenosis of the coronary artery originally supplying the collateralized area.

1. In the late 1980s Canty and the senior author reported findings in a canine circumflex ameroid preparation.[53] An apparent mismatch between resting flow and function became evident during the early phase of collateral development, that is, resting flow in the collateralizing circumflex bed remained at normal or near-normal levels while regional function fell below control values. The mismatch presumably represented activity-related episodes of stunning. At a later stage of collateralization, flow and function appeared to be matched at levels below their control values. However, this possibly hibernating state was relatively short-lived as collateral development continued.

2. More recently, Shen et al[54] have reported studies in a porcine ameroid preparation that convincingly demonstrate frequent episodes of stunning during the development of collaterals over a 3-week period. Although acknowledging that a coexistent hibernating process cannot be excluded, these investigators suggest that most of the reversible dysfunction observed in preparations such as this reflects chronic stunning rather than hibernation. Because the degree of collateralization that can be achieved is substantially less in porcine than in canine preparations, the porcine preparation has the potential to provide a

longer period of flow limitation (thereby improving the chances of detecting and studying any hibernation process). Conversely, chronic porcine ameroid preparations exhibit a small-to-moderate degree of myocardial scarring, which must be accounted for in evaluating flow and function.

3. In a clever alternative approach, Mills et al[6] have capitalized on an approach suggested by Millard[55] by placing a clip that is only slightly occlusive on the anterior descending artery of young pigs and studying them up to 32 weeks later. The clip becomes increasingly restrictive as the animal grows, producing a gradually developing stenosis that presumably avoids the difficulties that ensue when one attempts to narrow an artery of a mature animal to a "critical" degree. Mills et al found anterior descending flow to be systematically less than circumflex flow under resting conditions, even though a moderate degree of flow reserve persisted in the anterior descending bed. In addition, myocardial O_2 consumption in the anterior descending bed was reduced in relation to historical controls without coronary stenosis. Ongoing studies by Fallavollita et al[56,57] support the view that this can be a useful model. This group recently has reported relative reductions in resting subendocardial and full-thickness flow, associated with increased uptake of ^{18}F-2-deoxyglucose (FDG), in viable severely hypokinetic myocardium.[56] These findings are accompanied by induction of the 70-kd family of heat shock proteins, a presumably protective response.[57]

4. Some laboratories are utilizing the repeated brief occlusion method of collateral development developed by Fujita et al.[58,59] Although time-consuming, this approach has the potential advantage of minimizing stunning outside the experimental laboratory during collateral development. The usual intent is to develop collaterals to the point at which local arterial pressure is maintained at a predetermined level when the native artery is occluded, for example, 35–40 mm Hg, and then to occlude the artery permanently. In our experience decreases in resting regional function occur frequently during the period of collateralization.[60] The frequency with which these decreases represent hibernation, rather than stunning caused by arterial spasm and/or transient thrombus formation while the animal is outside the laboratory, is not clear.

5. Liedtke and coworkers have employed a porcine model in which observations are made in acute studies performed a few days after applying a partial external arterial constriction.[61–63] Studies in this preparation have focused on metabolic changes in response to the stenosis.

6. As noted earlier, Heyndrickx et al[33] have reported that it requires 1–2 weeks for abnormalities in ^{11}C-acetate metabolism to clear following a 1-hour reduction in flow sufficient to abolish systolic WT in chronically instrumented dogs. The same is true for ^{11}C-palmitate. Acetate and palmitate recovery patterns paralleled those of regional function and were interpreted as reflecting prolonged impairment of fatty acid β-oxidation and overall oxidative metabolism, despite the restoration of normal flow. Although myocardial necrosis was not evident at postmortem, the original ischemic stimulus was associated with transient elevations in plasma creatine kinase. As also noted earlier, Buxton et al interpret ^{11}C-acetate data in reversibly injured segments similarly in their canine infarction model.[32]

7. Chen et el recently have expanded on short-term hibernation protocols by sustaining a moderate flow reduction in pigs for 24 hours.[64] Myocardium subjected to the flow limitation showed acute metabolic, functional, and structural adaptations, which were in most cases reversible over the subsequent week.

Structural Changes and Possible Mechanisms Underlying Reversible Dysfunction

A structural component of long-term adaptive responses was suggested by Flameng and colleagues in the early 1980s on the basis of biopsy specimens obtained during bypass graft surgery from areas of human hearts thought to represent reversibly dysfunctional myocardium.[65,66] Structural changes have received increasing attention in the past few years[67,68] and recently have been reviewed by Vanoverschelde et al[69] and Elsasser et al.[70] The changes described include reductions in contractile filament material and sarcoplasmic reticulum, accumulation of glycogen, and the appearance of numerous small mitochondria. Recent electron microscopic studies in experimental animals indicate that at least some changes of this type can develop within hours to days.[64,71]

Bolli has provided a comprehensive review of mechanisms possibly underlying myocardial stunning.[2] These relate importantly to effects of postischemic reperfusion as well as ischemia itself. Studies of mechanisms underlying beneficial adaptations, that is, hibernation, remain hampered by the limitations of available animal models. A few points not mentioned previously are of interest.

Studies of excitation-contraction coupling and calcium handling have focused on calcium exchange at the sarcolemma and sarcoplasmic reticulum and on myofilament responsiveness to calcium. In studies of calcium handling in isovolumically contracting isolated ferret heart preparations, Marban's laboratory found that modest reductions in perfusion pressure (and therefore flow) cause reductions in developed pressure and the intracellular calcium transient without a decrease in intracellular pH or an increase in tissue lactate or inorganic phosphorus concentration.[40,72] These data were taken to indicate that a decrease in systolic calcium release may underlie the reduced contractile function in the "acute" hibernation response. When global ischemia was used to produce myocardial stunning in the same preparation, calcium transients were increased, suggesting an increased availability of cytoplasmic activator calcium. These latter data were taken to indicate that the defect in contractile function in stunning may result from a decreased responsiveness of myofilaments to calcium. A more recent study from this group supports this concept in that characteristics of stunned myocardium were mimicked by proteolytic damage to myofibrils.[73]

As summarized by Mubagwa,[74] measurements of calcium uptake by sarcoplasmic reticulum in stunned myocardium have given variable results. Using an alternate approach to implicate sarcoplasmic reticular dysfunction, Frass et al[75] have reported increases in messenger RNA (mRNA) levels for calcium ATPase, phospholamban, and calsequestrin in stunned porcine myocardium. They suggest that this is a regeneratory response stemming from damage to the corresponding calcium-regulating proteins. A recent study in an open-chest porcine model of short-term hibernation by Luss et al reported unchanged levels of mRNA for calcium ATPase and phospholamban during an 85-minute period of flow reduction and at 30 minutes of reperfusion.[76] Preliminary reports from Abraham et al[77] and our own laboratory[78] also failed to show increased mRNA levels for phospholamban, calcium ATPase, or calsequestrin within 2 hours following periods of moderate flow reduction. In our studies, mRNA for phospholamban was reduced systematically at 24 hours following flow reduction[78] and may have reflected an adaptive response. Possible adrenergic-related alterations in signal transduction have been studied in a porcine ameroid model by Hammond et al.[79] An additional area possibly relating flow and function is endothelial-myocyte coupling, that is, the influence of endothelial products on myocyte contractile behavior.[80]

Williams and Benjamin,[81] Yellon and Latchman,[82] Mestril and Dillman,[83] Knowlton,[84] and Das et al[85] have reviewed studies of heat shock proteins as they relate to ischemic stimuli. Increases in mRNA and levels of the heat shock protein HSP-70 can be induced by both reversible and irreversible ischemia and can reduce the degree of injury produced by ischemic stimuli. Overexpression of HSP-70 in transgenic mice also has a protective effect against ischemia.[86,87] Protective effects of heat shock proteins may relate in part to adverse effects of reperfusion following an ischemic period; that is, they may reduce the extent of reperfusion injury. Their role (if any) in the reduction of metabolic demand characteristic of short-term hibernation is unclear. Although increases in mRNA for heat shock protein and other stress proteins can occur quickly, that is, within an hour; delayed changes in gene expression also seem likely. The possibility that chronic hibernation involves long-term changes in gene expression, with synthesis of new classes of proteins, is of great interest.

Global Responses to Regional Flow Limitation

Pryzklenk et al have reported that preconditioning effects of regional ischemia can be global in extent; that is, a brief circumflex occlusion preceding a prolonged anterior descending occlusion in dogs caused a reduction in the size of the infarction produced by the anterior descending occlusion.[88] Although the basis for this effect was unclear, possibilities were felt to include a global alteration in fatty acid metabolism or adenosine release, global effects mediated through cardiac afferent nerves, and coupling through gap junctions. Similarly, ischemia-induced elevations in heat shock proteins have been reported to extend to nonischemic as well as ischemic areas of the left ventricle.[89] The possibility that early adaptive responses to regional ischemia and/or flow reduction are, at least in some cases, evident globally deserves further study.

Resting Flow in Viable Hypocontractile Myocardium—Normal or Reduced?

Measurements of coronary blood flow continue to be reported in milliliters per minute or milliliters per minute per gram, depending on the technique used. Techniques using diffusible tracers, for example, inert gases and positron-emitting radionuclides, provide average values per unit weight of tissue, expressed as milliliters per minute per gram (or milliliters per minute per 100 g). Approaches using intracoronary Doppler probes provide values of velocity; if luminal diameter at the probe site also is measured, total flow (milliliters per minute) through the sampled artery can be calculated. Similarly, coronary sinus thermodilution provides values of total flow (milliliters per minute) through whatever portion of the coronary venous system is sampled. When attempting to distinguish between stunning and hibernation, measurements of flow per unit weight are advantageous in that they avoid confounding differences in total flow arising from differences in size of the sampled ventricular segment.

Our experience and that of Cannon's group, dating back to the mid-1970s, has been that resting flow per unit weight in the left ventricle is reduced frequently in coronary patients.[90–95] In our laboratory, measurements of resting flow in the anterior left ventricular (LV) myocardium of patients with high-grade stenoses of the anterior descending coronary artery averaged only 64% of LV flows in patients with atypical chest pain and normal coronary arteriograms and ventriculograms.[93,95] Cannon's values of regional flow in patients with left anterior descending disease were similar.[94]

During this same period several laboratories reported defects in resting ^{201}Tl scans in coronary patients that improved within a few hours.[96–98] The transient defects presumably represented areas of viable myocardium in which blood flow was lower than in adjacent areas of the ventricle. Berger et al[97] found that most of these defects improved following revascularization, substantiating the view that they represented viable but hypoperfused myocardium.

Measurements in our laboratory[91] and that of Cannon[92] also indicated that reductions in resting LV flow occur globally as well as regionally in patients with widespread disease. Because the magnitude of these reductions could not be explained reasonably by myocardial scarring, we raised the possibility that myocardial metabolic demand was reduced chronically as an adaptation to inflow limitation.[91] Chen et al subsequently provided data indicating that LV wall thickness and mass are increased systematically in coronary disease and suggested that reductions in resting flow per gram result from systematically lower values of wall stress under resting conditions.[99] Reductions in contractile function also had been suggested by videodensitometric measurements of anterior wall function in Mayo Clinic patients with left main or proximal anterior descending stenoses.[100] An additional study from our laboratory demonstrated reduced resting flow in dysfunctional collateral-dependent myocardium, also suggesting the possibility of a long-term reduction in local O_2 demand.[101]

The data in the last few paragraphs support the view that resting flow frequently is reduced in viable myocardium. However, the data were all acquired in patients undergoing cardiac catheterization at least 15 years ago, and information about regional function is limited. Most recent measurements of resting flow have been performed using PET. Conclusions about the "normality" or "abnormality" of resting flow in reversibly hypocontractile myocardium have varied. In a 1996 editorial accompanying a study of Sun et al,[8] Rahimtoola reanalyzed five PET studies including 66 patients in whom resting flow in hibernating areas measured using $^{13}NH_3$ could be compared with resting flow in regions of the same hearts having normal systolic function.[102] He concluded that resting flow is reduced in hibernating myocardium. More recently, Heusch has reviewed 15 PET studies including 263 patients in whom resting flow measured with PET in hibernating areas could be compared with resting flow in regions with normal systolic function.[12] He concludes: "The majority of these studies clearly indicate a significant reduction in resting regional myocardial blood flow in those dysfunctional areas classified as hibernating myocardium as compared with intraindividual normal remote areas, with an average reduction in flow from baseline by 20%–30%." However, as noted by Sun et al [8] and others, there is no question that many hypocontractile areas that improve their performance following revascularization do not show discernible reductions in resting flow by PET or radionuclide scans. Interestingly, as pointed out by Schelbert,[103] resting flows in his group's original 1986 PET paper[11] were reduced in one-third and normal in two-thirds of myocardial segments which demonstrated improved contractile function after revascularization. In studies of patients undergoing biopsy of hypocontractile myocardium at the time of surgical revascularization, Maes et al reported that[13] NH_3 flows were one-third less in biopsied areas showing preserved uptake of fluorodeoxyglucose than in reference areas supplied by arteries with <50% stenosis.[67] The biopsied areas showed the ultrastructural changes described earlier and exhibited significant recovery of wall motion a few months after revascularization.

Technical issues that influence resting flow measurements continue to be debated. Apparent reductions in flow measured with PET and other radionuclide techniques may sometimes be an artifact of partial volume effects in hypocontractile tissue. Important additional issues relate to (1) limitations in measurement accuracy at resting levels of flow, (2) the variability of resting flow in healthy volunteers,[102,104] and (3) the inability to localize measurements to the inner portion of the myocardial wall. Although imaging measurements can be made to correlate with radioactive microsphere measurements over a wide range of flow in experimental animals, confidence limits for individual measurements remain quite wide; that is, 95% confidence limits are as much as 50% of resting flow. These limits confound the identification of modest reductions of flow in individual patients. In addition, when testing for differences in flow between patient groups, they

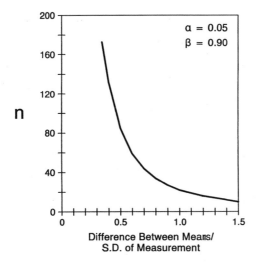

Figure 3. Size of patient groups needed to provide a 90% probability of identifying a group difference in a parameter such as coronary blood flow at $p = 0.05$. The abscissa represents the quotient of the actual difference in group means and the standard deviation of the measurement technique used to quantify the parameter being evaluated. For example, if one were designing a study to identify a 20% difference in resting flow in two patient groups and the standard deviation of the flow measurement technique was 25%, each group should include 34 patients. As measurement variability increases, the likelihood of an "underpowered" study increases sharply. Reprinted with permission from Reference 105.

also require larger-size groups than often appreciated (Fig. 3).[105] Finally, measurements of full-thickness flow may underestimate or fail to identify reductions in subendocardial perfusion having an important role in reduced contractile function.[12,56,102]

We conclude that resting flow in reversibly hypocontractile myocardium is variable, often being reduced and often within the normal range for the measurement technique used. Thus, hypocontractile myocardium that shows improved function following revascularization can reflect either hibernation or stunning (as traditionally defined) or some combination of the two.

Conclusions

Although the characterization of reversibly hypocontractile myocardium as hibernating or stunned has been useful in calling attention to beneficial as well as injurious responses to flow limitation, limitations of the dichotomous characterization are increasingly apparent. Most individual situations no doubt reflect a combination of beneficial adaptive processes, transient postischemic injury, and ultrastructural changes—all of which can vary in degree and temporal patterns of expression and remain incompletely understood. An improved understanding of mechanisms underlying reversibly hypocontractile myocardium will continue to be facilitated by studies in preparations in which it can be established that irreversible myocardial injury has been avoided or at least minimized to some quantifiable degree. As our understanding of the complex responses to flow limitation continues to increase, hopefully it will result in improved methods for recognizing and preserving viable myocardium—whether it be stunned, hibernating, or something else!

References

1. Ross J Jr. Myocardial perfusion-contraction matching. Implications for coronary heart disease and hibernation. *Circulation* 1991;83:1076–1083.
2. Bolli R. Myocardial "stunning" in man. *Circulation* 1992;86:1671–1691.
3. Heyndrickx GR, Millard RW, McRitchie RJ, et al. Regional myocardial functional and electrophysiological alterations after brief coronary artery occlusion in conscious dogs. *J Clin Invest* 1975;56:978–985.
4. Sambuceti G, Parodi O, Marcassa C, et al. Alteration in regulation of myocardial blood flow in one-vessel coronary artery disease determined by positron emission tomography. *Am J Cardiol* 1993;72:538–543.
5. Parodi O, Sambuceti G, Roghi A, et al. Residual coronary reserve despite decreased resting blood flow in patients with critical coronary lesions. A study by technetium-99m human albumin microsphere myocardial scintigraphy. *Circulation* 1993;87:330–344.
6. Mills I, Fallon JT, Wrenn D, et al. Adaptive responses of coronary circulation and myocardium to chronic reduction in perfusion pressure and flow. *Am J Physiol* 1994;266:H447–H457.
7. Berman M, Fischman AJ, Southern J, et al. Myocardial adaptation during and after sustained, demand-induced ischemia: Observations in closed-chest, domestic swine. *Circulation* 1996;94:755–762.
8. Sun KT, Czernin J, Krivokapich J, et al. Effects of dobutamine stimulation on myocardial blood flow, glucose metabolism, and wall motion in normal and dysfunctional myocardium. *Circulation* 1996;94:3146–3154.
9. Diamond GA, Forrester JS, deLuz PL, et al. Post-extrasystolic potentiation of ischemic myocardium by atrial stimulation. *Am Heart J* 1978;95:204–209.
10. Rahimtoola SH. A perspective on the three large multicenter randomized clinical trials of coronary bypass surgery for chronic stable angina. *Circulation* 1985;72:V123–V135.
11. Tillisch J, Brunken R, Marshall R, et al. Reversibility of cardiac wall-motion abnormalities predicted by positron tomography. *N Engl J Med* 1986;314:884–888.
12. Heusch G. Hibernating myocardium. *Physiol Rev* 1998;78:1055–1085.
13. Wijns W, Vatner SF, Camici PG. Hibernating myocardium. *New Engl J Med* 1998;339:173–181.
14. Triana JF, Li XY, Jamaluddin U, et al. Postischemic myocardial "stunning." Identification of major differences between the open-chest and the conscious dog and evaluation of the oxygen radical hypothesis in the conscious dog. *Circ Res* 1991;69:731–747.
15. Li XY, McCay PB, Zughaib M, et al. Demonstration of free radical generation in the "stunned" myocardium in the conscious dog and identification of major differences between conscious and open-chest dogs. *J Clin Invest* 1993;92:1025–1041.
16. Sherman AJ, Harris KR, Hedjbeli S, et al. Proportionate reversible decreases in systolic function and myocardial oxygen consumption after modest reductions in coronary flow: Hibernation versus stunning. *J Am Coll Cardiol* 1997;29:1623–1631.
17. Pagani M, Vatner SF, Baig H, et al. Initial myocardial adjustments to brief periods of ischemia and reperfusion in the conscious dog. *Circ Res* 1978;43:83–92.
18. Matsuzaki M, Gallagher KP, Kemper WS, et al. Sustained regional dysfunction produced by prolonged coronary stenosis: Gradual recovery after reperfusion. *Circulation* 1983;68:170–182.
19. Neill WA, Ingwall JS. Stabilization of a derangement in adenosine triphosphate metabolism during sustained, partial ischemia in the dog heart. *J Am Coll Cardiol* 1986;8:894–900.
20. Heyndrickx GR, Baig H, Nellens P, et al. Depression of regional blood flow and wall thickening after brief coronary occlusions. *Am J Physiol* 1978;234:H653–H659.
21. Laxson DD, Homans DC, Dai XZ, et al. Oxygen consumption and coronary reactivity in postischemic myocardium. *Circ Res* 1989;64:9–20.
22. Stahl LD, Weiss HR, Becker LC. Myocardial oxygen consumption, oxygen supply/demand heterogeneity, and microvascular patency in regionally stunned myocardium. *Circulation* 1988;77:865–872.
23. Dean EN, Shlafer M, Nicklas JM. The oxygen consumption paradox of "stunned myocardium" in dogs. *Basic Res Cardiol* 1990;85:120–131.

24. Vinten-Johansen J, Gayheart PA, Johnston WE, et al. Regional function, blood flow, and oxygen utilization relations in repetitively occluded-reperfused canine myocardium. *Am J Physiol* 1991;261:H538–H547.
25. Schaper W, Schott RJ, Kobayashi M. Reperfused myocardium: Stunning, preconditioning, and reperfusion injury. In: Heusch G, ed. *Pathophysiology and Rational Pharmacology of Myocardial Ischemia*. Darmstadt: Steinkopff-Verlag, 1990:175–197.
26. Liedtke AJ, DeMaison L, Eggleston AM, et al. Changes in substrate metabolism and effects of excess fatty acids in reperfused myocardium. *Circ Res* 1988;62:535–542.
27. McFalls EO, Duncker DJ, Krams R, et al. Recruitment of myocardial work and metabolism in regionally stunned porcine myocardium. *Am J Physiol* 1992;263:H1724–H1731.
28. McFalls EO, Pantely GA, Ophuis TO, et al. Relation of lactate production to postischaemic reduction in function and myocardial oxygen consumption after partial coronary occlusion in swine. *Cardiovasc Res* 1987;21:856–862.
29. Smith HJ. Depressed contractile function in reperfused canine myocardium: Metabolism and response to pharmacological agents. *Cardiovasc Res* 1980;14:458–468.
30. Lamping KA, Gross GJ. Improved recovery of myocardial segment function following a short coronary occlusion in dogs by nicorandil, a potential new antianginal agent, and nifedipine. *J Cardiovasc Pharmacol* 1985;7:158–166.
31. Lange R, Ware J, Kloner RA. Absence of a cumulative deterioration of regional function during three repeated 5 or 15 minute coronary occlusions. *Circulation* 1984;69:400–408.
32. Buxton DB, Mody FV, Krivokapich J, et al. Quantitative assessment of prolonged metabolic abnormalities in reperfused canine myocardium. *Circulation* 1992;85:1842–1856.
33. Heyndrickx GR, Wijns W, Vogelaers D, et al. Recovery of regional contractile function and oxidative metabolism in stunned myocardium induced by 1-hour circumflex coronary artery stenosis in chronically instrumented dogs. *Circ Res* 1993;72:901–913.
34. Gayheart PA, Vinten-Johansen J, Johnston WE, et al. Oxygen requirements of the dyskinetic myocardial segment. *Am J Physiol* 1989;257:H1184–H1191.
35. Chiu WC, Kedem J, Scholz PM, et al. Regional asynchrony of segmental contraction may explain the "oxygen consumption paradox" in stunned myocardium. *Basic Res Cardiol* 1994; 89:149–162.
36. Buxton DB. Dysfunction in collateral-dependent myocardium. Hibernation or repetitive stunning? *Circulation* 1993;87:1756–1758.
37. Fedele FA, Gewirtz H, Capone RJ, et al. Metabolic response to prolonged reduction of myocardial blood flow distal to a severe coronary artery stenosis. *Circulation* 1988;78:729–735.
38. Marshall RC. Correlation of contractile dysfunction with oxidative energy production and tissue high energy phosphate stores during partial coronary flow disruption in rabbit heart. *J Clin Invest* 1988;82:86–95.
39. Delyani JA, Van Wylen DG. Endocardial and epicardial interstitial purines and lactate during graded ischemia. *Am J Physiol* 1994;266:H1019–H1026.
40. Kitakaze M, Marban E. Cellular mechanism of the modulation of contractile function by coronary perfusion pressure in ferret hearts. *J Physiol* 1989;414:455–472.
41. Bristow JD, Arai AE, Anselone CG, et al. Response to myocardial ischemia as a regulated process. *Circulation* 1991;84:2580–2587.
42. Pantely GA, Malone SA, Rhen WS, et al. Regeneration of myocardial phosphocreatine in pigs despite continued moderate ischemia. *Circ Res* 1990;67:1481–1493.
43. Arai AE, Pantely GA, Anselone CG, et al. Active downregulation of myocardial energy requirements during prolonged moderate ischemia in swine. *Circ Res* 1991;69:1458–1469.
44. Schulz R, Guth BD, Pieper K, et al. Recruitment of an inotropic reserve in moderately ischemic myocardium at the expense of metabolic recovery. A model of short-term hibernation. *Circ Res* 1992;70:1282–1295.
45. Arai AE, Grauer SE, Anselone CG, et al. Metabolic adaptation to a gradual reduction in myocardial blood flow. *Circulation* 1995;92:244–252.
46. Ito BR. Gradual onset of myocardial ischemia results in reduced myocardial infarction. Association with reduced contractile function and metabolic downregulation. *Circulation* 1995; 91:2058–2070.

47. Keller AM, Cannon PJ. Effect of graded reductions of coronary pressure and flow on myocardial metabolism and performance: A model of "hibernating" myocardium. *J Am Coll Cardiol* 1991;17:1661–1670.

48. Kroll K, Kinzie DJ, Gustafson LA. Open-system kinetics of myocardial phosphoenergetics during coronary underperfusion. *Am J Physiol* 1997;272:H2563–H2576.

49. Schaefer S, Schwartz GG, Wisneski JA, et al. Response of high-energy phosphates and lactate release during prolonged regional ischemia in vivo. *Circulation* 1992;85:342–349.

50. Schaefer S, Carr LJ, Kreutzer U, et al. Myocardial adaptation during acute hibernation: Mechanisms of phosphocreatine recovery. *Cardiovasc Res* 1993;27:2044–2051.

51. Berman M, Fischman AJ, Southern J, et al. Myocardial adaptation during and after sustained, demand-induced ischemia. Observations in closed-chest, domestic swine. *Circulation* 1996; 94:755–762.

52. Kozlowski K, Sherman A, Evans D, et al. Myofibrillar creatine kinase activity is reduced in both short-term hibernation and myocardial stunning. *FASEB J* 1998;12:A1113. Abstract.

53. Canty JM Jr, Klocke FJ. Reductions in regional myocardial function at rest in conscious dogs with chronically reduced regional coronary artery pressure. *Circ Res* 1987;61:II107–H116.

54. Shen YT, Vatner SF. Mechanism of impaired myocardial function during progressive coronary stenosis in conscious pigs. Hibernation versus stunning? *Circ Res* 1995;76:479–488.

55. Millard RW. Induction of functional coronary collaterals in the swine heart. *Basic Res Cardiol* 1981;76:468–473.

56. Fallavollita JA, Perry BJ, Canty JM, Jr. ^{18}F-2-deoxyglucose deposition and regional flow in pigs with chronically dysfunctional myocardium; evidence for transmural variations in chronically hibernating myocardium. *Circulation* 1997;95:1900–1909.

57. Canty JM Jr, Fallavollita JA, Perry BJ, et al. Transmural induction of mRNA for HSP-70 in hibernating myocardium. *Circulation* 1995;92:I654. Abstract.

58. Fujita M, McKown DP, McKown MD, et al. Changes in coronary flow following repeated brief coronary occlusion in the conscious dog. *Heart Vessels* 1986;2:87–90.

59. Fujita M, McKown DP, McKown MD, et al. Evaluation of coronary collateral development by regional myocardial function and reactive hyperaemia. *Cardiovasc Res* 1987;21:377–384.

60. Klocke FJ, Davis, CA III, Srinivasan G, et al. Delayed reduction in regional myocardial function following repeated brief ischemia: A chronic canine model of myocardial hibernation. *Circulation* 1993;88:I188. Abstract.

61. Bolukoglu H, Liedtke AJ, Nellis SH, et al. An animal model of chronic coronary stenosis resulting in hibernating myocardium. *Am J Physiol* 1992;263:H20–H29.

62. Liedtke AJ, Renstrom B, Nellis SH, et al. Myocardial metabolism in chronic reperfusion after nontransmural infarction in pig hearts. *Am J Physiol.* 1993;265:H1614–H1622.

63. Liedtke AJ, Renstrom B, Nellis SH, et al. Mechanical and metabolic functions in pig hearts after 4 days of chronic coronary stenosis. *J Am Coll Cardiol* 1995;26:815–825.

64. Chen C, Chen L, Fallon JT, et al. Functional and structural alterations with 24-hour myocardial hibernation and recovery after reperfusion; a pig model of myocardial hibernation. *Circulation* 1996;94:507–516.

65. Flameng W, Suy R, Schwarz F, et al. Ultrastructural correlates of left ventricular contraction abnormalities in patients with chronic ischemic heart disease: Determinants of reversible segmental asynergy postrevascularization surgery. *Am Heart J* 1981;102:846–857.

66. Flameng W, Wouters L, Sergeant P, et al. Multivariate analysis of angiographic, histologic and electrocardiographic data in patients with coronary artery disease. *Circulation* 1984;70:7–17.

67. Maes A, Flameng W, Nuyts J, et al. Histological alterations in chronically hypoperfused myocardium. Correlation with PET findings. *Circulation* 1994;90:735–745.

68. Depre C, Vanoverschelde JL, Melin JA, et al. Structural and metabolic correlates of the reversibility of chronic left ventricular ischemic dysfunction in humans. *Am J Physiol* 1995; 268:H1265–H1275.

69. Vanoverschelde JL, Wijns W, Borgers M, et al. Chronic myocardial hibernation in humans; from bedside to bench. *Circulation* 1997;95:1961–1971.

70. Elsasser A, Schlepper M, Klovekorn WP, et al. Hibernating myocardium: An incomplete adaptation to ischemia. *Circulation* 1997;96:2920–2931.

71. Decker RS, Decker ML, Sherman AJ, et al. Myofibrillar disassembly in hibernating and stunned canine myocardium. *Circulation.* Abstract. 1998;98:I816

72. Marban E. Myocardial stunning and hibernation. The physiology behind the colloquialisms. *Circulation* 1991;83:681–688.

73. Gao WD, Atar D, Liu Y, et al. Role of troponin I proteolysis in the pathogenesis of stunned myocardium. *Circ Res* 1997;80:393–399.

74. Mubagwa K. Sarcoplasmic reticulum function during myocardial ischaemia and reperfusion. *Cardiovasc Res* 1995;30:166–175.

75. Frass O, Sharma HS, Knoll R, et al. Enhanced gene expression of calcium regulatory proteins in stunned porcine myocardium. *Cardiovasc Res* 1993;27:2037–2043.

76. Luss H, Boknik P, Heusch G, et al. Expression of calcium regulatory proteins in short-term hibernation and stunning in the in situ porcine heart. *Cardiovasc Res* 1998;37:606–617.

77. Abraham S, Young RF, Canty JM Jr. Post-ischemic dysfunction following short-term hibernation is not associated with increased mRNA for sarcoplasmic reticulum regulatory proteins. *Circulation* 1996;94:I186. Abstract.

78. Sherman AJ, Kozlowski KA, Harris KR, et al. Early alterations in sarcoplasmic reticular gene expression in viable reversibly hypocontractile myocardium. *Circulation* 1997;96:I197. Abstract.

79. Hammond HK, Roth DA, McKirnan MD, et al. Regional myocardial downregulation of the inhibitory guanosine triphosphate-binding protein (Giα2 and beta-adrenergic receptors in a porcine model of chronic episodic myocardial ischemia. *J Clin Invest* 1993;92:2644–2652.

80. Shah AM, Lewis MJ. Modulation of myocardial contraction by endocardial and coronary vascular endothelium. *Trends Cardiovasc Medicine* 1993;3:98–103.

81. Williams RS, Benjamin IJ. Stress proteins and cardiovascular disease. *Mol Biol Med* 1991;8: 197–206.

82. Yellon DM, Latchman DS. Stress proteins and myocardial protection. *J Mol Cell Cardiol* 1992;24:113–124.

83. Mestril R, Dillmann WH. Heat shock proteins and protection against myocardial ischemia. *J Mol Cell Cardiol* 1995;27:45–52.

84. Knowlton AA. The role of heat shock proteins in the heart. *J Mol Cell Cardiol* 1995;27:121–131.

85. Das DK, Maulik N, Moraru II. Gene expression in acute myocardial stress. Induction by hypoxia, ischemia, reperfusion, hyperthermia and oxidative stress. *J Mol Cell Cardiol* 1995; 27:181–193.

86. Marber MS, Mestril R, Chi SH, et al. Overexpression of the rat inducible 70-kD heat stress protein in a transgenic mouse increases the resistance of the heart to ischemic injury. *J Clin Invest* 1995;95:1446–1456.

87. Plumier JC, Ross BM, Currie RW, et al. Transgenic mice expressing the human heat shock protein 70 have improved post-ischemic myocardial recovery. *J Clin Invest* 1995;95:1854–1860.

88. Przyklenk K, Bauer B, Ovize M, et al. Regional ischemic "preconditioning" protects remote virgin myocardium from subsequent sustained coronary occlusion. *Circulation* 1993;87: 893–899.

89. Knowlton AA, Brecher P, Apstein CS. Rapid expression of heat shock protein in the rabbit after brief cardiac ischemia. *J Clin Invest* 1991;87:139–147.

90. Cannon PJ, Dell RB, Dwyer EM Jr. Regional myocardial perfusion rates in patients with coronary artery disease. *J Clin Invest* 1972;51:978–994.

91. Klocke FJ, Bunnell IL, Greene DG, et al. Average coronary blood flow per unit weight of left ventricle in patients with and without coronary artery disease. *Circulation* 1974;50:547–559.

92. Cannon PJ, Schmidt DH, Weiss MB, et al. The relationship between regional myocardial perfusion at rest and arteriographic lesions in patients with coronary atherosclerosis. *J Clin Invest* 1975;56:1442–1454.

93. Klocke FJ. Coronary blood flow in man. *Prog Cardiovasc Dis* 1976;19:117–166.

94. Cannon PJ, Weiss MB, Casarella WJ. Studies of regional myocardial blood flow: Results in patients with left anterior descending coronary artery disease. *Semin Nucl Med* 1976;6:279–303.

95. Klocke FJ. Measurements of coronary blood flow and degree of stenosis: Current clinical implications and continuing uncertainties. *J Am Coll Cardiol* 1983;1:31–41.

96. Wackers FJ, Lie KI, Liem KL, et al. Thallium-201 scintigraphy in unstable angina pectoris. *Circulation* 1978;57:738–742.

97. Berger BC, Watson DD, Burwell LR, et al. Redistribution of thallium at rest in patients with stable and unstable angina and the effect of coronary artery bypass surgery. *Circulation* 1979;60:1114–1125.
98. Gewirtz H, Beller GA, Strauss HW, et al. Transient defects of resting thallium scans in patients with coronary artery disease. *Circulation* 1979;59:707–713.
99. Chen PH, Nichols AB, Weiss MB, et al. Left ventricular myocardial blood flow in multivessel coronary artery disease. *Circulation* 1982;66:537–547.
100. St John Sutton MG, Frye RL, Smith HC, et al. Relation between left coronary artery stenosis and regional left ventricular function. *Circulation* 1978;58:491–497.
101. Arani DT, Greene DG, Bunnell IL, et al. Reductions in coronary flow under resting conditions in collateral-dependent myocardium of patients with complete occlusion of the left anterior descending coronary artery. *J Am Coll Cardiol* 1984;3:668–674.
102. Rahimtoola SH. Hibernating myocardium has reduced blood flow at rest that increases with low-dose dobutamine. *Circulation* 1996;94:3055–3061.
103. Schelbert HR. Metabolic imaging to assess myocardial viability. *J Nucl Med* 1994;35:8S–14S.
104. Camici PG, Wijns W, Borgers M, et al. Pathophysiological mechanisms of chronic reversible left ventricular dysfunction due to coronary artery disease (hibernating myocardium). *Circulation* 1997;96:3205–3214.
105. Klocke FJ, Frank MW. Principles of myocardial perfusion. In: DJ Skorton, BR Brundage, GL Wolf, HR Schelbert, eds. *Marcus' Cardiac Imaging*, 2nd ed. Philadelphia, PA: WB Saunders; 1996:8–19.

Preconditioning

James M. Downey, PhD
and Michael V. Cohen, MD

Introduction

An elusive goal of cardiology has been the identification of interventions that can limit the amount of myocardial necrosis caused by a coronary occlusive event. A major complication of acute myocardial infarction is loss of ventricular mass. Because the heart cannot regenerate myocardium, patients with myocardial infarction are left with a permanent deficit in pumping ability. Thrombolysis addresses this problem by dissolving clots thus producing reperfusion of the ischemic segments, but it rarely can be instituted early enough to prevent substantial tissue loss. As a result an adjunct intervention has been sought that would preserve viability until reperfusion can be instituted. Ischemic preconditioning has emerged as a model for such an intervention. If the mechanism of preconditioning can be understood and duplicated pharmacologically, then infarct size and the associated incidence of congestive heart failure in patients experiencing acute coronary thrombosis should be reduced substantially.

Ischemic preconditioning was first described in 1986 by Murry et al.[1] They noted that infarct size resulting from a 40-minute coronary occlusion in dogs could be reduced markedly if they first "preconditioned" the heart with a sublethal ischemic insult. In their protocol they used four cycles of 5 minutes of coronary occlusion with each cycle followed by 5 minutes of reperfusion. They found that the heart adapted itself within minutes to become resistant to ischemia-induced infarction. This phenomenon, now known as "classic" or "early" ischemic preconditioning, has been documented in dog,[1,2] rat,[3,4] rabbit,[5,6] and pig[7] hearts as well as in human isolated myocytes[8] and atrial muscle.[9] It is not possible to test directly whether in vivo human hearts can be preconditioned against infarction, but there is circumstantial evidence, albeit controversial, for preconditioning's presence in man.[10,11] Preconditioning's protection appears to be biphasic. Although the protection from ischemic preconditioning wanes quickly, there is now evidence that a "second window" of protection, sometimes called "late" preconditioning, appears 24 hours following a preconditioning episode and lasts for as long as 4 days.[12]

Preconditioning's Natural History

In the rabbit[5,13] and dog[2] a single 5-minute period of ischemia followed by 5 or 10 minutes of reperfusion is sufficient to put the heart into the preconditioned state. Multiple

From Dilsizian V (ed). *Myocardial Viability: A Clinical and Scientific Treatise.* Armonk, NY: Futura Publishing Co., Inc.; © 2000.

cycles of ischemia offer no more protection against infarction than a single cycle,[2,13] indicating either an all-or-none or more likely a saturating type of kinetic. Two 2-minute occlusions do not elicit protection in the rabbit, while a single 5-minute occlusion does,[5] suggesting that in the rabbit heart a relatively sharp threshold for protection exists somewhere between 2 and 5 minutes of ischemia. However, in man, there is evidence that as little as 90 seconds of coronary occlusion occurring during the course of routine angioplasty may be sufficient to precondition the heart.[10,14,15]

Preconditioning does not protect against all aspects of ischemia/reperfusion injury. Preconditioning reportedly attenuates both ischemia- and reperfusion-induced arrhythmias in dog[16] and rat.[17,18] However, we and others have been unable to observe an antiarrhythmic effect in open-chest pig or rabbit (J. M. Downey and M. V. Cohen, personal observation, 1999). Classical preconditioning offers little protection against stunned myocardium.[19] However, the second window of protection is associated with a strong antistunning effect.[20] Preconditioning has a clear beneficial effect on postischemic mechanical function in the isolated rat heart.[21–23] But in other models including the dog and the isolated rabbit heart (J. M. Downey and M. V. Cohen, personal observation, 1999) such protection has not been very reproducible. Preconditioning's effect on postischemic function of human atrial strips has shown better reproducibility.[9] It is the authors' opinion that the preconditioning-induced improvement in postischemic ventricular function in the rat and human atrial models is the result of a combination of reduction in myocyte necrosis and stunning. Why such a clear effect is not seen in rabbit or canine myocardium is unknown.

The early window of protection is quite short. Reports vary but the protection wears off in about 1 hour in most models.[5,13,24] Interestingly, a second window of protection can be seen 24 hours after preconditioning,[12,25,26] which is assumed to result from synthesis of cytoprotective proteins, although the latter hypothesis has not been proven. This late phase of preconditioning protects the myocardium against infarction,[12,25–28] stunning,[20,29] and arrhythmias.[30] In our hands the anti-infarct effect of the second window is less potent than that of classical preconditioning.[31]

Models for the Anti-Infarct Effect
of Preconditioning

Currently, we use several different models to measure preconditioning's anti-infarct effect. In the first the whole heart is exposed to a period of regional ischemia and reperfusion. The heart may be in situ in which case it is innervated and perfused with blood or, in the case of the rat and rabbit, may be removed from the host and perfused with a buffered salt solution. Infarction in the isolated rabbit heart has been found to be very similar to that in the in situ heart.[32] The isolated heart has obvious advantages when it is to be treated pharmacologically because the dose and schedule of the agent can be controlled precisely in the perfusate. On the other hand, the in situ model more closely mimics the clinical situation.

A second model involves isolated cardiomyocytes. There are two categories. In the first, the cells are incubated in hypoxic buffer, which may[33] or may not[8] include metabolic blockers, and the rate of cell death is assessed by either staining with vital dyes or measuring the appearance of cytosolic enzymes in the medium. Ganote[34] has introduced a slightly different version of this model, which we have used extensively. In this latter model cells in suspension are centrifuged gently into a pellet, most of the supernatant removed, and oxygen excluded with a layer of mineral oil. The cells quickly consume the residual oxygen in the pellet resulting in a hypoxic environment. The advantage of this model is that metabolic waste products and cytokines can accumulate in the pellet making the milieu very similar to that existing in ischemic tissue. While these nonbeating cells die very slowly in the pellet, they experience a rapid and predictable increase in osmotic fragility. Interestingly, preconditioning delays appearance of the latter. Aliquots of cardiomyocytes are removed from the pellet at regular intervals with a pipette and the osmotic fragility is measured by incubating the cells in hypotonic buffer. It is thought that this fragility contributes to necrosis because the ischemic myocyte is subjected to severe osmotic swelling.[35] We have found the pellet model to be an excellent mimic of the infarct model. Cellular models not only eliminate the effects of noncardiac tissue, but, because of their small volume, allow experiments with exotic agents and techniques that might be too expensive or otherwise impossible to use in a whole heart.

Protection Is Triggered by Receptors

Early studies revealed that classical preconditioning does not involve opening of collaterals,[1] induction of antioxidants,[36] synthesis of protective proteins,[37] or changes in mitochondrial adenosine triphosphatases (ATPases).[38] The first breakthrough came when it was demonstrated that protection was receptor mediated. During ischemia numerous agents are released by the myocardium including adenosine, catecholamines, angiotensin II, bradykinin, prostanoids, and endothelin.[39] In 1991 we reported that adenosine played an important role in ischemic preconditioning.[40] Adenosine is produced by the heart when there is a net catabolism of ATP. Removal of the high-energy phosphates from ATP leaves adenosine monophosphate (AMP). AMP is dephosphorylated by $5'$-nucleotidase to produce free adenosine, which can exit the cell easily. Once in the interstitial space adenosine can bind to surface receptors on the cardiomyocyte. We observed that adenosine receptor blockers aborted preconditioning's protection in rabbits but had little effect on nonpreconditioned hearts.[40] Furthermore, a 5-minute intracoronary infusion of either adenosine or $R(-)\text{-}N^6\text{-}(2\text{-phenylisopropyl})$ adenosine (R-PIA), a selective agonist for the adenosine A_1 receptor, in lieu of the preconditioning ischemia mimicked protection. It was concluded that adenosine, acting through its A_1 receptors, triggered preconditioning.

Protein Kinase C Appears to be Part of the Signal Transduction Pathway for Preconditioning

Current evidence suggests that adenosine receptors elicit protection by activating protein kinase C (PKC). PKC inhibitors have been shown to abort the protection from an ischemic preconditioning protocol in rabbit,[41,42] rat,[43,44] and dog[45] hearts (see Fig. 1). The same was seen in rabbit[46] and more importantly human[8] cardiomyocytes. Also, experiments similar to those shown in Figure 1 revealed that direct activators of PKC such as phorbol esters or diacylglycerols can mimic preconditioning in a variety of models[42,44,47] including human myocytes[8] and atrium.[48] If the hypothesis that PKC is an integral part of preconditioning's signal transduction pathway is correct, then any receptor that couples to PKC in the cardiomyocyte should be capable of mimicking preconditioning's anti-infarct effect. PKC-coupled receptors on the cardiomyocyte include the angiotensin AT_1,[49] α_1-adrenergic,[50] bradykinin B_2,[51] and endothelin ET_1[52] receptors. All have been shown to mimic preconditioning's protection in ischemic myocardium.[22,53–57] The only thing all of these receptors appear to have in common is their coupling to PKC.

However, it should be noted that attempts to confirm the PKC hypothesis in the dog[58] and pig[59,60] have, to date, not been universally successful. This failure may be

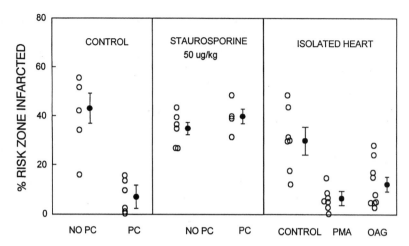

Figure 1. Infarct size expressed as percent infarction of the risk zone is shown on the vertical axis for rabbit hearts undergoing 30 minutes of regional myocardial ischemia. Each open circle represents an individual animal while closed circles represent group means. Note that preconditioning (PC) with a single 5-minute coronary occlusion markedly reduces infarct size (left panel). Blockade of protein kinase C (PKC) by staurosporine abolished preconditioning's protection but had no effect on infarction in nonpreconditioned hearts (middle panel). The right panel reveals that intracoronary infusion of 4β-phorbol-12-myristate-13-acetate (PMA) or the diacylglycerol 1-oleoyl-2-acetyl-*sn*-glycerol (OAG) mimicked preconditioning. Both of these are direct activators of PKC. Adapted with permission from Reference 42.

related to technical problems encountered in trying to block cardiac PKC in such a large animal. But more recent investigations in the pig have demonstrated that combined infusion of a PKC antagonist and a tyrosine kinase blocker (see below) effectively aborts protection.[61] Therefore, at least in this species, there may be redundant, parallel pathways with at least one involving PKC which ultimately ensure protection from preconditioning. The same may be true for canine myocardium.

Another point of controversy has been the lack of direct biochemical evidence for activation of PKC in preconditioned myocardium.[62] It currently is not possible to measure directly PKC's activity in a cell because its activity is modulated by stimulating cofactors such as diacylglycerol, calcium, and phosphatidylserine, which are altered during processing of the tissue. However, most isoforms of PKC physically bind to docking proteins called receptors for activated C kinase (RACKs)[63] during their activation. The RACKs are specific for the various PKC isozymes, so that only one isozyme can dock at a given RACK and each RACK can bind only one isozyme species. This docking can be seen as a translocation from the cytosol to the particulate fraction in a cell homogenate. Several studies have looked for such translocations in preconditioned myocardium, and have identified them in intact rat[44,64-66] and rabbit[67] hearts and isolated rat neonatal cardiomyocytes.[68,69] However, it must be acknowledged that at least one study in dogs examining translocation of total PKC activity[58] and one in rabbit cardiomyocytes searching for specific isozyme translocation[70] failed to detect any movement from cytosol to particulate fraction. But it is likely that technical considerations account for both of these failures. In an exhaustive study in rabbit myocardium Ping et al.[67] demonstrated that several cycles of brief coronary occlusion and reperfusion caused translocation of 2 of the 11 PKC isozymes present in rabbit heart, ϵ and η. In a subsequent study we used isozyme-specific RACK peptide antagonists to demonstrate that interference with docking of the PKC-ϵ isozyme to its RACK blocked preconditioning's protective effect in rabbit cardiomyocytes.[71] Thus there is now evidence that preconditioning is dependent on activation of a single isozyme, or at most a few specific ones.

There are alternative hypotheses, and other second messengers have been proposed to mediate preconditioning's protection. Parratt[72] has proposed that cyclic guanosine monophosphate (cGMP) is responsible for the antiarrhythmic effect of preconditioning in dogs and Lochner and her colleagues[73] have proposed that changes in cyclic AMP (cAMP) may mediate the preservation of postischemic function in the rat heart.

Multiple Mediators Ensure That Ischemia Will Precondition the Heart

The PKC hypothesis of preconditioning further broadens the possibilities of pharmacologic application because many agonists of PKC-coupled receptors in addition to adenosine are released by the ischemic myocardium.[39] This causes the preconditioning mechanism to be highly redundant. It can be shown in rabbit heart that bradykinin[53] and opioid receptors[74] participate equally with adenosine to trigger the protective state. For example, the bradykinin receptor antagonist HOE 140 will block protection from a single 5-minute occlusion, which is just above the threshold for protection. However, protection returns if three 5-minute cycles of ischemia are used,[53] which presumably is related to increased stimulation of the remaining receptors. Similar behavior is seen with opioid receptors.[74] Other potential triggers, angiotensin II,[54] norepinephrine,[55] and endothe-

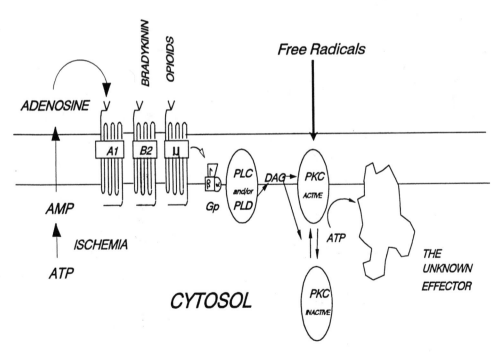

Figure 2. A proposed signal transduction pathway for ischemic preconditioning. Cell surface receptors through their G-proteins activate phospholipases, which produce diacylglycerol, which in turn activates PKC. PKC acts as a summing point for the signals from all of the activated receptors. In addition free radicals contribute by direct activation of PKC. PKC then protects by phosphorylating some as yet unidentified protein [possibly the K_{ATP}^+ channel via the p38 mitogen- activated protein kinase (MAPK) cascade].

lin,[57] appear to be released in quantities too small to have a measurable effect in the rabbit. In other species these proportions may be different. Adenosine appears to be a physiological trigger in man.[15,75] Although adenosine was felt initially not to be a physiological trigger in rat,[4,76] its release by ischemic myocardium in amounts much greater than in the rabbit requires significantly higher doses of an adenosine antagonist to block the protection of ischemic preconditioning.[77] An additional trigger is the variety of free radicals generated when the heart is reperfused at the end of the preconditioning ischemia. Free radicals are known to stimulate directly PKC[78] and can induce preconditioning.[79] In the rabbit model a free-radical scavenger also can block preconditioning's protection from a single 5-minute occlusion but not from multiple preconditioning cycles.[80] Figure 2 shows a simple diagram of the signal transduction pathways that we propose.

Tyrosine Kinases

Recent experiments have shed light on the signal transduction pathway beyond PKC used in ischemic preconditioning. PKC is a serine/threonine kinase that phosphorylates substrate proteins at either a serine or a threonine residue. At least one tyrosine kinase is present in the rabbit's signal transduction pathway because tyrosine kinase blockers abort protection in preconditioned hearts but have no effect on infarction in the nonpreconditioned heart.[81] Furthermore, the tyrosine kinase must be downstream of PKC because blockade of tyrosine kinases with either genistein or lavendustin A could block protection from direct activation of PKC by a phorbol ester.[81] A prime suspect for the tyrosine kinase is the activator of the 38-kd mitogen-activated protein kinase (p38 MAPK). This kinase

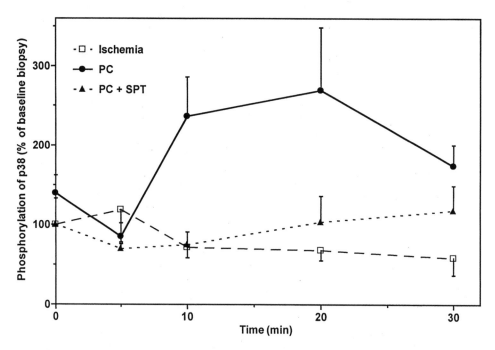

Figure 3. Phosphorylation of tyrosine 182 of p38 MAPK. This tyrosine residue must be phosphorylated to activate p38 MAPK. Note that p38 MAPK is only phosphorylated during ischemia if the heart has been preconditioned previously. Blockade of protection abolishes this increased phosphorylation. Reproduced with permission from Reference 88.

often is referred to as a stress-activated MAPK because it is activated during cellular stresses.[82,83] The p38 MAPK is activated by phosphorylation of both tyrosine 182 and threonine 180 residues. Once activated, it in turn phosphorylates MAPK activated protein (MAPKAP) kinase 2. MAPKAP kinase 2 then phosphorylates heat shock protein (HSP)-27, which, when phosphorylated, promotes cytoskeletal actin filament polymerization.[84,85] Thus, activation of p38 MAPK ultimately could result in strengthening of the cytoskeleton. Alternatively, MAPKAP kinase 2 could act to open ATP-sensitive potassium (K_{ATP}^+) channels.

Maulik et al.[86,87] have found that ischemic preconditioning of the rat heart is associated with increased quantities of phosphorylated p38 MAPK, MAPKAP kinase 2, and HSP-27. Figure 3 reveals that p38 MAPK is phosphorylated at its tyrosine activation site during ischemia but only if the heart has been preconditioned previously. Furthermore, when protection in ischemically preconditioned hearts is blocked by an adenosine receptor antagonist, phosphorylation of p38 MAPK during ischemia is no longer observed.[88] When p38 MAPK in isolated myocytes was activated directly with anisomycin (a bacterial product which activates both p38 MAPK and c-Jun N-terminal kinase [JNK]), the protection of ischemic preconditioning was mimicked.[88] Conversely, Figure 4 shows that blockade of p38 MAPK with SB 203580 completely abolishes preconditioning's protection in the isolated myocyte model.[88] Similar data have been reported in the intact rat heart.[89]

As previously noted combined blockade of PKC and tyrosine kinase is required to abort the protection of ischemic preconditioning in the porcine heart.[61] And in the rat the protective effect of multiple cycles of brief ischemia could be blocked only by combined kinase antagonist administration, whereas either individually was able to merely attenuate

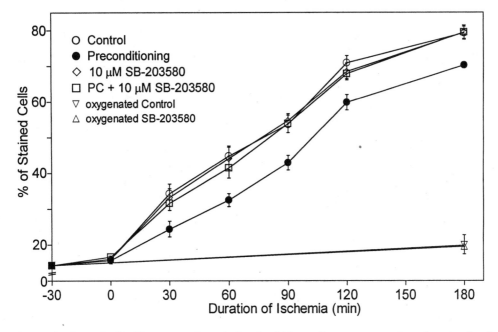

Figure 4. Osmotic fragility curves from isolated rabbit cardiomyocytes undergoing simulated ischemia. Every 30 minutes cells are removed from the pellet and placed in hypotonic (85 mOsm) buffer with trypan blue stain. Note that an increasing number of myocytes suffer membrane failure (stain blue) as simulated ischemia progresses. Preconditioning shifts the relationship downward so that the increase in fragility is delayed markedly. Inhibition of p38 MAPK with SB 203580 abolishes preconditioning's protection but has no effect on the nonpreconditioned cells. Reproduced with permission from Reference 88.

protection.[90,91] It is noteworthy that difficulty demonstrating roles for PKC[58] and tyrosine kinase[92] in preconditioning's signaling pathway in canine myocardium may stem from the failure to block both simultaneously. The presence of parallel, redundant pathways may be the organism's way of ensuring that a trigger of preconditioning will actually result in protection. In the rabbit it appears that PKC and tyrosine kinase are instead in series with the latter being downstream.[93] However, even in the rabbit redundancy is apparent. Whereas PKC blockers can prevent protection from a single preconditioning cycle, that blockade can be overcome if the heart is instead preconditioned with multiple cycles of ischemia.[94,95]

What Is Preconditioning's End Effector?

The signal transduction pathway must act by phosphorylating some protein(s), which then becomes directly responsible for preconditioning's cardioprotective effect. The identity of this end effector is not yet known, although there have been several suggestions. The K^+_{ATP} channel has been proposed repeatedly as the end effector. Several investigations have demonstrated that K^+_{ATP} channel openers can mimic preconditioning,[2,96–98] while channel blockers can abort the expected protection following brief ischemia.[2] A problem with the K^+_{ATP} hypothesis arises from the observation that K^+_{ATP} blockers do not prevent preconditioning's protection in all animal models, most notably the rat[21] in which preconditioning's protection is clearly PKC dependent.[43,47] However, in many models including human atrial trabeculae muscle[48] investigators have been able to demonstrate that it is possible to both block preconditioning's protection with glibenclamide, a K^+_{ATP} channel antagonist, and mimic the effect of preconditioning with K^+_{ATP} openers. Unpublished studies from our laboratory using patch clamp measurements reveal that the p38 MAPK activator anisomycin also opens K^+_{ATP} channels in rabbit cardiomyocytes.

It is unclear why opening of K^+_{ATP} channels should be so protective. They could be exerting their effect on volume regulation of the myocytes because opening of potassium channels is thought to reduce swelling.[99] Originally, the K^+_{ATP} openers were thought to act by conserving energy because they shorten the action potential, which should reduce calcium entry.[2] However, K^+_{ATP} openers appear to protect equally well in nonbeating myocytes,[100] which have no action potentials, and further can protect in intact hearts at doses which have no effect on the duration of the action potential.[97,98]

Recently it has become apparent that there are 2 distinct populations of K^+_{ATP} channels in the myocardial cell. Sarcolemmal and mitochondrial channels have different reactivities and different properties. Whereas pinacidil and glibenclamide will close both at the concentrations generally employed, diazoxide will open mitochondrial channels with at least a 2000-fold greater selectivity,[101,102] and 5-hydroxydecanoate (5HD) is a potent closer of mitochondrial channels.[103,104] Furthermore the new compound HMR 1883 will close surface[105] but not mitochondrial (E. Marban, personal communication, 1999) K^+_{ATP} channels. Use of these tools has enabled one to focus on the relative importance of sarcolemmal and mitochondrial channels in preconditioning. Diazoxide protects ischemic rat[104] and rabbit[106] hearts and isolated rabbit cardiomyocytes,[102] while 5HD blocks the protection of ischemic preconditioning.[102,104,106] Additionally HMR 1883 has no effect on the infarct-sparing action of preconditioning.[107] Therefore, it appears that the mitochondrial, not sarcolemmal, K^+_{ATP} channel is responsible for preconditioning's myocardial protection.

Armstrong and Ganote have noted that during ischemia myocytes experience a predictable increase in their osmotic fragility and propose that the latter is the result of changes in the cytoskeletal structure.[108] Additionally, they have observed that preconditioning myocardial cells with glucose-deficient medium or adenosine analogs causes them to be more resistant to osmotic swelling at any time during ischemia.[34] Cells are filled with osmotically active proteins. To avoid swelling, the cell pumps out sodium making extracellular sodium a counterbalancing osmolyte. During ischemia the sodium pumps fail and the sodium gradient collapses.[109] Furthermore, each mole of ATP is converted to 1 mole of AMP plus 2 moles of P_i. Thus, the osmotic pull of ATP is tripled. The net result is severe swelling in deeply ischemic tissue. Indeed, the mechanical disruption from swelling has even been proposed to be the lethal ischemic event.[35,108] Preconditioning could exert its final effect by strengthening the cell's cytoskeleton. An attractive hypothesis is that p38 MAPK promotes actin polymerization through the heat stress protein HSP-27.[88,110] In this paradigm protection does not derive from actual expression of HSP-27, but rather from phosphorylation of the constitutively expressed fraction.

Kitakaze and colleagues have proposed that increased 5'-nucleotidase activity is responsible for preconditioning's protection.[111] This enzyme dephosphorylates AMP to adenosine, which is free to leave the cardiomyocyte. The theory holds that preconditioned hearts produce more adenosine during ischemia, which then protects them by an as yet unidentified mechanism. Unfortunately, most investigators have found that preconditioned hearts actually produce and release less adenosine than their nonpreconditioned counterparts.[112–114] Furthermore, augmenting adenosine levels by two orders of magnitude with an adenosine deaminase inhibitor during regional ischemia in a canine model failed to mimic preconditioning's protection.[115] Thus it has been difficult to demonstrate a cause-and-effect relationship between the increased 5'-nucleotidase activity and preconditioning's protection.

Murry et al.[112] have proposed that protection is related to slower ATP utilization in ischemic myocardium, which would suggest that a metabolic enzyme is involved. Unfortunately, preserved ATP in the preconditioned heart has not been a universal finding. In preconditioned rat heart ATP actually falls more rapidly than in nonpreconditioned hearts.[116] It has not yet been proven that the K_{ATP}^+ channel or any other proposed channel, protein, or enzyme is the elusive end-effector. One must still be receptive to other suggestions. In fact Diaz et al.[117] recently presented very convincing data that opening of a chloride rather than potassium channel is responsible for the protection. Certainly, identification of the end effector must receive high priority because our understanding of preconditioning will be incomplete without it.

Pharmacologic Preconditioning

Preconditioning the heart with ischemia would not be feasible clinically except possibly during coronary angioplasty[10,14,15,75] or revascularization surgery.[11] The hope has been that a pharmacologic agent could be used instead to confer this protection. This would seemingly not be difficult because a large number of receptor agonists have been identified that can precondition the heart. The major drawback to the receptor agonist approach is that pretreatment appears to be an absolute requirement. Apparently, the changes responsible for protecting the heart must be in place very early in ischemia because none of the agents mentioned above has been found to be protective when administered after ischemia has started. The nonpreconditioned heart becomes awash with adenosine within minutes of a coronary occlusion but this adenosine fails to be protective. Only if the adenosine receptors are stimulated several minutes prior to ischemia will protection occur. Unfortunately, aside from the cardiac catheterization laboratory or surgical settings, there are few situations where the physician is able to anticipate an impending coronary occlusion.

We have explored the possibility of chronic prophylactic treatment with A_1-selective adenosine agonists but have found that tolerance to these agonists develops within 3 days.[118] Tolerance appeared to be the result of either down-regulation or decreased sensitivity of the adenosine receptor itself.[119] This observation raises another concern.

Could patients with a large ischemic burden also become tolerant to their own endogenously released adenosine? We chronically instrumented rabbits with a coronary balloon occluder and inflated the balloon with resulting coronary occlusion for 5 minutes every 30 minutes for 3 days.[120] Indeed, after 3 days of repeated coronary occlusions these animals also could no longer be protected by the 5-minute ischemic preconditioning protocol suggesting that such a tolerance had developed. Therefore, adenosine-based drugs may well prove to be ineffective in patients who have a history of frequent angina.

Finally, most of the agonists to the receptors identified as capable of preconditioning the heart cause severe peripheral effects, which would prevent their intravenous use. However, we have demonstrated that an intravenous cocktail of norepinephrine and adenosine, which generally have opposing hemodynamic effects and whose combination causes only minimal bradycardia, can protect the ischemic heart.[121] Two additional exceptions are adenosine A_1 agonists, which cause moderate but tolerable bradycardia and hypotension at protective doses, and opioids. High-dose opioids infused into the coronary circulation clearly precondition isolated rabbit hearts.[74] The rat heart also could be protected with intravenous morphine,[122] although we were unable to protect in situ rabbit hearts with an intravenous infusion of this agent.[74] It is unknown whether humans can be preconditioned with intravenous opioids.

Recently, we have examined a new class of compounds, the phosphatase inhibitors. In cell signaling substrate proteins are phosphorylated by kinases and the phosphate group is subsequently removed by a phosphatase. In the cell there are many phosphatases present, each with its own substrate specificity. Thus inhibition of a phosphatase should have an effect similar to that of stimulation of the associated kinase. Ganote noted some time ago that okadaic acid, a protein phosphatase 2A inhibitor, was very protective of cardiomyocytes during simulated ischemia.[123] Recently, we have tested fostriecin, a highly selective inhibitor of protein phosphatase 2A, in our isolated rabbit heart model.[124] As expected fostriecin was as protective as ischemic preconditioning in the reduction of infarct size. A comparable protective effect also has been observed in rabbit and pig cardiomyocytes.[125] Furthermore, when fostriecin infusion was started in the isolated rabbit heart model 10 minutes after ischemia had begun, protection was still evident.[124] It is not known at which step fostriecin acts to confer this protection, but protein phosphatase 2A is known to affect p38 MAPK activity.[82] The requirement for pretreatment with receptor agonists such as adenosine is believed to result from delays in the signal transduction pathways. As a result the end effector fails to be activated in time to protect the nonpreconditioned heart. Apparently, intervention at a point further down the signal transduction pathway bypasses the delays, and protection can be achieved even when the triggering agent is given after the onset of ischemia. Fostriecin has been used in man[126] with little long-term toxicity and thus could form the basis of an important new therapy.

Preconditioning in Humans

Ikonomidis[8] has studied cultures of human ventricular cardiomyocytes. Ischemia was simulated by placing the cells in phosphate buffer flushed with 100% nitrogen. Separate cultures were preconditioned with a period of anoxia followed by reoxygenation. Cell death was assessed by inability to exclude trypan blue. Preconditioning reduced the number of dead cells following both 90 minutes of simulated ischemia and 90 minutes of ischemia + 30 minutes of reoxygenation, but no effect on the ATP content was found during either ischemia or reperfusion. Ikonomidis et al. also found that addition of an adenosine receptor blocker abolished preconditioning's protective effect, while incubation of the myocytes in adenosine or the A_1-selective adenosine agonist R-PIA induced protection similar to that of simulated ischemic preconditioning. Finally, PKC blockade with calphostin C abolished preconditioning's protection and a phorbol ester mimicked it.

Walker[9] has induced preconditioning in human right atrial trabeculae. Ischemia was simulated by incubating the muscle in hypoxic, substrate-free medium and rapidly pacing it for 90 minutes followed by 120 minutes of reoxygenation. Preconditioning with 3 minutes of simulated ischemia followed by 10 minutes of reoxygenation caused a greater recovery of developed tension after 120 minutes of reoxygenation. Exposure of the cells to R-PIA resulted in a similar protective effect.[9] Preincubation of atrial trabeculae with the K_{ATP}^+ channel opener cromakalim or the PKC activator 1,2-dioctanoyl-*sn*-glycerol also improved postischemic function.[48] Preconditioning's protection was blocked by the PKC antagonist chelerythrine and the K_{ATP}^+ blocker glibenclamide.[48] Cleveland[127] also demonstrated that human ventricular trabeculae (removed from explanted hearts at the time of cardiac transplantation and thus possibly abnormal) could be preconditioned with phenylephrine or adenosine to cause improved mechanical function and preservation of tissue creatine kinase-MB following 30 minutes of simulated ischemia and 60 minutes of reperfusion. Thus human myocardial tissue also can be preconditioned by brief ischemic episodes and the cellular mechanisms appear to be identical to those seen in rabbit heart.

For obvious reasons it has been more difficult to document the existence of preconditioning in the intact human heart. Several approaches have been used. Yellon obtained biopsies from the anterior free wall of the left ventricle during coronary artery bypass surgery.[11] Hearts were preconditioned with two episodes of 3 minutes of global ischemia during cross-clamping of the aorta. Each ischemic period was followed by 2 minutes of reperfusion. During this preconditioning protocol the hearts were paced. These preliminary cross-clamping periods were absent in control hearts. All patients experienced 10 minutes of global ischemia caused by cross-clamping of the aorta with electrical ventricular fibrillation. Myocardial biopsies were analyzed for ATP content. ATP content after 10 minutes of ischemia was higher in the preconditioned group (12.0 ± 1.1 μmol/g dry weight) compared with controls (6.8 ± 0.2 μmol/g dry weight, $p < 0.05$). This study suggested that ischemic preconditioning slows the rate of ATP depletion during ischemia in the human heart, and that this preservation of ATP represented protection of the ischemic tissue. However, these same investigators repeated the protocol in another patient cohort and could not detect any evidence of ATP preservation in preconditioned myocardium.[128] In the latter study Jenkins and colleagues[128] noted that serum troponin T was modestly higher in nonpreconditioned patients following revascularization surgery, a possible indication of protection, but others have observed greater creatine kinase MB release following cardioplegic arrest in patients having undergone preconditioning than in controls.[129]

Deutsch and colleagues[10] examined the electrocardiogram (ECG) tracing recorded in angioplasty patients during serial balloon inflations. They noted that the ST segment rose more rapidly during the first coronary occlusion than in subsequent occlusions and attributed this change to possible preconditioning. Less pain and coronary sinus lactate production also were observed during the later occlusions. However, Cribier et al[14] and more recently Billinger and co-workers[130] suggested that the change in ST segments may have reflected improved collateral flow in the subsequent coronary occlusions rather than any preconditioning effect. The ST segment therefore was examined in the ischemic pig heart, which has a negligible collateral circulation. Indeed ST-segment shifts evolved much more slowly once the heart had been preconditioned.[131] A similar observation was made in preconditioned rabbit heart, and blockade of protection with an adenosine receptor blocker also abolished the beneficial effect of ischemic preconditioning on the ST segment.[132] Thus we were initially encouraged that a reduced rate of rise of the ST segment during ischemia was a true property of the preconditioned heart, and could be used to indicate a preconditoned state in man.

Investigators then began to use this response of S-T segments to multiple coronary occlusions to indicate which pharmacologic agents administered to patients before the first balloon inflation might be preconditioning-mimetics. Tomai and colleagues[133] reported that the K_{ATP}^+ blocker glibenclamide could abolish changes in the altered ST segments during serial balloon inflations in angioplasty patients. A similar effect on the ST segment was seen when the adenosine receptor blocker bamiphylline was given to patients during angioplasty.[134] Conversely, intracoronary adenosine in angioplasty patients caused changes in the ST segment, consistent with those seen with ischemic preconditioning.[15,75]

However, more recent investigations in the rabbit heart have demonstrated a dissociation between myocardial cardioprotection and declining maximum S-T segment voltage recorded during sequential coronary occlusions (M. Birincioglu, X.-M. Yang, J. M. Downey, and M. V. Cohen, unpublished data, 1999). Whereas the infarct-sparing effect of preconditioning appears to be associated with opening of mitochondrial K_{ATP}^+ channels, it is opening of sarcolemmal K_{ATP}^+ channels which results in the lessening of S-T segment elevation during the second and subsequent coronary occlusions. With ischemic preconditioning apparently both populations of channels open simultaneously. When these channels are manipulated pharmacologically, however, it cannot be assumed that modification of the S-T segment voltage implies anything about the state of protection of the heart. Thus this consideration in addition to uncertainty concerning changes in coronary collateral flow during sequential coronary artery occlusions makes the value of ECG monitoring in these angioplasty patients problematic.

Finally, population studies, principally retrospective, have been conducted to determine the prognostic significance of brief episodes of chest pain and therefore presumed myocardial ischemia prior to infarction. Kloner et al[135] examined the Thrombolysis in Myocardial Infarction (TIMI) database and found that patients who had one or more episodes of angina prior to an acute myocardial infarction had a lower incidence of both in-hospital mortality and congestive heart failure than those who did not report any antecedent angina. They concluded that the anginal attacks preceding the coronary thrombotic event preconditioned and thus protected the hearts. This conclusion has been echoed by others.[136–139]

But several considerations perhaps diminish enthusiasm for this position. Firstly, the presence of coronary collateral vessels has infrequently been considered because of lack of coronary angiography. Yet Hirai et al.[136,140] noted that coronary collaterals were more frequent in those with preceding angina, and regional left ventricular function was better in those with more developed collaterals. Secondly, those individuals with preinfarction angina lyse the thrombus occluding the coronary artery and reestablish distal flow faster than those without angina.[141] Reperfusion occurs approximately 21 min sooner after initiation of infusion of the thrombolytic agent in those with prior angina. Reasons for this difference are uncertain, but more rapid reperfusion might result in less infarction which could translate into an improved clinical course without any consideration of the preconditioning phenomenon. Finally, at least one study has demonstrated clinical benefits of preinfarction angina only in those younger than 65 years,[142] thus limiting general applicability of any protective mechanism. Hence, it is unclear whether these population studies have yet proved unequivocally that ischemic preconditioning exists in humans.

Second Window of Protection

A substantial body of evidence has documented that preconditioning's early protective phase is followed by a delayed phase of protection occurring many hours later. This delayed phase of protection has been termed the second window of protection.[12] The second window of protection was first noted in 1993 in open-chest rabbit[25] and canine[26] models as an anti-infarct effect appearing 24 hours after a preconditioning stimulus consisting of repetitive cycles of coronary occlusion. This anti-infarct effect subsequently has been confirmed in other open-chest rabbit studies[143,144] and also has been observed 24 hours after preconditioning in chronically instrumented conscious rabbits.[31] More recent work from Yellon's laboratory suggests that the delayed anti-infarct effect of a single preconditioning episode lasts for 3 days in the rabbit.[145]

Several lines of evidence suggest that the protection could be related to the appearance of new proteins or to alterations in protein activity by posttranslational mechanisms. A large number of proteins including proto-oncogenes, intracellular antioxidants, and heat shock proteins appear after sublethal ischemia. The slow onset of appearance (12–24 hours) and subsequent duration of the second window (24–72 hours) would be consistent with gene expression. The myocardial content of HSP-70i is elevated 24 hours after preconditioning and has been correlated with protection.[25] Hoshida et al.,[146] on the other hand, have proposed that protection is related to the expression of manganese superoxide dismutase (SOD). Although overexpression of HSP-70 can cause protection of murine hearts,[147] it has yet to be proven that either HSP-70 or Mn SOD is responsible for the protection of the second window of preconditioning. A third possibility is nitric oxide synthase (NOS). Bolli's group reports that NO acts as a trigger for the antistunning[148] as well as anti-infarct[27] effects seen 24 hours after ischemic preconditioning in the rabbit. More importantly, NOS inhibitors given just prior to the ischemic insult on the 2nd day also abolish the antistunning[29] and anti-infarct[28] effects, suggesting that protection involves increased production of NO. Induction of NOS would be the logical explanation.

The attractiveness of the second window is that it might be more amenable to prophylactic therapy. The cell signaling pathways that trigger the second window appear to be similar to those used by classical preconditioning. Yellon's group has shown that a single bolus of the adenosine A_1 receptor agonist 2-chloro-N^6-cyclopentyladenosine (CCPA) significantly protects the myocardium against infarction from a subsequent lethal ischemic insult 24–72 hours after the CCPA bolus.[143] PKC also appears to be involved. PKC inhibitors given just prior to the preconditioning stimulus abort the protection against both infarction[144] and stunning[149] in the rabbit.

Conscious, instrumented rabbits that were preconditioned 1 day prior to coronary occlusion also experienced a reduction of ischemia-induced ventricular fibrillation.[31] Vegh's group also has reported a delayed antiarrhythmic effect following pacing-induced preconditioning in dog heart.[30] They found that the antiarrhythmic protection was almost completely lost by 48 hours, which is in contrast to the anti-infarct effect in the rabbit, which extends to 72 hours.[145]

It is unknown whether second window protection occurs in humans, but it does not appear to occur in all species. Bolli failed to protect the pig heart against either infarction or stunning 24 hours after preconditioning.[150] However, a second window phenomenon could explain why Kloner saw a decreased mortality in infarct patients with antecedent angina even when the anginal episode was days prior to the coronary occlusion.[135] Ottani et al[137] selected patients with a history of angina in the 24-hour period prior to infarction. The mean time between the last episode of angina and onset of infarction was approximately 11 hours, a time that clearly falls outside the time frame of experimentally defined classic preconditioning. Yet the patients in whom angina heralded the infarction had a better prognosis than those without angina. In the study by Nakagawa et al.[138] patients in the group that showed benefit had their last episode of angina a mean of 25 hours before onset of infarction. Although the greatest benefit was seen in patients who had experienced angina closer to the onset of infarction, none of these patients experienced their last episode of angina within the time frame of classic preconditioning (60–90 minutes).

Conclusions

Ischemic preconditioning demonstrates that preservation of ischemic myocardium is at least theoretically possible. Already, research in this area has identified a wide variety of agents that can be used to precondition the heart pharmacologically. In situations such as surgery or angioplasty in which ischemia is anticipated, it is possible to protect the heart with one of the receptor agonists or even ischemia itself. As limited access myocardial revascularization grafting[151] gains in popularity, preconditioning mimetics should play an increasingly important role because standard cardioplegia cannot be used in this setting. However, the largest target population is still patients presenting with acute myocardial infarction. Treatment could be prophylactic periodic treatment with an A_1-selective adenosine agonist that might keep high-risk patients in the second window of protection.[152] The other approach would be identification of agents that can protect even after ischemia has begun. These might include a phosphatase inhibitor such as fostriecin. Because of its relatively mild side effects fostriecin or similar agent probably could be administered by emergency medical service personnel to any patient suspected of having a coronary thrombosis. As our knowledge of preconditioning's mechanism grows, more and more strategies for protecting the ischemic myocardium are sure to emerge.

References

1. Murry CE, Jennings RB, Reimer KA. Preconditioning with ischemia: A delay of lethal cell injury in ischemic myocardium. *Circulation* 1986;74:1124–1136.
2. Gross GJ, Auchampach JA. Blockade of ATP-sensitive potassium channels prevents myocardial preconditioning in dogs. *Circ Res* 1992;70:223–233.
3. Yellon DM, Alkhulaifi AM, Browne EE, et al. Ischaemic preconditioning limits infarct size in the rat heart. *Cardiovasc Res* 1992;26:983–987.
4. Liu Y, Downey JM. Ischemic preconditioning protects against infarction in rat heart. *Am J Physiol* 1992;263:H1107–H1112.
5. Van Winkle DM, Thornton JD, Downey DM, et al. The natural history of preconditioning: Cardioprotection depends on duration of transient ischemia and time to subsequent ischemia. *Coron Artery Dis* 1991;2:613–619.
6. Toombs CF, Wiltse AL, Shebuski RJ. Ischemic preconditioning fails to limit infarct size in reserpinized rabbit myocardium: Implication of norepinephrine release in the preconditioning effect. *Circulation* 1993;88:2351–2358.
7. Schott RJ, Rohmann S, Braun ER, et al. Ischemic preconditioning reduces infarct size in swine myocardium. *Circ Res* 1990;66:1133–1142.
8. Ikonomidis JS, Shirai T, Weisel RD, et al. Preconditioning cultured human pediatric myocytes requires adenosine and protein kinase C. *Am J Physiol* 1997;272:H1220–H1230.
9. Walker DM, Walker JM, Pugsley WB, et al. Preconditioning in isolated superfused human muscle. *J Mol Cell Cardiol* 1995;27:1349–1357.
10. Deutsch E, Berger M, Kussmaul WG, et al. Adaptation to ischemia during percutaneous transluminal coronary angioplasty: Clinical, hemodynamic, and metabolic features. *Circulation* 1990;82:2044–2051.
11. Yellon DM, Alkhulaifi AM, Pugsley WB. Preconditioning the human myocardium. *Lancet* 1993;342:276–277.
12. Yellon DM, Baxter GF. A "second window of protection" or delayed preconditioning phenomenon: Future horizons for myocardial protection? *J Mol Cell Cardiol* 1995;27:1023–1034.
13. Miura T, Adachi T, Ogawa T, et al. Myocardial infarct size-limiting effect of ischemic preconditioning: Its natural decay and the effect of repetitive preconditioning. *Cardiovasc Pathol* 1992;1:147–154.

14. Cribier A, Korsatz L, Koning R, et al. Improved myocardial ischemic response and enhanced collateral circulation with long repetitive coronary occlusion during angioplasty: A prospective study. *J Am Coll Cardiol* 1992;20:578–586.

15. Kerensky RA, Kutcher MA, Braden GA, et al. The effects of intracoronary adenosine on preconditioning during coronary angioplasty. *Clin Cardiol* 1995;18:91–96.

16. Vegh A, Szekeres L, Parratt JR. Protective effects of preconditioning of the ischaemic myocardium involve cyclo-oxygenase products. *Cardiovasc Res* 1990;24:1020–1023.

17. Hagar JM, Hale SL, Kloner RA. Effect of preconditioning ischemia on reperfusion arrhythmias after coronary artery occlusion and reperfusion in the rat. *Circ Res* 1991;68:61–68.

18. Shiki K, Hearse DJ. Preconditioning of ischemic myocardium: Reperfusion-induced arrhythmias. *Am J Physiol* 1987;253:H1470–H1476.

19. Ovize M, Przyklenk K, Hale SL, et al. Preconditioning does not attenuate myocardial stunning. *Circulation* 1992;85:2247–2254.

20. Sun J-Z, Tang X-L, Knowlton AA, et al. Late preconditioning against myocardial stunning: An endogenous protective mechanism that confers resistance to postischemic dysfunction 24 h after brief ischemia in conscious pigs. *J Clin Invest* 1995;95:388–403.

21. Asimakis GK, Inners-McBride K, Medellin G, et al. Ischemic preconditioning attenuates acidosis and postischemic dysfunction in isolated rat heart. *Am J Physiol* 1992;263:H887–H894.

22. Banerjee A, Locke-Winter C, Rogers KB, et al. Preconditioning against myocardial dysfunction after ischemia and reperfusion by an α_1-adrenergic mechanism. *Circ Res* 1993;73:656–670.

23. Zhai X, Lawson CS, Cave AC, et al. Preconditioning and post-ischaemic contractile dysfunction: The role of impaired oxygen delivery vs extracellular metabolite accumulation. *J Mol Cell Cardiol* 1993;25:847–857.

24. Murry CE, Richard VJ, Jennings RB, et al. Myocardial protection is lost before contractile function recovers from ischemic preconditioning. *Am J Physiol* 1991;260:H796–H804.

25. Marber MS, Latchman DS, Walker JM, et al. Cardiac stress protein elevation 24 hours after brief ischemia or heat stress is associated with resistance to myocardial infarction. *Circulation* 1993;88:1264–1272.

26. Kuzuya T, Hoshida S, Yamashita N, et al. Delayed effects of sublethal ischemia on the acquisition of tolerance to ischemia. *Circ Res* 1993;72:1293–1299.

27. Qiu Y, Rizvi A, Tang X-L, et al. Nitric oxide triggers late preconditioning against myocardial infarction in conscious rabbits. *Am J Physiol* 1997;273:H2931–H2936.

28. Takano H, Manchikalapudi S, Tang, X-L, et al. Nitric oxide synthase is the mediator of late preconditioning against myocardial infarction in conscious rabbits. *Circulation* 1998;98:441–449.

29. Bolli R, Manchikalapudi S, Tang X-L, et al. The protective effect of late preconditioning against myocardial stunning in conscious rabbits is mediated by nitric oxide synthase: Evidence that nitric oxide acts both as a trigger and as a mediator of the late phase of ischemic preconditioning. *Circ Res* 1997;81:1094–1107.

30. Kaszala K, Vegh A, Papp JG, et al. Time course of the protection against ischaemia and reperfusion-induced ventricular arrhythmias resulting from brief periods of cardiac pacing. *J Mol Cell Cardiol* 1996;28:2085–2095.

31. Yang X-M, Baxter GF, Heads RJ, et al. Infarct limitation of the second window of protection in a conscious rabbit model. *Cardiovasc Res* 1996;31:777–783.

32. Ytrehus K, Liu Y, Tsuchida A, et al. Rat and rabbit heart infarction: Effects of anesthesia, perfusate, risk zone, and method of infarct sizing. *Am J Physiol* 1994;267:H2383–H2390.

33. Gottlieb RA, Gruol DL, Zhu JY, et al. Preconditioning in rabbit cardiomyocytes: Role of pH, vacuolar proton ATPase, and apoptosis. *J Clin Invest* 1996;97:2391–2398.

34. Armstrong S, Ganote CE. Preconditioning of isolated rabbit cardiomyocytes: Effects of glycolytic blockade, phorbol esters, and ischaemia. *Cardiovasc Res* 1994;28:1700–1706.

35. Jennings RB, Reimer KA. Lethal myocardial ischemic injury. *Am J Pathol* 1981;102:241–255.

36. Turrens JF, Thornton J, Barnard ML, et al. Protection from reperfusion injury by preconditioning hearts does not involve increased antioxidant defenses. *Am J Physiol* 1992;262:H585–H589.

37. Thornton J, Striplin S, Liu GS, et al. Inhibition of protein synthesis does not block myocardial protection afforded by preconditioning. *Am J Physiol* 1990;259:H1822–H1825.
38. Jennings RB, Reimer KA, Steenbergen C. Effect of inhibition of the mitochondrial ATPase on net myocardial ATP in total ischemia. *J Mol Cell Cardiol* 1991;23:1383–1395.
39. Cohen MV, Downey JM. Myocardial preconditioning promises to be a novel approach to the treatment of ischemic heart disease. *Annu Rev Med* 1996;47:21–29.
40. Liu GS, Thornton J, Van Winkle DM, et al. Protection against infarction afforded by preconditioning is mediated by A_1 adenosine receptors in rabbit heart. *Circulation* 1991;84:350–356.
41. Liu Y, Cohen MV, Downey JM. Chelerythrine, a highly selective protein kinase C inhibitor, blocks the antiinfarct effect of ischemic preconditioning in rabbit hearts. *Cardiovasc Drugs Ther* 1994;8:881–882.
42. Ytrehus K, Liu Y, Downey JM. Preconditioning protects ischemic rabbit heart by protein kinase C activation. *Am J Physiol* 1994;266:H1145–H1152.
43. Li Y, Kloner RA. Does protein kinase C play a role in ischemic preconditioning in rat hearts? *Am J Physiol* 1995;268:H426–H431.
44. Mitchell MB, Meng X, Ao L, et al. Preconditioning of isolated rat heart is mediated by protein kinase C. *Circ Res* 1995;76:73–81.
45. Kitakaze M, Hori M, Morioka T, et al. α_1-Adrenoceptor activation increases ecto-5′-nucleotidase activity and adenosine release in rat cardiomyocytes by activating protein kinase C. *Circulation* 1995;91:2226–2234.
46. Armstrong S, Downey JM, Ganote CE. Preconditioning of isolated rabbit cardiomyocytes: Induction by metabolic stress and blockade by the adenosine antagonist SPT and calphostin C, a protein kinase C inhibitor. *Cardiovasc Res* 1994;28:72–77.
47. Speechly-Dick ME, Mocanu MM, Yellon DM. Protein kinase C: Its role in ischemic preconditioning in the rat. *Circ Res* 1994;75:586–590.
48. Speechly-Dick ME, Grover GJ, Yellon DM. Does ischemic preconditioning in the human involve protein kinase C and the ATP-dependent K^+ channel? Studies of contractile function after simulated ischemia in an atrial in vitro model. *Circ Res* 1995;77:1030–1035.
49. Sadoshima J-i, Izumo S. Signal transduction pathways of angiotensin II-induced c-*fos* gene expression in cardiac myocytes in vitro: Roles of phospholipid-derived second messengers. *Circ Res* 1993;73:424–438.
50. Talosi L, Kranias EG. Effect of α-adrenergic stimulation on activation of protein kinase C and phosphorylation of proteins in intact rabbit hearts. *Circ Res* 1992;70:670–678.
51. Minshall RD, Nakamura F, Becker RP, et al. Characterization of bradykinin B_2 receptors in adult myocardium and neonatal rat cardiomyocytes. *Circ Res* 1995;76:773–780.
52. Irons CE, Murray SF, Glembotski CC. Identification of the receptor subtype responsible for endothelin-mediated protein kinase C activation and atrial natriuretic factor secretion from atrial myocytes. *J Biol Chem* 1993;268:23417–23421.
53. Goto M, Liu Y, Yang X-M, et al. Role of bradykinin in protection of ischemic preconditioning in rabbit hearts. *Circ Res* 1995;77:611–621.
54. Liu Y, Tsuchida A, Cohen MV, et al. Pretreatment with angiotensin II activates protein kinase C and limits myocardial infarction in isolated rabbit hearts. *J Mol Cell Cardiol* 1995;27:883–892.
55. Thornton JD, Daly JF, Cohen MV, et al. Catecholamines can induce adenosine receptor-mediated protection of the myocardium but do not participate in ischemic preconditioning in the rabbit. *Circ Res* 1993;73:649–655.
56. Tsuchida A, Liu Y, Liu GS, et al. α_1-Adrenergic agonists precondition rabbit ischemic myocardium independent of adenosine by direct activation of protein kinase C. *Circ Res* 1994;75:576–585.
57. Wang P, Gallagher KP, Downey JM, et al. Pretreatment with endothelin-1 mimics ischemic preconditioning against infarction in isolated rabbit heart. *J Mol Cell Cardiol* 1996;28:579–588.
58. Przyklenk K, Sussman MA, Simkhovich BZ, et al. Does ischemic preconditioning trigger translocation of protein kinase C in the canine model? *Circulation* 1995;92:1546–1557.
59. Vogt AM, Htun P, Arras M, et al. Intramyocardial infusion of tool drugs for the study of molecular mechanisms in ischemic preconditioning. *Basic Res Cardiol* 1996;91:389–400.

60. Vahlhaus C, Schulz R, Post H, et al. No prevention of ischemic preconditioning by the protein kinase C inhibitor staurosporine in swine. *Circ Res* 1996;79:407–414.
61. Vahlhaus C, Schulz R, Post H, et al. Prevention of ischemic preconditioning only by combined inhibition of protein kinase C and protein tyrosine kinase in pigs. *J Mol Cell Cardiol* 1998;30:197–209.
62. Brooks G, Hearse DJ. Role of protein kinase C in ischemic preconditioning: Player or spectator? *Circ Res* 1996;79:627–630.
63. Mochly-Rosen D. Localization of protein kinases by anchoring proteins: A theme in signal transduction. *Science* 1995;268:247–251.
64. Yoshida K-i, Kawamura S, Mizukami Y, et al. Implication of protein kinase C-α, δ, and ϵ isoforms in ischemic preconditioning in perfused rat hearts. *J Biochem* 1997;122:506–511.
65. Miyawaki H, Ashraf M. Ca^{2+} as a mediator of ischemic preconditioning. *Circ Res* 1997;80:790–799.
66. Kawamura S, Yoshida K-I, Miura T, et al. Ischemic preconditioning translocates PKC-δ and -ϵ, which mediate functional protection in isolated rat heart. *Am J Physiol* 1998;275:H2266–H2271.
67. Ping P, Zhang J, Qiu Y, et al. Ischemic preconditioning induces selective translocation of protein kinase C isoforms ϵ and η in the heart of conscious rabbits without subcellular redistribution of total protein kinase C activity. *Circ Res* 1997;81: 404–414.
68. Gray MO, Karliner JS, Mochly-Rosen D. A selective ϵ-protein kinase C antagonist inhibits protection of cardiac myocytes from hypoxia-induced cell death. *J Biol Chem* 1997;272: 30945–30951.
69. Goldberg M, Zhang HL, Steinberg SF. Hypoxia alters the subcellular distribution of protein kinase C isoforms in neonatal rat ventricular myocytes. *J Clin Invest* 1997;99:55–61.
70. Armstrong SC, Hoover DB, Delacey MH, et al. Translocation of PKC, protein phosphatase inhibition and preconditioning of rabbit cardiomyocytes. *J Mol Cell Cardiol* 1996;28:1479–1492.
71. Liu GS, Cohen MV, Mochly-Rosen D, et al. Protein kinase C-ϵ is responsible for the protection of preconditioning in rabbit cardiomyocytes. *J Mol Cell Cardiol* 1999;31.
72. Parratt J. Endogenous myocardial protective (antiarrhythmic) substances. *Cardiovasc Res* 1993;27:693–702.
73. Moolman JA, Genade S, Tromp E, et al. A comparison between ischemic preconditioning and anti-adrenergic interventions: cAMP, energy metabolism and functional recovery. *Basic Res Cardiol* 1996;91:219–233.
74. Miki T, Cohen MV, Downey JM. Opioid receptor contributes to ischemic preconditioning through protein kinase C activation in rabbits. *Mol Cell Biochem* 1998;186:3–12.
75. Leesar MA, Stoddard M, Ahmed M, et al. Preconditioning of human myocardium with adenosine during coronary angioplasty. *Circulation* 1997;95:2500–2507.
76. Li Y, Kloner RA. The cardioprotective effects of ischemic "preconditioning" are not mediated by adenosine receptors in rat hearts. *Circulation* 1993;87:1642–1648.
77. Headrick JP. Ischemic preconditioning: Bioenergetic and metabolic changes and the role of endogenous adenosine. *J Mol Cell Cardiol* 1996;28:1227–1240.
78. Gopalakrishna R, Anderson WB. Ca^{2+}- and phospholipid-independent activation of protein kinase C by selective oxidative modification of the regulatory domain. *Proc Natl Acad Sci* 1989;86:6758–6762.
79. Tritto I, D'Andrea D, Eramo N, et al. Oxygen radicals can induce preconditioning in rabbit hearts. *Circ Res* 1997;80:743–748.
80. Baines CP, Goto M, Downey JM. Oxygen radicals released during ischemic preconditioning contribute to cardioprotection in the rabbit myocardium. *J Mol Cell Cardiol* 1997;29:207–216.
81. Baines CP, Wang L, Cohen MV, et al. Protein tyrosine kinase is downstream of protein kinase C for ischemic preconditioning's anti-infarct effect in the rabbit heart. *J Mol Cell Cardiol* 1998;30:383–392.
82. Rouse J, Cohen P, Trigon S, et al. A novel kinase cascade triggered by stress and heat shock that stimulates MAPKAP kinase-2 and phosphorylation of the small heat shock proteins. *Cell* 1994;78:1027–1037.
83. Waskiewicz AJ, Cooper JA. Mitogen and stress response pathways: MAP kinase cascades and phosphatase regulation in mammals and yeast. *Curr Opin Cell Biol* 1995;7:798–805.

84. Landry J, Huot J. Modulation of actin dynamics during stress and physiological stimulation by a signaling pathway involving p38 MAP kinase and heat-shock protein 27. *Biochem Cell Biol* 1995;73:703–707.

85. Guay J, Lambert H, Gingras-Breton G, et al. Regulation of actin filament dynamics by p38 map kinase-mediated phosphorylation of heat shock protein 27. *J Cell Sci* 1997;110:357–368.

86. Maulik N, Watanabe M, Zu Y-L, et al. Ischemic preconditioning triggers the activation of MAP kinases and MAPKAP kinase 2 in rat hearts. *FEBS Lett* 1996;396:233–237.

87. Maulik N, Yoshida T, Zu Y-L, et al. Ischemic preconditioning triggers a tyrosine kinase-dependent signal transduction process involving p^{38} MAP kinases and MAPKAP kinase 2. *J Mol Cell Cardiol* 1997;29:A171. Abstract.

88. Weinbrenner C, Liu G-S, Cohen MV, et al. Phosphorylation of tyrosine 182 of p38 mitogen-activated protein kinase correlates with the protection of preconditioning in the rabbit heart. *J Mol Cell Cardiol* 1997;29:2383–2391.

89. Maulik N, Yoshida T, Zu Y-L, et al. Ischemic preconditioning triggers tyrosine kinase signaling: A potential role for MAPKAP kinase 2. *Am J Physiol* 1998;275:H1857–H1864.

90. Tanno M, Tsuchida A, Hasegawa T, et al. Both protein kinase C (PKC) and tyrosine kinase contribute to cardioprotection by repetitive preconditioning in rats. *J Mol Cell Cardiol* 1998;30:A312. Abstract.

91. Fryer RM, Schultz JEJ, Hsu AK, et al. Importance of PKC and tyrosine kinase in single or multiple cycles of preconditioning in rat hearts. *Am J Physiol* 1999;276:H1229–H1235.

92. Kitakaze M, Node K, Funaya H, et al. Tyrosine kinase is not involved in the infarct size-limiting effect of ischemic preconditioning in the canine heart. *Circulation* 1997;96(suppl I):I574. Abstract.

93. Iliodromitis EK, Miki T, Liu GS, et al. The PKC activator PMA preconditions rabbit heart in the presence of adenosine receptor blockade: Is 5′-nucleotidase important? *J Mol Cell Cardiol* 1998;30:2201–2211.

94. Sandhu R, Diaz RJ, Mao GD, et al. Ischemic preconditioning: Differences in protection and susceptibility to blockade with single-cycle versus multicycle transient ischemia. *Circulation* 1997;96:984–995.

95. Miura T, Miura T, Kawamura S, et al. Effect of protein kinase C inhibitors on cardioprotection by ischemic preconditioning depends on the number of preconditioning episodes. *Cardiovasc Res* 1998;37:700–709.

96. Grover GJ, Dzwonczyk S, Parham CS, et al. The protective effects of cromakalim and pinacidil on reperfusion function and infarct size in isolated perfused rat hearts and anesthetized dogs. *Cardiovasc Drugs Ther* 1990;4:465–474.

97. Yao Z, Gross GJ. Effects of the K_{ATP} channel opener bimakalim on coronary blood flow, monophasic action potential duration, and infarct size in dogs. *Circulation* 1994;89:1769–1775.

98. Grover GJ, D'Alonzo AJ, Parham CS, et al. Cardioprotection with the K_{ATP} opener cromakalim is not correlated with ischemic myocardial action potential duration. *J Cardiovasc Pharmacol* 1995;26:145–152.

99. Hallows KR, Knauf PA. Principles of cell volume regulation. In: Strange K, ed. *Cellular and Molecular Physiology of Cell Volume Regulation*. Boca Raton: CRC Press; 1994:3–29.

100. Armstrong SC, Liu GS, Downey JM, et al. Potassium channels and preconditioning of isolated rabbit cardiomyocytes: Effects of glyburide and pinacidil. *J Mol Cell Cardiol* 1995;27:1765–1774.

101. Garlid KD, Paucek P, Yarov-Yarovoy V, et al. The mitochondrial K_{ATP} channel as a receptor for potassium channel openers. *J Biol Chem* 1996;271:8796–8799.

102. Liu Y, Sato T, O'Rourke B, et al. Mitochondrial ATP-dependent potassium channels: Novel effectors of cardioprotection? *Circulation* 1998;97:2463–2469.

103. McCullough JR, Normandin DE, Conder ML, et al. Specific block of the anti-ischemic actions of cromakalim by sodium 5-hydroxydecanoate. *Circ Res* 1991;69:949–958.

104. Garlid KD, Paucek P, Yarov-Yarovoy V, et al. Cardioprotective effect of diazoxide and its interaction with mitochondrial ATP-sensitive K^+ channels: Possible mechanism of cardioprotection. *Circ Res* 1997;81:1072–1082.

105. Gögelein H, Hartung J, Englert HC, et al. HMR 1883, a novel cardioselective inhibitor of the ATP-sensitive potassium channel. Part I: Effects on cardiomyocytes, coronary flow and pancreatic β-cells. *J Pharmacol Exp Ther* 1998;286:1453–1464.

106. Baines CP, Liu GS, Birincioglu M, et al. Ischemic preconditioning depends on interaction between mitochondrial K_{ATP} channels and actin cytoskeleton. *Am J Physiol* 1999;276: H1361–H1368.

107. Yang X-M, Downey JM, Cohen MV. HMR 1883, a surface K_{ATP} channel antagonist, blocks protection from diazoxide: Diazoxide's specificity for mitochondrial K_{ATP} is questionable. *Circulation* 1999;100 (Suppl I):I000. Abstract.

108. Ganote C, Armstrong S. Ischaemia and the myocyte cytoskeleton: Review and speculation. *Cardiovasc Res* 1993;27:1387–1403.

109. Van Emous JG, Nederhoff MGJ, Ruigrok TJC, et al. The role of the Na^+ channel in the accumulation of intracellular Na^+ during myocardial ischemia: Consequences for post-ischemic recovery. *J Mol Cell Cardiol* 1997;29:85–96.

110. Huot J, Houle F, Marceau F, et al. Oxidative stress-induced actin reorganization mediated by the p38 mitogen-activated protein kinase/heat shock protein 27 pathway in vascular endothelial cells. *Circ Res* 1997;80:383–392.

111. Kitakaze M, Hori M, Takashima S, et al. Ischemic preconditioning increases adenosine release and 5′-nucleotidase activity during myocardial ischemia and reperfusion in dogs: Implications for myocardial salvage. *Circulation* 1993;87:208–215.

112. Murry CE, Richard VJ, Reimer KA, et al. Ischemic preconditioning slows energy metabolism and delays ultrastructural damage during a sustained ischemic episode. *Circ Res* 1990;66: 913–931.

113. Van Wylen DGL. Effect of ischemic preconditioning on interstitial purine metabolite and lactate accumulation during myocardial ischemia. *Circulation* 1994;89:2283–2289.

114. Goto M, Cohen MV, Van Wylen DGL, et al. Attenuated purine production during subsequent ischemia in preconditioned rabbit myocardium is unrelated to the mechanism of protection. *J Mol Cell Cardiol* 1996;28:447–454.

115. Silva PH, Dillon D, Van Wylen DGL. Adenosine deaminase inhibition augments interstitial adenosine but does not attenuate myocardial infarction. *Cardiovasc Res* 1995;29:616–623.

116. Kolocassides KG, Seymour A-ML, Galiñanes M, et al. Paradoxical effect of ischemic preconditioning on ischemic contracture? NMR studies of energy metabolism and intracellular pH in the rat heart. *J Mol Cell Cardiol* 1996;28:1045–1057.

117. Diaz RJ, Losito VA, Mao GD, et al. Chloride channel inhibition blocks the protection of ischemic preconditioning and hypo-osmotic stress in rabbit ventricular myocardium. *Circ Res* 1999;84:763–775.

118. Tsuchida A, Thompson R, Olsson RA, et al. The anti-infarct effect of an adenosine A_1-selective agonist is diminished after prolonged infusion as is the cardioprotective effect of ischaemic preconditioning in rabbit heart. *J Mol Cell Cardiol* 1994;26:303–311.

119. Hashimi MW, Thornton JD, Downey JM, et al. Loss of myocardial protection from ischemic preconditioning following chronic exposure to $R(-)-N^6$-(2-phenylisopropyl)adenosine is related to defect at the adenosine A_1 receptor. *Mol Cell Biochem* 1998;186:19–25.

120. Cohen MV, Yang X-M, Downey JM. Conscious rabbits become tolerant to multiple episodes of ischemic preconditioning. *Circ Res* 1994;74:998–1004.

121. Cohen MV, Thornton JD, Thornton CS, et al. Intravenous co-infusion of adenosine and norepinephrine preconditions the heart without adverse hemodynamic effects. *J Thorac Cardiovasc Surg* 1997;114:236–242.

122. Schultz JEJ, Rose E, Yao Z, et al. Evidence for involvement of opioid receptors in ischemic preconditioning in rat hearts. *Am J Physiol* 1995;268:H2157–H2161.

123. Armstrong SC, Ganote CE. Effects of the protein phosphatase inhibitors okadaic acid and calyculin A on metabolically inhibited and ischaemic isolated myocytes. *J Mol Cell Cardiol* 1992;24:869–884.

124. Weinbrenner C, Baines CP, Liu G-S, et al. Fostriecin, an inhibitor of protein phosphatase 2A, limits myocardial infarct size even when administered after onset of ischemia. *Circulation* 1998;98:899–905.

125. Armstrong SC, Kao R, Gao W, et al. Comparison of in vitro preconditioning responses of isolated pig and rabbit cardiomyocytes: Effects of a protein phosphatase inhibitor, fostriecin. *J Mol Cell Cardiol* 1997;29:3009–3024.

126. Moore MJ, Erlichman C, Pillon L, et al. A phase I study of fostriecin in a daily ×5 schedule. *Proc Am Assoc Cancer Res* 1995;36:239. Abstract.
127. Cleveland JC Jr, Wollmering MM, Meldrum DR, et al. Ischemic preconditioning in human and rat ventricle. *Am J Physiol* 1996;271:H1786–H1794.
128. Jenkins DP, Pugsley WB, Alkhulaifi AM, et al. Ischaemic preconditioning reduces troponin T release in patients undergoing coronary artery bypass surgery. *Heart* 1997;77:314–318.
129. Perrault LP, Menasché P, Bel A, et al. Ischemic preconditioning in cardiac surgery: A word of caution. *J Thorac Cardiovasc Surg* 1996;112:1378–1386.
130. Billinger M, Fleisch M, Eberli FR, et al. Is the development of myocardial tolerance to repeated ischemia in humans due to preconditioning or to collateral recruitment? *J Am Coll Cardiol* 1999;33:1027–1035.
131. Shattock MJ, Lawson CS, Hearse DJ, et al. Electrophysiological characteristics of repetitive ischemic preconditioning in the pig heart. *J Mol Cell Cardiol* 1996;28:1339–1347.
132. Cohen MV, Yang X-M, Downey JM. Attenuation of ST segment elevation during repetitive coronary occlusions truly reflects the protection of ischemic preconditioning and is not an epiphenomenon. *Basic Res Cardiol* 1997;92:426–434.
133. Tomai F, Crea F, Gaspardone A, et al. Ischemic preconditioning during coronary angioplasty is prevented by glibenclamide, a selective ATP-sensitive K^+ channel blocker. *Circulation* 1994;90:700–705.
134. Tomai F, Crea F, Gaspardone A, et al. Effects of A_1 adenosine receptor blockade by bamiphylline on ischaemic preconditioning during coronary angioplasty. *Eur Heart J* 1996;17:846–853.
135. Kloner RA, Shook T, Przyklenk K, et al. Previous angina alters in-hospital outcome in TIMI 4: A clinical correlate to preconditioning? *Circulation* 1995;91:37–45.
136. Hirai T, Fujita M, Yamanishi K, et al. Significance of preinfarction angina for preservation of left ventricular function in acute myocardial infarction. *Am Heart J* 1992;124:19–24.
137. Ottani F, Galvani M, Ferrini D, et al. Prodromal angina limits infarct size: A role for ischemic preconditioning. *Circulation* 1995;91:291–297.
138. Nakagawa Y, Ito H, Kitakaze M, et al. Effect of angina pectoris on myocardial protection in patients with reperfused anterior wall myocardial infarction: Retrospective clinical evidence of "preconditioning." *J Am Coll Cardiol* 1995;25:1076–1083.
139. Kloner RA, Shook T, Antman EM, et al. Prospective temporal analysis of the onset of preinfarction angina versus outcome: An ancillary study in TIMI-9B. *Circulation* 1998;97:1042–1045.
140. Hirai T, Fujita M, Yoshida N, et al. Importance of ischemic preconditioning and collateral circulation for left ventricular functional recovery in patients with successful intracoronary thrombolysis for acute myocardial infarction. *Am Heart J* 1993;126:827–831.
141. Andreotti F, Pasceri V, Hackett DR, et al. Preinfarction angina as a predictor of more rapid coronary thrombolysis in patients with acute myocardial infarction. *New Engl J Med* 1996;334:7–12.
142. Abete P, Ferrara N, Cacciatore F, et al. Angina-induced protection against myocardial infarction in adult and elderly patients: A loss of preconditioning mechanism in the aging heart? *J Am Coll Cardiol* 1997;30:947–954.
143. Baxter GF, Marber MS, Patel VC, et al. Adenosine receptor involvement in a delayed phase of myocardial protection 24 hours after ischemic preconditioning. *Circulation* 1994;90:2993–3000.
144. Baxter GF, Goma FM, Yellon DM. Involvement of protein kinase C in the delayed cytoprotection following sublethal ischaemia in rabbit myocardium. *Br J Pharmacol* 1995;115:222–224.
145. Baxter GF, Goma FM, Yellon DM. Characterisation of the infarct-limiting effect of delayed preconditioning: Timecourse and dose-dependency studies in rabbit myocardium. *Basic Res Cardiol* 1997;92:159–167.
146. Hoshida S, Kuzuya T, Fuji H, et al. Sublethal ischemia alters myocardial antioxidant activity in canine heart. *Am J Physiol* 1993;264:H33–H39.
147. Marber MS, Mestril R, Chi S-H, et al. Overexpression of the rat inducible 70-kD heat stress protein in a transgenic mouse increases the resistance of the heart to ischemic injury. *J Clin Invest* 1995;95:1446–1456.

148. Bolli R, Bhatti ZA, Tang X-L, et al. Evidence that late preconditioning against myocardial stunning in conscious rabbits is triggered by the generation of nitric oxide. *Circ Res* 1997; 81:42–52.

149. Qiu Y, Tang X-L, Rizvi A, et al. Protein kinase C mediates late preconditioning against myocardial stunning in conscious rabbits. *Circulation* 1996;94(suppl I):I184. Abstract.

150. Qiu Y, Tang X-L, Park S-W, et al. The early and late phases of ischemic preconditioning: A comparative analysis of their effects on infarct size, myocardial stunning, and arrhythmias in conscious pigs undergoing a 40-min coronary occlusion. *Circ Res* 1997;80:730–742.

151. Cooley DA. Limited access myocardial revascularization: A preliminary report. *Tex Heart Inst J* 1996;23:81–84.

152. Dana A, Baxter GF, Walker JM, et al. Prolonging the delayed phase of myocardial protection: Repetitive adenosine A_1 receptor activation maintains rabbit myocardium in a preconditioned state. *J Am Coll Cardiol* 1998;31:1142–1149.

Part III

Vascular Biology and Cellular Physiology

Chapter 5

Experimental Models Useful in Evaluating Myocardial Viability*

James T. Willerson, MD
and H. Vernon Anderson, MD

Introduction

Thrombotic occlusion of a coronary artery, with subsequent acute myocardial infarction or sudden lethal arrhythmia, is the most common cause of death in western industrial countries. Experimental animal models with thrombotic occlusive disease in coronary arteries have been developed to simulate the clinical condition. These models may be used to develop methods for detecting viable and irreversibly injured myocardium with the expectation that these methods might be useful in humans for the same purposes. These animal models, used with and without lysis of thrombi after varying periods of coronary artery occlusion should be valuable for these purposes. Admittedly, there is not as yet any perfect model to simulate the human situation exactly, that is, an atherosclerotic plaque with an ulcerated endothelial surface or one of chronic myocardial ischemia. However, at least six different and useful models of arterial thrombosis or mechanical occlusion have been developed that should be useful in the development of methods to detect myocardial viability: (1) electrical injury, (2) copper coil, (3) Folts' (cyclic flow) model, (4) thrombin injection, (5) vessel eversion, and (6) temporary occlusion of a coronary artery for varying periods of time followed by reperfusion. Each of these models is described in this chapter.

Electrical Injury Model

In the early 1950s, Sawyer and Pate at the Naval Medical Research Institute noted that abnormal electrical potentials developed in aortic walls that suffered crush injury.[1,2] They found that the normal electrical potential difference across the wall of the aorta and its major branches was $-3--15$ mV, with the lumen being negative compared with the external adventitial surface. Crush injury reversed the electrical potential at the injury site,

---

* This chapter is modified from Anderson HV, Willerson JT. Experimental models of thrombosis. In: Loscalzo J, AI Schafer AI, eds. *Thrombosis and Hemorrhage*. Boston, Ma: Blackwell Scientific Publications; 1994:385–393.

From Dilsizian V (ed). *Myocardial Viability: A Clinical and Scientific Treatise*. Armonk, NY: Futura Publishing Co., Inc.; © 2000.

and the injured luminal surface rose to 2–5 mV. This injury and this new electrical potential were associated with thrombus development at the injured site. With these observations as background, Sawyer and Pate constructed a needle electrode, which they advanced through the walls of aortas and positioned in their lumens (Fig. 1). The exterior end of the electrode was connected to the positive pole of a 9-V battery. Small metal rings were placed around the aorta and connected through potentiometers to the negative battery pole. They could, thereby, simulate the effects of crush injury by establishing a positive electrical potential on the inner surface of an otherwise normal artery. This reverse electrical potential difference also caused thrombosis, if sufficient current was applied. The smallest current causing complete thrombosis of an aorta in their studies was 50 μA and required approximately 270 minutes (4½ hours). Histological examination indicated that the electrically induced thrombus was no different from that developing after crush injury. In 1961 Salazar described a modification of this technique that did not require surgery.[3] A catheter was introduced through the carotid artery of a dog and positioned under fluoroscopic guidance in the left coronary ostium. A wire electrode was advanced out of the tip of the catheter into one of the major coronary arteries. This wire, which extended from the catheter, was connected to the positive pole of a voltage source. The negative pole was connected through potentiometers to the chest wall. The coronary arterial lumen then could be made positive in charge compared with the adventitial surface. Currents of 200–300 μA for 2–3 hours were required to produce thrombosis. Currents <200 μA inconsistently produced thrombus, whereas currents >500 μA produced a burn injury of the endothelial surface. This catheter technique was used by several investigators for acute studies in anesthetized animals.[4]

In 1980, Romson et al[5] described a modification of the electrical injury model that has become the accepted technique for both acute and some chronic studies. In this experimental preparation (Fig. 2), a 25-gauge stainless steel hypodermic needle tip is inserted directly through the coronary arterial wall, such that the tip protrudes into the arterial lumen. Two or three shallow sutures in the epicardium secure the needle tip. A 28- or 30-gauge silver-coated copper wire with Teflon insulation is attached to the needle tip. The coronary artery just proximal to the needle tip insertion site is gently dissected free of surrounding epicardial tissue over several millimeters length. Either an electromagnetic or Doppler ultrasound flow probe is attached around this exposed artery proximal to the needle tip. Occasionally, a snare or clamp is placed around the coronary artery just distal to the needle tip to impede flow selectively through the vessel (Fig. 3). For acute studies, the needle tip wire is connected immediately to the positive pole of a 9-V battery by a potentiometer. The negative terminal of the battery is connected with a wire to any subcutaneous site. The potentiometer is adjusted to deliver 50–200 μA current. Blood flow in the artery is monitored continuously through the flow probe. Several variables related to thrombosis can be studied using this model: (1) documenting occurrence of thrombotic occlusion (flow signal of zero), (2) measuring elapsed time until occlusion, (3) documenting restoration of vessel patency (flow returns to preocclusion value), (4) documenting occurrence and time of vessel reocclusion, and (5) documenting cyclic declines and restorations of blood flow caused by repetitive accumulation and dislodgement of platelet aggregates (the so-called cyclic flow variations).[6,8–12] In general, rapidity of initial thrombus formation in this model is a function of two influences: first, the amount of electric current delivered and second, the degree of constriction by a clamp or snare. Higher currents and more tightly constricted arteries develop thrombus more quickly (approximately 30 minutes), while lower currents and less or no constriction require longer times, that is, often approximately 3–4 hours. The rationale for use of a clamp or snare is that it more closely mimics the human situation of a stenotic coronary artery with some stimulus to acute thrombosis.

One advantage of this model over others described later is that it also can be used for chronic studies.[6,8] After placing the flow probe, the needle electrode, and a constrictor (if this addition is desired) the wires can be exteriorized and connected to appropriate monitoring equipment. Animals then can have their chests closed and subsequently recover and be ambulatory. When the investigator is ready, the coronary artery electrode can be connected to a current course and thrombus initiated. Thus, acute coronary thrombosis in awake, unsedated animals can be modeled with this technique.

Copper Coil Model

In 1951, Stone and Lord[13] published an account of the superior thrombogenic effects of magnesium and magnesium-aluminum wire coils in dog aortas. In 1964, Blair and his colleagues[14] described a modification of Stone and Lord's technique that advanced the model into coronary arteries. Anesthetized dogs had their hearts exposed with thoracotomies. A short segment of the left anterior descending (LAD) coronary artery in each dog was gently dissected free from epicardial tissue. A spiral-shaped length of wire was inserted directly into the exposed LAD artery by twisting it in like a screw. The

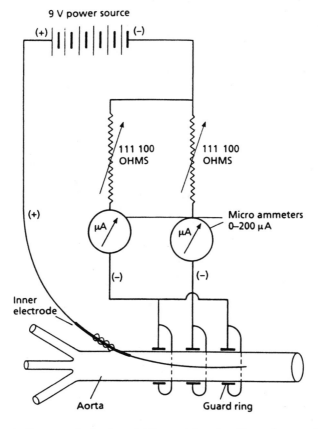

Figure 1. Schematic diagram of animal model for studying the effects of reversed electrical potentials on thrombus formation in aortas. Originally, this was developed as a model of crush injury. The needle electrode introduced into the lumen of the aorta, along with the metal rings surrounding a portion of the aorta, when connected to a 9-V battery made the lumen positive in charge compared with the adjacent wall. If sufficient current was delivered, thrombosis occurred. Reproduced with permission from Reference 1.

advantages of this technique are that no fluoroscopy equipment is required and occlusive thrombosis usually occurs gradually over 7–10 days. The gradual formation of thrombus is an advantage over current-induced coronary artery ligation models because it avoids the higher incidence of ventricular fibrillation that often accompanies acute ligation.

In 1972, Kordenat and colleagues[15] described another modification of the coil model, which, with minor adaptations, has become the standard technique. This method involves formation of small coils of wire around an 18-gauge needle. Magnesium and magnesium-aluminum were used originally, but subsequently these were replaced with copper wire. The wrapping of the coil can be varied to achieve different lengths of coil with selected numbers of turns (Fig. 4). The coil must be inserted under fluoroscopic guidance. A large-bore catheter is inserted into the animal through either the carotid or femoral artery. The catheter is directed to the ostium of the left coronary artery. A small inner catheter or a coronary guide wire then is advanced out of this larger catheter and manipulated into the desired coronary artery. The coil slides over this smaller wire into the artery. The catheters are subsequently removed. Another adaptation made has been to place a Doppler or electromagnetic flow probe on the proximal part of the coronary artery to monitor flow.

The copper coil model has been used extensively to evaluate thrombolytic agents.[16,17] Thrombus formation is rapid, and complete arterial occlusion usually occurs within 10–20 minutes. Thus, the copper coil model is used primarily for acute studies. A clamp or snare usually is not added to the artery because the coil alone is a powerful stimulus to thrombosis. Although the thickness of the wire creates some degree of stenosis of the lumen, this is not considered to be an important mechanism by which thrombosis is promoted. Similarly, the amount of local endothelial trauma caused by the presence of

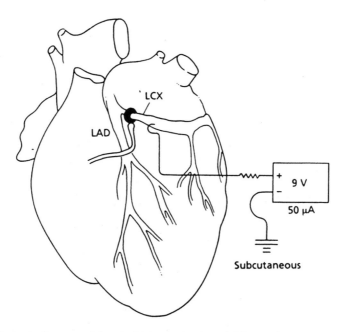

Figure 2. Schematic diagram of electrical injury animal model for producing acute coronary artery thrombosis. A 25-gauge stainless steel needle attached to a 28- or 30-gauge wire is inserted through the arterial wall into the lumen. The needle/wire is anchored with an epicardial suture. An electromagnetic or Doppler ultrasound flow probe is placed on the coronary artery proximal to the needle. The wire is connected to the positive terminal of a 9-V battery. The negative terminal of the battery is connected to any subcutaneous site. Abbreviations: LAD, left anterior descending artery; LCX, left circumflex artery. Reproduced with permission from Reference 6.

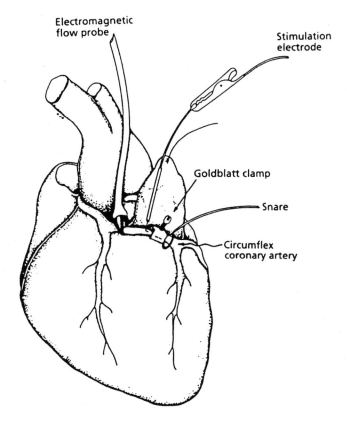

Electromagnetic
flow probe

Stimulation
electrode

Goldblatt clamp

Snare

Circumflex
coronary artery

Figure 3. Schematic diagram of one variation of electrical injury animal model for producing acute coronary artery thrombosis. In addition to a flow probe and an electrode, a clamp and a snare are added distally. The snare can be used to occlude blood flow transiently, thereby hastening development of thrombus at the needle tip electrode. The clamp can be used to add a fixed stenosis to the artery, thereby mimicking more closely the usual human coronary situation. Reproduced with permission from Reference 7.

the coil is not considered a major stimulus for thrombosis. Rather, the existence of a relatively large area of positive charges on the metallic coil surface apparently is the mechanism by which platelets, fibrin, and other blood elements are attracted and adhere. Turbulence and stasis of blood flow in the deep interstices between the coil windings is another mechanism promoting thrombosis.

Folts' (Cyclic Flow) Model

In 1976, Folts and colleagues[18] made the important observation that repetitive cycles of blood flow reduction, followed by sudden restorations to full flow, occur in partially obstructed canine coronary arteries injured by squeezing or pinching. These cycles (Fig. 5) were presumed to be caused by the repetitive accumulation and dislodgement of platelet aggregates at the site of an arterial stenosis with endothelial injury. Subsequent research has shown that this indeed is the process generating cyclic flow reductions.[19,20] The exact rheological conditions required to produce cyclic flows involve both the turbulence and the stasis produced by partial arterial constriction of significant length (approximately 3 mm), along with exposure of subendothelial elements by arterial injury at or near the constricted region. The model is created by exposing the heart and gently dissecting free from surrounding tissue a segment of one major coronary artery. Either an electromagnetic or Doppler flow probe is placed on the proximal portion of the exposed artery. Cushioned forceps are used to pinch the artery distal to the flow probe. A hard, plastic disk with a center hole and slit is used to provide external constriction. The central holes of the disks should be made in various diameters. Variation in size between individual arteries requires the experimenter to try first one and then another constrictor until the proper hole size is found that reduces flow appropriately. Other approaches to achieve appropriate partial constriction involve positioning either a length of tapered nylon fishing line or an angioplasty catheter balloon between a loose plastic collar and the external arterial surface. The plastic collar provides support while the tapered nylon line is manipulated backward or forward and then fixed when the experimenter achieves the desired degree of partial occlusion. With the other system, the angioplasty balloon is inflated partially and externally compresses the artery in order to achieve the desired partial occlusion effect.[19]

More recently, the Folts' model has been extended to a chronic, awake, and unsedated canine preparation.[20,21] With properly applied vascular injury, cyclic flows develop immediately after injury but then fade away. Animals are allowed to recover and are returned to their housing. Several days later (ie, 2–3 days) cyclic flows usually return but can be prevented by chronic administration of selected antiplatelet agents. This new model offers some additional insights into chronic influences of platelets and platelet aggregates on injured arterial walls. In particular, platelets adhering to arterial walls at sites of injury are known to release various mediators that play a role in thrombosis, dynamic vasoconstriction, and proliferation of medial smooth muscle cells, which occurs after angioplasty, and is thought to be the basis for restenosis. Prevention of cyclic flows in dogs

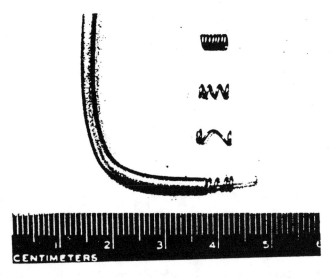

Figure 4. Photograph of copper coils and other items used to produce acute coronary thrombosis in dogs. The coils can be made with various numbers of turns of wire. A large guiding catheter contains both a coil and a small central tube or guide wire. The large guiding catheter is positioned under fluoroscopic guidance in the coronary ostium, and then the smaller guide wire is directed out of the larger catheter into the desired coronary artery. Finally, the coil slides into the coronary artery over the guide wire and lodges at the level where the outer diameter of the coil equals the inner diameter of the artery. The smaller guide wire and larger catheter then are removed. Reproduced with permission from Reference 15.

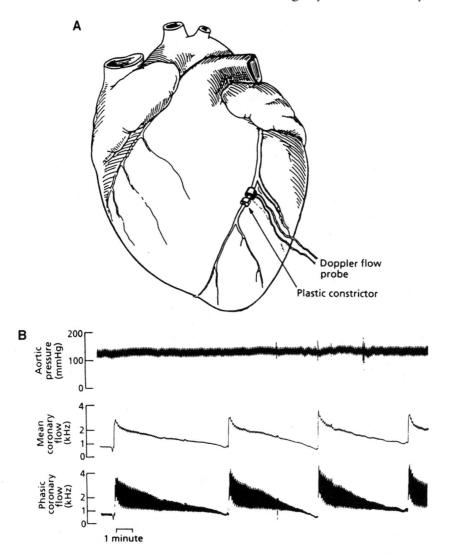

Figure 5. (**A**) Schematic diagram of the Folts' model for producing coronary artery cyclic flow variations. The midportion of a large epicardial coronary artery is injured by pinching or squeezing. A plastic constrictor that reduces but does not occlude coronary blood flow is placed onto the artery at the injured zone. (**B**) Representative tracings from a Folts' model in a canine coronary artery. The upper tracing is aortic pressure. The middle tracing is mean coronary flow velocity from the Doppler ultrasound flow probe. The lower tracing is phasic coronary flow velocity from the same probe. These cycles of gradual declines in coronary blood flow over several minutes followed by sudden restorations of flow are caused by repetitive accumulation and dislodgement of platelet aggregates at sites of coronary artery stenosis with endothelial injury. Reproduced with permission from Reference 41.

in the days after coronary arterial injury correlates with reduction in the degree of neointimal proliferation.[22] However, this chronic cyclic flow model also may be very limited for studies of acute thrombosis. Another variation in this model is the use of transluminal balloon dilatation angioplasty at the coronary arterial site just distal to the flow probe. Angioplasty injures the arterial wall from the inside, mimicking the human situation, and then replacement of a plastic constrictor at the injured arterial site provides a residual stenosis. Cyclic flows develop in this model just as with the external forceps injury method, and histologically the arterial wall response appears to be similar.[22]

The cyclic flows in the Folts' model and its variants are caused by periodic accumulations and dislodgements of platelet aggregates and dynamic vasoconstriction at the injured and stenotic site. If not dislodged manually, occasionally the flow will remain at zero and not be restored. Therefore, shaking the platelet plug loose is sometimes required. Once they have developed, cyclic flows usually will continue undiminished for at least 3 hours.

Thrombin Injection Model

Gold and Collen modified a venous thrombosis technique to include coronary arterial and femoral arterial applications.[23–25] A segment of LAD coronary artery, including a side branch, is gently dissected free from surrounding tissue (Fig. 2). An electromagnetic or Doppler flow probe is placed on the artery proximal to the side branch. A variable constrictor is placed on the distal portion of the exposed segment. The side branch is cannulated with a small-bore plastic tube attached to a needle. The exposed segment of artery is injured by pinching it with forceps. Snares then are placed to isolate the entire exposed segment temporarily and occlude flow. Using the cannulated side branch, a mixture of whole blood and thrombin (10 U) is injected into the injured and static segment of artery. After approximately 5 minutes of occlusion the proximal snare is released, and approximately 2 minutes later, the distal snare is released. This leaves an injured and stenotic coronary artery with occlusive thrombus present. The effects of various agents on restoration of flow can be studied. The flow probe provides continuous monitoring of blood flow status.

Everted Segment Model

Gold and his colleagues have developed yet another model of arterial thrombosis.[23–26] This model relies on an arterial stenosis to reduce flow, along with exposure to the blood stream of subendothelial (nonendothelial) tissues (Fig. 3). The heart is exposed by thoracotomy. A segment of the left circumflex coronary artery is gently dissected free from surrounding tissue. An electromagnetic or Doppler ultrasound flow probe is placed around the proximal portion of the exposed segment. A plastic snare is placed around the distal portion of the exposed segment to create partial obstruction. A 1-cm section of artery between the flow probe and constrictor then is isolated with microvascular clamps, excised, everted inside out, and then reattached in position using 7–0 nylon sutures. The microvascular clamps then are removed. This procedure places the adventitial surface of the everted section into contact with blood flowing through the artery. The combination of reduced blood flow due to the constrictor, along with an abnormal nonendothelial surface, creates total thrombotic occlusion within approximately 5 minutes.

Transient Occlusion of Coronary Artery

An additional experimental model used to study myocardial ischemia/infarction and of potential use in evaluating myocardial viability is a model of transient coronary artery occlusion followed by reperfusion with the coronary artery occlusion provided by a reversible snare occluder placed proximally or more distally on a coronary artery. The occluding device often is a snare occluder placed around a portion of a coronary artery that has been carefully dissected away from surrounding tissue. The occluder can be tightened down and the artery occluded for periods of several minutes to several hours and then the occlusion released allowing reperfusion. This reversible occlusion can be used in acute or chronic models allowing one to study the effects of acute ischemia/infarction in awake, unsedated animals and the insult of acute occlusion and reperfusion in the days or weeks after the occlusive event.[27–29] When the coronary artery occlusion is maintained for more than 30–40 minutes prior to reperfusion, the reperfused myocardium contains a variable mixture of ischemic but viable and irreversibly injured myocardium. One may study the effects of acute and chronic ischemia on regional ventricular function and contractile reserve using ultrasonic crystals placed in multiple segments of the left ventricle (LV) to "ma" segmental wall thickening (WT) or subendocardial length changes correlating the functional observations with other evaluations of myocardial viability.[27–29]

Histological Detection of Irreversibly Injured Myocardium

Irreversibly injured myocardium can be detected using triphenyltetrazolium chloride (TTC) staining. Viable myocardium stains brick red with this stain and irreversibly injured myocardium fails to take up the TTC. Light and electron microscopy can be used to confirm the presence of irreversibly injured myocardium.

Coronary Artery Occlusion by Thrombosis

The five experimental models of arterial thrombosis that are described here all have a number of similar features. They all utilize an electromagnetic or Doppler ultrasound flow probe to provide continuous monitoring of flow within the subject artery. Basically, they all are acute models requiring open thoracotomy and monitoring of continuously anesthetized animals. Although the electrical injury model can be closed and the animals allowed to recover, with thrombosis created at a later desired time in awake and unsedated animals, it is not clear that this would have any substantial differences for studies dealing with the phenomena of acute thrombosis and thrombolysis. Similarly, the Folts' model can be closed and the animals allowed to recover. This permits chronic monitoring of coronary flow in awake, unsedated animals with coronary stenosis and endothelial injury and a chronic model of the effects of platelets and platelet products at sites of endothelial injury and stenosis. This model also allows both acute and chronic therapies to be evaluated.

The major differences among the five models relates to the character of the occluding thrombus that forms. Because thrombosis is an interaction between aggregating platelets and fibrin formed from the coagulation cascade, these elements appear to develop in relative proportions. Thus, some models produce relatively platelet-rich thrombi, while others produce relatively fibrin-rich thrombi. The Folts' model probably is the most platelet-rich thrombus model of the group, while the thrombin injection and copper coil models probably are the most fibrin-rich. The other two models (electrical injury and everted vessel segment) appear to be intermediate in platelet-rich and fibrin-rich compositions. Because thrombolytic agents achieve their effects by activating the enzyme plasminogen and thereby lysing strands of fibrin, these agents are highly effective in fibrin-rich models but less effective in platelet-rich models. For example, in one study[30] using both the relatively platelet-rich electrical injury model and the relatively fibrin-rich copper coil model, the fibrinolytic agent, recombinant tissue-type plasminogen activator (rt-PA) was given to both groups of animals. Successful reperfusion was achieve in 100% (18 of 18) of the copper coil arteries (fibrin-rich), but in only 79% (19 of 24) of the electrically injured ones (platelet-rich). Agents that interfere with platelet function, such as thromboxane receptor antagonists,[31] serotonin receptor antagonists,[32] glycoprotein IIb-IIIa receptor antagonists,[33] and others, are more effective in platelet-rich models but less effective in fibrin-rich models. It also has been demonstrated that reocclusion after successful thrombolysis, in all models, usually is preceded by a period of cyclic flow variations, which appear to be predominantly a platelet-mediated process.[21,22,25] Histological studies of reoccluding thrombus have confirmed their platelet-rich composition.[26,34] Antiplatelet agents, when added to thrombolytic agents, attenuate or eliminate these cyclic flows and prevent or delay reocclusion.[25,26,31,32]

Another important factor is thrombus age. Platelet-rich thrombi, which often are present early in thrombus formation and growth, gradually accumulate more fibrin as the coagulation process becomes activated and progresses.[35] Thus, what begins as a platelet-rich thrombus, perhaps at that phase more sensitive to antiplatelet agents but less sensitive to fibrinolytic agents, gradually may shift its responsiveness as its character changes. Furthermore, fibrin-rich thrombi also change as they age as factor XIII–dependent cross-linkages form between recently deposited fibrin strands.[36] In one study, using a copper coil (fibrin-rich) model of canine coronary thrombosis, significant differences were found in thrombolysis related to thrombus age.[37] In dogs with occlusive thrombi present for 30 minutes prior to treatment with rt-PA, 5 of 6 (83%) could be reperfused successfully. However, when occlusive thrombi were present for 180 minutes prior to treatment, only 1 of 7 (15%; $p < 0.05$) could be reperfused. Addition of heparin to rt-PA equalized the ability successfully to lyse thrombi—5 of 7 for 30-minute thrombi compared with 4 of 7 for 180-minute thrombi. However, there was still a significant delay in time to successful reperfusion using rt-PA and heparin—15 ± 3 minutes for 30-minute thrombi compared with 38 ± 5 minutes for 180-minute thrombi ($p < 0.01$). In another study, using the Folts' model (platelet-rich), there also were time-related differences.[38] When cyclic flow variations had been established in canine coronary arteries for only 30 minutes, either heparin or a specific thrombin antagonist (MCI-9038) was equally effective in abolishing them (12 of 18 = 66% versus 5 of 7 = 71%). However, when the cyclic flows had been established for 180 minutes before treatment, 0 of 7 dogs treated with heparin and only 1 of 7 dogs treated with MCI-9038 had these cyclic flows abolished.

These animal models have highlighted the complex and important interactions that occur between platelet activation and the coagulation pathways. Arterial thrombosis begins with the deposition, activation, and aggregation of platelets. Platelet aggregates serve as substrates to initiate and accelerate thrombin activation, ultimately producing fibrin. Although thrombolysis can degrade the fibrin meshwork of a clot, platelets and platelet aggregates, if left uninhibited, remain active and activate more platelets, interfere with the fibrinolytic state, and cause rethrombosis.[39,40] Appreciation of this phenomenon in recent years has led to an explosion of combination therapies directed both at thrombolytic as well as antiplatelet activities. These experimental models used with appropriate inhibitors of thrombosis should allow the further development of imaging techniques and possibly other interventions capable of detecting viable and irreversibly injured myocardium.

References

1. Sawyer PN, Pate JW. Bioelectric phenomena as an etiologic factor in intravascular thrombosis. *Am J Physiol* 1953;175:103–107.
2. Sawyer PN, Pate JW, Weldon CS. Relations of abnormal and injury electric potential differences to intravascular thrombosis. *Am J Physiol* 1953;175:108–112.

3. Salazar AE. Experimental myocardial infarction: Induction of coronary thrombosis in the intact closed-chest dog. *Circ Res* 1961;9:1351–1356.

4. Moschos CB, Lahiri K, Lyons M, et al. Relation of microcirculatory thrombosis to thrombus in the proximal coronary artery: Effect of aspirin, dipyridamole, and thrombolysis. *Am Heart J* 1973;86:61–68.

5. Romson JL, Haack DW, Lucchesi BR. Electrical induction of coronary artery thrombosis in the ambulatory canine: A model for in vivo evaluation of anti-thrombotic agents. *Thromb Res* 1980;17:841–853.

6. Shea MJ, Driscoll EM, Romson JL, et al. The beneficial effects of nafazatrom (BAYg6575) on experimental coronary thrombosis. *Am Heart J* 1984;107:629–637.

7. Bush LR, Shebuski RJ. In vivo models of arterial thrombosis and thrombolysis. *FASEB J* 1990;4:3087.

8. Schumacher WA, Lee EC, Lucchesi BR. Augmentation of streptokinase-induced thrombolysis by heparin and prostacyclin. *J Cardiovasc Pharmacol* 1985;7:739–746.

9. Fitzgerald DJ, Fitzgerald GA. Role of thrombin and thromboxane A_2 in reocclusion following coronary thrombolysis with tissue-type plasminogen activator. *Proc Natl Acad Sci U S A* 1989;86:7585–7589.

10. Mickelson JK, Simpson PJ, Cronin M, et al. Antiplatelet antibody [7E3 F(ab')2] prevents rethrombosis after recombinant tissue-type plasminogen activator-induced coronary artery thrombolysis in a canine model. *Circulation* 1990;81:617–627.

11. Jackson CV, Crowe VG, Craft TJ, et al. Thrombolytic activity of a novel plasminogen activator, LY 210825, compared with recombinant tissue-type plasminogen activator in a canine model of coronary artery thrombosis. *Circulation* 1990;82:930–940.

12. Shebuski RJ, Stabilito IJ, Sitko GR, et al. Acceleration of recombinant tissue-type plasminogen activator-induced thrombolysis and prevention of reocclusion by the combination of heparin and a Arg-Gly-Asp-containing peptide bitistatin in a canine model of coronary thrombosis. *Circulation* 1990;82:169–177.

13. Stone P, Lord JW. An experimental study of thrombogenic properties on magnesium and magnesium-aluminum wire in the dog's aorta. *Surgery* 1951;30:987–993.

14. Blair E, Nygren E, Cowley RA. A spiral wire technique for producing gradually occlusive coronary thrombosis. *J Thorac Cardiovasc Surg* 1964;48:476–485.

15. Kordenat RK, Kezdi T, Stanley EL. A new catheter technique for producing experimental coronary thrombosis and selective coronary visualization. *Am Heart J* 1972;83:360–364.

16. Bergmann SR, Fox KAA, Ter-Pogossian MM, et al. Clot-selective coronary thrombolysis with tissue-type plasminogen activator. *Science* 1983;220:1181–1183.

17. Cercek B, Lew AS, Hod H, et al. Enhancement of thrombolysis with tissue-type plasminogen activator by pre-treatment with heparin. *Circulation* 1986;74:583–587.

18. Folts JD, Crowell EB, Rowe GG. Platelet aggregation in partially obstructed vessels and its elimination with aspirin. *Circulation* 1976;54:365–370.

19. Folts JD. An in vivo model of experimental arterial stenosis, intimal damage, and periodic thrombosis. *Circulation* 1991;83(suppl IV):3–14.

20. Willerson JT, Golino P, Eidt J, et al. Specific platelet mediators and unstable coronary artery lesions. *Circulation* 1989;80:198–205.

21. Anderson HV, Yao SK, Murphree SS, et al. Cyclic coronary artery flow in dogs after coronary angioplasty. *Coron Artery Dis* 1990;1:717–723.

22. Willerson JT, McNatt J, Yao SK, et al. Frequency and severity of cyclic flow alterations and platelet aggregation predict the severity of neointimal proliferation following experimental coronary stenosis and endothelial injury. *Proc Natl Acad Sci U S A* 1991;88:10624–10627.

23. Flameng W, Vanhaecke J, Stump DC, et al. Coronary thrombolysis by intravenous infusion of recombinant single chain urokinase-type plasminogen activator or recombinant urokinase in baboons: Effect on regional on blood flow, infarct size and hemostasis. *J Am Coll Cardiol* 1986;8:118–124.

24. Yasuda T, Gold HK, Fallon JT, et al. A canine model of coronary artery thrombosis with superimposed high grade stenosis for the investigation of rethrombosis after thrombolysis. *J Am Coll Cardiol* 1989;13:1409–1414.

25. Gold HK, Yasuda T, Jang IK, et al. Animal models for arterial thrombolysis and prevention of reocclusion. *Circulation* 1991;83(suppl IV):26–40.

26. Jang IK, Gold HK, Ziskind AA, et al. Differential sensitivity of erythrocyte-rich and platelet-rich arterial thrombi to lysis with recombinant tissue-type plasminogen activator. *Circulation* 1989;79:920–928.

27. Sasayama S, Franklin D, Ross J Jr, et al. Dynamic changes in left ventricular wall thickness and their use in analyzing cardiac function in the conscious dog. *Am J Cardiol* 1976;38:870–879.

28. Roan PG, Scales F, Saffer S, et al. Functional characterization of left ventricular segmental responses during the initial 24H and 1WK after experimental canine myocardial infarction. *J Clin Invest* 1979;63:1074–1088.

29. Bush LR, Buja LM, Samowitz W, et al. Recovery of left ventricular segmental function after long-term reperfusion following temporary coronary occlusion in conscious dogs. Comparison of 2- and 4-hour occlusions. *Circ Res* 1983;53:248–263.

30. Haskel EJ, Adams SP, Feigen LP, et al. Prevention of reoccluding platelet-rich thrombi in canine femoral arteries with a novel peptide antagonist of platelet glycoprotein IIb/IIIa receptors. *Circulation* 1989;80:1775–1782.

31. Ashton JH, Ogletree ML, Michel IM, et al. Cooperative mediation by serotonin S$_2$ and thromboxane A$_2$ prostaglandin H$_2$ receptor activation of cyclic flow variations in dogs with severe coronary artery stenoses. *Circulation* 1987:952–959.

32. Golino P, Buja LM, Ashton JH, et al. Effect of thromboxane and serotonin receptor antagonists on intracoronary platelet deposition in dogs with experimentally stenosed coronary arteries. *Circulation* 1988;78:701–711.

33. Yasuda T, Gold HK, Leinbach RC, et al. Lysis of plasminogen activator-resistant platelet-rich coronary artery thrombus with combined bolus injection of recombinant tissue-type plasminogen activator and antiplatelet GP IIb/IIIa antibody. *J Am Coll Cardiol* 1990;16:1728–1735.

34. Gold HK, Leinbach RC. Strategy of thrombolytic therapy. In: Haber E, Braunwald E, eds. *Thrombolysis: Basic Contributions and Clinical Progress.* St. Louis, Mo: Mosby-Year Book; 1991:207–223.

35. Coller BS. Role of platelets in thrombolytic therapy. In: Haber E, Braunwald E, eds. *Thrombolysis: Basic Contributions and Clinical Progress.* St. Louis, Mo: Mosby-Year Book; 1991:155–178.

36. Verstraete M. Biology and chemistry of thrombosis. In: Haber E, Braunwald E, eds. *Thrombolysis: Basic Contributions and Clinical Progress.* St. Louis, Mo: Mosby-Year Book; 1991:13–16.

37. Yao SK, McNatt J, Anderson HV, et al. Thrombin inhibition enhances recombinant tissue-type plasminogen activator-induced thrombolysis and delays reocclusion. *Am J Physiol* 1992;262:H374–H379.

38. Eidt J, Allison P, Noble S, et al. Thrombin is an important mediator of platelet aggregation in stenosed canine coronary arteries with endothelial injury. *J Clin Invest* 1989;84:18–27.

39. Coller BS. Platelets and thrombolytic therapy. *N Engl J Med* 1990;322:33–42.

40. Fujii S, Abendschein DR, Sobel BE. Augmentation of plasminogen activator inhibitor type 1 activity in plasma by thrombosis and thrombolysis. *J Am Coll Cardiol* 1991;18:1547–1554.

41. Anderson HV, Willerson JT. Experimental models of thrombosis. In: Loscalzo J, AI Schafer AI, eds. *Thrombosis and Hemorrhage.* Boston, Ma: Blackwell Scientific Publications; 1994:385–393.

Chapter 6

Essential Fuels for the Heart and Mechanical Restitution

Heinrich Taegtmeyer, MD, DPhil,
and Raymond R. Russell III, MD, PhD

Introduction

Intermediary metabolism of energy-providing substrates in the heart has the dubious reputation of extraordinary complexity. However, the central hypothesis is quite simple. It states that the sum of metabolic pathways is more than the sum of the individual enzyme-catalyzed steps. In heart muscle this hypothesis is best illustrated by the convergence of energy transfer on adenosine triphosphate (ATP).[1] In the course of 1 day the human heart produces and uses 5 kg of ATP, which is more than 10 times its own weight.[2]

The hypothesis also seems to be reflected in the term "energy charge" in studies of myocardial energetics, which has been defined by Atkinson as

$$\text{energy charge} = \frac{[\text{ATP}] + \frac{1}{2}[\text{ADP}]}{[\text{ATP}] + [\text{ADP}] + [\text{AMP}]}.$$

Energy charge is a linear measure of the metabolic energy stored in the adenine nucleotide system.[3] According to Atkinson a "system is fully charged when all the adenylate is converted to ATP and fully discharged when only AMP is present." Over the years much work on myocardial energy metabolism has centered on implicating changes in energy charge as a cause of contractile dysfunction.[4-6] However, the term energy charge (and the static measurements it entails) has to be distinguished from the free energy change of ATP hydrolysis. A decrease in the free energy change of ATP hydrolysis, rather than a fall in the absolute amount of ATP, is considered one of the main causes of contractile failure in anoxic myocardium.[7]

The interactions of myocardial metabolism and contractile function are still incompletely understood.[8] Although it is well known that in isolated mitochondria respiration is driven by the concentration of adenosine diphosphate (ADP),[9] such a control has yet to be established in the organ as a whole. In working hearts subjected to dynamic changes in workload and O_2 consumption, the estimated cytosolic ADP concentration, as measured by ^{31}P nuclear magnetic resonance (NMR) spectroscopy, does not show any change over

The authors' work was supported in part by National Institutes of Health grants RO1–43133 (HT) and 5T32DK07058–20 (RR).

From Dilsizian V (ed). *Myocardial Viability: A Clinical and Scientific Treatise.* Armonk, NY: Futura Publishing Co., Inc.; © 2000.

a wide range of cardiac power.[10–15] Other investigators have proposed that respiration is controlled by either the intramitochondrial redox state[16] or intramitochondrial free $[Ca^{2+}]$.[17] Neither hypothesis can be tested in the intact heart with methods currently available. In light of these difficulties it is reasonable to explore the regulation of cardiac energy metabolism from a new and less worn perspective.

Four Principles

Our understanding of the control of regulation of cardiac metabolism is guided by four principles (Table 1).

The first principle describes energy metabolism as a system in flux[18] and defines the heart as both a consumer and a provider of energy.[2] The heart consumes energy through the regulated combustion of substrates and captures energy for a fleeting moment in the form of ATP and/or phosphocreatine. ATP is hydrolyzed by the contractile apparatus, by ion pumps, and by enzymes of biosynthetic pathways. The result of normal contractile function in the heart is the provision of substrates and oxygen to the rest of the body. The rate of ATP production (5 kg of ATP per day in the human heart, see previous text) exceeds the amount of ATP in the heart by several orders of magnitude.[2] Because of the enormous energy requirements of the heart and the comparatively small stores of ATP, it is not surprising to find the heart to be a sensitive indicator of energy transfer. Specifically, impaired flux through metabolic pathways rapidly results in impaired contractile function of the heart.

The second principle arises from the first principle and defines the heart as an organ that responds to changes in workload with changes in the rate of substrate utilization. An acute increase in workload results in enhanced breakdown of the endogenous substrates glycogen and triglycerides. Figure 1 shows that rates of glucose uptake do not change in an isolated working rat heart when the workload of the heart is double [Fig. 1(A)]. Instead, the increased energy requirement is met by utilization of glycogen and triglycerides [Fig. 1(B)]. With glucose as the only exogenous substrate in this experiment (Fig. 1) the increase in energy demand must necessarily be supplied by utilization of endogenous reserves. The in vitro findings in perfused rat heart correspond to similar observations in dog heart obtained by ^{13}C-NMR spectroscopy in vivo.[19] A decrease in workload to a subphysiological level results in a decrease in substrate uptake, which can be tracked by the glucose tracer analog $[^{18}F]$2-deoxy-2-fluoro-D-glucose.[20]

The third principle defines the heart as a metabolic omnivore.[21] Like the human body, the heart derives energy from the oxidation of different substrates. Work spanning almost the entire length of this century and culminating in measurements of arteriovenous (coronary sinus) differences of substrates and metabolites across the heart has established that heart muscle oxidizes glucose and lactate, fatty acids, ketone bodies, and even certain amino acids. The driving forces of fuel selection in vivo are relatively simple: As the physiological state of the body changes, so change the various substrates in the blood and with it the preferred substrate for respiration. The exception to this rule is the preferential oxidation of glycogen on acute adrenergic stimulation of the heart.[22]

Table 1
Control and Regulation of Cardiac Metabolism: Four Principles

1. The heart is consumer and provider of energy.
2. All is in flux: Changes in workload cause changes in the rate of substrate utilization.
3. Heart muscle is considered an omnivore.
4. Efficient energy transfer occurs through a series of moiety-conserved cycles.

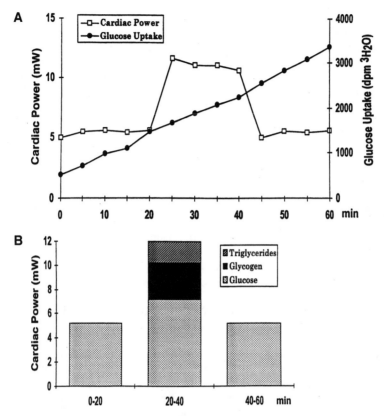

Figure 1. (**A**) Glucose uptake and work job; effects of an acute increase in workload on cardiac power and glucose uptake shown by a representative experiment of an isolated working rate heart perfused at low (1–20 minutes and 40–60 minutes) and high (20–40 minutes) workload with Krebs Henseleit buffers and glucose (10 mmol/L) as the only substrate. Glucose uptake was measured by the release of ^3H_2O from $[2\text{-}^3H]$-glucose. Cardiac power ($\square$) was calculated from cardiac output and mean aortic pressure. (**B**) Shows the relative contribution of exogenous (glucose) and endogenous (glycogen and triglycerides) substrates to energy production. Cardiac power was calculated from the caloric equivalent of glucose oxidation. Hearts ($n = 4$) from fed rats were perfused with Krebs Henseleit buffer containing glucose (10 mmol/L) and freeze-clamped at 20, 40, and 60 minutes, for measurement of glycogen and triglycerides. Statistical data are omitted for clarity.

A metabolic "hierarchy" in the isolated, substrate-controlled, perfused heart was established when Randle and his coworkers observed that fatty acid utilization suppresses glucose oxidation.[23] Randle described a blood phase and a cellular phase of a "glucose-fatty acid cycle," drawing attention to the turnover of triglycerides on the one hand and to the inhibition of glucose oxidation by fatty acids on the other hand. The importance of these seminal observations for the control of fuel homeostasis was recognized immediately and resulted in a productive era in cardiac metabolism. Much of the work that followed concentrated on defining the regulatory sites in metabolic pathways and on exploring their operational control.[24,25]

Although the concept of the glucose-fatty acid cycle has never been questioned seriously, subsequent work by Randle[26] and by others[27–29] suggested that the suppression of glucose utilization by fatty acids may not be as exclusive or as complete as originally proposed. Nearly 30 years ago Randle and his coworkers also suggested that fatty acids inhibit glucose oxidation more than glycolysis and glycolysis more than glucose uptake. Glucose utilization is regulated on several levels by fatty acid utilization. Fatty acid oxidation results in increases in both the acetylated form of coenzyme A (acetyl-CoA) and citrate, which inhibit pyruvate dehydrogenase and phosphofructokinase, respectively.

Fifteen years ago we found that glucose also partially inhibits the oxidation of long-chain fatty acids.[29] The inhibition of fatty acid oxidation through malonyl-CoA and its inhibitory effect on carnitine palmitoyl transferase has been defined on a molecular basis.[30] The key regulatory step appears to be carboxylation of acetyl-CoA through acetyl-CoA carboxylase,[31] which, in turn, is regulated by an adenosine monophosphate (AMP)-dependent protein kinase.[32] These findings emphasize the principle that substrate preference will change with substrate supply.

In this context it is of interest that under extreme conditions (ie, when lactate levels in the plasma rise to very high values with strenuous exercise) lactate replaces all the other fuels for respiration.[33,34] These in vivo observations are supported by observations in isolated working hearts in vitro: Glucose or lactate can support the full work output of an isolated working rat heart. By contrast, with ketone bodies as the only substrate contractile performance rapidly declines.[29]

The reason for a substrate effect on contractile function in the heart becomes obvious in the fourth principle, which defines efficient energy transfer through moiety-conserved cycles. This principle is based on three simple observations: (1) metabolic pathways are for the most part not linear, (2) products are recycled, and, (3) cycles provide greater efficiency than linear pathways.

The importance of moiety-conserved cycles is understood easily by comparing the energy expenditure of a runner and of a cyclist. To cover the same distance in the same amount of time, the cyclist uses less than one-third of the energy used by the runner.[35] The only difference between running and riding a bicycle is, of course, the interposition of two wheels or two moiety-conserved cycles. Just as the interposition of cycles confers a mechanical advantage to the runner, so do cycles offer a biochemical advantage to metabolism.

Cycling and recycling also is a general biological principle that functions at many levels. Table 2 shows a partial listing of moiety-conserved cycles in the cardiovascular system, starting with the body as a whole and ending with intracellular signaling pathways. Four examples are discussed in support of the general hypothesis that moiety-conserved cycles improve the efficiency of energy transfer.

The most obvious example of a moiety-conserved cycle is the circulation of blood. Blood picks up O_2 and eliminates CO_2, but changes in the moiety (ie, red blood cells) are, by comparison to metabolic processes, infinitely slow. However, acute blood loss requires acute replenishment of blood to secure the survival of the whole organism. Another

---

Table 2

Examples of Moiety-Conserved Cycles in the Cardiovascular System

1. Circulation
2. Actin-myosin cross-bridges
3. Ca^{2+} release and reuptake
4. Adenosine triphosphate-adenosine diphosphate (ATP-ADP), phosphocreatine-creatine
5. Citric acid cycle
6. Phosphorylation/dephosphorylation of enzymes
7. Coenzyme A (CoA)
8. Oxidized nicotinamide-adenine dinucleotide (NAD^+/NADH), oxidized flavin adenimine dinucleotide (FAD^+/FADH)
9. H^+ gradient
10. Glucose transporters
11. Carnitine palmitoyl transferase
12. Second messengers [cyclic adenosine monophosphate (cAMP) and cyclic guanosine monophosphate (GMP)]
13. Signal transduction pathways (G-proteins, etc.)

example is the attachment and detachment of the actin and myosin filaments in the process of cross-bridge cycling.[36] A third example is hydrolysis and resynthesis of ATP. Finally, there is a series of interconnected cycles of substrate metabolism, beginning with the cycling of CoA between its free (CoASH) and acetylated (acetyl-CoA) form, continuing with the citric acid cycle, and the capture of reducing equivalents through the cycling of oxidized nicotinamide-adenine dinucleotide (NAD^+) to the reduced form of NAD^+ (NADH) and the buildup and collapse of the proton gradient, and ending with ATP synthesis from ADP and inorganic phosphate (P_i) in the respiratory chain. ADP arises from hydrolysis of ATP in the contractile process mentioned and brings together a mechanical cycle (cross-bridge formation) and a chemical cycle.

Depletion of the Citric Acid Cycle

The cycle of all cycles in the interconnected network of energy transfer within the myocardial cell is, of course, the citric acid cycle, discovered more than 60 years ago by Krebs and Johnson.[37] The evolutionary advantage of the citric acid cycle is that the reaction sequences of the cycle make efficient use of substrates.[38] It has always been assumed that the citric acid cycle responds directly to the energy needs of the cell and that the quality of the substrate does not affect flux through the cycle, because the vast majority of substrates are converted to acetyl-CoA before entering the cycle.

With this background, we determined the rate-limiting steps of the citric acid cycle in an organ with a high rate of energy turnover, and we perfused the isolated working rat heart at a high workload with ketone bodies as the only substrate. We chose ketone bodies because they are the least regulated of all oxidizable substrates in the heart and have direct access to the mitochondrial matrix (Fig. 2). Ketone bodies also do not undergo β-oxidation and are not substrates for triglyceride synthesis. In the mitochondrial matrix ketone bodies also are converted to acetyl-CoA by a process that is less regulated than the conversion of fatty acids to acetyl-CoA.

Unexpectedly, in a system imposing a physiological workload on the heart, cardiac contractile function declines rapidly during ketone body oxidation.[29] Function returns

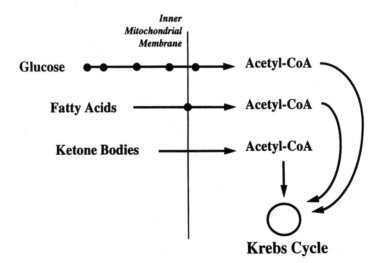

Figure 2. Metabolic scheme highlighting the major regulatory sites (●) in the metabolism of glucose, fatty acids, and ketone bodies to acetyl-CoA. Note the unimpeded access of ketone bodies to the mitochondrial matrix (right side of the figure).

Table 3

Intramitochondrial Concentrations of CoASH, 2-Oxoglutarate, and NAD$^+$ for Mitochondria Oxidizing Either Pyruvate or Acetoacetate

Substrate	State-3 Respiration (natomes O$_2$/ min per mg)	CoASH (mmol/L)	2-Oxoglutarate (mmol/L)	NAD$^+$ (mmol/L)
Pyruvate (5 mmol/L) + malate (5 mmol/L)	292.0 ± 17.8	0.108 ± 0.022	0.128 ± 0.012	0.187 ± 0.011
Acetoacetate (5 mmol/L) + malate (5 mmol/L)	151.7 ± 25.3*	0.046 ± 0.011*	0.205 ± 0.017	0.409 ± 0.095*

Values are means ± SEM for four hearts.
* $P < 0.001$. See Reference 37 for further details.

just as rapidly to control values after the addition of glucose. Similar results can be obtained with pyruvate as second substrate.[39] These observations have resulted in the general hypothesis that in the substrate-controlled, perfused working heart, the quality of the fuel for respiration affects the contractile performance of the heart. The concept of a metabolically induced contractile abnormality is strengthened by the observation that the contractile dysfunction is corrected by the addition of a second substrate, which appears to supply a missing ingredient. In essence, contractile function is lost because of the loss of an efficient moiety-conserved cycle and the question becomes whether the addition of the second substrate somehow helps to restore the cycle.

The decline in contractile function is the result of insufficient rates of ketone body oxidation to support cardiac work. The site of inhibition is the reaction catalyzed by the enzyme 2-oxoglutarate dehydrogenase, as suggested by the accumulation of 2-oxoglutarate, and glutamate as well as acetyl-CoA and acetoacetyl-CoA. At the same time, there is a fall in succinyl-CoA and free coenzyme A.[40] The decline in contractile function, the rise in 2-oxoglutarate and glutamate, and the fall in succinyl-CoA and free CoASH is reversed by the provision of the precursors of CoA, pantothenic acid (15 μmol/L), and cysteine (0.2 mmol/L).[40]

Table 3 lists the intramitochondrial concentrations of CoASH, 2-oxoglutarate, and NAD$^+$ for rat heart mitochondria oxidizing either pyruvate or acetoacetate in the presence of malate.[40] The state-3 rate of respiration for mitochondria using acetoacetate is approximately half that for mitochondria oxidizing pyruvate, which is consistent with inhibition of 2-oxoglutarate dehydrogenase.[41] The fall in intramitochondrial [CoASH] with acetoacetate compared with pyruvate (-57%) is in the same order of magnitude as the K$_{mCoA}$ value of 2-oxoglutarate dehydrogenase for CoASH,[42] and changes in intramitochondrial [2-oxoglutarate] mirror the changes found in the whole heart.[43] Table 3 also shows an increase in intramitochondrial [NAD$^+$] with acetoacetate. Taken together, these findings are consistent with decreased state-3 respiration and therefore decreased oxidative energy production that results from inhibition of 2-oxoglutarate dehydrogenase through sequestration of free CoASH.

Anaplerosis

The inhibition of the citric acid cycle at the level of 2-oxoglutarate dehydrogenase not only affects efficient energy transfer but also provides an opportunity to test the hypothesis that replenishment of the citric acid cycle restores energy transfer and, hence, normal contractile function in the heart. Kornberg, in his work with *Escherichia coli* (*E. coli*), has termed replenishment of a metabolic cycle "anaplerosis." In the case of bacteria, depletion of the glyoxylate cycle inhibits their growth. The stunted growth is reversed by the provision of anaplerotic substrate.[44] In the case of the citric acid cycle, anaplerotic precursors increase the pool of oxaloacetate available for condensation with acetyl-CoA to form citrate and thereby allow oxidative phosphorylation to support contractile function. In other words, anaplerotic pathways are the means by which moiety-conserved cycles can be replenished in pathological conditions.

As mentioned, the isolated working rat heart, perfused at a near-physiological workload, has proven to be a sensitive model for the assessment of energy transfer and citric acid cycle function. Although changes in citric acid cycle flux and anaplerosis antedate the functional decline in isolated working rat hearts utilizing acetoacetate,[45] the decline of function is either prevented or quickly reversed on addition of anaplerotic substrate.[39,45,46] Perhaps the most elegant demonstration of anaplerosis in the working rat

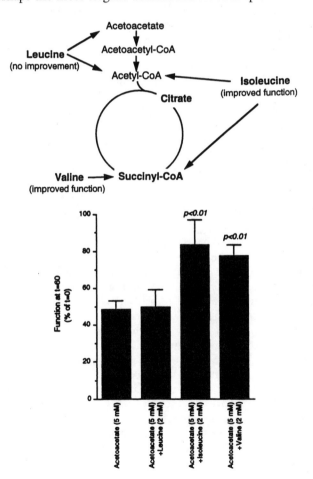

Figure 3. (**Top**) A metabolic scheme of the metabolism of the branched-chain amino acids leucine, isoleucine, and valine. Note that while both valine and isoleucine contribute succinyl-CoA to the citric acid cycle through anaplerosis, leucine only contributes acetyl-CoA. (**Bottom**) Pressure-volume work following 60 minutes of perfusion of hearts utilizing acetoacetate (5 mmol/L) either alone or with leucine (2 mmol/L), isoleucine (2 mmol/L), or valine (2 mmol/L) as a competing substrate.

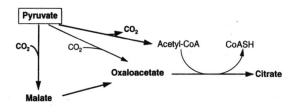

Figure 4. Metabolic scheme indicating the carboxylation and decarboxylation pathways of pyruvate metabolism in heart muscle. Note that pyruvate is both decarboxylated (via the pyruvate dehydrogenase complex) and carboxylated [via oxidized nicotinamide-adenine-dinucleotide phosphate ($NADP^+$)-dependent malic enzyme and pyruvate carboxylase].

heart depleted of citric acid cycle intermediates by perfusion with acetoacetate comes from the demonstration of functional improvement with some (isoleucine and valine), but not all (leucine), branched-chain amino acids (Fig. 3). Heart muscle contains the enzymatic machinery for the catabolism of branched-chain amino acids.[47] As shown in Figure 3 (top), valine and isoleucine enter the citric acid cycle via succinyl-CoA (an anaplerotic substrate), but leucine enters the citric acid cycle via acetyl-CoA (not an anaplerotic substrate).

Another (and quantitatively probably more important) anaplerotic substrate is pyruvate, which can be either decarboxylated to acetyl-CoA or carboxylated to malate or oxaloacetate in the heart (Fig. 4).[39,48–51] The functional importance of anaplerosis through pyruvate carboxylation is, again, best shown in the citric acid cycle depleted, acetoacetate perfused, isolated working rat heart. Although the cardiac power output after 60 minutes of perfusion in hearts utilizing acetoacetate alone had fallen by 44% of the initial value, the addition of pyruvate resulted in a stable performance with no fall in the work output. Inhibition studies and isotopic labeling studies in the same model support the idea that enrichment of malate by pyruvate improves function by increasing the production of reducing equivalents in the span of the citric acid cycle from malate to 2-oxoglutarate.

Because contractile failure in hearts oxidizing ketone bodies is caused by sequestration of free CoASH, which can be reversed by the addition of anaplerotic substrates that enrich the citric acid cycle, we also found that the addition of propionyl-L-carnitine (2 mmol/L) can improve the performance of working hearts oxidizing acetoacetate (7.5 mmol/L).[46] The addition of propionyl-L-carnitine in the presence of acetoacetate resulted in a sustained improvement in the work output of the heart to a level comparable with the mechanical performance of hearts perfused with glucose as the only substrate. However, the addition of propionate (2 mmol/L) or L-carnitine (2 mmol/L) alone in the presence of acetoacetate (7.5 mmol/L) had negligible effects on contractile function. Propionyl-L-carnitine increased the uptake of acetoacetate by 130% without a change in the release of β-hydroxybutyrate, indicating that the rate of acetoacetate oxidation was increased. With propionyl-L-carnitine there was no accumulation of citric acid cycle intermediates in the span from citrate to 2-oxoglutarate. However, there was an increase in the tissue content to malate. The improvement most likely is caused by anaplerosis, which allows enhanced rates of acetoacetate oxidation and citric acid cycle flux.

Integration: Moiety-Conserved Cycles, the Control of Respiration, and Cardiac Function

The present hypothesis concerning the importance of moiety-conserved cycles has to be viewed in the wider context of proposed mechanisms of the control of respiration.

These mechanisms are not mutually exclusive. As reviewed by Brown,[9] the views on the mechanisms by which energy transfer and mitochondrial respiration are thought to be controlled have undergone several revisions over the last few decades. All these views provide correct, yet incomplete, explanations for the control of respiration. Work with isolated mitochondria[52] has led to the concept that mitochondrial respiration and ATP synthesis are controlled by the ATP demand of ATP-utilizing reactions. The "near-equilibrium hypothesis" of Klingenberg[53] and of Erecinsca and Wilson[54] emphasizes that the whole of oxidative phosphorylation from mitochondrial NADH to cytosolic ATP operates close to equilibrium, apart from cytochrome oxidase, which is far from equilibrium. Consequently, mitochondrial respiration and ATP synthesis are controlled by the triad of mitochondrial $[NADH]/[NAD^+]$ ratio, the phosphorylation potential, and any effectors of cytochrome oxidase (such as pH or P_{O_2}). The possible control of energy transfer by changes in the "free energy charge,"[3] discussed earlier, is based on the general observation that ATP, ADP, and AMP act as allosteric effectors of glycolytic enzymes, matrix dehydrogenases, and ATP-utilizing pathways. Likewise, the proposed control of energy transfer by cellular Ca^{2+} levels,[55,56] is based on the observation that Ca^{2+} acts as an activator of several key matrix dehydrogenases in the mitochondria. Others[57] have advanced the idea that the control of mitochondrial respiration of ATP synthesis is shared by a number of reactions and pathways and that the distribution of control changes under different metabolic conditions. Such changes in the control point for a metabolic pathway have been suggested in recent studies of myocardial glycolysis in perfused rat heart.[58]

Our own studies in the isolated working rat heart have confirmed the well-established concept that, even in the setting of high rates of energy transfer, metabolite levels control enzyme activities and enzyme activities control metabolite levels. Efficient energy transfer occurs through moiety-conserved cycles. We have demonstrated that not all substrates are created equal (Fig. 5). Although heart muscle is capable of oxidizing both fatty acids and carbohydrates, the citric acid cycle requires replenishment of its intermediates from carbohydrates.[59]

The importance of the citric acid cycle for energy transfer in an organ with high rates of energy turnover cannot be overestimated. As Efraim Racker[60] put it, "The efficiency of the energy budget is increased by this device by a factor of 2.5, a rather distinct advantage in the survival of struggling organisms."

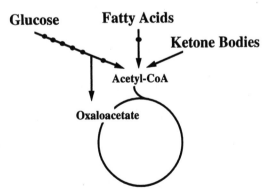

Figure 5. Metabolic scheme highlighting the differences of glucose, fatty acids, and ketone bodies in their respective pathways of oxidative metabolism. Filled circles (●) represent the major regulatory sites. Although highly regulated, glucose provides both substrates for the citrate synthase reaction, while β-oxidation of fatty acids and ketone bodies supply acetyl-CoA only. Pyruvate carboxylation to oxaloacetate and anaplerosis of the citric acid cycle is essential for the unimpeded flow of energy through this moiety-conserved cycle.

Depletion and Replenishment of Moiety-Conserved Cycles in Ischemic Heart Muscle

Although an association of hypoglycemia with cardiac enlargement and heart failure has been observed in newborn infants,[61] it can be argued that depletion of the citric acid cycle does not occur in vivo, where the heart is always exposed to more than one substrate and where blood glucose levels are relatively constant. Indeed, early studies that investigated myocardial substrate utilization in human disease found (with the notable exception of ischemic heart disease) no correlation between disease state and substrate utilization.[21,62]

There is one important clinical situation where depletion and replenishment of the citric acid cycle come into focus. This situation is myocardial ischemia and reperfusion.

While arrested, hearts oxidizing [2-^{13}C] acetate exhibit increased contributions from anaplerotic sources for citric acid cycle intermediate formation.[14] We have shown that under hypoxic conditions the opposite occurs.[63] Heart muscle uses glutamate and produces succinate (Fig. 6, top). This short pathway is linked to substrate level phosphorylation of guanosine diphosphate (GDP). Others have demonstrated, in addition, a dramatic fall in aspartate with ischemia.[49] Although the depletion of citric acid cycle intermediates with ischemia has been known for some time, it is only now becoming apparent that replenishment of the depleted cycle (Fig. 6, bottom) may be a salient feature of the return of function in viable, reperfused myocardium although the evidence is for the most part still indirect.[64-68] Substrate competition studies in postischemic myocardium have shown that glucose utilization (and oxidation) early during reperfusion may be

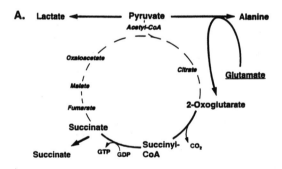

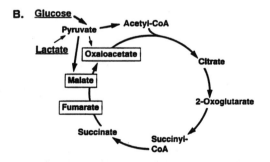

Figure 6. The citric acid cycle during ischemia (**A**) and reperfusion with glucose and lactate as the main energy providing substrates (**B**). Note the depletion of intermediates downstream from succinate and the replenishment of the same intermediates through anaplerosis from pyruvate carboxylation. Reproduced with permission from Rference 72.

crucial for functional recovery.[69,70] Independent studies with amino acid precursors have yielded similar results.[71]

The scheme presented in Figure 6 (bottom) provides a rationale for metabolic support of the reversibly ischemic, reperfused heart muscle through anaplerosis and pyruvate carboxylation. The scheme is not inconsistent with the observations that increased flux through pyruvate dehydrogenase improves cardiac performance on reperfusion[72,73] without increasing flux through the glycolytic pathway.[74] It can be stated again, that in reperfused heart muscle not all substrates are created equal.[75] A very plausible mechanism for the beneficial effect of glucose-insulin-potassium (GIK) in refractory left ventricular contractile failure after hypothermic ischemic arrest of the heart[76] is enhanced glucose utilization and pyruvate carboxylation by the reperfused myocardium. Glucose and lactate are converted to pyruvate and restore contractile function through replenishment of a depleted citric acid cycle and restoration of flux through a series of moiety-conserved cycles. It seems that the greater the failure of left ventricular function, the more the heart must rely on anaplerosis.[77]

Summary

Intermediary metabolism of energy-providing substrates in the heart has the dubious reputation of extraordinary complexity. This chapter examines the hypothesis that efficient transfer of energy requires the coordinated operation of a series of moiety-conserved cycles. The effects of depletion and replenishment of the citric acid cycle on contractile function of the isolated working heart serve as an example. Because ischemia depletes the citric acid cycle of some of its intermediates, their replenishment may become important for the return of contractile function with reperfusion.

Acknowledgments: We thank Dr. Gary Goodwin for critical comments and Rachel Ralston for typing the manuscript.

References

1. Lipmann F. Metabolic generation and utilization of phosphate bond energy. *Adv Enzymol* 1941;1:99–165.
2. Taegtmeyer H. Energy metabolism of the heart: From basic concepts to clinical applications. *Curr Prob Cardiol* 1994;19:57–116.
3. Atkinson DE. *Cellular Energy Metabolism and Its Regulation.* New York: Academic Press; 1977.
4. Pool PE, Covell JW, Chidsey CA, et al. Myocardial high energy phosphate stores in acutely induced hypoxic heart failure. *Circ Res* 1966;19:221–229.
5. Wilson DP, Nishiki K, Erecinska M. Energy metabolism in muscle and its regulation during individual contraction-relaxation cycles. *Trends Biochem Sci* 1981;6:16–19.
6. Clarke K, O' Conner AJ, Willis RJ. Temporal relation between energy metabolism and myocardial function during ischemia and reperfusion. *Am J Physiol* 1987;253:H412–H421.
7. Kammermeier H, Schmidt P, Jungling E. Free energy charge of ATP-hydrolysis: A causal factor of early hypoxic failure of the myocardium? *J Mol Cell Cardiol* 1982;14:267–277.
8. Osbakken MD. Metabolic regulation of in vivo myocardial contractile function: Multiparameter analysis. *Mol Cell Biochem* 1994;133/134:13–37.
9. Brown GC. Control of respiration and ATP synthesis in mammalian mitochondria and cells. *Biochem J.* 1992;284:1–13.
10. Jacobus WE, Moreadith RW, Vandegaer KM. Mitochondrial respiratory control. Evidence against the regulation of respiration by extramitochondrial phosphorylation potentials or by [ATP]/[ADP] ratios. *J Biol Chem* 1982;257:2397–2402.
11. Balaban RS, Kantor HL, Katz LA, et al. Relation between work and phosphate metabolite in the in vivo paced mammalian heart. *Science* 1986;232:1121–1123.

12. Kupriyanov VV, Lakomkin VL, Kapelko VI, et al. Dissociation of adenosine triphosphate levels and contractile function in isovolumic hearts perfused with 2-deoxyglucose. *J Mol Cell Cardiol* 1987;19:729–740.

13. Balaban RS. Regulation of oxidative phosphorylation in the mammalian cell. *Am J Physiol* 1990;258:C377–C389.

14. Lewandowski ED. Nuclear magnetic resonance evaluation of metabolic and respiratory support of work load in intact rabbit hearts. *Circ Res* 1992;70:576–582.

15. Scholz TD, Laughlin MR, Balaban RS, et al. Effect of substrate on mitochondrial NADH, cytosolic redox state, and phosphorylated compounds in isolated hearts. *Am J Physiol* 1995; 268:H82–H91.

16. Sato K, Kashiwaya Y, Keon CA, et al. Insulin, ketone bodies, and mitochondrial energy transduction. *FASEB J* 1995;9:651–658.

17. McCormack JG, Halestrap AP, Denton RM. Role of calcium ions in reperfusion of mammalian intramitochondrial metabolism. *Physiol Rev* 1990;70:391–425.

18. Holmes FL. *Between Biology and Medicine: The Formation of Intermediary Metabolism.* Berkeley, Calif: University of California at Berkeley; 1992.

19. Robitaille PML, Rath DP, Abduljalil AM, et al. Dynamic ^{13}C NMR analysis of oxidative metabolism in the canine myocardium. *J Biol Chem* 1993;268:26296–26301.

20. Nguyễn VTB, Mossberg KA, Tewson TJ, et al. Temporal analysis of myocardial glucose metabolism by ^{18}F-2-deoxy-2-fluoro-D-glucose. *Am J Physiol* 1990;259:H1022–H1031.

21. Bing RJ. The metabolism of the heart. *Harvey Lect* 1955;50:27–70.

22. Randle PJ, Garland PB, Hales CN, et al. The glucose fatty-acid cycle. Its role in insulin sensitivity and the metabolic disturbances of diabetes mellitus. *Lancet* 1963;1:785–789.

23. Goodwin GW, Ahmad F, Doenst T, et al. Energy provision from glycogen, glucose and fatty acids upon adrenergic stimulation of isolated working rat heart. *Am J Physiol* 1998;274: H1239–H1247.

24. Neely JR, Morgan HE. Relationship between carbohydrate and lipid metabolism and the energy balance of heart muscle. *Ann Rev Physiol* 1974;36:413–439.

25. Randle PJ, Tubbs PK. Carbohydrate and fatty acid metabolism. In: Berne R, Sperelakis V, Geiger S, eds. *Handbook of Physiology. The Cardiovascular System.* Bethesda, Md: American Physiological Society; 1979:805–844.

26. Randle PJ, Garland PB, Hales CN, et al. Interactions of metabolism and the physiological role of insulin. *Rec Prog Horm Res* 1966;22:1–41.

27. Keul J, Doll E, Keppler D. *Energy Metabolism of Human Muscle.* Basel, Germany: Karger; 1972.

28. Gertz EW, Wisneski JA, Neese R. Myocardial lactate extraction: Multidetermined metabolic function. *Circulation* 1980;61:256–261.

29. Taegtmeyer H, Hems R, Krebs HA. Utilization of energy providing substrates in the isolated working rat heart. *Biochem J* 1980;186:701–711.

30. Lopaschuk GD, Collins-Nakai R, Olley PM, et al. Plasma fatty acid levels in infants and adults after myocardial ischemia. *Am Heart J* 1994;128:61–67.

31. Saddik M, Gamble J, Witters LA, et al. Acetyl-CoA carboxylase regulation of fatty acid oxidation in the heart. *J Biol Chem* 1993;268:25836–25845.

32. Carling D, Aguan K, Woods A, et al. Mammalian AMP-activated protein kinase is homologous to yeast and plant protein kinases involved in the regulation of carbon metabolism. *J Biol Chem* 1994;269:11442–11448.

33. Drake AJ, Haines JR, Noble MM. Preferential uptake of lactate by the normal myocardium in dogs. *Cardiovasc Res* 1980;14:65–72.

34. Kaijser L, Berglund B. Myocardial lactate extraction and release at rest and during heavy exercise in healthy men. *Acta Physiol Scan* 1992;144:39–45.

35. Bursztein S, Elwyn DH, Askanazi J, et al. *Energy Metabolism, Indirect Calorimetry and Nutrition.* Philadelphia, Pa: Williams and Wilkins; 1989.

36. Rayment I, Holden HM, Whittacker M, et al. Structure of actin-myosin complex and its implications for muscle contraction. *Science* 1993;261:58–65.

37. Krebs HA, Johnson WA. The role of citric acid in intermediate metabolism in animal tissues. *Enzymologia* 1937;4:148–156.

38. Baldwin JE, Krebs HA. The evolution of metabolic cycles. *Nature* 1981;291:381–382.

39. Russell RR, Taegtmeyer H. Pyruvate carboxylation prevents the decline in contractile function of rat hearts oxidizing acetoacetate. *Am J Physiol* 1991;261:H1756–H1762.
40. Russell RR, Taegtmeyer H. Coenzyme A sequestration in rat hearts oxidizing ketone bodies. *J Clin Invest* 1992;89:968–973.
41. Unitt JF, McCormack JG, Reid D, et al. Direct evidence for a role of intramitochondrial Ca^{2+} in the regulation of oxidative phosphorylation in the stimulated rat heart. *Biochem J* 1989;262: 1293–1301.
42. Read G, Crabtree B, Smith GH. The activities of 2-oxoglutarate dehydrogenase and pyruvate dehydrogenase in hearts and mammary glands from ruminants and non-ruminants. *Biochem J* 1977;164:349–355.
43. Taegtmeyer H. On the inability of ketone bodies to serve as the only energy providing substrate for rat heart at physiological work load. *Basic Res Cardiol* 1983;78:435–450.
44. Kornberg HL. Anaplerotic sequences and their role in metabolism. *Essays Biochem* 1966;2:1–31.
45. Russell RR, Taegtmeyer H. Changes in citric acid cycle flux and anaplerosis antedate the functional decline in isolated rat hearts utilizing acetoacetate. *J Clin Invest* 1991;87:384–390.
46. Russell RR, Mommessin JI, Taegtmeyer, H. Propionyl-L-carnitine-mediated improvement in contractile function of rat hearts oxidizing acetoacetate. *Am J Physiol* 1995;268:H441–H447.
47. Livesay G, Lund P. Determination of branched-chain amino and keto acids with leucine dehydrogenase. *Methods Enzymol* 1988;106:3–10.
48. Peuhkurinen KJ, Hassinen IE. Pyruvate carboxylation as an anaplerotic mechanism in the isolated perfused rat heart. *Biochem J* 1982;202:67–76.
49. Peuhkurinen KJ, Nuutinen EM, Pietilainen EP, et al. Role of pyruvate carboxylation in the energy-linked regulation of pool sizes of tricarboxylic acid-cycle intermediates in the myocardium. *Biochem J* 1982;208:577–581.
50. Sundqvist KE, Heikkila J, Hassinen IE, et al. Role of $NADP^+$-linked malic enzymes as regulators of the pool size of tricarboxylic acid-cycle intermediates in the perfused rat heart. *Biochem J* 1987;243:853–857.
51. Sundqvist KE, Hiltunen JK, Hassinen IE. Pyruvate carboxylation in the rat heart. Role of biotin-dependent enzymes. *Biochem J* 1989;257:913–916.
52. Chance B, Williams GR. Respiratory enzymes in oxidative phosphorylation: III. The steady state. *J Biol Chem* 1955;217:409–427.
53. Klingenberg, M. Fur Reversibilitat der oxidativen phosphorylierung. *Biochem Z* 1961;335: 231–272.
54. Erecinska M, Wilson DF. Regulation of cellular energy metabolsim. *J Membr Biol* 1982;70:1–14.
55. Denton RM, McCormack JG. On the role of the calcium transport cycle in the heart and other mammalian mitochondria. *FEBS Lett* 1980;119:1–8.
56. Hansford RG. Control of mitochondrial substrate oxidation. *Curr Top Bioenerg* 1980;10:217–278.
57. Tager JM, Wanders RJ, Groen AK, et al. Control of mitochondrial respiration. *FEBS Lett* 1983;151:1–9.
58. Kashiwaya Y, Sato K, Tsuchiya N, et al. Control of glucose utilization in working perfused rat heart. *J Biol Chem* 1994;269:25502–25514.
59. Krebs HA. Some aspects of the regulation of fuel supply in omnivorous animals. *Adv Enzyme Regul* 1972;10:397–420.
60. Racker E. Energy cycles in health and disease. *Curr Top Cell Regul* 1981;18:361–375.
61. Amatayakul O, Cumming GR, Haworth JC. Association of hypoglycemia with cardiac enlargement and heart failure in newborn infants. *Arch Dis Child* 1970;45:717–720.
62. Bing RJ. Biochemical basis of myocardial failure. *Hosp Pract* 1983;9:93–112.
63. Taegtmeyer H. Metabolic responses to cardiac hypoxia: Increased production of succinate by rabbit papillary muscles. *Circ Res* 1978;43:808–815.
64. Bunger R, Mallet RT, Hartman DA. Pyruvate-enhanced phosphorylation potential and inotropism in normoxic and postischemic isolated working heart. Near-complete prevention of reperfusion contractile failure. *Eur J Biochem* 1989;180:221–233.
65. Mallet RT, Hartman DA, Bünger R. Glucose requirement for postischemic recovery of perfused working heart. *Eur J Biochem* 1990;188:481–493.

66. Weiss RG, Gloth ST, Kalil-Filho R, et al. Indexing tricarboxylic acid cycle flux in intact hearts by carbon-13 nuclear magnetic resonance. *Circ Res* 1992;70:392–408.

67. Jessen ME, Tovarik TE, Jeffrey FM, et al. Effects of amino acids on substrate selection, anaplerosis, and left ventricular function in the ischemic perfused rat heart. *J Clin Invest* 1993;92:831–839.

68. Goodwin GW, Taegtmeyer H. Metabolic recovery of the isolated working rat heart after brief global ischemia. *Am J Physiol* 1994;267:H462–H470.

69. Fralix TA, Steenbergen C, London RE, et al. Metabolic substrates can alter postischemic recovery in preconditioned ischemic heart. *Am J Physiol* 1992;263:C17–C23.

70. Tamm C, Benzi RH, Papageorgiou I, et al. Substrate competition in postischemic myocardium. Effect of substrate availability during reperfusion on metabolic and contractile recovery in isolated rat hearts. *Circ Res* 1994;75:1103–1112.

71. Shug AL, Madsen D, Dobbie R, et al. Protection of mitochondrial and heart function by amino acids after ischemia and cardioplegia. *Life Sci* 1994;54:557–567.

72. Lopaschuk GD, Spafford MA, Davies NJ, et al. Glucose and palmitate oxidation in isolated working rat hearts reperfused after a period of transient global ischemia. *Circ Res* 1990;66:546–553.

73. McVeigh JJ, Lopaschuk GD. Dichloroacetate stimulation of glucose oxidation improves recovery of ischemic rat hearts. *Am J Physiol* 1990;259:H1079–H1085.

74. Taegtmeyer H. Metabolic support for the postischaemic heart. *Lancet* 1995;345:1552–1555.

75. Lewandowski ED, White LT. Pyruvate dehydrogense influences postischemic heart function. *Circulation* 1995;91:2071–2079.

76. Gradinak S, Coleman,GM, Taegtmeyer H, et al. Improved cardiac function with glucose-insulin-potassium after coronary bypass surgery. *Ann Thorac Surg* 1989;48:484–489.

77. Jeffrey FMH, Storey CJ, Malloy CR. Predicting functional recovery from ischemia in the rat myocardium. *Basic Res Cardiol* 1992;87:548–558.

Nitric Oxide and Energetics of the Heart:

Physiology and Pathophysiology

Joanne S. Ingwall, PhD

Introduction

Nitric oxide (NO) is one of the most important in vivo regulators of biological processes. Since being named the "molecule of the year in 1992,"[1] much has been learned about its synthesis and function in almost every tissue in the body. The rapidly growing number of meetings, presentations, and publications on this subject shows that NO is the subject of active investigation. The molecule functions in normal physiology and in pathophysiology. Physiological functions for endogenously derived NO include smooth muscle relaxation, platelet inhibition, neurotransmission, cell adhesion, cell lysis, and hormonal release. Pathophysiological roles of NO produced in relatively large amounts also have been described, for example, for the lung. Although slow to reveal its secrets, it is now known that NO has several functions in intact muscle, including physiological regulation of vascular biology and a pathophysiological role on the energetics of myocytes. The chemistry, physiology, and pathophysiology of NO and the heart have been reviewed in detail elsewhere.[2] The recent review by Kelly, Balligand, and Smith[3] focusing on cardiac function is especially recommended. Here a brief summary of the chemistry, physiology, and pathophysiology of NO with a focus on energetics of muscle is presented.

Fundamentals

NO is a free radical gas, NO˙ in equilibrium with the closely related redox forms NO^- and NO^+. With a molecular weight of only 30 dal/mol (for reference, molecular oxygen is 32 dal/mol), NO is readily diffusible. The half-life of NO is 0.1–5 seconds.

Nitric Oxide Synthesis

The synthesis of NO˙ is complex (Fig. 1). A guanidino nitrogen of the amino acid L-arginine undergoes a multistep oxidation in the presence of molecular oxygen to form

This work was suppported in part by National Heart, Lung, and Blood Institute grant SCOR HL 52320.

From Dilsizian V (ed). *Myocardial Viability: A Clinical and Scientific Treatise.* Armonk, NY: Futura Publishing Co., Inc.; © 2000.

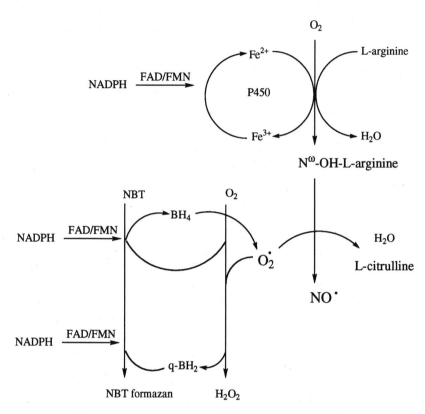

Figure 1. Simplified pathway for nitric oxide (NO') synthesis from O_2 and L-arginine. Essential cofactors are nicotinamide-adenine-dinucleotide phosphate (NADPH), the flavoproteins flavin adenine dinucleotide (FAD) and flavin mononucleotide (FMN), H_4 biopterin, and thiol moieties. See text for more detailed description.

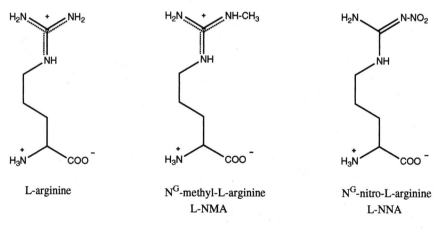

Figure 2. Chemical structure of L-arginine and two arginine derviatives commonly used to study NO synthesis in cells and tissues.

citrulline and NO˙. Obligatory cofactors are the reduced form of nicotinamide-adenine-dinucleotide phosphate (NADPH), the flavoproteins flavin adenine dinucleotide (FAD) and flavin mononucleotide (FMN), H_4 biopterin, and thiol moieties. Citrulline can be salvaged to form arginine and in this way fuels the cycle. Based on the known chemistry and specificity for L-arginine of the NO synthesis pathway, synthetic inhibitors have been designed. These include derivatives of arginine such as the alkyl-substituted derivative N^G-methyl-L-arginine (L-NMA) and the nitro derivative, N^G-nitro-L-arginine(L-NNA) (Fig. 2).

Nitric Oxide Synthases

The enzyme that catalyzes NO synthesis is NO synthase (NOS). There are at least three NOS isoenzymes, products of separate genes, which share 50%–60% homology at both the nucleotide and the amino acid levels.[4] The C-terminal domain, which functions as a reductase, is homologous to cytochrome P-450 reductase. The N-terminal domain, which functions as an oxygenase, contains a heme group. These two domains are linked by a calmodulin-binding domain. The binding of calcium to the calmodulin domain serves as a molecular switch to increase the binding of calmodulin to NOS and thus activate NO synthesis.[5-7] Consensus sequences for sites of cyclic adenosine monophosphate (cAMP)-dependent protein kinase phosphorylation and for binding of NADPH, FAD, and FMN also have been identified.

The original nomenclature for the NOSs designated them by where they were first discovered: neuronal (nNOS), now called NOS1, and large-vessel endothelial cells (eNOS), now called NOS3. An inducible NOS (iNOS) or NOS2 is induced by cytokines and lipopolysaccharides. The iNOS is Ca^{2+}-insensitive because it has a higher affinity for binding calmodulin.

Localization of Nitric Oxide Synthases

It is now known that the NOS isoenzymes are present in many cell types. In heart, histochemical staining for NOS1 has been found in atria, epicardial coronary arteries, and in conduction cells.[8] The NOS2, the cytokine-inducible Ca^{2+}-insensitive NOS, accumulates in ventricular myocytes[9] as well as vascular smooth muscle cells, microvascular endothelium, endocardial endothelium, fibroblasts, and infiltrating inflammatory cells. NOS3 is expressed in the endothelium of the endocardium and of the coronary vasculature, in myocytes, and in conduction cells. NOS3 expression in atrial and ventricular myocytes appears to be constitutive.[10]

NOSs exist in functional or actual compartments within cells by binding to other proteins and to membranes. NOSs undergo a variety of posttranslational modifications, including phosphorlyation, myristoylation, and palmitoylation, which may govern their movements between particulate and cytosolic compartments within the cell. Particularly interesting is evidence showing that acylated NOS3 is localized to caveolae, structures that contain proteins involved in signaling cascades.[11] The possibility that NOS may be involved directly with protein trafficking and control of signal transduction pathways is under active study. In this way, NOSs could play roles in both spatial and temporal events within the cell.

Regulation of Nitric Oxide Synthase

Regulation of NOS expression and activity is complex, differing for the three isozymes and even for the same isozyme in different cell types. An example of up-regulation is increased NOS expression caused by higher levels of cyclic guanosine monophosphate (cGMP), which were caused by increased NO in vascular endothelial cells.[12] An example of down-regulation is the loss of activity by the binding of NO to labile moieties in NOS itself.[13] The regulation of NOS2 expression and activity is the subject of intense study. Direct and indirect regulation of the cytokine-inducible Ca^{2+}-insensitive NOS occurs, for example, via multiple cytokine-responsive elements, neurotransmitter and peptide signaling pathways, various cAMP stimulators, insulin, etc. Kelly et al[3] review the evidence for and against activation of NOS3 by beating, β-adrenergic agonists, muscarinic cholinergic agonists, and inflammatory cytokines. NOS3 regulation is likely to be regulated differently in myocytes and endothelial cells.

Molecular and Cellular Targets

Because NO is readily diffusible, once it is made, it can effect whatever molecular target is near. Table 1 lists some of the reactive targets for NO. Molecular oxygen is itself a target, forming NO_2, which goes on to form NO_2^-, and NO_3^-. NO reacts with the free radical superoxide O_2^- to form the reactive species peroxynitrite $ONOO^-$. NO reacts with iron, including iron in heme moieties, to form $Fe^{2+}NO$ complexes. Amino, thiol, diazo, and tyrosyl groups in proteins are all targets.

Based on this chemistry, many of the macromolecular targets of NO in cells can be understood. For example, activation of the signal transduction protein guanylyl cyclase occurs via NO binding to its heme. Binding of NO to heme proteins may be one mechanism whereby NO is "disarmed." As another example, inhibition of creatine kinase and some of the glycolytic proteins including glyceraldehyde phosphate dehydrogenase by NO most likely occurs by binding to labile reactive —SH groups. A recent review by Gross and Wolin[2] describes many of the molecular targets of NO. The macromolecular targets include receptors, signal transduction proteins, cytosolic proteins such as the glycolytic proteins and creatine kinase, nuclear proteins such as those involved in DNA synthesis and mitochondrial proteins, particularly those involved in the electron transport chain. Some of these targets are involved in the physiological regulation of the cell, while others are likely to be important only when NO synthesis is massive because of induction of NOS, while still others may be only test tube anomalies.

There now is good evidence that NO plays a role in regulating the activity of proteins essential for maintaining normal adenosine triphosphate (ATP) synthesis rates in muscle. NO plays a role in both the physiological control of ATP synthesis and the several important pathologies when NO production is high due to induction of NOS2 (Fig. 3). These are summarized below.

Table 1

Molecular Targets of Nitric Oxide

1. O_2, $O_2^{\bullet -}$
2. Fe and other transition metals (eg, guanyl cyclase and hemoglobin)
3. Amines and thiols (eg, creatine kinase)
4. Diazo groups
5. Tyrosyl groups

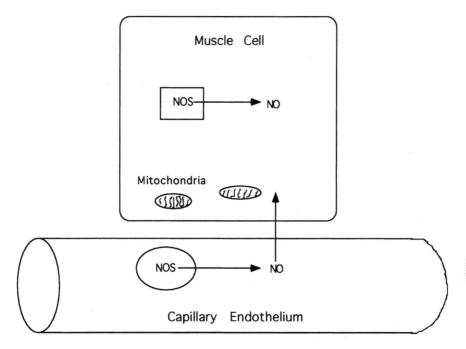

Figure 3. Cartoon showing that NO produced by NO synthase (NOS) in the capillary endothelium can diffuse to target cells to exert physiological control. NO produced within the muscle cells also functions in this way. Under conditions where inducible NOS (iNOS) is induced, NO concentrations are likely to be high, exerting pathophysiological effects on cardiac function.

Physiology: Control of Respiration

Mitochondria

Although the identity of the inhibitor was not known at the time, the first report showing that NO could alter the primary pathway for ATP synthesis in cells was published by Granger and Lehninger in 1982.[14] They showed that mitochondrial respiration was inhibited in a leukemia cell line injured by exposure to cytotoxic macrophages (the source of NO). Moreover, they identified the precise molecular targets responsible for the inhibition: complex I [nicotinamide-adenine dinucleotide (NADH)-coenzyme Q reductase] and complex II (succinate-coenzyme Q reductase) in the electron transport chain (Fig. 4). We now know that it was NO produced by the toxic macrophages that inhibited respiration by binding to the Fe-S target in these two protein complexes. The Fe-S center of aconitase[15] in the Krebs cycle and the heme of cytochrome oxidase in the electron transport chain also are targets of NO (Fig. 4). Other enzymes are unaffected. These discoveries illustrate the important principle that the targets of NO are specific, not ubiquitous. Specificity is caused by availability (NO must be near to the target) and, given equal availability, to the relative binding affinity of the various candidate target moieties for NO and its related molecules. In this case affinity for NO binding of the Fe-S groups is much greater than the affinity for NO of the other potentially reactive targets (eg, sulphydryls present in all proteins).

These experiments were performed using permeabilized cells (to allow measurement and manipulation of mitochondrial function) and thus ensure that NO was near to the

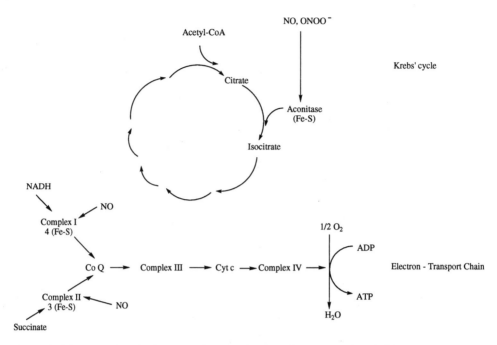

Figure 4. Two mitochondrial targets: diagram showing that NO (and probably ONOO⁻ as well) can bind to aconitase in the Krebs cycle and two protein complexes in the electron transport chain, namely, complex I and complex II. As a result of this binding, mitochondrial respiration can be inhibited.

target proteins in the mitochondria. Could respiration be controlled by NO in this way in vivo?

Whole Animal Oxygen Consumption

The work of Shen and Hintze and their colleagues [16–18] studying whole body oxygen consumption in the dog has provided good evidence that NO produced in physiological amounts via the constitutive NOSs in the capillary enothelium most likely contributes to the regulation of oxygen consumption in skeletal muscle (Fig. 3). Shen et al[16] showed that supplying a NOS inhibitor to resting dogs increased both total body oxygen extraction and total body oxygen consumption. This unexpected result suggested that NO produced by the capillary endothelium partially inhibits oxygen consumption. If so, constitutive NO production could serve as a brake for oxygen consumption, much like phospholamban serves as a brake for Ca^{2+} release by the sarcoplasmic reticulum in the heart. In this way, there always would be a reserve for new ATP synthesis when needed. Moreover, for a given level of work, such a regulatory role for NO would create a more "efficient" ratio of ATP production by oxygen consumption and work. This would be analogous to negative feedback control of an individual enzyme.

These initial observations were supported by additional experiments in which complex I, one of the target sites for the control of respiration, was inhibited by barbituates prior to blocking the release of NO.[16] As predicted, this maneuver prevented the increase in oxygen consumption caused by inhibiting NO synthesis.

Exercise induces NO synthesis through the physical force of shear stress to the vessel wall. Studying treadmill exercise in the conscious dog, Shen et al showed that inhibiting

NO production by the capillary endothelium during exercise also led to increased oxygen extraction and consumption.[18] This was the case for four different levels of exercise. Taken together, all of these results support a physiological role of NO linking the circulation and the target parenchymal cell. Other groups studying skeletal muscle using similar approaches have found comparable results.[19] More recent experiments show similar findings for the heart.[20–21]

Pathophysiology

Although low levels of NO produced by the endothelium are likely to contribute to the efficiency of ATP production and ensure an energy reserve under physiological conditions, it is now clear that NOS is induced in cardiomyocytes under pathophysiological conditions (Fig. 3). Given its high chemical reactivity, it is likely that high concentrations of NO produced by iNOS contributes to impaired contractile function and even increases susceptibility to cell injury. Two recent reports merit particular mention. Depre et al have shown that nonvasoactive concentrations of NOS inhibitors protect against ischemic injury in isolated perfused rabbit hearts, suggesting that NO and/or its related compounds impair critical reactions needed for cell viability.[22] Haywood et al studying biopsy specimens obtained from ventricles of failing human hearts showed that iNOS is induced in heart failure.[23] Using immunohistochemistry, they found diffuse cytosolic staining of iNOS in hearts failing because of a variety of causes.

Under conditions where iNOS is induced dramatically, it is likely that NO functions to alter macromolecular function in two distinct ways. First, many proteins are chemically modified, altering their activities. Second, excessive activation of the soluble guanylate cyclase would lead to high levels of cGMP, which in turn effects many target pathways in the cell. In this way protein function can be modified (eg, by phosphorylation) as a result of control by the guanylate cyclase signaling pathway. Depending on the protein, either of these mechanisms for regulation can occur and could lead to either activation or inhibition. In either case, normal metabolism may not be maintained.

An example of how excessive NO supply can inhibit the activity of a specific enzyme and impact on cardiac contractile performance has been shown recently by our group.[24] In experiments designed to determine the effects of high-NO supply on cardiac contractile performance both at baseline and under conditions of inotropic challenge, we made the surprising observation that supplying NO using a donor that spontaneously generates NO [S-nitrosoacetylcysteine (SNAC)] to isolated perfused rat hearts had no effect on baseline function but markedly blunted contractile reserve. Although the heart rate and developed pressure product (RPP) increased ~75% in normal hearts challenged with high concentrations of Ca^{2+}, essentially there was no increase in RPP when the hearts were perfused with SNAC at concentrations that produced submaximal vasodilatation.

^{31}P nuclear magnetic resonance (NMR) spectroscopy experiments of these hearts provided a clue explaining why the contractile reserve of the hearts was blunted. During inotropic challenge in the rat heart, the ATP concentration remained constant but the phosphocreatine (PCr) concentration fell. This is because creatine kinase catalyzyes the transfer of a phosphoryl group from PCr to ATP. In NO-supplied hearts during inotropic challenge, the opposite pattern was observed: ATP fell but PCr was little changed. Because PCr participates in no other reaction than creatine kinase, these results show that high concentrations of NO inhibit creatine kinase activity. Other experiments showed that creatine kinase activity indeed was inhibited in NO-supplied hearts, most likely by chemically modifying of one of the critical cysteines in this enzyme. Other work has shown that inhibiting creatine kinase activity by other chemical modifiers contributes to decreased contractile reserve of the heart,[25] supporting the hypothesis that inhibiting creatine kinase activity by NO led to the observed decrease in contractile reserve. Whether this also occurs under in vivo conditions, where the production of NO is likely to be less than achieved under these experimental conditions, is not known. This example may serve as a paradigm showing how NO modification of reactive —SH groups in many proteins could function to decrease contractile function and metabolitic events in the heart in important pathophysiological conditions such as heart failure and ischemia.

Acknowledgments: I thank Dr Weiqun Shen for his help preparing this chapter and to Karen Shore for preparing the figures.

References

1. Culotta E, Kushland DE Jr. NO news is good news. *Science* 1992;258:1862–1865.
2. Gross SS, Wolin MS. Nitric oxide: Pathophysiological mechanisms. *Annu Rev Physiol* 1995; 57:737–769.
3. Kelly RA, Balligand J-L, Smith TW. Nitric oxide and cardiac function. *Circ Res* 1996;79:363–380.
4. Nathan C, Xie Q-W. Regulation of biosynthesis of nitric oxide. *J Biol Chem* 1994;269:13725–13728.
5. Su Z, Blazing MA, Fan D, et al. The calmodulin-nitric oxide synthase interaction: Critical role of the calmodulin latch domain in enzyme activation. *J Biol Chem* 1995;270:29117–29122.
6. Abu-Soud HM, Loftus M, Stuehr DJ. Subunit dissociation and unfolding of macrophage NO synthase: Relationship between enzyme structure, prosthetic group binding, and catalytic function. *Biochemistry* 1995;34:11167–11175.
7. Siddhanta U, Wu C, Abu-Soud HM, et al. Heme iron reduction and catalysis by nitric oxide synthase heterodimer containing one reductase and two oxygenase domains. *J Biol Chem* 1996;271:7309–7312.
8. Ursell PC, Mayes M. Anatomic distribution of nitric oxide synthase in the heart. *Int J Cardiol* 1995;50:217–223.
9. Schulz R, Nava E, Moncada S. Induction and potential biological relevance of a Ca^{2+} -independent nitric oxide synthase in the myocardium. *Br J Pharmacol* 1992;105:575–580.
10. Balligand J-L, Kelly RA, Marsden PA, et al. Control of cardiac muscle cell function by an endogenous nitric oxide signalling system. *Proc Natl Acad Sci U S A* 1993;90:347–351.
11. Shaul PW, Smart EJ, Robinson LJ, et al. Acylation targets endothelial nitric oxide synthase to plasmalemmal caveolae. *J Biol Chem* 1996;271:6518–6522.
12. Ravichandran LV, Johns RA. Up-regulation of endothelial nitric oxide synthase mRNA expression by cyclic guanosine 3',5'-monophosphate. *FEBS Lett* 1995;374:295–298.
13. Colasanti M, Persichini T, Menegazzi M, et al. Induction of nitric oxide synthase mRNA expression: Suppression by exogenous nitric oxide. *J Biol Chem* 1995;270:26731–26733.
14. Granger DL, Lehninger AL. Sites of inhibition of mitochondrial electron transport in macrophage-injured neoplastic cells. *J Cell Biol* 1982;95:527–535.
15. Stadler J, Billiar TR, Curran RD, et al. Effect of exogenous and endogenous nitric oxide on mitochondrial respiration of rat hepatocytes. *Am J Physiol* 1991;260:C910–C916.
16. Shen W, Xu X, Ochoa M, et al. Role of nitric oxide in the regulation of oxygen consumption in conscious dogs. *Circ Res* 1994;75:1086–1095.
17. Shen W, Hintze TH, Wolin MS. Nitric oxide. An important signaling mechanism between vascular endothelium and parenchymal cells in the regulation of oxygen consumption. *Circulation* 1995;92:3505–3512.
18. Shen W, Zhang X, Zhao G, et al. Nitric oxide production and NO synthase gene expression contribute to vascular regulation during exercise. *Med Sci Sports Exerc* 1995;27:1125–1134.
19. King CE, Melinshyn MJ, Mewburn JD, et al. Canine hind-limb blood flow and oxygen uptake after inhibition of EDRF/NO synthesis. *L Appl Physiol* 1994;76:1166–1177.
20. Xie Y-W, Shen W, Zhao G, et al. Role of endothelium-derived nitric oxide in the modulation of canine myocardial mitochondrial respiration in vitro. *Circ Res* 1979;9:381–387.
21. Zhang X, Xie Y-W, Xu X, et al. ACE inhibitors promote nitric oxide accumulation to modulate myocardial oxygen consumption. *Circulation* 1997;95:176–182.

22. Depre C, Vanoverschelde J-L, Goudemant J-F, et al. Protection against ischemic injury by nonvasoactive concentrations of nitric oxide synthase inhibitors in the perfused heart. *Circulation* 1995;92:1911–1918.
23. Haywood GA, Tsao PS, von der Leyen HE, et al. Expression of inducible nitric oxide synthase in human heart failure. *Circulation* 1996;93:1087–1094.
24. Gross WL, Bak MI, Ingwall JS, et al. Nitric oxide inhibits creatine kinase and regulates rat heart contractile reserve. *Proc Natl Acad Sci U S A* 1996;93:5604- 5609.
25. Tian R, Ingwall JS. Energetic basis for reduced contractile reserve in isolated rat hearts. *Am J Physiol* 1996;270:H1207–H1216.

Chapter 8

Channels, Ischemia, and Stunning: Cellular Electrophysiology and Intercellular Communication

Marc Ovadia, MD, and Peter R. Brink, PhD

All knowledge available . . . suggests that the interference with metabolic activity . . . produce[s] effects remarkably similar to those produced by the elevation of K^+ in the external milieu. A considerable burden of proof lies upon the investigators who advance mechanisms other than the one suggested by this fact. BF Hoffman and PK Cranefield, Electrophysiology of the Heart *(1960).*

Introduction

Stunning is the presence of contractile reserve in the absence of contractile function, without overt ischemia. Frequently observed instances of stunning include (1) the hypo-contractile state of heart muscle reperfused after transient occlusion of arterial supply and (2) the prolonged hypocontractile state of the rewarmed perfused heart after cardioplegia. Though not ischemia, stunning typically exists subsequent to ischemia, and in certain clinical settings undiagnosed ischemia and infarction may be additional factors in the causation of the observed hypocontractile or acontractile state of heart muscle that is attributed to stunning.

The most familiar state characterized by reduced contractile function is acute ischemia. In acute ischemia, function returns as perfusion returns toward normal. Beyond the scope of this chapter are hibernation and preconditioning, states in which ischemia has altered the degree to which cardiac contractility is reduced in response to reduction in flow (the degree is greater in the first case and lesser in the latter) in a manner that persists for a longer or shorter time.

The challenge of cellular investigations of stunning and ischemia is not limited to the lack of a useful cellular model of ischemia or stunning. Additional difficulties include the indeterminate site of effects of ischemia and other insults (vascular versus myocardial, channels versus pumps, extramitochondrial versus mitochondrial, cytoplasmic versus nuclear, *de novo* versus replacement protein synthesis[1-3]), the diverse physiologic implications—both for cellular electrophysiology and for excitation-contraction coupling, and the unquantitated contribution of irreversible biochemical degradation of enzymes and

From Dilsizian V (ed). *Myocardial Viability: A Clinical and Scientific Treatise.* Armonk, NY: Futura Publishing Co., Inc.; © 2000.

structural protein elements in the causation of the observed phenomena. A further problem is the possible coexistence of stunning and ischemia in many clinical manifestations of these processes.

It is the purpose of this chapter to review channels biophysics relevant to the electrophysiology of stunning and ischemia. Implications for excitation-contraction coupling will be noted but excitation-contraction coupling will not be reviewed specifically. The reader who is a clinician may be introduced for the first time to channels phenomenology.

Although whole animal models have been the chief model used for experimentation in this field, the physiological states of ischemia and stunning, while defined only at the organ level, are caused by cellular changes due to vascular effects (interruption of flow) at a tissue level. Experimentation at the level of the organ or tissue excludes the possibility of recordings from cells or subcellular compartments. The chapter shall focus on data derived from the latter types of study.

The organization of the chapter will be (1) to review phenomena, (2) to survey the channels that exist in the heart, with emphasis on human data, discussing channel by channel the possible relevance of each channel to ischemia and stunning, and (3) to summarize the likely mechanisms of ischemia and stunning based on the available data.

Attention will be limited to intrinsic myocardial channels or pores and effects referable to high ion fluxes. Excluded are transporters and slow effects of low fluxes or isoform turnover (eg, of contractile or channel proteins). Such phenomena would be observed over a longer timescale than the opening and closing of channels with rapid shifts in cellular potential. Excluded also are the membrane attack complex (MAC) pore (part of the complement cascade) and mitochondrial channels because the one is not present and the others probably are not implicated in the phenomenology of clinical ischemia and stunning. Despite the insult the tissue is sufficiently intact that MAC pores and mitochondrial effects are absent. Also excluded is a direct discussion of vascular and neuronal transporters and channels. However, it is known that during ischemia adenosine triphosphate (ATP) depletion in the sympathetic nerve terminal leads to reversal of a neuronal uptake transporter with consequent massive release of norepinephrine and significant effects on myocardial tissue; this underlies the cardioprotective action of the drug amiloride.

Ischemia and Stunning: Review of Phenomena

Ischemia is characterized electrophysiologically at the cellular level by a less negative resting potential, reduced action potential upstroke and amplitude, shortened action potential duration, and an initial increase followed by a rapid decrease in the conduction velocity. This occurs at a time when the whole organ exhibits decreased or absent contraction with both specific and nonspecific electrocardiographic (ECG) changes. These findings are observed in the context of acidosis and hypoxia and are fairly rapid in occurrence. Among the additional changes seen in ischemia are reduced phosphocreatine, reduced intracellular ATP concentration $[ATP]_i$, elevated extracellular potassium concentration[†] $[K]_o$, impairment of oxidative phosphorylation, and increased axial resistance.

Stunning has not been characterized at the cellular level. At the whole organ level initially there is increased followed by reduced contractility at a time when clinical electrophysiology appears normal and perfusion is reduced only mildly. If the human or animal survives, recovery of function occurs in hours to days.

[†] The notation $[K]_e$ also appears in the literature but will not be used further in this chapter.

Myocardial Channels

A channel is an intermolecular (or intramolecular) pore through an oligomeric integral membrane protein of sarcolemma or another biological membrane. Opening of the pore permits equilibration of ions according to concentration gradients and the electrical potential difference across that membrane.

In aqueous solutions far from electrodes, electrical conduction is simply the motion of ions (eg, Na^+, K^+, Ca^{2+}, and Cl^- with or without their hydration shells) from one point to another. Thus, measurement of the electrical conductance of a channel (in units of siemens or picosiemens $= 10^{-12}$ siemens) reflects the actual ion flux through the channel for an applied voltage.[‡]

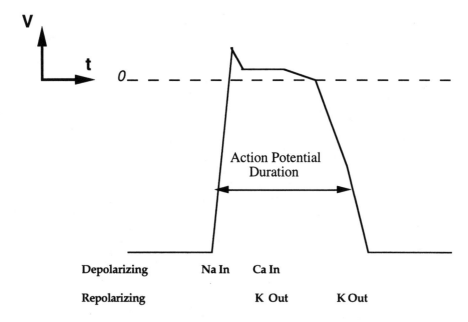

Figure 1. This diagram of the action potential in the ventricular myocyte correlates the identity of the ionic current with the membrane potential (depolarization and repolarization). The y axis is intracellular potential and the x axis represents time. The action potential upstroke is caused by an inward sodium (cation) current. The influx of positively charged ions (cations—sodium ions at this time) has a depolarizing effect on the myocyte. The intracellular potential started out negative with respect to the outside but because of this inward Na^+ current ("Na In") the potential becomes less negative and then positive. At this point active currents include both (1) outward K^+ (cation) currents ("K Out"), which would lead to repolarization of the cell if they were unopposed, and (2) inward Ca^{2+} (cation) current, a depolarizing current like the sodium current. The latter Ca^{2+} current tends to prolong the action potential duration (indicated with the horizontal arrow) while the outward K^+ currents tend to shorten the action potential duration. In this diagram the repolarizing potassium current eventually wins out, persisting when the calcium current is gone and leading to repolarization (return to a negative resting potential) of the myocyte. An inward cation current depolarizes the heart cell and an outward cation current repolarizes it. Not depicted here are several currents including the chloride (Cl^-, an anion) currents of the myocyte, because of their uncertain significance. To anion currents, an opposite rule applies. An inward anion (negatively charged ion such as Cl^- with or without its hydration shell) current is repolarizing.

[‡] The equations governing conductance through a channel across a biological membrane are the diffusion equation, the Nernst equation, Maxwell's equations, and Einstein's relation.

The relevant membranes where channels exist include the membrane of the sarcoplasmic reticulum and the sarcolemma. Familiar channels include the sarcolemmal channels that underlie the action potential, including the sodium channel, the L-type calcium channel of the sarcolemma, and certain K^+ channels involved in repolarization (Fig. 1). Possibly unfamiliar channels include the chloride channels of the sarcolemma, the ryanodine receptor (RyR) of the sarcoplasmic reticulum (a calcium channel), and the gap junction channel connecting the cytoplasm of pairs of adjacent myocytes.

The most important channel for heart muscle contraction is the calcium channel of the sarcoplasmic reticulum—the RyR—and therefore we shall review this channel of the sarcoplasmic reticulum first and then proceed to the channels of the sarcolemma.

Nonsarcolemmal Channels: Channels of the Sarcoplasmic Reticulum

Ryanodine Receptor (RyR)

The RyR is the calcium release channel of the sarcoplasmic reticulum (SR). The sarcoplasmic reticulum is the chief source of calcium for excitation-contraction coupling in normal adult tissues, via the RyR (Fig. 2). A different source of calcium for contraction appears to exist in immature animals; species differences exist as well.

There are at least three isoforms (different protein forms) of the RyR, localized chiefly according to tissue type. These are RyR1, RyR2, and RyR3. The RyR2 is the RyR of the sarcoplasmic reticulum of working heart muscle.[4,5]

The RyR exists as a tetramer (each subunit, 564 kd; Fig. 3) and as a heterooctamer when activated, where each subunit is associated with a FK-506 binding protein,[6] characteristic of the physiological state of the channel.

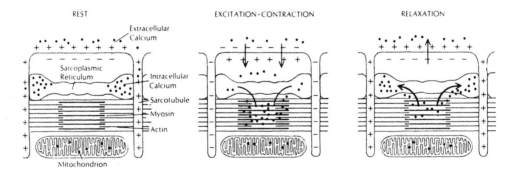

Figure 2. In the adult heart at rest extracellular calcium (black dots outside the heart cell) is seen outside the sarcolemmal membrane. Intracellular calcium is sequestered chiefly in the sarcoplasmic reticulum (black dots in the sarcoplasmic reticulum) awaiting delivery to the contractile apparatus. With depolarization of the cell membrane and excitation of the cell, there is rapid entry of extracellular calcium. The appearance of this calcium at the cytosolic surface of the sarcoplasmic reticulum triggers release of the intracellular calcium stores and activation of contraction. The calcium leaves the lumen of the sarcoplasmic reticulum to enter the cytosol via the ryanodine receptor (RyR). This is the name of the calcium channel of the sarcoplasmic reticulum. Reproduced with permission from Reference 146.

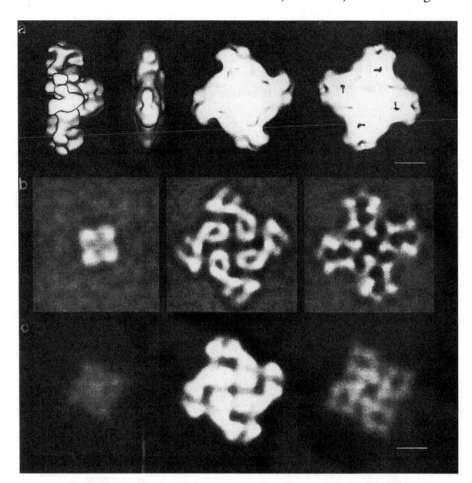

Figure 3. RyR structure. Three-dimensional reconstructions of the RyR (the calcium release channel of the sarcoplasmic reticulum) determined from electron micrographs of frozen-hydrated and negatively stained specimens. (**A**) The first two images in this row are side views of the RyR. Leftward is the side that faces the cytoplasm and rightward in the first image is the protrusion that crosses the membrane of the sarcoplasmic reticulum. The third and fourth images are front and back views, showing, respectively, the side of the RyR facing the interior of the sarcoplasmic reticulum, and the side facing the cytoplasm. (**B** and **C**) Sections through the RyR parallel to the plane of the membrane of the sarcoplasmic reticulum, by reconstruction of frozen-hydrated (B) and negatively stained (C) RyRs. The three sections are at comparable levels in B and C. The first section is in a plane parallel to the plane of the membrane of the sarcoplasmic reticulum and approximately at this plane. The next two sections are both in planes on the cytoplasmic side of the membrane of the sarcoplasmic reticulum. These images, the first of their kind, show the fourfold symmetry of the protein about a central axis. The central axis is the single pore, surrounded by the four identical protein subunits that together make up the RyR. The depiction is of RyR1. The bar is 10 nm (100 Å). Reproduced with permission from Reference 147.

In experimental preparations the channel of the RyR has a low-conductance state and a high-conductance state that is relevant physiologically. The latter state has been documented in lipid bilayer experiments to be a cation channel of 106 picosiemens in Ca^{2+} (Fig. 4). By multiple reopenings at its highest reported conductance state, this channel underlies the calcium current (Fig. 5). There also are subconductance states that appear to be important in its regulation.

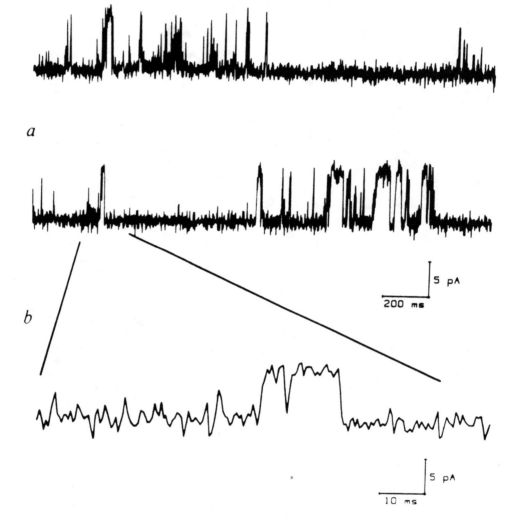

Figure 4. Single channel recording of the RyR, the calcium release channel of the sarcoplasmic reticulum. Current tracings, where upward deflections correspond to a cation (eg, calcium) current going from the lumen of the sarcoplasmic reticulum to the cytosol (ie, to the cytoplasm or myoplasm of the heart muscle cell). Single square openings are observed, all to the same height. This is typical for a single channel recording of multiple reopenings of a channel. The height of opening is the unitary conductance (scaled by the voltage difference across the channel). (Rabbit sarcoplasmic reticulum vesicles, Ba^{2+} as charge carrier. This figure was the first published tracing of RyR calcium channel.) Reproduced with permission from Reference 85.

Permeation selectivity (permselectivity) of this channel is unusual in that in the absence of divalent cations, the channel conducts group Ia monovalent cations with little selectivity (K^+, Na^+, etc.) but in the presence of divalent cations the former conductances are minimal in comparison. It conducts all of the alkaline earth divalents well (permeability equal $Ca^{2+} \sim Mg^{2+}$). A small degree of inward rectification (enhanced SR lumen-to-cytosol cationic conductance) may be conferred by endogenous polyamines in living tissue.

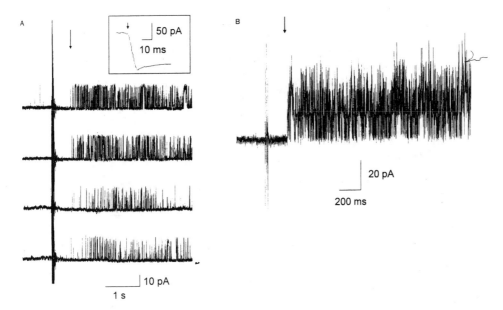

Figure 5. RyR activation by calcium RyR's incorporated into a lipid bilayer (phosphatidylethanol-amine) are exposed to a Ca^{2+} pulse (arrow) and open their channels. (**A**) Single channel incorporated into a lipid bilayer. The four data sweeps were acquired under identical experimental conditions. At the arrow, $[Ca^{2+}]$ concentration on the cytosolic side of the channel is increased from 0.1 to 100 μmol/L. This triggers opening and multiple reopenings of the channel. The y axis is current across the lipid bilayer; upward is sarcoplasmic reticulum luminal-to-cytosolic Ca^{2+} current. There is a 40-mV potential difference across the channel, luminal side positive. (**B**) Calcium current elicited from five RyR channels incorporated into the same lipid bilayer, under the same conditions as in A. Note the simultaneous opening of at least three of the channels and the multiple reopenings. These data show clearly the RyR (the calcium release channel of the sarcoplasmic reticulum) openings triggered by calcium. Reproduced with permission from Reference 148.

The open probability is reduced by caffeine (after brief increase), increased by Ca^{2+} bound either at a cytosolic or at a luminal (SR) site (which significantly modulates Ca^{2+} release for excitation-contraction coupling[7]), by ATP, and by EMD4100 and is relatively unaffected by Mg^{2+}. It is gated by ruthenium red and modified or closed by ryanodine and procaine. A mechanism of adaptation has been described as well, which probably is responsible for the time-dependent variation in the effect of caffeine. Phosphorylation may increase conductance [cyclic adenosine monophosphate (cAMP)-dependent protein kinase and Ca^{2+}-calmodulin–dependent protein kinase II]. Speculatively, kinases also may act via removal of inhibition of Ca^{2+} release associated with the binding of sorcin, a ubiquitous protein that appears to be a potent inhibitor of RyR channel opening.[8]

The mechanism of ryanodine is that ryanodine energetically stabilizes an ordinarily absent (or infrequent) lower conductance subconductance state and turns off other regulatory mechanisms (perhaps because this subconductance state is not tied mechanistically to such regulatory gating mechanisms; Fig. 6). By removing the finely tuned amplificatory response to Ca^{2+} or other signals without abolishing Ca^{2+} conductance, this has the effect of increasing mean cytoplasmic $[Ca^{2+}]$ and reducing its oscillations. If the Ca^{2+} concentration in the cytoplasm is conceived of in analogy to an electrical signal, then cellular homeostasis depends on the mean of the signal being clamped at near 0, and muscle contraction depends on oscillations (analogous to AC current) of appropriate frequency and configuration, for example, proper sine waves rather than narrow spikes. Ryanodine, in this analogy, removes the oscillatory (AC component) changes and lets the

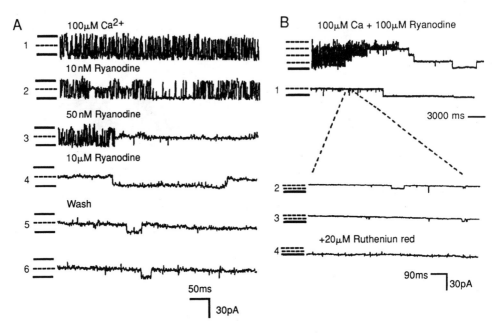

Figure 6. Ryanodine effects on the RyR. Demonstration of subconductance states in the calcium release channel of the sarcoplasmic reticulum (the RyR). Current traces of the RyR (RyR1) in lipid bilayers. (**A**) (1) Basal state shows unitary conductance with multiple rapid reopenings of the channel after exposure to 100 μmol/L Ca^{2+}. Note that there is a single channel that opens (openings are upward deflections) always to the same current level and then closes down very quickly. (2) This preparation, which contains a single channel, now has been exposed to a low concentration of the alkaloid ryanodine (0.01 μmol/L) from the cytosolic surface. For the first time, a current level other than the unitary conductance is observed. Solid lines show the closed state conductance and the unitary conductance, dashed line shows the new conductance state. This is a subconductance state of the channel. Note that when the (single) channel opens to the subconductance state, the opening is longer than when it opens to the unitary conductance state. Evidently, the opening and closing of this subconductance state is governed differently than the opening and closing to the unitary conductance state; mechanistically, the channel acts as if it is "locked open" in the subconductance state for longer periods of time. (3) Exposure to a higher concentration of the alkaloid (0.05 μmol/L). About one-third of the way into the tracing, the channel opens into its subconductance state. This one opening lasts through the end of the tracing. (4) A higher concentration of the alkaloid. A long opening into the subconductance state ends, there is a long closed period and then the channel opens again into the subconductance state with its long openings and closings. (5 and 6) Perfusion with Ca^{2+}-free buffer and repeated exposure to 100 μmol/L Ca^{2+} fail to restore the channel to its basal state. The channel appears to be locked open in its subconductance state by the alkaloid ryanodine. In summary, A is a nice demonstration of subconductance states and how their gating properties (opening and closing kinetics) typically differ from those of the unitary conductance state of the channel. It should not be concluded that it is necessary to add a foreign substance to observe subconductance state behavior. The alkaloid ryanodine merely stabilizes a subconductance state intrinsically present in the channel. Subconductance states are common in ion channels and obviously are important in their regulation. (**B**) Shows that the calcium release channel of the sarcoplasmic reticulum (the RyR) in fact has multiple subconductance states, brought out here by ryanodine. In the last panel ruthenium red is shown to close the channel. Reproduced with permission from Reference 149.

DC component deviate from 0 and in fact progressively increase in time. This abolishes contraction and leads to a Ca^{2+} overload state in the cytosol that by various mechanisms may be deleterious to the cell.

In normal cardiac function, RyR calcium channel opening is activated by cytoplasmic Ca^{2+}, whose source is the L-type channel of the sarcolemma [so-called calcium-induced calcium release (CICR)]. The increased local $[Ca^{2+}]_i$ increases the open probability of the RyR channel and brings on the state of multiple reopenings and interaction with FK-506.12BP, which stabilizes this high-conductance state with rapid gating (in some ways the opposite effect to ryanodine), a mechanism well documented for RyR1 but possibly true as well for RyR2.[9] Between the L-type calcium channel of the sarcolemma and the RyR (whose conductance is triggered by local increase in the calcium concentration because of the influx of calcium from the L-type calcium channel) there appears to exist a privileged communication. Thus the calcium concentration rises first (because of calcium influx through the L-type calcium channel) in some sort of sequestered space that extends to the cytoplasmic aspect of the RyR.

The FK-506 binding protein involved in the regulation of the channel is one of the soluble FK-506 receptors, FK-506.12BP. This is a *cis-trans* peptidyl-prolyl isomerase whose function in other cells where it is expressed (eg, T cells) is related to Ca^{2+} concentration. There FK-506 and similar agents (eg, rapamycin) bind to the protein, removing it from the RyR; and this complex is an inhibitor of calcineurin, a phosphatase important in T-cell activation. All that is known about its function in the heart cell is that it appears to stabilize energetically the high-conductance-subconductance state of the RyR.

As noted previously, the RyR of working heart muscle is RyR2. The RyR3 isoform also exists in heart but appears to be localized to the conduction tissue. RyR1 is the RyR of skeletal muscle. Mutations in RyR1 are associated with the predisposition to malignant hyperthermia via an effect on skeletal muscle. The brain channels include as well RyR3, which may be involved in nonspecific cell death mechanisms including excitotoxicity (reviewed below). RyR2 also is found in neural tissues. Structurally, the RyR of heart is similar to the RyRs of other tissues, with important points of difference, including absence of sensitivity to Mg^{2+}, the lack of a direct functional coupling with the L-type calcium channel of the sarcolemma (the dihydropyridine receptor) as exists in skeletal muscle RyR RyR1, and reduced caffeine sensitivity (in comparison with RyR3). Functionally, the RyR

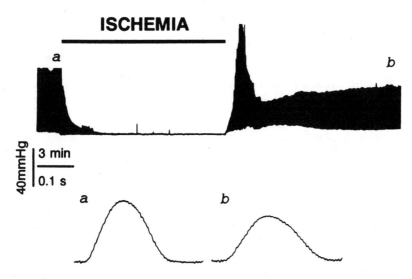

Figure 7. Stunning in the isolated perfused ferret heart. The upper panel shows a continuous record of isovolumic left ventricular (LV) pressure before, during, and after 15-minute ischemia. Reperfusion leads to a period of arrhythmia punctuated with potentiated beats, after which contractile pressure reaches a quasi steady-state value distinctly lower than control. Two systoles are displayed in the lower panel at a different timescale, one sampled before (**A**) and one sampled after (**B**) ischemia. The postischemic depression of pressure generation apparent in B is stunning. Reproduced with permission from Reference 14.

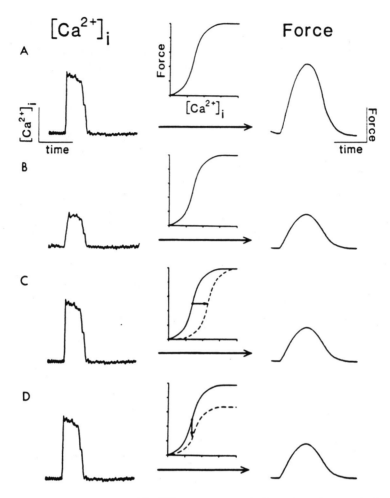

Figure 8. Schematic representation of $[Ca^{2+}]_i$ versus time (left) force (far right) and the $[Ca^{2+}]_i$-force relation (middle). (**A**) Control. (**B**) Effect of decreasing the amplitude of the $[Ca^{2+}]_i$ transient, other things being equal. (**C**) Effect of a shift in myofilament sensitivity (Compare control relation, drawn as a solid curve, to the shifted, dashed curve). (**D**) Effect of a decrease in maximal Ca^{2+}-activated force. By way of anticipation, the Marban data support a combination of C and D as the mechanism of stunning, with no component of B. Reproduced with permission from Reference 12.

Figure 9. Time course of intracellular calcium concentration in normal and stunned myocardium in the postischemic ferret model. Myocardium is loaded with the fluorinated (^{19}F) nuclear magnetic resonance (NMR) Ca^{2+} indicator 5,5'-difluoro-1,2-bis(2-aminophenoxy)-ethane-N,N,N',N'-tetraacetic acid (5F-BAPTA). According to the chemical equation $bound_{5F-BAPTA} = Ca^{2+} + free_{5F-BAPTA}$ and the equilibrium constant $[Ca^{2+}]_i$ $[free_{5F-BAPTA}]/[bound_{5F-BAPTA}] = K_d = 0.285$ $\mu mol/L$, it is possible to calculate $[Ca^{2+}]_i$ from the NMR spectroscopic signals corresponding to $[bound_{5F-BAPTA}]$ and to $[free_{5F-BAPTA}]$, which appear at 8 and 2 ppm, respectively. The equation is rewritten $[Ca^{2+}]_i = K_d \cdot [bound_{5F-BAPTA}]/[free_{5F-BAPTA}]$. Thus the time course of $[Ca^{2+}]_i$ (**C**) is determined from gated NMR spectra for diastole (**A**) and systole (**B**) from control (left) and stunned (right) data. The ratio of signal at 8 ppm to that at 2 ppm clearly increases in systole as compared with diastole, both for control and for stunned hearts. $[Ca^{2+}]_i$ is proportional to this ratio and curves C are thereby constructed. It is seen that the calcium transient in stunned muscle is

continued

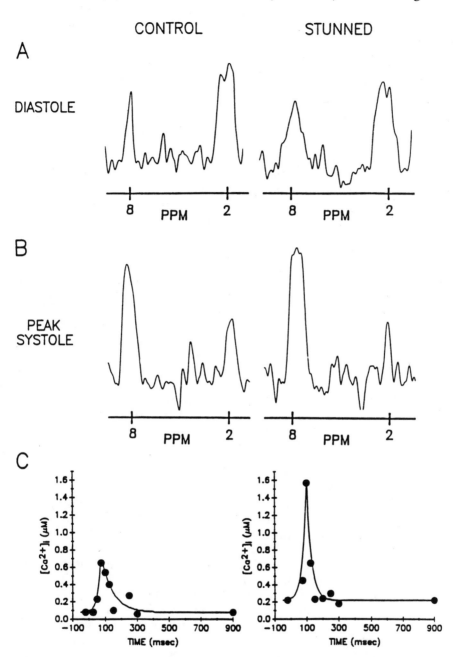

CONTROL   STUNNED

A

DIASTOLE

8   PPM   2   8   PPM   2

B

PEAK
SYSTOLE

8   PPM   2   8   PPM   2

C

Figure 9. *(continued)* similar to or greater than that of control muscle. These data have been interpreted to show that the availability of activator Ca^{2+} is not decreased and indeed may be increased in stunned myocardium. This technique of intracellular $[Ca^{2+}]$ determination involves supraphysiological total $[Ca^{2+}]$ concentration because of the low dissociation constant of 5F-BAPTA. The total Ca is increased to an arbitrary endpoint of four times normal, though a priori 10–11 times normal might be more appropriate given conservative assumptions based on the dissociation constant and the system. Also, reduction of temperature and probenecid are used to limit 5F-BAPTA extrusion; yet it is not known whether there exist differential effects subsequent to these interventions on control versus stunned cells. These different considerations open the possibility of unquantitated artifact and biased $[Ca^{2+}]_i$ signal sampling. Reproduced with permission from Reference 13.

can take the place of other Ca^{2+} release channels in tissues that ordinarily lack RyR's as Ca^{2+} release channel.

The fundamental phenomenon of CICR is effectuated by Ca^{2+}-induced opening of the RyR2, where the Ca^{2+} that activates the RyR entered the cell via the sarcolemmal L-type calcium channel (the dihydropyridine receptor).

The effects of ischemia and stunning on the structure and function of the RyR remain obscure but may not be significant.

In ischemia the Ca^{2+} transient is reduced, presumably consequent to reduced L-type Ca channel current, and the RyR plays no primary role. (Similar results may apply to hibernation; a discussion of that process is beyond the scope of the present chapter.)

To understand stunning, it is useful to review a series of investigations of Marban and coworkers where these investigators used a postischemic ferret whole-heart preparation as well as an isolated rat trabecula preparation to model stunning[10-20] (Fig. 7). The models permit hemodynamic comparison of postischemic with normal myocardium with determination of pH and $[Ca^{2+}]_i$ by nuclear magnetic resonance (NMR) spectroscopy or fluorometry. After appropriate loading with an NMR indicator of intracellular Ca^{2+} [bis-(o-aminophenoxy)-N,N,N',N'-tetraacetic acid (5F-BAPTA)] in the ferret model, it is possible to quantitate intracellular calcium transients with high temporal resolution (regrettably at the cost of foregoing the possibility of maintaining the tissue in the physiological range of Ca^{2+} concentrations, because the calcium indicator 5F-BAPTA requires supraphysiological total Ca^{2+} concentrations for use). A similar model also has been used to study the effect of hypoxia on myocardial function.

The studies sought to distinguish the mechanism of stunning-related depression of contractile function of the left ventricle, based on the hypothesis that depressed function was caused by one of the following three mechanisms: reduced activator Ca^{2+}, reduced maximal Ca^{2+}-activated force, or reduced myofilament sensitivity to Ca^{2+} (Fig. 8). The first possible mechanism is translatable into a hypothesis that can be framed within the scope of the present chapter; that is, is the L-type Ca^{2+}-current-induced RyR2 Ca^{2+} transient depressed in this model of stunning?

In brief, the findings are that the peak cytosolic $[Ca^{2+}]$ in the postischemic model is not reduced; in fact it is either identical to or higher than control (Figs. 9 and 10). The Marban data suggest that the aggregate conductance may not be reduced significantly in stunning or early stunning. Additional points to note, in using those data, include the lack of documented full recovery of contractile function in their class of models (though the protocol was not designed to document complete similarity to clinical stunning), the presence of some degree of Ca^{2+} paradox, and the appearance of reduced maximal Ca^{2+}-activated force (though preload is not controlled in these experiments) as well as other abnormalities of the force-$[Ca^{2+}]$ curve. The latter two findings are of uncertain interpretation; reduced myofilament sensitivity is possible. Other possibilities include degradation of contractile proteins, poorly coordinated contraction, or loss of excited tissue mass. However, the key finding of normal activator Ca^{2+} reduces the likelihood that any significant abnormality of the L-type Ca^{2+} channel and RyR2 coordinated function exists in stunning in all heart cells, at least in the early stages of stunning.

Similar experiments conducted in hypoxia implicate reduced $[ATP]_i$ and acidosis in the loss of contractile function in no-flow ischemia.

Hyperkalemia (elevated $[K^+]_o$) and the mild elevations of resting potential are not believed to have significant effects on RyR function.

It is interesting to note that in isolated sarcoplasmic reticulum, lipophilic substances induce a Ca^{2+} conductance. This may be relevant to ischemia and stunning, because increased lipids and lipid metabolite concentrations are present in and around the cell from the onset of ischemia.[21] However, this conductance has not been demonstrated to

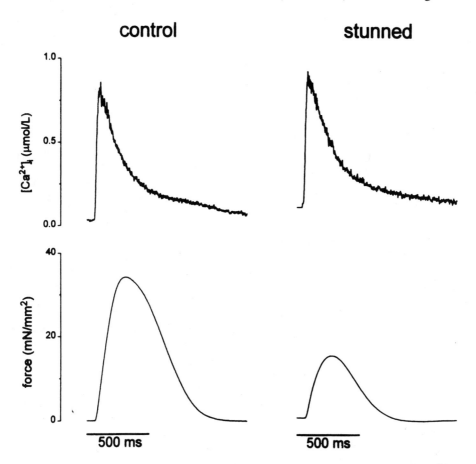

Figure 10. Myocardial stunning in an isolated rat trabeculae model. Intracellular Ca^{2+} transients and force development from a control heart (left) and a stunned heart (right). The trabeculae were kept in Krebs' buffer at 1 mmol/L $[Ca^{2+}]_o$. Peak values for force per unit area were 39.9 mN/mm² in the control and 18.8 mN/mm² in the stunned trabecula. Peak $[Ca^{2+}]_i$ transients were 0.81 μmol/L in the control and 0.88 μmol/L in the stunned trabeculae. Despite a remarkable similarity of the amplitude and configuration of the Ca^{2+} transient, force generation was depressed significantly in the stunned trabeculae as compared with the control trabeculae. The control had never been subjected to ischemia. The technique of intracellular $[Ca^{2+}]$ determination involved Fura-2 loading via the gap junction after microiontophoretic application to a single cell. Therefore, the calcium concentration versus time curves reflect only coupled cells, a factor of uncertain significance but possibly artifactually biasing the sampling. Reproduced with permission from Reference 150.

be related to the RyR. Experiments conducted in other systems demonstrate no excess conductance from sarcoplasmic reticulum in relation to lipid perfusion.

As the source of cytoplasmic calcium in adult cardiac tissue, this channel is involved in late stages of Ca^{2+} overload believed to mediate progression to cell death. This is a component of the late phase of stunning and will be discussed later.

Although not within the scope of this chapter, in ischemic preconditioning a speculative role exists for the RyR: a transient reduction of RyR channels may offset a deficiency in oxalate-supported Ca^{2+}-adenosine triphosphatase (ATPase) activity or excessive leak.

Cl^- Channels of the Sarcoplasmic Reticulum

Three chloride channels of the sarcoplasmic reticulum have been documented in cardiac and skeletal muscle preparations.[22-24] Unlike the familiar Na^+, Ca^{2+}, and K^+ channels of the sarcolemma, which are cation channels, chloride (Cl^-) channels are anion channels and have different characteristics.

The smallest of the three channels is a 50- to 75-picosiemens channel[23,25,26] at negative cytosolic potentials in lipid bilayers with short brief openings and flicker with apparent voltage dependence.[25] Its structure is unknown. In the physiological state it is activated by extrasarcoplasmic reticular [Cl^-], that is, intracellular (cytosolic) chloride concentration [Cl^-]. The channel has the noteworthy property of poor permeation selectivity and admits cations including Ca^{2+}.[23] Permeation selectivity is 1:0.3 Cl^-:Ca^{2+}. Indeed it may function as a calcium channel more important for basal Ca^{2+} conductance than the RyR itself; in the absence of RyR stimulation it appears responsible for a greater Ca^{2+} conductance than the RyR. It does not appear to be involved in volume regulation or charge neutralization. Ca^{2+} may traverse the channel in association with two Cl^- ions. Pharmacologic blockers include ruthenium red and clofibric acid but it is not affected by anthracene-9-carboxylic acid nor by diphenylaminecarboxylate or 4,4'-diisothiocyano-stilbene-2,2'-disulfonic acid (DIDS), typical blockers of Cl^- channels.[23] Its conductance is distinct from that of the RyR but may or may not represent a current pathway entirely independent of the RyR; it may share a final common conductance problem with RyR, the site of ruthenium red block.

The next largest of the channels is a 70- to 116-picosiemens channel, structure unknown,[24] with long open times and rectification that would favor Cl^- sarcoplasmic reticulum to cytosolic transit (outward rectifying in lipid bilayers where *cis* chamber is cytosol). Its chloride conductance is very sensitive to rundown but is reactivated by phosphorylation [protein kinase A (PKA)].[24] It is not [Ca^{2+}]$_i$ or voltage dependent. Pharmacologic blockers include DNDS.

The largest of the channels governs a 200- to 400-picosiemen Cl^- conductance, structure unknown, permeation selectivity unknown. Voltage dependence has been reported.[27]

Although not studied in ischemia and stunning, the presence of a clofibric acid-sensitive Ca^{2+}-conducting anion channel not regulated by Ca^{2+} or (indirectly) by voltage raises the question of whether there exists a high-conductance pathway for egress of Ca^{2+} from the sarcoplasmic reticulum independent of the normal oscillatory Ca^{2+} RyR excitation-contraction mechanism. Such a pathway may be of great significance in later phases of stunning.

Sarcolemmal Channels

L-Type Calcium Channel (Dihydropyridine Receptor)

The L-type Ca^{2+} channel of cardiac tissue is a voltage-gated calcium channel that admits depolarizing calcium current and thereby prolongs the action potential duration. In cardiac tissue this increase in cytosolic [Ca^{2+}]$_i$ triggers opening of the RyR (CICR), which leads to contraction of the myocyte.

The L-type calcium channel is composed of several subunits: the α_1-subunit ($\sim$170 kd), the $\alpha_2\delta$ ($\sim$140 kd), and the β ($\sim$55 kd); in skeletal muscle γ-subunit ($\sim$33 kd) is present as well (Fig. 11). In this it is like all other sarcolemmal Ca channels, of which six are known to date: the L-type, the T-type, the P-type, the N-type, the R-type, and the

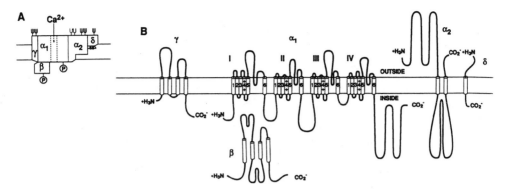

Figure 11. Subunit structure of L-type Ca^{2+} channel. (**A**) Model of the L-type channel derived from biochemical experiments. (**B**) Transmembrane folding models of the Ca^{2+} channel subunits derived from primary structure determination and analysis. Cylinders represent predicted α-helical segments in the transmembrane region of the α_1-, α_2-, δ-, and γ-subunits and in the peripherally associated β-subunit. The transmembrane folding pattern for the α_1-subunit is derived in analogy with the current models for the structures of Na^+ and K^+ channels. The α_1-subunit is the pore. (P, sites of cAMP-dependent protein phosphorylation; ψ, N-linked glycosylation.) This figure is based on the model for the first L-type channel successfully analyzed, that of the skeletal muscle. Reproduced with permission from Reference 151.

putative Q-type.[28] These are distinguished by their tissue distribution, ligands, and pharmacologic blockers, as well as by differing voltage gating characteristics. All have these coimmunoprecipitating subunits; in rare tissue types an additional constituent polypeptide has been found.[29]

The α_1-subunit constitutes the channel itself and in expressed systems can function as a pore even in isolation.[30] This subunit (α_{1C} in cardiac muscle) has four homologous repeating segments (repeats), each composed of six transmembrane segments with a charged moiety likely constituting the voltage sensor and another segment constituting part (one-fourth) of the lining of the pore. The structure bears substantial homology to those of the voltage-sensitive K^+ channels and the Na^+ channel, although in the K^+ channel the four repeats surrounding the channel pore lie on separate polypeptides. Like the voltage-gated K^+ channels, the sarcolemmal Ca^{2+} channels are exemplars of a gene superfamily subclassified by (cDNA) sequence homology. In the classification of Numa, the cardiac L-type channel is identified as class C, in contradistinction to the skeletal muscle channel (class Sk) and the neuronal (and pancreatic) L-type channel (class BIV). In other classifications encountered in the literature, the cardiac is Snutch class C or Perez-Reyes class 2.

The unitary conductance of the cardiac L-type calcium channel appears to be 6.9 picosiemens at physiological Ca^{2+} concentrations (Fig. 12) and is characterized by brief openings. It is a voltage-gated current activating at relatively high (depolarized) voltages. The current is characterized in cardiac tissue by rapid activation kinetics and relatively rapid apparent inactivation of a component of the whole-cell current. Skeletal L-type Ca current activates more slowly. The skeletal isoform also inactivates much more slowly (though still not as slowly as the L-type neuronal channel).

A component of the current in whole-cell studies appears as a sustained current. The basis of the sustained inward current is multiple reopenings of the channel (Fig. 12). Because the brief openings tend to be clustered either early or late the subpopulation of channels where the openings are clustered early can produce the appearance of a peak followed by inactivation. The remainder of the channels produce the sustained inward current, by their multiple reopenings.[31]

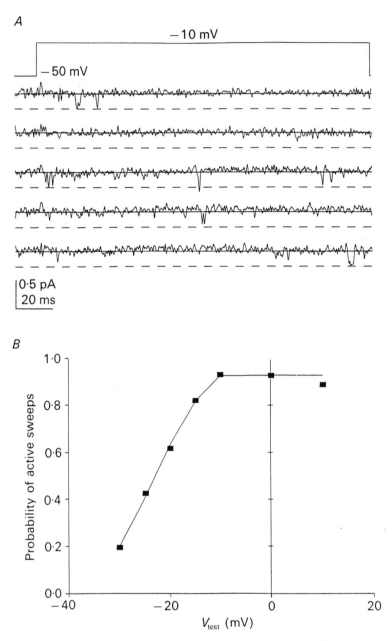

Figure 12. Cardiac L-type Ca^{2+} channel current. (**A**) Single channel current through L-type Ca^{2+} channel during depolarizations to −10 mV in the guinea pig heart. Openings are represented by deflections downward. Note multiple reopenings of the same channel during the same current pulse. each opening is brief. Summation of the late openings among the approximately 28 000 L-type Ca^{2+} channels in the typical ventricular myocyte are what underlie the sustained or "pedestal" inward current. (**B**) Probability of at least one opening per depolarizing pulse at test pulse (v_{test}) voltages from −30 mV to +10 mV. Ca^{2+} is the charge carrier; these data are derived with $[Ca^{2+}]_i$ in the physiological range. Reproduced with permission from Reference 31.

The open probability of the cardiac L-type calcium channel is increased by depolarizations from potentials to -40 to -60 mV, which encompasses the normal membrane potential range of activation of the channel. Phosphorylation at α_{1C}- and β-subunit sites has varying effects. Palmitoyl-L-carnitine increases open probability but may decrease single channel conductance in a later phase; arachidonic acid also depresses L-type channel conductance but by an undetermined mechanism. Pharmacologic agents that function as channel openers include Bay K 2644, FPL64176, and $+-(S)$-202–791.[32] The channel is blocked pharmacologically by agents of the 1,4-dihydropyridine class (eg, nimoldipine and nifedipine) as well as by drugs of phenylalkylamine (eg, verapamil, D600, its methoxy, and D800, a quaternary derivative) and benzothiazepine types; the latter two classes bind to a different site than the 1,4-dihydropyridines. Block by phenylalkylamines and dihydropyridines is not specific to Ca^{2+} channels; the delayed rectifier K^+ channel is blocked by the former and Na^+ (and some K^+) channels by the latter, reflecting perhaps their related structures noted above. Ca^{2+}-dependent inactivation is well described. Another condition of cardiac L-type channel inactivation is exposure to Cd^{2+}.

This channel extends the period of inward current and in cardiac tissue admits the Ca^{2+} that initiates excitation-contraction coupling by secondarily triggering Ca^{2+} release from the sarcoplasmic reticulum (Fig. 2). In a remarkable piece of work Tanabe[30,33] constructed chimeric L-type Ca^{2+} channel proteins to investigate the determinants of cardiac in comparison to skeletal gating. In control and in muscle tissue from $mdg/mdg-$ mice (skeletal L-type calcium channel-deficient) repleted with skeletal cDNA, normal excitation-contraction coupling was restored that was $[Ca^{2+}]_i$ independent, typical for normal skeletal muscle, and skeletal L-type calcium channel current (slow activation and slow inactivation of whole cell current) was confirmed. In contrast, the insertion and expression of the cardiac gene led to a form of excitation-contraction coupling alien to the normal skeletal muscle cell, with contraction dependent on Ca^{2+} entry, implying CICR from an intracellular store induced by the channel. These data further imply that the L-type calcium channel protein isoform is what determines cardiac as opposed to skeletal muscle behavior, and that the RyR isoform does not have the property of specifying tissue characteristics. In the expressed $mdg/mdg-$ system, the same research group made the further observation that myotubes from constructs that included one or more of skeletal or cardiac internal repeats behaved in one of only two ways: either like normal skeletal excitation-contraction coupling if the first internal repeat was skeletal, that is, $[Sk]$-$[X]$-$[X]$-$[X]$, (where X can be skeletal Sk or cardiac C with no effect on phenotype) or like normal cardiac excitation-contraction coupling with CICR from an internal calcium store, if the first internal repeat was cardiac, that is, $[C]$-$[X]$-$[X]$-$[X]$. The experiments show that a specific moiety of the L-type channel protein subunit (the first internal repeat) can confer the characteristic properties (eg, cardiac) of excitation-contraction coupling on the excitable cell. Skeletal excitation-contraction coupling does not use a Ca^{2+} signal; rather a direct protein-protein interaction of the L-type calcium channel with the RyR occurs.

The relevance of the myocardial L-type Ca^{2+} channel to ischemia and stunning is unclear. The effects probably are indirect and minor. By actions on nonmyocyte tissues, specifically the smooth muscle of the cardiac vasculature, the role of this channel in modulating ischemia is of course well documented, as is the action of blockers of this channel in avoiding ischemia.[34] In the heart muscle cell pharmacologic blockade of this channel is hypothesized to limit buildup of intracellular Ca^{2+} and thereby reduce stunning. The data argue that the contribution of this effect is mild in early stunning.

T-Type Ca^{2+} Channel

Although in cardiac tissue the ubiquitous L-type channel is of greatest importance, T-type channels also have been found to be present in many regions. It has similar heteromultimeric composition. Its α_1-subunit is the α_{1G}.

The T-type channel is a calcium channel with lower single channel conductance ($\sim$8 picosiemens in high $[Ca^{2+}]$ and 4–5 picosiemens in 10 mmol/L $[Ca^{2+}]$[35]) than the L-type channel, with faster activation and inactivation and insensitivity to 1,4-dihydropyridine agents and Cd^{2+}. The channel is blocked nonspecifically by amiloride (which also blocks epithelial Na^+ channels), octanol (which also blocks gap junctions and other channels), mibefradil (Ro 40–5967), and Ni^{2+}. It is activated by lesser depolarizations from normal resting potential than are necessary for opening L-type channels, and because of steady-state inactivation, there is no available T-type current at moderately depolarized potentials ($>$-50 mV). It is the only low-voltage–activated calcium channel described to date, distinguishing it from types L, N, P, R, and Q.

It is unlikely to be important in normal cellular electrophysiology of working myocardium for humans and higher animals. It has not been investigated in ischemia or stunning.

P-Type Ca^{2+} Channel

The message for P-type channels has been documented in cardiac tissue but its α_{1A}-subunit mRNA is distributed most generally in the brain and particularly in cerebellar Purkinje cells. The P-type channel (Numa class BI, Snutch class A, Perez-Reyes class 4; 16 picosiemens with Ba^{2+} as charge carrier) is characterized by high-voltage–activation kinetics, similar to L-type channels but with complete insensitivity to typical L-type channel blockers, for example, 1,4-dihydropyridines. Indeed, as concentrations of blockers such as nitrendipine are increased, Na^+ channels are blocked nonspecifically at concentrations where P-type channels remain unaffected. It is insensitive to ω-conotoxin.

P-type channels are blocked specifically by ω-agatoxin (ω-Aga-IVA) and blocked partially by ω-Aga-IIIA. Although the channel itself has not yet been observed by electrophysiological techniques, the presence of P-type channel message in cardiac tissue (rabbit) was first documented by Mori[36] and later by Starr.[37] Expression and function have not been studied in ischemia and stunning.

P-type channels are found more commonly in neural tissue. Indeed, in neurons all Ca^{2+} channel types have been observed, including a fourth N-type channel, blocked by ω-conotoxin (ω-CTx-IVA), a fifth R-type channel, partially blocked by ω-Aga-IIIA and mibefradil, and the putative Q-type, less sensitive than the P-type to ω-Aga-IVA. The N-type channel governs the bulk of Ca^{2+} current of intracardiac neurons.[38] These will not be discussed further at this time.

K^+ Channels

A diverse set of K currents exists. Important ones among these include the inward rectifier K channel i_{K1} (associated with the h1RK1 or Kir2.1 channel), the delayed rectifier currents i_{Kr} and i_{Ks}, the transient outward current, and the ATP-sensitive K current $i_{K,ATP}$ (associated with the KCNJ5 channel). However, there exist more channels than currents.[39–43] It is difficult in 2000 to assign with certainty the currents to the responsible channels for human heart, because of important species differences, as well as topographical, study-to-study, and possibly developmental differences.

Inward Rectifier (i_{K1}, hIRK1, HH-1RK1, and Kir2.1). The inward rectifier current (i_{K1}, i_{bg}, $i_{K,rec}$, and Kir2.1) is an inward K^+ current active during repolarization.[44] In repolarization, the current is active subsequent to two other potassium currents that will be discussed shortly, i_{to} and i_K[45-47] (Fig. 13).

It is a tetramer that has two rather than six transmembrane loops. Its structure differs from that of other K^+ channels, specifically from that of the voltage-gated K^+ channels, which among the K^+ channels most resemble the L-type Ca^{2+} channel already discussed. It is structurally related to two other K^+ channels, those underlying the ATP-sensitive K^+ channel ($i_{K,ATP}$) and the muscarinic receptor–gated K^+ channel ($i_{K,Ach}$). (The same direction of current physiologically characterizes one delayed rectifier, the hERG channel, though the molecular basis for this physiology is different, resembling that of certain neuronal channels, but not the cardiac channels of this Kir group.)

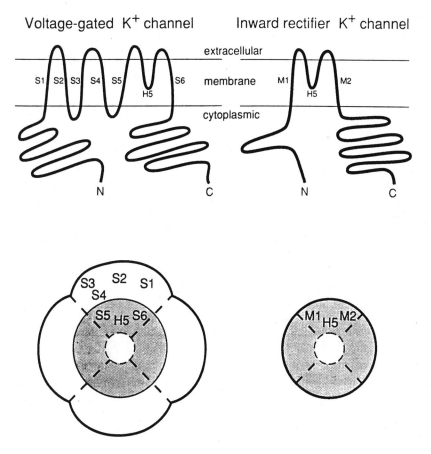

Figure 13. This figure contrasts voltage-gated K^+ channel structure (**left**) with the structure of the inward rectifier K^+ channel. Although both channel types have four subunits, the transmembrane topology is very different. In the voltage-gated K^+ channels (**right**), which resemble very closely the L-type Ca^{2+} as well as the Na^+ channels, there are six membrane spanning domains, with an inner shell consisting of the S5, H5, and S6 segments that contribute to the pore. An outer shell consists of the S1, S2, S3, and S4 α-helical membrane-spanning segments. By contrast, in the inward rectifier K^+ channel no structure resembling the latter segments appears to exist. Transmembrane segments are limited to the M1, M2, and H5 segments; the latter is the chief constituent of the pore. Reproduced with permission from Reference 96.

At physiological $[K^+]_o$ in guinea pig it is a 3.6- to 10-picosiemens inward channel at potentials more negative than the K^+ equilibrium potential, and it is strongly inwardly rectifying. Channels of this class have a conductance varying as the square root of the $[K^+]$[48,48a] and consistent with this, when studied at high $[K^+]$ the single channel conductance increases to 32 picosiemens.

The channel has multiple subconductance states (Fig. 14) and two distinct gating modes.

Cs^+ is an open channel blocker. The current is reduced in conditions of reduced $[ATP]_i$. In the normal functioning of the channel, rectification occurs because of spermine (and other polyamines) and Mg^{2+} binding.

Certain properties of this current are important at the time of the action potential plateau, that is, at depolarized potentials. In contradistinction to the familiar delayed rectifier K^+ channel of invertebrate neurophysiology, the channels underlying the i_{K1} have characteristics that prolong action potential duration, specifically reduced permeation of K^+ ions at depolarized potentials.

This is the channel chiefly responsible for the resting membrane K^+ conductance of cardiac muscle and determines the resting potential of the tissue, which is the basis for its relevance to ischemia and stunning. Its current is active during the resting phase and in repolarization subsequent to i_{to} and i_K; in light of the reduced delayed rectifier current in human tissue in normal physiology[49]; it may be the most important channel in late repolarization and the resting phase. It appears to be gated by Cs^+ and Ba^{2+} and its current is reduced in conditions of reduced $[ATP]$ intracellularly,[50] unlike the ATP-

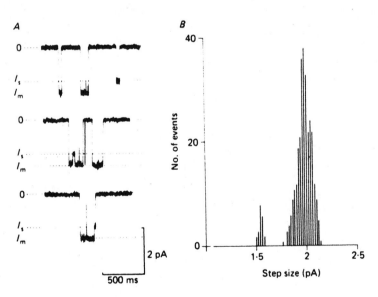

Figure 14. The most common subconductance state of the inward rectifier K^+ channel in guinea pig heart cells. (**A**)Recording with 145 mmol/L KCl in the patch pipette. The patch membrane potential was −80 mV. The dotted line marked 0 indicate the zero current level (channel closed). The current jumps to two other levels as indicated by the two other dotted lines. The main level I_m is observed most frequently; this larger step-size value represents the main conductance state of the channel. The current level I_s is a subconductance state. It is the subconductance state most frequently observed, occurring either as a single step (upper trace), as a step from and back to the main level (middle trace), or at the end (lower trace) or beginning of a sojourn at the main level. (**B**) Distribution of current levels from data such as A. The number of events represents the number of main and sublevel amplitudes observed irrespective of the way in which the current reached the level. Reproduced with permission from Reference 48.

sensitive K^+ channel. The G-protein $G_{\gamma s}$ may reduce its conductance via activation of a phosphatase, though other reports document reduced conductance caused by β-adrenergic activation, with guanosine triphosphate $(GTP_{\gamma s})$ and $G_{i\alpha}$ (acetylcholine stimulation) causing reversal of this.

A human inward rectifier hIRK1 has been cloned and studied at high $[K^+]$. It is reported to have a single channel conductance of 28 picosiemens[51] with similar current-voltage relations; a similar channel has been recorded from atrial myocytes[52] in humans (Fig. 15). Noteworthy are the long openings of this channel, lasting as long as seconds.

This class of channels has not been shown to play a major direct role in ischemia and stunning, though similar channels in nervous tissue play a role mediating excitotoxicity (see below). That polyamines accumulate in cell injury is a fact of no significance for this channel, though it may be important for other channels gated by binding of these polycationic amino acid catabolites. However, by passively setting the resting potential, this channel is involved indirectly in an important sequence of changes (important to the Na^+ channel) that occur in ischemia subsequent to the increase in $[K^+]_o$.

i_{Kto} (i_{qr}). The transient outward current of the cardiac myocyte has been demonstrated to be carried partly by K^+ ions. At least two channels underlie this repolarizing current, which is active at depolarized potentials. It is 4-aminopyridine sensitive in part i_{to1} and is known to be regulated by phosphorylation. The channel apears to be in the Kv4.3 group of voltage-gated K^+ channels. It resides primarily in the epicardium and is responsible for the slight dip toward hyperpolarized potentials early in the action potential plateau. It is not responsible for modulation of action potential duration in ischemia.

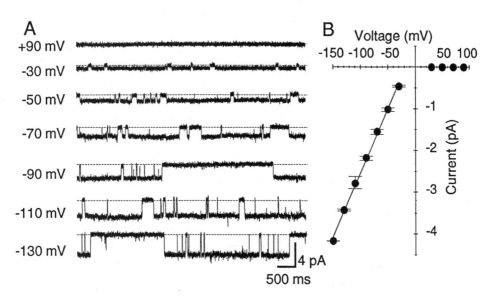

Figure 15. Single channel currents from HH-IRK1 expressed in *Xenopus* oocytes. (**A**) Single channel current recordings from a cell-attached patch held at the indicated voltages. (**B**) Single channel current versus voltage relation. The points on the x axis signify the absence of outward current at potentials positive to the K^+ equilibrium potential. This behavior is consistent with an inwardly rectifying channel, and this human channel is believed to be the cardiac inward rectifier channel. Note the long openings. Reproduced with permission from Reference 51.

Delayed Rectifier K Currents i_K (i_{Kr} and i_{Ks}). A plethora of channels have been identified that may underlie components of this current,[53-61] which is of uncertain significance in normal human electrophysiology[49] but is extremely important in that it is the locus of effect of drugs (eg, Vaughan Williams class III antiarrhythmic agents such as amiodarone) and of some mutations that underlie the congenital long QT syndrome. This current activates at depolarized potentials (Fig. 16). In normal tissue there are at least two distinct whole-cell currents that contribute to i_K, namely, i_{Kr} and i_{Ks}, distinguishable by kinetics as well as by antiarrhythmic drug sensitivity (eg, E-4031). (A developmentally modulated ultrarapid component i_{Kur} may exist as well.) The current is viewed classically as exhibiting the pattern of rectification where outward cation currents are enhanced (in contrast to the opposite behavior observed in the previously described inward rectifier channel, which has been called "anomalous rectification").

Several distinct and well-characterized channels exist in heart that appear to govern components of this current. KvLQT1/minK ia a heteromer that underlies the slow component i_{Ks}, and hERG (KvLQT2,erg1; possibly also modulated by minK association) underlies the rapidly activating current i_{Kr}. Possibly distinct channels homologous to *Drosophila* (fruit fly) *shaker*, termed Kv1.5 channels, further include the fHK (identical to the hPCN.1 and HK_2 channels) and the HK_1 channels. In atrium alone, a fifth well-characterized channel i_{RAK} is found.

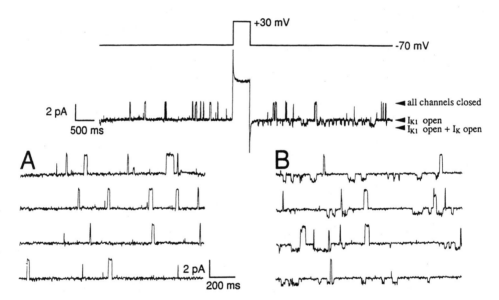

Figure 16. Delayed rectifier channel. This channel recording demonstrates a protocol to elicit voltage-gated K^+ channel activity on a background of inward rectifier (i_{K1}, a K^+ channel that is not voltage gated) channel opening with very high i_{K1} channel open probability. Single channel currents recorded from a cell-attached patch of rabbit cardiac myocyte membrane at -70 mV before and directly after a depolarizing pulse step to $+30$ mV (pulse of 500-millisecond duration). Channel openings are seen as downward deflections. (**Top**) Voltage protocol with example of original current tracing. I_{K1}, inward rectifier current; I_K, delayed rectifier current. (**A**) Four current tracings before a depolarizing step with only I_{K1} channel activity. (**B**) Four current tracings directly after a depolarizing step. Voltage-gated channel activity is now present, seen as openings of smaller current amplitude (downward implies channel opening) that are initially frequent and then fewer and fewer. This is a voltage-gated channel with inactivation. Note the different kinetics as well as amplitudes of the two channels: I_{K1}, inward rectifier currents characterized by extremely long opening and relatively large amplitude (in this protocol); I_K, by brief relatively small openings clustered in time after the voltage pulse. Reproduced with permission from Reference 152.

The channels all share the same basic topology with four identical subunits, each of which has six membrane-spanning domains (S1–6) with the pore localized between S5 and S6 (Fig. 13).The pore is formed chiefly by a highly conserved linker region between the S5 and S6 segments[62] (Fig. 17). Important modulation results from association with the minK (hISK) peptide, previously thought to represent a channel in its own right.[63–65]

The channels will be discussed separately as follows:

KvLQT1/minK. This channel is believed to underlie the slow delayed rectifier. Mutations in either peptide cause the typically autosomal recessive long QT syndrome, type I. These mutations are the most important cause of the long QT syndrome.

hERG (KvLQT2,erg1). This is an important distinct human delayed rectifier channel.[66–68] Mutations in this channel have been proven to underlie some cases of autosomal dominant long QT syndrome (Romano-Ward variant). Structurally, the channel is similar to the *Drosophila* $i_{K,eag}$ channel. It exhibits increased open probability when extracellular potassium concentration $[K^+]_o$ is elevated. It exhibits inward rectification [sic] caused by unusual voltage-dependent inactivation kinetics.[69,70] Rapid inactivation facilitates inward rectification by timing channel opening with a period of net inward electrochemical gradient. Pharmacologic blockers of this channel differ from those of other K^+ channels (Fig. 18). It is important in ischemia and stunning because of the increased outward current in the presence of elevated $[K^+]_o$, which enhances repolarization in the presence of a pathological accumulation of extracellular K^+, as occurs in ischemia. This could be an independent contributing factor to action potential shortening in ischemia.

Kv1.5: fHK (hPCN.1, HK_2). This was the first cardiac channel described that is a member of the class of voltage-gated K channels bearing homology to the K^+ channel superfamily whose characteristics were first sketched out in *Drosophila* the fruit fly. *Drosophila* K^+ channels include multiple families related to the gene prod-

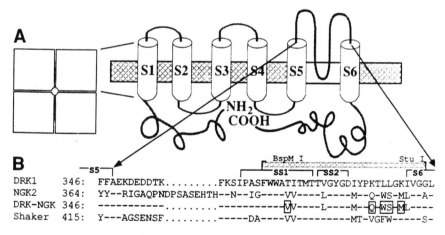

Figure 17. This figure from Hartmann's fundamental experimental proof that the linker region between the S5 and the S6 segments is part of the pore in the voltage-gated K^+ channels. (**A**) A model of the structure of a voltage-gated K^+ channel. On the left (the subdivided square) are depicted the four identical subunits arranged around a central pore. On the right is a single subunit with its six transmembrane segments and their connecting loops. (**B**) Changes in this linker region characteristically change the biophysical properties of permeation according to the source of the sequence placed in this region. This constitutes proof that this linker region between S5 and S6 is part of the pore of the voltage-gated K^+ channel, whether in *Shaker* channels in *Drosophila* or in the corresponding delayed rectifier channels in human heart.

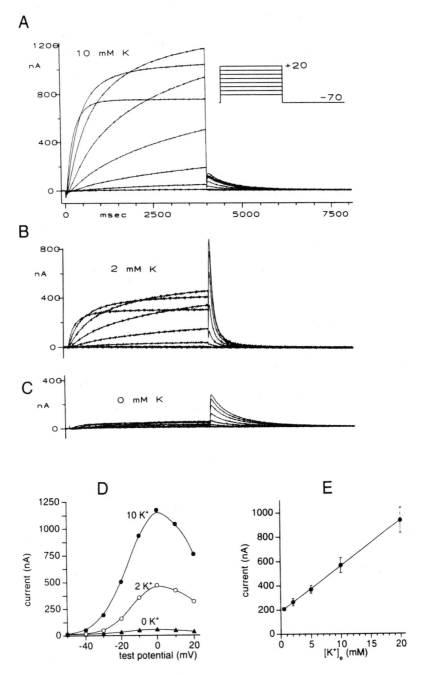

Figure 18. The hERG channel current and its modulation by extracellular K^+ concentration $[K^+]_o$. *The hERG channel is one of the channels underlying i_{Kr}*, the delayed rectifier current. (**A**, **B**, and **C**) Show the current time course in response to 4-second pulses to a test potential between -50 and $+20$ mV in a *Xenopus* oocyte expressing the hERG channel. (An expression plasmid containing the human hERG cDNA was used.) External $[K^+]_o$ was varied. The currents seen are outward repolarizing currents. It clearly is seen that the current is greater with increased extracellular $[K^+]_o$. This evidently is paradoxical, because as the extracellular $[K^+]_o$ goes up, there is reduced chemical driving force $[K]_{in}$-$[K]_{out}$; thus the increased current implies recruitment of more channels (or

continued

ucts of *Shak, Shab, Shaw,* and *Shal*[71,72](for nomenclature see Chandy[73]). The Kv1.5: fHK channel is a voltage-gated channel with tetrameric structure. It is blocked pharmacologically. Significantly, its conductance is reduced by increased $[Ca^{2+}]_i$ with the effect of action potential prolongation and possibly altered contractility under such conditions as may be relevant to late stunning. This channel has not been studied directly in ischemia and stunning.

Kv1.5: HK_1. This too is a homologue of the *Drosophila Shaker* K channel, a tetrameric voltage-gated channel where each polypeptide chain has been documented to be characterized by an N-terminal globular tail that can nestle in the channel pore thereby inactivating the channel (so-called ball-and-chain inactivation). No significant physiological differences from the HK_2 channel have been proven to date.

i_{RAK}. The i_{RAK} channel is a K^+ selective delayed rectifier channel cloned originally from rat atrium.[74] It may be identical to RBK2, NGK1, and Kv1.2. Its single channel conductance is 18 picosiemens when phosphorylated, with a 12-picosiemens subconductance state. In the native state, its conductance levels are 8.8 and 12 picosiemens. Phosphorylation increases open probability. No significance in ischemia and stunning is known, but the fact that catecholamines mediate increased open probability would be consistent with shortened action potential with β-adrenergic activation. Whether a homologous channel exists in ventricle is unknown.

Adenosine Triphosphate–Sensitive K Channel ($i_{K,ATP}$, K_{ATP}-1, KCNJ5, hBIR, and SUR1/Kir6.2).

The observation of shortening of action potential duration, fundamental in the electrophysiology of ischemia,[75] far antedates the attempts to elucidate its biophysical basis. In whole-tissue preparations hypoxia or metabolic uncoupling (using cyanide or 2,4-dinitrophenol) shortens action potential duration, and this effect is considered to be identical to that observed in ischemia.

The sarcolemmal ATP-sensitive K^+ channel ($i_{K,ATP}$) may be involved in the causation of action potential shortening.[76,77] This is a sarcolemmal K^+ channel with structural characteristics that place it in the inward rectifier channel class.[77–84] It also bears similarity to the muscarinic receptor–gated K channel ($i_{K,Ach}$ and GIRK). Four subunits constitute the channel itself. The pore (H5 region) appears to be sandwiched between two membrane spanning regions (M1 and M2). An additional component of the functional channels is the sulfonylurea receptor SUR1,[84] a member of the ATP-binding cassette superfamily of proteins. Each subunit of the functional channel is a dimer of the Kir6.2 protein with SUR1.

Usually closed, the ATP-sensitive sarcolemmal K channel exhibits an 80-picosiemens conductance on reduction of $[ATP]_i$[76,85,86] (Fig. 19), an effect that can effectuate action potential shortening. This unitary conductance is considerably higher than that of the inward rectifier K^+ channel. The ATP-sensitive K^+ channel is responsible for whole-cell currents up to 0.5 microsiemens with reversal potential of ~ -85 mV, consistent with K^+ selectivity. The density of channels is 10–100 times greater than the density of delayed rectifier or inward rectifier channels.

Single channel studies and extrapolations have shown that $[ATP]_i$ modulation changes opening probability of the 80-picosiemen unitary conductance. It is not voltage

Figure 18. *(continued)* increased open time, unlikely for other reasons). The clinical implication of this is twofold: (1) in hypokalemia, this important repolarizing current is reduced leading to longer action potentials, longer QT, and dispersion of refractoriness and arrhythmia and (2) in ischemia, when $[K^+]_o$ is increased, this channel will predominate among the normal repolarizing channels and will provide repolarizing current to avoid action potential lengthening. (**D**) Shows current voltage relation (outward current is upward). It clearly displays the rectification property of this channel. (**E**) Shows the current as a function of $[K^+]_o$. The linearity of the curve without saturation supports the notion that additional identical channels are recruited at higher $[K^+]_o$.

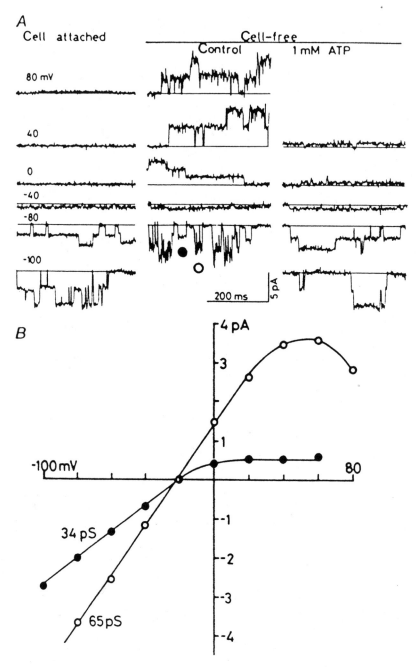

Figure 19. The ATP-sensitive K$^+$ channel i_{KATP}. Patch clamp recordings of cyanide-treated cardiac myocytes in asymmetrical KCl-containing solutions. (**A**) Recordings in cell-attached (**left**) and cell-free (inside-out) patch before (**middle**) and after (**right**) applying 1 mmol/L ATP to the inner surface of the membrane (●, inward rectifier channel; ○, the ATP-sensitive K$^+$ channels at −80 mV). The membrane potentials are indicated on the left of each trace in A. (**B**). Current voltage relations for each channel in A (●, inward rectifier channel; ○, the ATP-sensitive K$^+$ channel). The membrane potentials are indicated on the left of each trace in A. The external side of the membrane was taken as reference. Equilibrium potential for a K$^+$-selective channel may be calculated from the

(continued)

gated. Its gating kinetics are modulated by voltage and K^+-electrochemical gradient, with reduced bursting behavior and prolonged channel open times associated with decreasing membrane potential. Subconductance states have been observed, but their physiological significance and biophysical mechanism have not been investigated.

The channel is K^+-selective with relatively high conductance and is characterized by absence of prominent voltage gating in the physiological range of potentials, mild inward rectification at markedly depolarized potentials, and closure in the presence of ATP ($[ATP]_i > 1–2$ mmol/L) and ADP, but not AMP or adenosine. High lactate concentrations may shift the response in the direction of higher $[ATP]_i$. High intracellular $[Na^+]$ also closes the channel (in contrast to the effect of $[Na^+]$ on the Na^+-activated K^+ channel) but this effect is not important physiologically. Blockers include sulphonylureas (eg, glibenclamide), tetraethylammonium, 4-aminopyridine, diadenosine polyphosphates, nonhydrolyzable ATP analogs,[85] and 5-hydroxydecanoate.

Agents that increase conductance include cromakalim (BRL 34915), diazoxide, nicorandil, and pinacidil.[87]

A typical protocol for observing the conductance might be depolarization to 5 mV under condition of $[ATP]_i$ below 1–2 mmol/L; such a protocol establishes the presence of the outward current whose presence in this range abbreviates the action potential,[88–90] though the probability of channel opening is not in fact affected by the depolarization in this range. For activation of the channel, $[ATP]_i$ concentration that is low in the region of the channel is probably all that occurs[91]; the rest of the cytosol may enjoy a higher $[ATP]_i$ than that in the region of the channel. (This region may correspond to the juxtasarcolemmal "fuzzy space" whose existence is inferred from studies of Na^+-Ca^{2+} exchange[92,93]).

The suggestion that the ATP-sensitive K^+ channel is the sole mediator of action potential shortening from the very onset of ischemia probably must assume the existence of this separate subsarcolemmal region supporting a concentration gradient relative to the bulk of the cytosol. In clinical ischemia the phosphocreatine (PCr) pool is believed to be depleted only after the action potential shortens experimentally; therefore, although later action potential shortening may reasonably be ascribed to the ATP-sensitive K^+ channel without positing a low subsarcolemmal $[ATP]_i$ concentration relative to the bulk of cytosol, for channel opening the early occurrence of action potential shortening appears to require a lower $[ATP]_i$ concentration than is believed possible at that stage of ischemia. More data are required to resolve this issue, but lactate-mediated alteration of the $[ATP]_i$ threshold for channel opening may partly resolve this issue. Alternatively, other channels may be involved in the causation of action potential shortening.

Effects on ischemic myocardium of action potential shortening may include predisposition to reentry because of inhomogeneity of action potential duration and dispersion of refractoriness, as well as reduced contractile function, because reduced action potential duration reduces the magnitude of Ca^{2+} transients. Hence this is a most important channel in ischemia, both from the point of view of electrophysiology and that of excitation-contraction coupling.

The channel also probably is responsible in part for the development of local extracellular elevations of $[K]_o$, that lead to reduction in resting potential and reduction in Na^+ current availability.

Figure 19. *(continued)* Nernst equation $E_K = 2.303 \cdot (R \cdot T/F) \cdot \log([K_{electrode}]/[K_{bath}]) = -26$ mV at approximately 20°C. The channels both cross the x axis at this same point, which indicates that they are both K^+-selective channels. The traces in cell-attached recordings are typical for the inward rectifier K^+ channels, while in the cell-free patch an additional channel of larger current amplitude appeared. The larger events disappeared during application of 1 mmol/L ATP. Reproduced with permission from Reference 76.

In stunning its effects remain undefined. In early stunning, excited cells are likely to display shortened action potentials if this state reflects ischemia. However, the data appear to be divided on this point.[94]

In the related condition of ischemic preconditioning, the ATP-sensitive K$^+$ channel is believed to play a part, and this may in certain cases further affect the response of the myocyte to ischemia and stunning.[95]

Muscarinic Receptor–Gated K Channel ($i_{K,Ach}$, GIRK/GIRK4, and Kir3.1/Kir3.4).

This is a $G_{\beta\gamma}$-sensitive 35-picosiemens inwardly rectifying K channel of especial importance in atrium. Its structure is different from that of voltage-gated K channels in that it has two membrane-spanning regions M1 and M2 on each side of an H5 pore region, of which four are required to reconstitute a functional channel.[96,97] It is thus similar in structure to the inward rectifier channel discussed previously. Its structure is that of a heterotetramer of which two monomers come from each of two distinct classes of inward rectifier channel: Kir3.1 and Kir3.4.[98]

Its gating kinetics differ significantly from those of either of the two related channel peptides of which it is composed, with open times exceeding those of the other two channels by factors between 10:1 and 30:1. Modulation of gating by heteropolymers of channel peptide isoform is seen in only one other sarcolemmal channel, the gap junction, and may represent a primitive mode of biophysical modulation observable during the spontaneous molecular evolution of a new channel type.

This channel is of indirect importance in ischemia, in that it is the receptor on sinus node pacemaker cells for the vagally mediated parasympathetic stimulation in the familiar depressor reflexes that appear to mediate sinus slowing in inferior wall ischemia.

G_α binding directly to the channel has been described. Also described is a putative modulatory mechanism similar to the (related) inwardly rectifying channel; that is, the channel current is characterized by inward rectification caused by polyamine binding.

Na$^+$-Activated K$^+$-Channel ($i_{K,Na}$).

At intracellular Na concentrations of ~20 mmol/L, a K current is activated that probably is of limited physiological significance. A large channel (220 picosiemens) has been demonstrated to underlie this current[99]; remarkably, it has 12 subconductance states, of which two are highly stable. Amiodarone reduces open probability.

Na$^+$ Channel (hH1)

The Na$^+$ channel is the voltage-gated channel underlying the action potential upstroke in nonspecialized ventricular myocardium.[100]

The cardiac Na$^+$ channel is composed of an α-subunit, a polypeptide of molecular weight 260 kd, associated in heart with a β-subunit of 330 kd. The α-subunit constitutes the channel, and its sequence includes four homologous internal repeats that line the pore (Fig. 20). There is homology and functional similarity both to the skeletal muscle Na$^+$ channel, as well as to the neuronal channels at the nodes of Ranvier of myelinated axons.

It is a 7- to 11-picosiemens channel in Na$^+$-containing physiological solutions. In patch preparations, voltage steps from physiological resting potentials to depolarized potentials in the -35 to $+35$-mV range activate the channel and lead to the (sodium) inward current responsible for the upstroke of the action potential and depolarization of the cardiac cell (Fig. 21).

After activation, the channel cycles through an inactivated state. Hyperpolarization is required to make the channel available again for activation ("removal of inactivation"). Thus the available current is affected by resting membrane potential.

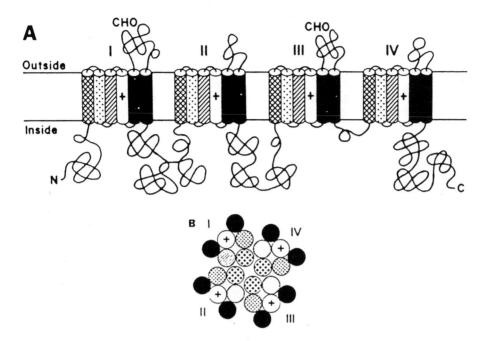

Figure 20. Sodium channel structure. (**A**) Proposed transmembrane topology of the sodium channel. (**B**) Proposed arrangement of the transmembrane segments viewed in cross section. In A, the four homology units spanning the membrane are displayed linearly. Segments S1–S6 in each repeat (I-IV) are shown as cylinders. Reproduced with permission from Reference 100.

The channel is characterized by multiple modes of inactivation, even in the absence of pharmacologic agents interacting with the channel.[101] One fast and several slow modes are described in preparations as diverse as invertebrate nerve, developing mammalian heart tissue, and the cardiac channel of the mature adult animal. Variant slow inactivation kinetics also are seen in the human channel in expressed systems (human α-subunit expressed in *Xenopus laevis*) when exposed to agents such as DPI 201–106; it is likely that this finding represents another manifestation of the same phenomenon.[102] The physiological significance of these modes is uncertain.

The cardiac sodium channel is distinguished from other Na^+ channels by its reduced tetrodotoxin sensitivity relative to the other Na^+ channels[103] and by its increased Cd^{2+} and Zn^{2+} sensitivity.[104] It also is closed by class I antiarrhythmic drugs. Pathological elevations of extracellular K concentration $[K^+]_o$ reduce available current via effects on resting membrane potential. Arachidonic acid and oleic acid (a polyunsaturated fatty acid increased in ischemia) reversibly depress Na^+ channel conductance. The channel mutation SCN5A (impaired inactivation, with a sustained noninactivating component) underlies a form of the congenital long QT syndrome (LQT3).

In ischemia, extracellular K^+ accumulation, acidosis, and hypoxia appear to be the three chief biochemical changes. The first two affect Na^+ channel behavior markedly and in such manner as to explain the behavior of the channel (and tissue electrophysiology) in ischemia.

K^+ accumulation in the clefts occurs within 5–7 minutes of the onset of ischemia. This reduces the resting potential of cardiac cells, reducing Na^+ current availability. Also reducing current availability is the binding of polyunsaturated fatty acids that result from membrane breakdown. These factors lead to reduced conduction velocity.

Acidosis, which also occurs soon after the onset of ischemia, also leads to reduction in conduction velocity by affecting Na^+ channel current.[105]

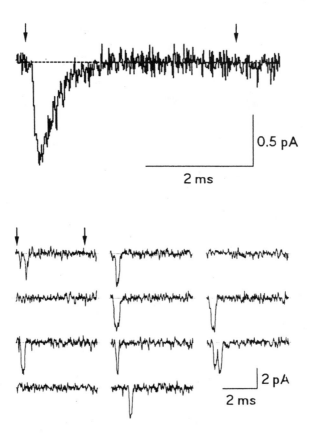

Figure 21. Single channel Na$^+$ current typical fast-inactivating Na$^+$ currents obtained from a patch with one and only one channel. (**Top**) Ensemble-averaged current from $n = 119$ sweeps (y axis, current (down-inward); x axis, time). Mice heart cells. (**Bottom**) Eleven selected traces. Arrows indicate beginning and ending of test pulses (not depicted) to -40 mV from a prepulse potential of -100 mV. Note that openings occurred exclusively during the first 2 milliseconds after the beginning of the pulse. Reproduced with permission from Reference 101.

Taken together, these biochemical changes appear to explain all Na$^+$ channel phenomena associated with ischemia.[106–108] However, Na$^+$ channels in preparations suitable for single channel investigation do not lend themselves to direct testing under conditions of ischemia.

Under conditions of stunning, limited data are available with respect to the sodium channel. If clinical stunning is always initiated by ischemia, then the first part of the period of stunning is ischemia, followed by a transition from ischemia to another hypo- or acontractile state. Under this hypothesis, channel physiology of the initial phase of stunning would be identical to that of ischemia. The biophysics of the subsequent period remains obscure, except for the likelihood of the following two hypotheses: in types of stunning where intracellular [Ca^{2+}] increase may occur, this may add to the depression of action potential upstroke once intracellular pH has been restored[105]; and acidosis (and increased intracellular Ca^{2+} if present) will reduce intercellular coupling, leading to microdesynchronization of action potential upstrokes on a tissue level during recovery from ischemia (stunning); therefore, action potential upstroke and $(dV/dt)_{max}$ will be reduced disproportionately in relation to the already reduced available inward Na$^+$ current.

Given the present state of knowledge, it is not possible to speculate on the range of channel characteristics modulated directly or indirectly by stunning and ischemia.

Adenosine Triphosphate–Activated Nonspecific Cation Channel

A poorly characterized ATP-activated nonspecific cation channel has been described in ventricular myocytes. ATP induces a rapidly desensitizing strongly rectifying inward current with reversal potential of 5 mV. The 2-methyl-thio-ATP and AMP-C-PP also appeared to activate the channel. Antibodies to a similar cloned *vas deferens* smooth muscle channel[109] appear to cross react with this channel, suggesting it may be a similar or identical channel.

Chloride Channels

Three chloride conductances appear to be well documented in cardiac muscle. One is a volume-sensitive conductance that probably is the mediator of regulatory volume decrease (RVD), the normal homeostatic response to abnormal cell swelling; one an important cAMP-sensitive conductance; and one less well described that may be a contributory conductance to the transient outward current. Accurate correlation of current with channel identity remains speculative at the present time; additional channels are present as well.

Regulatory Volume Decrease. This well-described chloride conductance of heart muscle appears to underlie RVD and has been investigated most comprehensively by Zhang.[110] This reportedly isoproterenol-insensitive current is induced by hypo-osmotic swelling and leads to reduction in cell volume by mediating an outward chloride conductance. It also can lead to cell depolarization. Osmotic gradient within a physiological range and hydraulic cell swelling induce this current (though the latter only in isolated atrial cells where concomitant frank blebbing was observed). It is likely to be operative in models of stunning, where after ischemia and reperfusion swelling and intracellular hyperosmolar states exist. Significantly, under such circumstance RVD currents are depolarizing and can bring cell membrane potential to threshold in experimental preparations, an effect that, if present clinically, could enhance a variety of cell detrimental mechanisms (and perhaps one cell-preserving mechanism, that of gap junction voltage gating).

The channel that underlies this current cannot be attributed with certainty in the present state of our knowledge, but it is likely to be associated with the single channel conductance that has been reported by Coronado and Latorre.[110a]

Cystic Fibrosis Transmembrane Regulator (i_{Cl}, Cyclic Adenosine Monophosphate–Sensitive Cl^- Conductance). The second well-described Cl^- conductance was reported by Bahinski, and analyzed further by Harvey and Hume.[111] In cardiomyocytes they reported a significant chloride conductance (symmetrical in the hands of Bahinski, mildly outwardly rectifying in the reports of Hume) readily induced by isoproterenol or forskolin (also by cAMP and the regulatory component of PKA) and abolished by acetylcholine. This current (affected by Na^+ in nonphysiological concentrations and by disulfonic acid stilbene derivatives and aromatic acids at usual concentrations for chloride channel inhibition) appears similar to other cAMP-dependent chloride conductances from other tissues. Recently, it has been identified definitively with the cystic fibrosis transmembrane regulator (CFTR) channel. This channel, with 12 transmembrane domains, two nucleotide binding domains, and a regulatory domain, governs this conductance in a plethora of tissues. It is a member of the ABC or "ATP-binding cassette" class of transport proteins. Mutations underlie cystic fibrosis. Because it is not voltage-gated, its most significant effects are likely during repolarization, and the channel causes a marked shortening of action potential duration under β-adrenergic stimulation (Fig. 22), reminiscent of effects seen in ischemic preparations and attributed to $i_{K,ATP}$ effects. That the latter attribution has always been rendered insecure by the space gradient paradox (that supraphysiological cytosolic gradients of ATP must be posited to account for the behavior of the channels in the face of known ATP concentrations to be higher than would permit significant activation of the channel) is an argument for a possible contributory significance of this chloride channel in these phenomena. Stilbene testing has not yet been reported in Langendorff or other models of ischemia to address this hypothesis, but because ischemia and stunning often are associated with elevated β-adrenergic species levels (physiological or pharmacologic) it is likely that part of action potential shortening in these conditions reflects chloride conductance, independently of whether the $i_{K,ATP}$ channel is activated and additive to $i_{K,ATP}$ effects. However, pharmacologic crossover effects may affect the L-type Ca^{2+} channel.[112] Ehara studied the single channel conductance of this channel.[112a]

The likely importance of this Cl^- channel was implicit in data from over a decade ago of Piwnica-Worms, showing a Cl^- flux (conductance plus transport) of twice the magni-

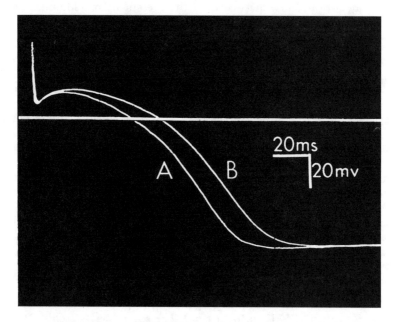

Figure 22. Demonstration of the effect of Cl^- channels on the action potential duration in chick heart cells. (**A**) Control state action potential. (**B**) $[Cl^-]_o$ reduced to zero by substitution of an impermeant anion. Note prolongation of the action potential (increase in action potential duration). The presence after Cl^- removal of an anion current that lengthens the action potential implies the presence of a significant inward Cl^- current shortening the action potential in the control state. [Substitution of Na-methanesulfonate and K-methanesulfonate for NaCl and KCl in extracellular (Earle's) solution in chick embryo polystrand preparation. Resting potential may be indeterminate to ± 1–2 mV because of liquid junction potentials.] Reproduced with permission from Reference 153.

tude of that of K^+.[112b] Unusual membrane phenomena affected by nonspecific disulfonic acid stilbene derivatives had been demonstrated several years previously as well.

It is significant that CFTR has not been identified in the myocytes of all mammals; for instance, it appears to be absent in rat.

i_{to2} Cl^- *Conductance.* The third putative Cl^- current has been documented by Zygmunt[112c] as the 4-aminopyridine resistant component of the transient outward current. It is Ca^+ transient dependent, but its single channel basis is not known.

Additionally, single channel properties have been described for two additional known chloride channels studied at the single channel level, that may be present in sarcolemma. Coulombe described in the heart a maxi Cl^- channel with conductance of 400 picosiemens. Expression cloning techniques have documented presence of ClC1 and ClC2, as well as ClC4, in cardiac tissue, though it is not known whether these are sarcolemmal.

Intercellular Channels

The gap junction is the intercellular channel that allows the propagation of action potentials from cell to cell, whether the cell types be pacemaker, conducting, or working myocytes. Both intracellular pH (pH_i) and intracellular $[Ca^{2+}]_i$ are thought to be important in the regulation of the gap junction–mediated intercellular pathway.[113,114] Elevation of either will result in the closure of gap junction channels and these ions appear to act synergistically as well in effecting channel closure.[113] Under normal physiological conditions calcium (free$[Ca^{2+}]_i = 100–200$ nmol/L) is able to diffuse through the gap junction channel[115,116] but this has not yet been shown directly in mammalian cardiac myocytes. It has been shown, though, in cell types that utilize the same type of gap junction channels as cardiac myocytes.[117,118] Considering the size and mobility of H^+ (or H_3O^+) it seems likely that it also can traverse the channel under normal physiological conditions where the H^+ concentration in the cytoplasm is on the order of 0.1 μmol/L. Thus these two ions are able to diffuse through the gap junction channel and, in addition, down-regulate channel open probability with increased concentration.[115] In effect, under conditions that are expected to arise in ischemia and stunning the response is to isolate and protect viable myocytes from those that are damaged.[114]

The structure and permselectivity of gap junction channels are unique relative to other known channel types (Fig. 23). Each of two closely apposed cells contributes half of the entire channel in the form of a hemichannel. Each hemichannel is composed of six connexin subunit proteins. The hemichannels of two adjacent cells then link together to form a channel that excludes the extracellular space and connects the interiors of the two cells such that K^+-mediated current flow can occur and thus allow action potential propagation. In addition, the diffusion from cell to cell of other solutes such as cAMP[119] can proceed, again with the exclusion of the extracellular domain.

There are at least 18 identified connexin subunit proteins.[120] Typically, as is the case for working myocardium, only one connexin type usually is made by cells; thus the hemichannels and gap junction channel they subtend are constructed of identical units. This type of construct is called a homotypic gap junction channel consisting of 12 identical subunits. Heterotypic gap junction channels are composed of two different connexins where all of one type comprise one of the two hemichannels and all of the other comprise the other hemichannel. Heteromeric gap junction channels are composed of at least two different connexins where different connexins are found in each hemichannel. Thus by definition a homomeric hemichannel is composed of only one connexin type.

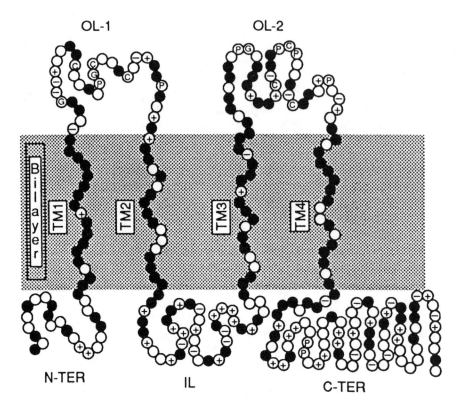

Figure 23. General topology of connexins. Based on hydrophobicity maps and on data from immunocytochemistry and partial proteolysis, connexins are believed to contain four transmembrane domains (TM), both N (N-TER) and C (C-TER) termini at the cytoplasmic side of the membrane, two outer loops (OL-1 and OL-2), and an inner loop (IL). Filled circles, hydrophobic residues; open circles, polar residues. Mapped here is the rat connexin 32 (Cx32). Reproduced with permission from Reference 154.

The major connexin type found in the working myocardium is the 43-kd species known as connexin 43 (Cx43). Other connexin forms are found within the adult heart but are not distributed as uniformly nor are they as ubiquitous as Cx43. They are Cx37, Cx40, and Cx45.[121-124] Cx40 is found in the atrium while Cx45 is found in the conducting system. Cx43 is found in all of these areas as well.

Cx45 appears in early development. Whether it forms homotypic channels or can form heteromeric and/or heterotypic channels with Cx43 remains speculative.[125] It is interesting to note that osteoblasts also make Cx43 and Cx45 and evidence from that system suggests that the two connexins can form heteromeric channels.[126]

To better understand how "mixed" channel forms might have an impact on cellular and tissue physiology, the homotypic characteristics must be defined first. Homotypic Cx43 is one of the most well-characterized gap junctions. In mammalian myocytes the unitary conductance of a single channel has been reported to be 60 picosiemens in 135 mmol/L K glutamate solution.[127] Human Cx43 in smooth muscle cells has a unitary conductance of 113 picosiemens in 165 mmol/L CsCl.[128] The permselectivity of Cx43 can be characterized as nonselective. Cx43 is able to allow the passage of many cations ($K \approx Cs > Na > TMA$ [tetramethylammonium]) and will allow the passage of anions as well.[115,129] Cx43 channels are weakly voltage dependent and the kinetics of voltage-dependent inactivation is slow.[128,130] The mean open time for human Cx43 is on the order 0.43–5.25 seconds while mean closed time is on the order of 0.21–1.49 seconds. The calculated open probability when there is no transjunctional voltage is $P_o = 0.95$. Thus the channel stays open for long time periods and spends most of its time in the open state, a veritable freeway.

The homotypic Cx45 gap junction channel has a unitary conductance of 25–35 picosiemens and will allow the passage of negatively charged dyes.[129,131] It has similar cation permselectivity ($K \approx Cs$) and while it allows the diffusion of Cl^- it is less anion permeant than Cx43. Cx45 voltage dependence is stronger (more sensitive) than Cx43. The kinetics are approximately five times more rapid.[131]

Both channels allow the passage of small cations and anions, which presumably include a number of second messengers. These properties appear to be important not only to tissue homeostasis but could be critical in dynamic responses of the myocardium.[115,127]

Other factors that are known to affect channel patency in Cx43 are specific lipid agents,[127,132] cAMP and cyclic guanosine monophosphate (cGMP).[127] The effects of these agents have not been demonstrated for Cx45 as yet.

The significance of mixed forms of heteromeric channel types can only be imagined at this juncture. If the heteromeric forms altered the voltage-dependent properties or responded differently to changes in $[Ca^{2+}]_i$ or pH_i or had dramatically different permselectivity properties, as the data of Koval[126] suggest, then understanding the distribution and behaviors of this channel population becomes of paramount importance in terms of understanding processes such as ischemia or stunning. If heteromeric channels had different sensitivities or lacked sensitivity to $[Ca^{2+}]_i$ or to second messengers such as cAMP then these channel types could well have an impact on the time course of sealing over or stunning.

As already indicated, the gap junction channel permits the longitudinal current flow from cell to cell necessary for the propagation of action potentials. The robustness of the channel in terms of the $[Ca^{2+}]_i$ and $[H^+]_i$ levels necessary to cause channel closures, the weak voltage dependence, and elongated mean open times make the channel an unlikely rate limiting step in early ischemia. In fact, the ability to pass Ca^{2+} could easily promote contractility in healthier regions surrounding a damaged area.

Another factor in action potential propagation centers on the fate of lipids and their influence on gap junctions. Ischemia is known to lead to increased levels of lipids in myocytes caused by membrane lipid breakdown.[21,133,134] In addition, gap junction channels are known to close in response to a number of lipophilic agents.[132] Further, there is an excellent correlation between the number of functioning gap junction channels and the ability to propagate action potentials from cell to cell.[125,128,135] A number of other factors also could be affecting conduction such as altered geometry.[136] The magnitude of lipid effects in adult heart have not been demonstrated clearly to be of physiological or pathophysiological significance but clearly it is a potentially important process to dissect in understanding ischemia and stunning. In neonates gap junction–mediated conduction is highly sensitive to lipophilic agents.[132,137] Could this be an example of a heteromeric Cx45/Cx43 channel with greater sensitivity to lipoid metabolic products?

The three parameters, $[Ca^{2+}]_i$, $[H^+]_i$, and lipophilic agents, are all able to affect gap junctions and, in principle if not in practice, alter action potential propagation. In addition, synergistic interaction of Ca^{2+} and H^+ and possibly lipid agents could be important with regard to sealing over processes. Indeed, these phenomena most likely underlie the sealing over effects observed in Purkinje cells[114] where with the death of adjacent cells, gap junction channels close, isolating normal from dying tissue. This latter case may be relevant to radionuclide imaging, and the known high sensitivity and specificity of thallium-201 (^{201}Tl) imaging early after myocardial infarction may be caused not by the lack of flow to an area but by lack of intercellular equilibration of intracellular ^{201}Tl. (This suggests the interesting and important hypothesis that even ^{201}Tl may underestimate viability under certain circumstances, ie, redistribution, but that this shortcoming may be rectified by reinjection.)

Second messengers such as cAMP, which increase gap junction membrane conductance and enhance contractile strength,[119] would be thought to act after rather than during an ischemic episode and in fact could be part of the phenomena of stunning. Increased contractile strength seen in stunning might be the result of the buildup of second messengers like cAMP in normal cells within or near an infarct. What would cause increased cAMP production in ischemic or peri-ischemic regions? Elevated extracellular catecholamines triggering a receptor-mediated activation of adenyl cyclase is one possibility. Those cells responding to extrinsic stimuli by the production of cAMP, for example, would experience enhanced contractile output and the cAMP also would diffuse down its concentration gradient from cell to cell. Thus those cells adjacent to a stimulated cell also would be recruited and further enhance contractile force. Healthy cells isolated by the protective action of sealing over also could produce cAMP in response to extrinsic stimuli. In theory once these cells reformed gap junction channels with other cells cAMP would diffuse rapidly into cells with lesser amounts. Again, an equivalent recruitment phenomena could occur.

Whether these effects are in fact protective in injury to the reversibly injured cells remains a matter of conjecture (see the next section). This effect also could underlie uncoupling within the heart in stunning where $[Ca^{2+}]_i$ may be elevated and lead to islands of perfused but nondepolarized cardiomyocytes during systole. The presence of such cells that either fail to contract or contract tardily and hence asynchronously, could lead also to increased stiffness as well as to reduction of contractile function.

Neural Analogs: Excitotoxic Cell Death

In excitable tissue, there exist several models of potentially reversible cell injury and malfunction not related necessarily to ischemia. The best studied of these phenomena is excitotoxicity,[138–141] the NMDA (N-methyl-D-aspartate) receptor–mediated destruction of cortical neurons that may underlie cell death in seizures and occur as a secondary phenomenon in trauma and ischemic stroke.[142–144]

As studied in cortical neuron cultures, the phenomenon is characterized by a two-stage process leading to cell death after stimulation by normal or supranormal amounts of glutamine, the most common neurotransmitter. This effect, mediated solely by the NMDA receptor, a ligand-gated Ca^{2+} channel, is characterized by an initial phase of Na^+ and Ca^{2+} influx that leads to cellular swelling, followed by a Ca^{2+} overload phase that is uniformly irreversible once established. The initial phenomenon, though generally characterized by a Ca^{2+} transient, need not always be. A pathological influx of ions may simply reflect disturbed homeostasis in this phase.

The second step is characterized by a Ca^{2+} influx, which stimulates calcium-dependent phospholipases, proteases, and endonucleases and leads to loss of membrane integrity with cellular demise. This latter phase can be imitated by exposure to Ca^{2+} ionophores and, interestingly, it can be blocked by Mg^{2+} at pharmacologic levels, as well as by dantrolene. It may be relevant that the brain RyR's include isoforms that are Mg^{2+} sensitive and dantrolene sensitive (this being the drug that aborts malignant hyperthermia by blocking the RyR in skeletal muscle), unlike the RyR2 cardiac isoform.

Less well-described similar phenomena in excitable tissues include acetylcholine-mediated injury of skeletal muscle and isoproterenol cardiomyonecrosis; neither phenomenon is well described at this time.

The example of neuronal excitotoxicity raises the question, Is there a cardiac process analogous to neuronal excitotoxicity? It appears that the answer to this question is, *yes*. In clinical ischemia as well as in stunning, a component of damage is probably the release of calcium from internal stores via the RyR, activated through the normal processes of gap junction mediated cell depolarization and L-type sarcolemmal Ca^{2+} channel mediated calcium influx, augmented by the pathological mechanisms of abnormal Ca^{2+} clearance mechanisms and pathologically augmented trans-sarcolemmal calcium influx.

Viewed in this way, several disparate channel phenomena are seen to act in concerted manner to limit the destructive advance of these "excitotoxic" cell processes. In ischemia the action potential shortening reduces the Ca^{2+} influx through the L-type Ca^{2+} channel and secondarily limits the magnitude of the RyR2 Ca^{2+} entry into the cytosol of the injured cell. Action potential shortening, mediated in a relatively early stage by the ATP-sensitive K channel (whether or not this is the first channel mediating this effect is immaterial to the present argument), is continued by contributions from the hERG channel, which among the ordinary repolarizing channels has its opening enhanced under conditions of accumulation of extracellular K. Elevated internal calcium concentration $[Ca^{2+}]_i$ and reduced pH mediate closure of the gap junctions, and this, along with elevated resting potential caused by increased external potassium concentration, conspires to render the working ventricular myocyte inexcitable; in certain forms of ischemia central neural reflexes slow the sinus rate for the entire heart. Under the assumption that excitotoxicity exists and plays a role in the phenomena of ischemia and stunning, these channel phenomena work to attenuate excitotoxic Ca^{2+} accumulation and cell death in the heart.

Ischemia and Stunning: Summary

We have reviewed in some detail the data on ion channels in heart muscle cells. At this point we integrate this information with the experimental facts of ischemia and stunning.

Ischemia is characterized by shortened action potential duration, less negative resting potential, reduced action potential upstroke and amplitude, shortened action potential duration, and an initial increase followed by a rapid decrease in the conduction velocity. The following findings occur in the context of acidosis and tissue hypoxia[145]:

Shortened Action Potential Duration. The $i_{K,ATP}$ channel opens. This occurs because of the reduction in $[ATP]_i$ and is enhanced by the reduced pH. The enormous conductance governed by the aggregate of the $i_{K,ATP}$ channels leads to a large outward K^+ repolarizing current that shortens action potential duration and increases extracellular K^+ concentration $[K^+]_o$. The reduced action potential duration shortens the period during which the L-type calcium channel is exposed to a depolarized potential, reducing the inward Ca^{2+} influx that, via the mechanism of CICR, will open the RyR2 and cause contraction. Contractility thereby is reduced in ischemia. Other channels contribute to action potential shortening in ischemia and may even precede the $i_{K,ATP}$ channel in contributing to this effect. The other channels include the hERG channel (important because of its continuing contribution to action potential shortening even after $[K^+]_o$ is increased), CFTR—the cAMP-sensitive Cl^- conductance (an inward anion current, ie, an inward current of negatively charged ions, having the same repolarizing effect as an outward current of cations such as $i_{K,ATP}$ or hERG), and the gap junction Cx43. Other mechanisms contribute to reduced contractility; detailed discussion of excitation-contraction coupling is beyond the scope of this review.

Less Negative Resting Potential. The increased extracellular potassium concentration $[K^+]_o$ alters the resting potential via the inward rectifier potassium channel i_{K1} (hIRK1) in accordance with the Nernst equation. During ischemia the $i_{K,ATP}$ channel contributes to diastolic membrane K^+ permeability as well. The gap junction equalizes the diastolic potentials of adjacent cells.

Reduced Action Potential Upstroke and Amplitude. There is less available sodium channel current partly because of the less negative resting potential and (less importantly) to the acidosis.

Increase Followed Decrease in Conduction Velocity. Conduction velocity depends on: (1) action potential sodium current for local depolarization of sarcolemma and (2) gap junction intercellular coupling to propagate the action potential from cell to cell. Less charge and less current are needed to depolarize a partially depolarized membrane (because the capacitance is constant). Because of the partially depolarized state of the ischemic sarcolemma caused by the increased $[K^+]_o$, the conduction velocity initially increases in ischemic tissue. Very soon, because of the reduced sodium channel current, the conduction velocity falls. Various factors, including (not independently) pH and $[Ca^{2+}]_i$, reduce gap junction conductance, leading to increased axial resistance, which reduces conduction velocity directly, and this also leads to microdesynchronization and altered geometry of the conductive pathways in the heart, altering the observed conduction velocity indirectly.

Thus the changes in physiology in ischemia have an ionic basis.

Stunning appears to have two stages, both with depressed myocardial function. In the antecedent period of ischemia (or other insult) that preceded and caused stunning, increased $[Ca^{2+}]_i$ and generation of free radicals set the stage for injury. The first phase of stunning reflects myofilament damage. Normal or near-normal function of the L-type Ca channel and the RyR (RyR2) appear likely; however, Ca^{2+} buildup may be occurring. An additional component of clinical stunning in this stage is residual ischemia masquerading as stunning. The second phase of stunning reflects further and progressive injury. A component of clinical stunning in this phase may be cellular uncoupling (reduced gap junction conductance) caused by increased $[Ca^{2+}]_i$ and lipid catabolites. Resolution (if the hemodynamic deterioration can be reversed and can be tolerated) will require replacement protein synthesis.

Stunning has not been characterized at the cellular level. At the whole-organ level initially there is increased followed by reduced contractility at a time when clinical electrophysiology appears normal and perfusion is reduced only mildly. If the human or animal survives, recovery of function occurs in hours to days.

This literature and the above discussion offer the following two plausible hypotheses about the origin of stunning: (1) an ischemic model of stunning, wherein slow reversal of the electrophysiological concomitants of ischemia paralyzes regions of myocardium most severely affected, compounded by some irreversible injury caused by ischemia or Ca^{2+} paradox and some degree of loss of coordination and perhaps frank loss of excitation of some areas, caused by one of several mechanisms (reduced conduction velocity, depolarization impairing the Ca^{2+} transient, and sealing over), and (2) a protein degradation hypothesis of the causation of stunning, with diffuse cell injury and myofilament loss and where free-radical injury and membrane lipid breakdown (as part of free-radical injury that assumes its full role in ischemia and infarction but which also may be secondary to the unbridled amplification by the RyR of an inappropriately elevated intracellular calcium concentration, with lipoxygenase activation and Ca^{2+} paradox amplification) are the necessary and sufficient cause of the bulk of the phenomena known as stunning.

Stunning is not a channels phenomenon. Even to the extent to which abnormal ionic concentrations are implicated in the pathogenesis of stunning, it is the steady-state concentrations rather than the rapid and oscillatory components that are etiologic.

A useful model for stunning is the neural analog of excitotoxicity, discussed in detail above, where the excitatory neurotransmitter glutamate acting via the NMDA receptor (a Ca^{2+} conductance) triggers a two-phase phenomenon leading to cell injury in the first phase and cell death in the second, via a mild, followed by a severe Ca^{2+} influx, where the first triggers enzyme activation that eventually may contribute to cell destruction via apoptosis. If this analogy is correct, and we believe that it may be, then in the cardiac myocyte the gap junction–mediated depolarizing current (that initiates cellular excitation and further Ca^{2+} buildup) is the analog of synaptic neuronal excitation, and after multiple mechanisms have contributed to Ca^{2+} influx, lipase activation stimulates membrane degradation that underlies subsidiary phenomena of stunning. Reversal involves new protein synthesis. The well-described sealing over phenomenon of the gap junction in tissue therefore represents an important homeostatic mechanism for reducing stunning (and ischemic) injury, perhaps the primary homeostatic mechanism for staving off apoptosis. Hypothetically, the explanation for the sensitivity of ^{201}Tl reinjection over ^{201}Tl redistribution may be related to this mechanism.

The enhanced hemodynamically deleterious effect of incessant supraventricular tachycardia on the heart, with hypofunction exceeding that predicted by hemodynamic alterations and lasting beyond the time of resolution of the tachycardia, suggests that repetitive rapid stimulation per se may create stunning. Perhaps this is the most pure example of cardiac excitotoxicity, because it occurs in the absence of hypotension and hypoperfusion.

Late stunning is reflective of different processes than early stunning.

Acknowledgments: The authors acknowledge the assistance of Sheila S. Lobel and Eleanor Licalsi in the preparation of this manuscript and the expertise of Katherine S. Zippert, Ellen Rothbaum, James Redman, and Debra Eisenberg of the Payson Memorial Library. M. Ovadia is a recipient of grants from the American Heart Association (9860018T-NY), the CFIDS Association, and E.G. & G. Instruments/Princeton Applied Research (Oak Ridge, Tenn). P. R. Brink is the recipient of grants from the National Institutes of Health (NIH).

References

1. Knoll R, Zimmermann R, Schaper W. Altered gene transcription following brief episodes of coronary occlusions. In: Sideman S, Beyar R, eds. *Molecular and Subcellular Cardiology: Effects of Structure and Function.* New York, NY: Plenum Press; 1995:175–183.
2. Knoll R, Zimmermann R, Berwing K, et al. Characterization of differential expressed genes following short coronary occlusions. *JMCC* 1995;A145.
3. Schaper W. Stunned myocardium, an opinioned review. *Basic Res Cardiol* 1995;90:273–275.
4. Smith JS, Coronado R, Meissner G. Sarcoplasmic reticulum contains adenosine nucleotide-activated calcium channels. *Nature* 1985;316:446–449.
5. Smith JS, Imagawa T, Ma J, et al. Purified ryanodine receptor from rabbit skeletal muscle is the calcium-release channel of sarcoplasmic reticulum. *J Gen Physiol* 199;92:1–26.
6. Jayaraman T, Brillantes A-M, Timerman AP, et al. FK506 Binding protein associated with the calcium release channel (ryanodine receptor). *J Biol Chem* 1992;267:9474–9477.
7. Lukyanenko V, Györke I, Györke S. Regulation of calcium release by calcium inside the sarcoplasmic reticulum in ventricular myocytes. *Pflügers Arch* 1996;432:1047–1054.
8. Lokuta AJ, Meyers MB, Sander PR, et al. Modulation of cardiac ryanodine receptors by sorcin. *J Biol Chem* 1997;272(40):25333–25338.
9. Xiao R-P, Valdivia HH, Bogdanov K, et al. The immunophilin FK 506-binding protein modulates Ca^{2+} release channel closure in rat heart. *J Physiol* 1997;500:2:343–354.
10. Koretsune Y, Corretti MC, Kusuoka H, et al. Mechanism of early ischemic contractile failure. *Circ Res* 1991;68:255–262.
11. Kusuoka H, Weisfeldt ML, Zweier JL, et al. Mechanism of early contractile failure during hypoxia in intact ferret heart: Evidence for modulation of maximal Ca^{2+}-activated force by inorganic phosphate. *Circ Res* 1986;59:270–282.
12. Kusuoka H, Porterfield JK, Weisman HF, et al. Pathophysiology, and pathogenesis of stunned myocardium. Depressed Ca^{2+} activation of contraction as a consequence of reperfusion-induced cellular calcium overload in ferret hearts. *J Clin Invest* 1987;79:950–961.
13. Kusuoka H, Koretsuna Y, Chacko VP, et al. Excitation-contraction coupling in postischemic myocardium. Does failure of activator Ca^{2+} transients underlie stunning? *Circ Res* 1990;66:1268–1276.

14. Kusuoka H, Marban E. Cellular mechanisms of myocardial stunning. *Annu Rev Physiol* 1992;54:243–256.
15. Marban E, Gao WD. Stunned myocardium: A disease of the myofilaments? *Basic Res Cardiol* 1995;90:269–272.
16. Marban E. Excitation-contraction coupling in hibernating myocardium. *Basic Res Cardiol* 1995;90:12–22.
17. Marban E. Myocardial stunning and hibernation. *Circulation* 1991;83:681–688.
18. Marban E, Kusuoka H, Yue DT, et al. Maximal Ca^{2+}-activated force elicited by tetanization of ferret papillary muscle and whole heart: Mechanism and characteristics of steady contractile activation in intact myocardium. *Circ Res* 1986;59:262–269.
19. Marban E, Kitakaze M, Koretsune Y, et al. Quantification of $[Ca^{2+}]_i$ in perfused hearts. *Circ Res* 1990;66:1255–1267.
20. Marban E, Koretsune Y, Kusuoka H. Disruption of intracellular Ca^{2+} homeostasis in hearts reperfused after prolonged episodes of ischemia. *Ann N Y Acad Sci* 1994;723:38–50.
21. Kako KJ. Membrane phospholipids and plasmalogens in the ischemic myocardium. *Can J Cardiol* 1986;2:184–194.
22. Al-Awqati Q. Chloride channels of intracellular organelles. *Curr Opin Cell Biol* 1995;7:504–508.
23. Sukhareva M, Morrissette J, Coronado R. Mechanism of chloride-dependent release of Ca^{2+} in the sarcoplasmic reticulum of rabbit skeletal muscle. *Biophys J* 1994;67:751–765.
24. Kawano S, Nakamura F, Tanaka T, et al. Cardiac sarcoplasmic reticulum chloride channels regulated by protein kinase A. *Circ Res* 1992;71:585–589.
25. Rousseau E. Single chloride-selective channel from cardiac sarcoplasmic reticulum studied in planar lipid bilayers. *J Membr Biol* 1989;110:39–47.
26. Rousseau E, Roberson M, Meissner G. Properties of single chloride selective channel from sarcoplasmic reticulum. *Eur Biophys J* 1988;16:143–151.
27. Tanifuji M, Sokabe M, Kasai M. An anion channel of sarcoplasmic reticulum incorporated into planar lipid bilayers: Single-channel behavior and conductance properties. *J Membr Biol* 1987;99:103–111.
28. Regan LJ, Sah DW, Bean BP. Ca^{2+} channels in rat central and peripheral neurons: High threshold current resistant to dihydropyridine blockers and omega-conotoxin. *Neuron* 1991;6:269–280.
29. McEnery MW, Snowman AM, Sharp AH, et al. Purified ω-conotoxin GVIA receptor of rat brain resembles a dihydropyridine-sensitive L-type calcium channel. *Proc Natl Acad Sci U S A* 1991;88:11095–11099.
30. Mikami A, Imoto K, Tanabe T, et al. Primary structure and functional expression of the cardiac dihydropyridine-sensitive calcium channel. *Nature* 1989;340:230–233.
31. Rose WC, Balke CW, Weir WG, et al. Macroscopic and unitary properties of physiological ion flux through L-type Ca^{2+} channels in guinea-pig heart cells. *J Physiol (Lond)* 1992;456:267–284.
32. Sanguinetti MC, Krafte S, Kass RS. Voltage-dependent modulation of Ca channel current in heart cells by Bay K8644. *J Gen Physiol* 1986;88:369–392.
33. Tanabe T, Beam KG, Powell JA, et al. Restoration of excitation-contraction coupling and slow calcium current in dysgenic muscle by dihydropyridine receptor complementary DNA. *Nature* 1988;336:134–139.
34. Kuriyama H, Kitamura K, Nabata H. Pharmacological and physiological significance of ion channels and factors that modulate them in vascular tissues. *Pharmacol Rev* 1995;47:387–573.
35. Balke CW, Rose WC, Marban E, et al. Macroscopic and unitary properties of physiological ion flux through T-type Ca^{2+} channels in guinea-pig heart cells. *J Physiol (Lond)* 1992;456:247–265.
36. Mori Y, Friedrich T, Kim M-S, et al. Primary structure and functional expression from complementary DNA of a brain calcium channel. *Nature* 1991;350:398–402.
37. Starr TVB, Prystay W, Snutch TP. Primary structure of a calcium channel that is highly expressed in the rat cerebellum. *Proc Natl Acad Sci U S A* 1991;88:5621–5625.
38. Jeong SW, Wurster RD. Calcium channel current in acutely dissociated intracardiac neurons from adult rats. *J Neurophysiol* 1997;77:1769–1778.

39. Backx PH, Marban E. Background potassium current active during the plateau of the action potential in guinea pig ventricular myoctes. *Circ Res* 1993;72:890–900.

40. Wang Z, Fermini B, Nattel S. Sustained depolarization-induced outward current in human atrial myocytes. *Circ Res* 1993;73:1061–1076.

41. Yue DT, Marban E. A novel cardiac potassium channel that is active and conductive at depolarized potentials. *Pflügers Arch* 1988;413:127–133.

42. Kim D, Clapham DE. Potassium channels in cardiac cells activated by arachidonic acid and phospholipids. *Science* 1989;244:1174–1176.

43. Shimoni Y, Clark RB, Giles WR. Role of an inwardly rectifying potassium current in rabbit ventricular action potential. *J Physiol* 1992;448:709–727.

44. Nichols CG, Lopatin AN. Inward rectifier potassium channels. *Annu Rev Physiol* 1997;59:171–191.

45. Kubo Y, Reuveny E, Slesinger PA, et al. Primary structure and functional expression of a rat G-protein-coupled muscarinic potassium channel. *Nature* 1993;364:802–806.

46. Kurachi Y. Voltage-dependent activation of the inward-rectifier potassium channel in the ventricular cell membrane of guinea-pig heart. *J Physiol (Lond)* 1985;366:365–385.

47. Matsuda H, Standfield, PR. Single inwardly rectifying potassium channels in cultured muscle cells from rat and mouse. *J Physiol* 1989;414:111–124.

48. Sakmann B, Trube G. Conductance properties of single inwardly rectifying potassium channels in ventricular cells from guinea-pig heart. *J Physiol (Lond)* 1984;347:641–657.

48a. Sakmann B, Trube G. Voltage-dependent inactivation of inward-rectifying single-channel currents in the guinea-pig heart cell membrane. *J Physiol* 1984;347:659–683.

49. Varró A, Nánási PP, Lathrop DA. Potassium currents in human atrial and ventricular cardiocytes. *Acta Physiol Scand* 1993;149:133–142.

50. Trube G, Hescheler J. Inward-rectifying channels in isolated patches of the heart cell membrane: ATP-dependence and comparison with cell-attached patches. *Pflügers Arch* 1984;401:178–184.

51. Raab-Graham KF. Molecular cloning and expression of a human heart inward rectifier potassium channel. *Neuroreport* 1994;5:2501–2505.

52. Heidbüchel H, Vereecke J, Carmeliet E. Three different potassium channels in human atrium. *Circ Res* 1990;66:1277–1286.

53. Rettig J, Heinemann SH, Wunder F, et al. Inactivation properties of voltage-gated K$^+$ channels altered by presence of β-subunit. *Nature* 1994;369:289–294.

54. Boyle WA, Nerbonne JM. A novel type of depolarization-activated K+ current in adult rat atrial myocytes. *Am J Physiol* 1991;260:H1236–H1247.

55. Carmeliet E. Use-dependent block and use-dependent unblock of the delayed rectifier K$^+$ current by Almokalant in rabbit ventricular myocytes. *Circ Res* 1993;73:857–868.

56. Honoré E, Barhanin J, Attali B, et al. External blockade of the major cardiac delayed-rectifier K$^+$ channel (Kv 1.5) by polyunsaturated fatty acids. *Proc Natl Acad Sci* 1994;91:1937–1944.

57. Wu MH, Su MJ, Lue HC. Inward rectifier and delayed outward potassium currents in isolated guinea-pig ventricular myocytes: Maturation and its role in repolarization. *Acta Paediatr Sin* 1992;33:363–371.

58. Stefani E, Toro L, Perozo E, et al. Gating currents of cloned shaker K$^+$ channels. Chapter 3. In: Peracchia C, ed. *Handbook of Membrane Channels. Molecular and Cellular Physiology.* San Diego, Calif: Academic Press, Inc.; 1994:29–40.

59. Shibasaki T. Conductance and kinetics of delayed rectifier potassium channels in nodal cells of the rabbit heart. *J Physiol (Lond)* 1987;387:227–250.

60. Sasaki Y, Ishii K, Nunoki K, et al. The voltage-dependent K$^+$ channel (Kv1.5) cloned from rabbit heart and facilitation of inactivation of the delayed rectifier current by the rat β subunit. *FEBS Lett* 1995;372:20–24.

61. Mays DJ, Foose JM, Philipson LH, et al. Localization of the Kv1.5 K$^+$ channel protein in explanted cardiac tissue. *J Clin Invest* 1995;96:282–292.

62. Lopez GA, Jan YN, Jan LY. Evidence that the S6 segment of the Shaker voltage-gated K$^+$ channel comprises part of the pore. *Nature* 1994;367:179–82.

63. Blumenthal EM, Kaczmarek LK. Inward rectification of the min K potassium channel. *J Membr Biol* 1993;136:23–29.

64. Varnum MD, Busch AE, Bond CT, et al. The min K channel underlies the cardiac potassium current I_{Ks} and mediates species-specific responses to protein kinase C. *Proc Natl Acad Sci* 1993;90:11528–11532.

65. Yang T, Kupershmidt S, Roden DM. Anti-minK antisense decreases the amplitude of the rapidly activating cardiac delayed rectifier K^+ current. *Circ Res* 1995;77:1246–1253.

66. Sanguinetti MC, Jiang C, Curran ME, et al. A mechanistic link between an inherited and an acquired cardiac arrhythmia: HERG encodes the IKr potassium channel. *Cell* 1995;81(2): 299–307.

67. Schreibmayer W, Dessauer CW, Vorobiov D, et al. Inhibition of an inwardly rectifying K^+ channel by G-protein α subunits. *Nature* 1996;380:624–627.

68. Trudeau MC, Warmke JW, Ganetzky B, et al. HERG a human inward rectifier in the voltage-gated potassium channel family. *Science* 1996;269:92–95.

69. Smith PL, Baukrowitz T, Yellen G. The inward rectification mechanism of the Herg potassium channel. *Nature* 1996;374:833–836.

70. Faravelli I, Arcangeli A, Olivotto M, et al. A HERG-like K^+ channel in rat F-11 DRG cell line: Pharmacological identification and biophysical characterization. *J Physiol (Lond)* 1996;496: 13–23.

71. Covarrubias M, Wei A, Salkoff L. Shaker, Shal, Shab, and Shaw express independent K^+ current systems. *Neuron* 1991;7:763–773.

72. Jan LY, Jan YN. Structural elements involved in specific K^+ channel functions. *Ann Rev Physiol* 1992;54:537–555.

73. Chandy KG, Douglas J, Gutman GA. Simplified gene nomenclature. *Nature* 1991;352:26.

74. Huang X-Y, Morielli AD, Peralta EG. Molecular basis of cardiac potassium channel stimulation by protein kinase A. *Proc Natl Acad Sci U S A* 1994;91:624–628.

75. Trautwein W, Gottstein U, Dudel J. Der Aktionβtrom der Myokardfaβer im Sauerstoffmangel. *Pflügers Arch* 1954;260:40–60.

76. Noma A. ATP-regulated K channels in cardiac muscle. *Nature* 1983;305:147–148.

77. Noma A, Shibasaki T. Membrane current through adenosine-triphosphate-regulated potassium channels in guinea-pig ventricular cells. *J Physiol* 1985;363:463–480.

78. Sakura H, Bond C, Warren-Perry M, et al. Characterization and variation of a human inwardly-rectifying K-channel gene (KCNJ6): A putative ATP-sensitive K-channel subunit. *FEBS Lett* 1995;367:193–197.

79. Tucker SJ, James MR, Adelman JP. Assignment of K_{ATP}-1, the cardiac ATP-sensitive potassium channel gene (KCNJ5), to human chromosome 11a24. *Genomics* 1995;28:127–128.

80. Ho K, Nichols CG, Lederer WJ, et al. Cloning and expression of an inwardly rectifying ATP-regulated potassium channel. *Nature* 1993;362:31–38.

81. Ashord MLJ, Bond CT, Blair TA, et al. Cloning and functional expression of a rat heart K_{ATP} channel. *Nature* 1994;370:456–459.

82. Kozlowski RZ, Ashford MLJ. ATP-sensitive K^+-channel run-down is Mg^{2+} dependent. *Proc R Soc Lond B Biol Sci* 1990;240:397–410.

83. Inagaki N, Tsuura Y, Namba N, et al. Cloning and functional characterization of a novel ATP-sensitive potassium channel ubiquitously expressed in rat tissues, including pancreatic islets, pituitary, skeletal muscle, and heart. *J Biol Chem* 1995;270:5691–5694.

84. Inagaki N, Gonoi T, Clement JP, et al. Reconstitution of I_{KATP}: An inward rectifier subunit plus the sulfonylurea receptor. *Science* 1995;270:1166–1170.

85. Kakei M, Noma A, Shibasaki T. Properties of adenosine-triphosphate-regulated potassium channels in guinea-pig ventricular cells. *J Physiol* 1985;363:441–462.

86. Kameyama M, Kiyosue T, Soejima M. Single channel analysis of the inward rectifier K channel in the rabbit ventricular cells. *Jpn J Physiol* 1983;33:1039–1056.

87. Standen NB, Quayle JM, Davies NW, et al. Hyperpolarizing vasodilators activate ATP-sensitive K^+ channels in arterial smooth muscle. *Science* 1989;245:177–180.

88. Taniguchi T, Noma A, Irisawa H. Modification of the cardiac action potential by intracellular injection of adenosine triphosphate and related substances in guinea pig single ventricular cells. *Circ Res* 1983;53:131–139.

89. Opie LH. Modulation of ischemia by regulation of the ATP-sensitive potassium channel. *Cardiovasc Drugs Ther* 1993;7:507–513.

90. Vereecke J, van Bogaert PP, Verdonck F. *Ionic Currents and Ischemia.* Leuven University Press; Leuven, Belgium,1990.

91. Friedrich M, Benndorf K, Schwalb M, et al. Effects of anoxia on K and Ca currents in isolated guinea pig cardiocytes. *Pflügers Arch* 1990;416:207–209.

92. Lederer WJ, Niggli E, Hadley RW. Sodium-calcium exchange in excitable cells: Fuzzy space. *Science* 1990;248:283.

93. Wendt-Gallitelli MF, Voigt T, Isenberg G. Microheterogeneity of subsarcolemmal sodium gradients. Electron probe microanalysis in guinea-pig ventricular myocytes. *J Physiol* 1993; 472:33–44.

94. Auchampach JA, Maruyama M, Cavero I, et al. Pharmacological evidence of a role of ATP-dependent potassium channels in myocardial stunning. *Circulation* 1992;86:311–319.

95. Armstrong SC, Liu GS, Downey JM, et al. Potassium channels and preconditioning of isolated rabbit cardiomyocytes: Effects of glyburide and pinacidil. *J Mol Cell Cardiol* 1995; 27:1765–1774.

96. Kubo Y, Baldwin TJ, Jan YN, et al. Primary structure and functional expression of a mouse inward rectifier potassium channel. *Nature* 1993;362:127–133.

97. Wickman K, Clapham DE. Ion channel regulation by G proteins. *Physiol Rev* 1995;75:865–885.

98. Krapivinsky G, Gordon EA, Wickman K, et al. The G-protein gated K^+ channel IKACH is a heteromultimer of two inwardly rectifying K^+ channel proteins. *Nature* 1995;374:135–141.

99. Kameyama M, Kakei M, Sato R, et al. Intracellular Na^+ activates a K^+ channel in mammalian cardiac cells. *Nature* 1984;309:254–256.

100. Numa S, Noda M. Molecular structure of sodium channels. *Ann N Y Acad Sc* 1986;479: 338–355.

101. Böhle T, Benndorf, K. Multimodal action of single Na^+ channels in myocardial mouse cells. *Biophys J* 1995;68:121–130.

102. Krafte DS, Davison K, Dugrenier N, et al. Pharmacological modulation of the human cardiac Na^+ channel. *Eur J Pharmacol* 1994;266:245–254.

103. Cohen C, Bean BP, Tsien RW. Tetrodotoxin block of sodium channels in rabbit Purkinje fibers: Interactions between toxin binding and channel gating. *J Gen Physiol* 1981;78:383–411.

104. Frelin C, Cognard C, Vigne P, et al. Tetrodotoxin-sensitive and tetrodotoxin-resistant Na+ channels differ in their sensitivity to Cd2+ and Zn2+. *Eur J Pharmacol* 1986;122:245–250.

105. Kagiyama Y, Hill JL, Gettes LS. Interaction of acidosis and increased extracellular potassium on action potential characteristics and conduction in guinea pig ventricular muscle. *Circ Res* 1982;51:614–623.

106. Shaw R, Rudy Y. Electrophysiological changes of ventricular tissue under ischemic conditions: A simulation study. *Comput Cardiol* 1994;641–644.

107. Luo CH, Rudy Y. A dynamic model of the cardiac ventricular action potential. I. Simulations of ionic currents and concentration changes. *Circ Res* 1994;74:1071–1096.

108. Luo CH, Rudy Y. A dynamic model of the cardiac ventricular action potential. II. Afterdepolarizations, triggered activity, and potentiation. *Circ Res* 1994;74:1097–1113.

109. Friel DD. An ATP-sensitive conductance in single smooth muscle cells from rat vas deferens. *J Physiol* 401;1988:361–380.

110. Zhang J, Rasmusson RL, Hall SK, et al. A chloride current associated with swelling of cultured chick heart cells. *J Physiol* 1993;472:801–820.

110a.Coronado R, Latorre R. Detection of k+ Cl- channels from calf cardiac sarcolemma in planar lipid bilayers. *Nature (London)* 1982;298:849–851.

111. Harvey RD, Clark CD, Hume JR. Chloride current in mammalian cardiac myocytes. Novel mechanism for autonomic regulation of action potential duration and resting membrane potential. *J Gen Physiol* 1990;95:1077–1102.

112. Walsh KB, Wang C. Effect of chloride channel blockers on the cardiac CFTR chloride and L-type calcium currents. *Cardiovasc Res* 1996;32:391–399.

112a.Ehara T, Ishihara K. Anion channels activated by adrenaline in cardiac myocytes. *Nature (London)* 1990;347:284–286.

112b.Piwnica-Worms D, Jacob R, Russell Horres C, et al. Transmembrane chloride flux in tissue-cultured chick heart cells. *J Gen Physiol* 1983;81:731–748.

112c.Zygmunt AC, Gibbons WR. Calcium-activated chloride current in rabbit ventricular myocytes. *Circ Res* 1991;68:424–437.

113. White BL, Doeller JE, Verselis VK, et al. Gap junctional conductance between pairs of ventricular myocytes is modulated synergistically by H^+ and Ca^{++}. *J Gen Physiol* 1990;95: 1061–1075.

114. Délèze, J. Calcium ions and the healing-over of heart fibres. In: Tuccardi B, Marchetti G, eds. *Electrophysiology of the Heart*. Oxford: Pergamon Press; 1965:147–178.

115. Brink PR. Gap junction channels and cell-to-cell messengers in myocardium. *J Cardiovasc Electrophysiol* 1991;2:360–366.

116. Brehm P, Lechleiter J, Smith S, et al. Intracellular signaling as visualized by endogenous calcium-dependent bioluminescence. *Neuron* 1989;3:191–198.

117. Moreno AP, Campos de Carvalho AC, Christ G, et al. Gap junctions between human corpus cavernosum smooth muscle cells: Gating properties and unitary conductance. *Am J Physiol* 1993;264(1 Pt 1):C80–C92.

118. Christ GJ, Spray DC, El-Sabbah M, et al. Gap junctions in vascular tissues. Evaluating the role of intercellular communication in the modulation of vasomotor tone. *Circ Res* 1996;79:631–646.

119. Tsien RW, Weingart R. Inotropic effect of cyclic AMP in calf ventricular muscle studied by a cut end method. *J Physiol (Lond)* 260–117-141.

120. Bennett MV, Zheng X, Sogin ML. The connexins and their family tree. *Soc Gen Physiol Ser* 1994;49:223–233.

121. Kanter HL, Saffitz JE, Beyer EC. Cardiac myocytes express multiple gap junction proteins. *Circ Res* 1992;70:438–444.

122. Davis LM, Rodefeld ME, Green K, et al. Gap junction protein phenotypes of the human heart and conduction system. *J Cardiovasc Electrophysiol* 1996;7:382–383.

123. Willecke K, Heynkes R, Dahl E, et al. Mouse connexin 37: Cloning and functional expression of a gap junction gene highly expressed in lung. *J Cell Biol* 1991;114:1049–1057.

124. Reed KE, Westphale EM, Larson DM, et al. Molecular cloning and functional expression of human connexin 37, an endothelial gap junction protein. *J Clin Invest* 1993;91:997–1004.

125. Brink PR, Cronin K, Banach K, et al. Evidence for heteromeric gap junction channels formed from rat connexin 43 and human connexin 37. *Am J Physiol* 1997;273:C1386–C1396.

126. Koval M, Geist ST, Westphale EM, et al. Transfected connexin 45 alters gap junction permeability in cells expressing endogenous connexin 43. *J Cell Biol* 1995;130:987–995.

127. Burt JM, Spray DC. Single-channel events and gating behavior of the cardiac gap junction channel. *Proc Natl Acad Sci, U S A* 1988;85:3431–3434.

128. Brink PR. Gap junction channel gating and permselectivity: Their roles in coordinated tissue function. *Clin Exp Pharmacol Physiol* 1996;23:1041–1046.

129. Veenstra RD, Wang HZ, Beblo DA, et al. Selectivity of connexin-specific gap junction does not correlate with channel conductance. *Circ Res* 1995;77:1156–1165.

130. Wang H-Z, Li J, Lemanski LF, et al. Gating of mammalian cardiac gap junction channels by transjunctional voltage. *Biophys J* 1992;63:139–151.

131. Veenstra RD, Wang H-Z, Beyer EC, et al. Selective dye and ionic permeability of gap junction channels formed by connexin 45. *Circ Res* 1994;75:483–490.

132. Burt JM, Minnich BN, Massey KD, et al. Influence of lipophilic compounds on gap junction channels. *Prog Cell Res* 1993;3:113–120.

133. McHowat J, Yamada KA, Wu J, et al. Recent insights pertaining to sarcolemmal phospholipid alterations underlying arrhythmogenesis in the ischemic heart. *J Cardiovasc Electrophyiol* 1993;4:288–310.

134. Yamada KA, McHowat J, Yan GX, et al. Cellular uncoupling induced by accumulation of long-chain acylcarnitine during ischemia. *Circ Res* 1994;74:83–95.

135. Cole WC, Picone JB, Sperelakis N. Gap junction uncoupling and discontinuous propagation in the heart. A comparison of experimental data with computer simulation. *Biophys J* 1988; 53:809–818.

136. Levine JH, Moore EN, Weisman HF, et al. Depression of action potential characteristics and a decreased space constant are present in postischemic, reperfused myocardium. *J Clin Invest* 1987;79:107–116.

137. Ovadia M, Burt JM. Developmental modulation of susceptibility to arrhythmogenesis in myocardial ischemia: Reduced sensitivity of adult vs. neonatal heart cells to uncoupling by lipophilic substances. *Circulation* 1991;84:II324.

138. Olney JW, Ho OL, Rhee V. Cytotoxic effects of acidic and sulphur containing amino acids on the infant mouse central nervous system. *Exp Brain Res* 1971;14:61–76.
139. Olney JW, Rhee V, Ho OL. Kainic acid: A powerful neurotoxic analogue of glutamate. *Brain Res* 1974;507–512.
140. Mody I, MacDonald JF. NMDA receptor-dependent excitotoxicity: The role of intracellular Ca^{2+} release. *TiPS* 1995;16:356–359.
141. Wisden W, Seeburg PH. Mammalian ionotropic glutamate receptors. *Curr Opin Neurobiol* 1993;3:291–298.
142. Choi DW. Ionic dependence of glutamate neurotoxicity. *J Neurosci* 1987;7:369–379.
143. Choi DW. Excitotoxic cell death. *J Neurobiol* 1992;23:1261–1276.
144. Steller H. Mechanisms and genes of cellular suicide. *Science* 1995;267:1445–1462.
145. Carmeliet E. Myocardial ischemia: Reversible and irreversible changes. *Circulation* 1984;70: 149–151.
146. Braunwald E. Pathophysiology of heart failure. Chapter 14. In: Braunwald E, ed. *Heart Disease. A Textbook of Cardiovascular Medicine*. Philadelphia, Pa: W. B. Saunders Co.; 1992: 393–414.
147. Radermacher M, Rao V, Grassucci R, et al. Cryo-electron microscopy and three-dimensional reconstruction of the calcium release channel/ryanodine receptor from skeletal muscle. *J Cell Biol* 1994;127:411–423.
148. Sitsapesan R, Montgomery RAP, Williams AJ. New insights into the gating mechanisms of cardiac ryanodine receptors revealed by rapid changes in ligand concentration. *Circ Res* 1995;77:765–772.
149. Zimanyi I. Pessah I. Pharmacology of ryanodine-sensitive Ca^{2+} release channels. Chapter 31. In: Peracchia C, ed. *Handbook of Membrane Channels. Molecular and Cellular Physiology*. San Diego, Calif: Academic Press, Inc.; 1994:475–494.
150. Gao WD, Atar D, Backx PH, Marban E. Relationship between intracellular calcium and contractile force in stunned myocardium. *Circ Res* 1995;76:1036–1048.
151. Catterall WA. Functional subunit structure of voltage-gated calcium channels. *Science* 1991; 253:1499–1500.
152. Veldkamp MW, van Ginneken ACG, Bouman LN. Single delayed rectifier channels in the membrane of rabbit ventricular myocytes. *Circ Res* 1993;72:865–878.
153. Piwnica-Worms D, Jacob R, Horres CR, et al. Transmembrane chloride flux in tissue-cultured heart cells. *J Gen Physiol* 1983;81:731–748.
154. Peracchia C. *Handbook of Membrane Channels. Molecular and Cellular Physiology*. San Diego, Calif: Academic Press, Inc.; 1994:362.

Part IV

Advances in Functional Imaging

New Methods for Measurement of Regional and Global Ventricular Function

Stephen L. Bacharach, PhD

_____

Introduction

The measurement of regional ventricular function is important in assessing viability.[1-7] Obviously, a region of the myocardium that thickens contains at least some viable tissue. Of course, the converse is not true—absence of thickening does not necessarily imply absence of viable tissue. In addition, global left ventricular (LV) function is a critical factor in influencing the treatment of many types of cardiac disease. The decision as to whether a patient with viable but ischemic tissue is a suitable candidate for surgical intervention often is influenced by the degree of global dysfunction that may be present. For these reasons, it is important to understand some of the newly developed nuclear-based techniques available for determining regional and global ventricular function.

Nuclear medicine procedures for many years have offered a well-accepted method for making quantifiable measurements of global LV function, and for making visual assessments of regional function. The principle tools for making such measurements have been planar gated bloodpool (GBP) imaging, either at equilibrium or, less commonly, during first transit of a bolus injection. Planar GBP imaging has served well to make reliable measurements of global LV function. The proportionality between counts and volume make the technique less susceptible to the errors found in geometric-based methods. However, the ability of the technique to make measurements of regional function always has been somewhat limited. These limitations stem primarily from the very nature of planar imaging, namely, the superimposition of counts from underlying and overlying tissue and the inability to view the ventricle perpendicular to its long axis. Therefore even the most common view—the modified left anterior oblique (LAO) view—still is suboptimal. Anterior and posterior walls overlap each other, as do the atria and the basal aspect of the LV cavity. The modified LAO view typically produces a very foreshortened perspective of the left ventricle,[8] and this view usually pushes the apex into the lower to middle portion of the LV cavity. When other views (eg, anterior or lateral) are used to try to separate out the surfaces of interest, still other structures interfere. Many years ago, GBP single photon emission computed tomography (SPECT) imaging was proposed to

_____

From Dilsizian V (ed). *Myocardial Viability: A Clinical and Scientific Treatise.* Armonk, NY: Futura Publishing Co., Inc.; © 2000.

overcome some of these limitations. Recently, the advent of multiheaded SPECT cameras coupled with the availability of large amounts of inexpensive computer memory has at last made gated SPECT imaging clinically feasible.[9–15]

Most GBP imaging (SPECT or planar) techniques are based on the fact that changes in counts over the cardiac cycle are proportional to changes in volume. This has made the technique extremely powerful for measures of global function, such as ejection fraction (EF). It also has meant that (apart from background considerations) the measurements of global function do not depend on accurate tracings of ventricular borders. Global measurements from techniques such as gated magnetic resonance imaging (MRI) or echocardiography require very accurate determinations of the endocardial borders during the cardiac cycle, because measurements of global function made with these techniques are based on geometry not on an inherent proportionality between counts and volume.

In GBP imaging, one directly images the bloodpool itself, rather than the myocardial walls whose contraction is expelling the blood from the LV cavity. For measurement of pump function, this is exactly the quantity of interest. The motion of the endocardial borders is of course responsible for the motion of the adjacent blood, so endocardial motion should track changes in bloodpool exactly. However, it also is often desired to be able to measure not just how the endocardial surface moves, but also how the myocardial wall thickens with time. In the past, such measurements were the exclusive province of echocardiography and MRI. Recently, however, gated tomographic myocardial imaging has been recognized as a viable alternative to these other methods.[11,16–22] The myocardial imaging agent might be technetium-99m (^{99m}Tc) sestamibi (MIBI) (using SPECT), ^{18}F-2-deoxyglucose (FDG) [with positron emission tomography (PET)], or other agents taken up by the myocardium, including ^{201}Tl. Tomographic gating of these myocardial agents allows simultaneous measurement of mechanical and biochemical function, for example, simultaneous measurement of perfusion and LV function.

The purpose of this chapter is to discuss both of these two new techniques: gated tomographic bloodpool imaging and gated tomographic myocardial imaging. The methods for implementing these modalities in clinical practice will be presented, and a discussion of the basic principles underlying each method will be given. The latter is especially important if the clinical advantages and limitations of each method are to be clearly understood.

Gated Bloodpool Tomography

GBP tomography was first described many years ago.[13–15] Only recently, however, has it become clinically practical because of the availability of multiheaded SPECT cameras. With such cameras, the acquisition time to achieve a clinically useful study is approximately 20–30 minutes. Because typically three views are taken during planar GBP imaging, planar imaging times typically are 15–25 minutes (eg, if 5–8 minutes are acquired per view)—not very different from imaging times with gated SPECT. For visualization of regional ventricular function (ie, regional wall motion), fewer counts may be needed in GBP SPECT than with planar imaging to achieve the same signal to noise (S/N) ratio, because of the reduction of background from over and underlying tissue achievable with SPECT. At rest there is ample data validating the utility of the technique. Although there probably is sufficient clinical need for rest-only studies to justify its use, there also is interest in trying to push the technique to its limits by imaging during pharmacologic stress or even during physical exercise. However, use of the technique during stress is as yet unproved except in research settings.[23]

GBP tomography also has been performed with PET, primarily using labeled carbon monoxide, either with an ^{15}O label (2-minute half-life) or with a ^{11}C label (20-minute half-life).[24,25] PET GBP can produce superb quality, quantitatively accurate images, but it is not clear that the additional information provided by PET, compared with SPECT, would ever justify the extra cost for this application.

Typical Single Photon Emission Computer Tomography Gated Bloodpool Acquisition

Radiolabeling of the bloodpool is identical to that used for planar GBP imaging. Typically, 25 mCi of ^{99m}Tc are used, with either in vitro or in vivo labeling techniques. Forty-millicurie doses have been tried for rapid dobutamine SPECT imaging, but in this case some care has to be taken to account for camera dead time.

With two-headed, 90° apart cameras, typically at least 60 projections (3° steps) should be taken over 180°. The optimal 180° span usually is considered to be 45° right anterior oblique (RAO) to 45° left posterior oblique (LPO).[26] As in all SPECT imaging, care should be taken to make sure that no regions in the plane of reconstruction that emit counts are excluded from the field of view (lest artifacts be produced). If a three-headed camera is used, the same minimum 3° steps are recommended, giving 120 projections. There is little data about the relative advantages of 360° versus 180° imaging for GBP SPECT. This issue has been investigated much more thoroughly for perfusion SPECT imaging, but even in that case there is still controversy as to which methodology is better. Several facts are agreed on, however. The 360° SPECT is most efficiently done with a three-headed camera, while 180° usually is performed with a 90° two-headed camera. Obviously, if the same number of angles and time per angle were used for three-headed 360° versus two-headed 180° imaging, then three-headed 360° imaging would require 30% more total imaging time than two-headed 180° imaging. However, the extra 30% acquisition time does not necessarily produce 30% more counts, because the posterior views of the heart have very reduced count rates (from the heart) because of attenuation. Also, two-headed 180° imaging, because all views are relatively close to the heart, can in theory produce images with slightly better spatial resolution. However, the resolution in 180° imaging often is less uniform than with 360° imaging; that is, for 180° imaging, the resolution is poorer in some directions than in others. This can cause small artifacts in perfusion imaging, but these may not be a significant deleterious factor in GBP imaging. The resolution is more homogeneous with 360° imaging, because conjugate view averaging is used. Finally, artifacts caused by inconsistent projections (which in turn are caused primarily by not performing corrections for attenuation and scatter) may be very slightly more pronounced for 180° than for 360° imaging. Again, it is unclear whether any of these differences are of clinical importance for GBP SPECT, and both modalities have been used successfully in clinical situations.

Electrocardiogram (ECG) gating in general can be performed in nearly the same way as with planar imaging. However, there are some important differences. First, the number of gates usually is limited, because of memory limitations (remember that a single 16-gate SPECT study requires the same space as 16-ungated SPECT studies). The influence of limited number of gating periods has been investigated thoroughly.[27] If ejection fraction is the only quantity of interest, these data show that at rest, approximately 60 milliseconds or less per gated frame should be used. This translates, for a heart rate of 70, to approximately 14 frames per cycle. This number of frames per cycle should be increased at lower heart rates (or, alternatively, kept the same and the end of the cycle truncated) and may be decreased at higher heart rates (as necessary to keep the time per frame 60 milliseconds or less, during a resting study). Using a smaller number of time points (ie, a larger time per frame) will introduce a small systematic underestimate in ejection fraction.[27] Depending on the circumstances, this bias may or may not be clinically important.

Heart rate irregularities can seriously affect gated SPECT studies. In nongated SPECT, each projection angle is acquired for the same length of time. To achieve a constant acquisition time per step in gated SPECT, one must collect a fixed number of cardiac cycles at each angle. This is because the total acquisition time for a particular frame (time point) in the cycle is the number of beats multiplied by the time per frame. If one or more beats is not within whatever beat length "window" may have been set, the SPECT camera pauses at that projection angle until the proper number of beats have occurred. For some camera/computer systems this means that changes in heart rate occurring during the study can seriously prolong the total acquisition. Systems that track changes in heart rate can reduce this problem. Other schemes of acquisition, including "phase mode" gating[28,29] and acquiring for a fixed time per step but correcting for varying number of beats are under investigation and may further improve the ease with which one can perform a gated SPECT study.

After acquisition, the data are reconstructed into transaxial slices, which then are reoriented into short-axis or long-axis views. In the past, most cardiac analysis (eg, nongated perfusion SPECT imaging) has been based on reorienting the cardiac data into short-axis slices. However, long-axis slices (Fig. 1) can offer several significant advantages over short-axis views (eg, significantly better visualization of the apex), while retaining the ability to perform quantitative analysis. This is especially important for gated SPECT bloodpool studies, but this observation also may make it worthwhile to rethink the conventional wisdom of short-axis analysis for other SPECT cardiac studies (eg, perfusion). There also has been some progress toward the development of methods for three-dimensional (3D) display of the gated data.[11,17,30] In principle, this would preserve the complete 3D nature of the data, and if suitable display devices were available, which

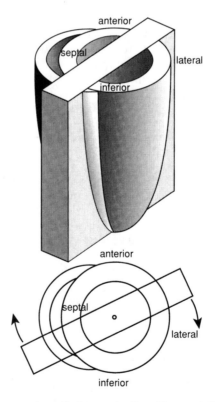

Figure 1. (**Top**) Illustrating creation of a long-axis slice. (**Bottom**) Schematic diagram showing how one long-axis slice (the rectangle) can be created from a stack of short-axis slices. To create a set of long-axis slices that encompass all walls of the heart (eg, as in Fig. 4), one might rotate the rectangle about the center of the heart as shown.

permitted real-time rotations of the LV bloodpool as it beat, such displays might result in improved visualization of regional function. Considerable developmental work still is needed to optimize such displays.

Global Function From Tomographic Gated Bloodpool

Tomographic GBP allows true 3D visualization of the beating heart. Despite the advantages of being able to compute regional function from the 3D data, measures of global function, for example, global EF, are still of great clinical importance, and it is therefore desirable to be able to compute such global indices from the 3D data set. At first one would think that the optimum way to compute global function from the 3D data would be to use the individual short-or long-axis tomograms. This is indeed possible, although quite tedious. Regions of interest (ROIs) could be drawn on each slice, at each time point, requiring drawing many times more ROIs than are necessary for analysis of planar studies. Drawing so many ROIs (either manually or automatically by computer) might well lead to significant variability in the analysis. Nonetheless, two methods have been suggested for using the SPECT slices in this way.[9,13,31] The first is to treat the data as though it were echocardiography or MRI data and carefully trace the endocardial borders (ie, the outer edge of the bloodpool) from each slice. The area of each slice multiplied by the slice thickness then is the volume of that slice. By adding up all such volumes from all slices, the volume of the LV may be calculated. Performing this summation at end diastole (ED) and at end systole (ES) allows EF to be computed, and, in addition, one obtains (in theory) the ED volume and the ES volume in absolute units (milliliters). This method makes no assumptions of proportionality between counts and volume and relies instead solely on geometry. Unfortunately, the volumes determined in this geometric manner are very sensitive to the exact definition of the border. Although echocardiography and possibly MRI may produce high enough resolution images to determine these endocardial borders accurately, it is not yet clear whether nuclear medicine images can be used to produce accurate, reliable, geometric estimates of absolute volume.

The second method of computing global function also involves drawing ROIs on each slice, but bases the computation of EF on the assumption that changes in counts are proportional to changes in volume. In this second method, the counts in each ROI are recorded at the desired time points (eg, ED and ES). If only relative changes in volume are needed (eg, EF) and not absolute volumes, the sum of all the counts at ED minus the sum of all counts at ES divided by the sum of all counts at ED yields a measure of ejection fraction. Because in the tomographic study background is very low, small variations in region size do not produce nearly as much change in EF as they would in a geometrically based method. In planar studies, there is of course no attenuation correction performed, which causes counts from the anterior portion of the LV cavity to be weighted slightly more heavily than counts from the posterior portion of the LV. Similarly, in a SPECT GBP that has not been corrected for attenuation (the usual case at this writing), there is a similar artificial weighting caused by attenuation. There is some evidence that this weighting causes only very small errors.[8] At first one might think that attenuation correction would be necessary to make use of a proportionality between counts and volume. However, it is easy to prove that as long as attenuation at a particular location can be assumed to be constant from ED to ES, attenuation correction is not necessary if one only wishes to compute the relative change in counts at that particular location. This means that regional pixel by pixel computations are immune to the effects of attenuation (and in fact it is possible to make use of this fact when computing global ejection fraction as well).

Although the counts-based method can be used to yield EF values, without the errors associated with the geometrical method, it cannot yield absolute volumes without knowledge of the proportionality constant between counts and volume. There is some data about how one might determine this factor for planar imaging, but to date no one has attempted such a determination for SPECT imaging, and such a measurement would seem to require accurate attenuation correction.

A third method for using tomographic GBP data to measure global EF recently has been proposed.[8] This method may well be the easiest to implement and may yield the most reliable and accurate values of global EF. This third method also is a counts-based method. It involves taking the gated short-axis slices, for example, and reprojecting them along the true long axis of the heart into a pseudoplanar study (Fig. 2). Why bother to acquire a tomographic study if one simply is going to reconvert it into a planar study? There are several reasons. First, it is possible to reproject the images so as to give a true long-axis view of the heart. It has been shown that conventional planar studies, even with a caudal tilt, deviate by an average of 60° from a true long-axis view, and that this deviation has significant impact on the accuracy and reproducibility of global ejection fractions (primarily because of overlap of the atrium with the left ventricle).[8] The true long-axis projection can be shown to have far less atrial overlap and permits better visualization of wall motion than an actual planar study. Second, when reprojecting, it is possible to mask out counts from over- and underlying tissue. Even if the masking is done crudely, by simply (and potentially automatically) placing a box around the entire heart, background has been shown to be reduced by a factor of about 2.5 compared with the background in planar images. At this reduced level of background activity, global EF becomes much less

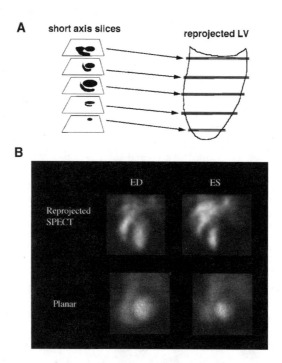

Figure 2. (**Top**) Schematic illustration of how a stack of short-axis slices are reprojected (ie, summed along one direction) to produce a planar, reprojected image. (**Bottom**) Actual planar end diastole and end systole images from a typical patient. The reprojected single photon emission computer tomography (SPECT) images have been reprojected from a SPECT short-axis set of slices, to give a true long-axis view, while the planar images below it were acquired with a planar gamma camera and therefore are considerably foreshortened. Note the larger background activity in the true planar images as compared with the reprojected SPECT images, because of masking, which was used to reduce background in the reprojected SPECT images (as described in text).

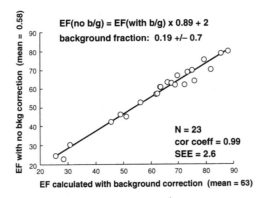

Figure 3. Ejection fraction (EF) from reprojected SPECT gated bloodpool (GBP) images, with and without background correction. Background fraction [background counts/left ventricular (LV) ED counts] with reprojected SPECT averages only 0.19. Even if no correction is made for background (ordinate) the EF values agree quite well with the background corrected Efs (abscissa). Note the excellent correlation and the low standard error of the estimate (SEE).

sensitive to LV ROI placement and very insensitive to background ROI placement. In fact, recent results indicate that it might be possible to ignore background completely when computing global EF from a reprojected GBP SPECT study (Fig. 3). In Figure 3, although EF is reduced slightly by ignoring background, there is very little variability introduced. Therefore a simple linear correction can be used to produce the "true" EF. If a similar comparison between EF with and without background correction were made for an actual planar study, the variability would be expected to be prohibitively large. Finally, by reprojecting the SPECT data, analysis is simplified considerably. Only two ROIs need be drawn (at ED and ES), and because of the improved S/N due to lower background in the reprojected images, compared with data acquired in planar mode, automatic methods of region drawing may behave much more reliably with reprojected images than with true planar images.

Reprojected SPECT EFs have been shown to be approximately 30% higher than planar EFs[8] (ie, a 50% EF by planar translates to approximately 65% EF by reprojected SPECT). These reprojected EF values are more consistent with the EF values that have been reported from other modalities (eg, MRI and biplane ventriculography). In addition, there is evidence that by using either the reprojected or slice-by-slice counts–based methods, one obtains more accurate and less variable values of global EF than could be obtained with planar imaging. If this reduction in variability is confirmed by further studies, the GBP SPECT method for computing global EF could have a significant clinical impact. For example, the potential reduction in variability of global EF by using GBP SPECT could improve the utility of global EF for clinical situations in which the reliable determination of small changes in EF over time are important (eg, assessment of adriamycin therapy).

Regional Function From Gated Bloodpool Single Photon Emission Computer Tomography

At this writing, the principle method for evaluating regional function from GBP SPECT is visual analysis (just as it is for planar imaging). The visual analysis might be performed by displaying cine images of the short-axis slices or of the long-axis slices (the latter may be preferred because the apex is better visualized). It also is possible to examine the reprojected images at several views (because any view is possible from the SPECT data set). It is not yet clear which method is best; however, one might imagine that displaying the SPECT slices (which have no superimposed counts) would give better results than reprojected images. There may be one circumstance when this is not true, namely, if very rapid (eg, pharmaceutical stress) acquisitions are required. In this case, limited counts may make cine SPECT slices difficult to read, while reprojected images, with their increased total counts, may produce more reliable visual readings.[23]

When visualization of cine images acquired from a planar camera are compared with those from GBP SPECT, frequently defects seen as being only mild on the planar images may be perceived as severe defects with GBP SPECT imaging. Which analysis is correct? By reprojecting the SPECT study into the equivalent planar view at the same angle as used by the planar gamma camera, it quickly becomes obvious that wall motion abnormalities can be masked easily by over- and underlying activity in the ventricle (eg, Fig. 4). The superimposition of regions of the LV with normal counts changes on top of regions with abnormal counts changes can transform a truly severe defect into an apparently mild one. This quite commonly occurs with defects at the apex, because in the foreshortened view used in planar studies, the apex is superimposed on the lower portion of the ventricular cavity. It also frequently occurs with anterior or inferior wall defects. SPECT avoids these difficulties.

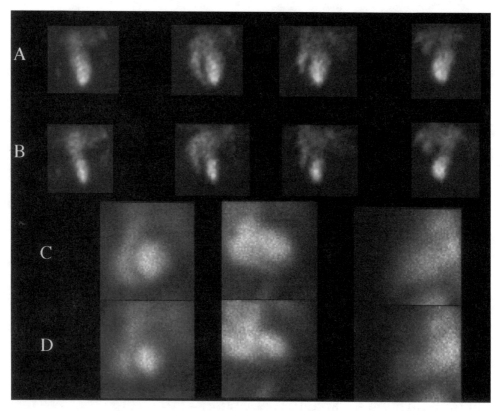

Figure 4. Long-axis GBP SPECT views at ED (row A), and ES (row B). The four long-axis views were created as in Figure 1. The first long axis view was made with the slicing rectangle positioned at 22.5° on Figure 1(bottom), and each of the other three long-axis views were spaced 45° apart. This subject has a severe apical wall motion defect, easily seen in the long-axis views but poorly visualized in the planar GBP images [left anterior oblique (LAO), anterior (Ant), and lateral (Lat)] shown in rows C (at ED) and D (at ES).

A decade or more ago, many attempts were made to quantify regional wall motion abnormalities from planar GBP studies by use of functional imaging. With the exception of phase imaging for the characterization of electrical conduction abnormalities, none of these functional imaging methods were adopted widely in clinical practice. One reason for their lack of success may be related again to the superimposition of counts inherent in planar cine sequences. It is possible that if these functional imaging methodologies were applied to SPECT cine sequences,[10,32,33] much better results would be obtained, perhaps allowing realization of the goal of replacing visualization of regional wall motion with objective quantitative evaluation. In the near future, it is expected that this speculation will be tested.

Gated Perfusion and Metabolic Imaging

Regional Function From Gated Perfusion/Metabolism Images

Pharmaceuticals such as Tc-labeled MIBI or FDG or ^{201}Tl are taken up by the myocardium. When one gates tomographic images (from either PET or SPECT cameras) acquired with such agents, the cardiac walls can be seen to move (and thicken) during the cardiac cycle. The resolution of either PET or SPECT imaging devices [realistically approximately 6–7 and 12–18 mm full-width half-maximum (FWHM), respectively] possibly may be too poor to permit quantitative measurements of regional myocardial thickening to be made by simple edge tracking, as is done in echocardiography and MRI. However, it has been observed that if a gated SPECT slice is displayed as a cine sequence, not only can the myocardial wall be observed to thicken, but it also appears to brighten from ED to ES. This effect is seen in Figure 5, in which a gated FDG PET transaxial slice is shown at ED and at ES. Clearly, there is increased intensity in the myocardium at ES compared with ED. In Figure 5 a profile of counts through the image at ED and ES also is shown, and one can observe the increase in the height of the profile at ES compared with ED. The effect is seen easily on the free and septal walls but also occurs in the right ventricular (RV) wall. There is a well-understood physical phenomenon—the partial volume effect—which can explain why this brightening occurs. By understanding the cause of the brightening, one can understand the advantages and limitations of trying to use this brightening as a method of quantifying myocardial thickening.

The partial volume effect and its influence on cardiac images is quite easy to understand. Imagine that one had a perfect SPECT camera (one with perfect resolution and which could correct perfectly for scatter and attenuation). If we imaged a patient with perfectly uniform myocardial uptake, a short-axis image of the patients heart might look like Figure 6(A). In Figure 5(A) it has been assumed that the uptake of pharmaceutical in the heart resulted in 100 U of brightness in the image and that the myocardial wall thickness was 12 mm. A profile (plot of counts versus distance) across one location of the heart would look as shown by the solid line in Figure 6(C); the measured activity is zero outside the heart and rises instantly up to 100 inside the myocardium. However, no SPECT camera has perfect resolution. Instead, a typical SPECT cardiac image might have 12–18 mm resolution. That is, the counts in the image would be blurred. Some of the 100 counts inside the myocardium of Figure 6(A) would be blurred to regions outside the myocardium, as shown in Figure 6(B). Note that the total counts remains the same— some of the counts that were previously inside the myocardium now are simply blurred outside the myocardial wall, as seen from the profile of Figure 6(C) (dotted line). If an ROI were drawn around Figure 6(A) at exactly the true anatomical myocardial border and then that ROI were applied to the blurred image of Figure 6(B), the counts from Figure

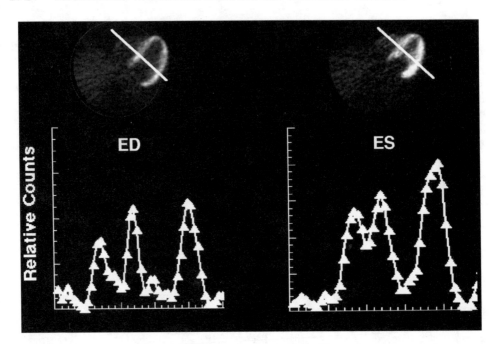

Figure 5. (Top) Gated positron emission tomography (PET) ^{18}F-2-deoxyglucose (FDG) images (transaxial) at ED and ES. **(Bottom)** Count profiles along the lines indicated in the ED and ES images. Brightness of the septal and free wall increases at ES compared with ED, and this is reflected also in the increase in the peak of the count profiles.

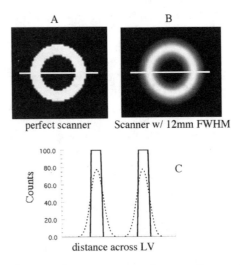

Figure 6. (A) An idealized short-axis image of a subject with a perfectly uniform uptake of myocardial activity, as might be imaged with a scanner with perfect resolution. **(B)** The same image but as would be seen if imaged with a 12-mm full-width half-maximum (FWHM) resolution SPECT scanner. **(C)** Profiles through images A and B; the solid line is a profile through A while the dotted line is a profile through image B. The blurring causes the peak counts of the profile to be reduced, because some counts are blurred outside the true anatomical border of the image.

6(B) would be lower than those from Figure 6(A) because some of the counts would have been blurred outside the true anatomical myocardial ROI. This reduction in counts is said to be caused by "the partial volume" effect. If the SPECT resolution were 12 mm FWHM, then the total counts in the ROI would drop by approximately 33% from Figure 6(A) to 6(B). Thus the "recovery" coefficient (the fraction of the true total number of counts recovered in the ROI at this resolution) associated with this ROI, this wall thickness, and this SPECT resolution, would be 67%. The thinner the wall, the larger the fraction of counts are blurred to regions outside the wall. Figure 7(A) plots the percentage of total counts in the anatomical ROI as a function of myocardial thickness for several different resolutions (FWHM). The poorer the resolution, the lower will be the recovery of counts. For each resolution, the percent of counts recovered increases with increasing

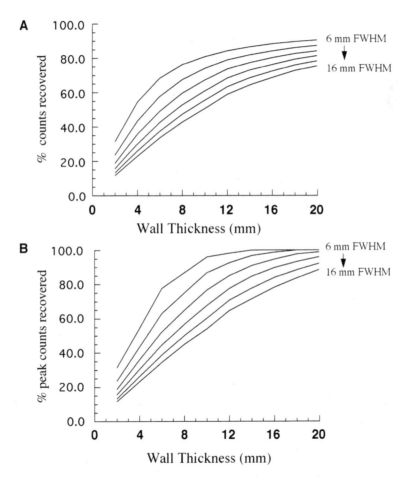

Figure 7. (A) The percentage of total counts in the anatomical regions of interest (ROI) as a function of myocardial thickness for several different resolutions (FWHM). The poorer the resolution, the poorer will be the recovery of counts. For each resolution, the percent of counts recovered increases with increasing wall thickness. For very thin walls, the increase is at first rapid and then flattens out as the wall gets thicker and thicker, as can be seen from A. (**B**) The percentage of peak recovered counts in the myocardium [the peak of the profile in Fig. 6(C)] as a function of wall thickness for several different imaging resolutions. A value of 90%, for example, means that the measured peak would be only 90% of the true peak counts. The general shape of this figure is quite similar to that in A. In A it is the mean counts in an anatomical ROI that are plotted, while in B it is the maximum counts in the region (ie, the peak of the profile).

wall thickness. For very thin walls, the increase is at first rapid and then flattens out as the wall gets thicker and thicker, as can be seen from Figure 7(A).

Clearly, the counts closest to the edge of the myocardial wall go down the most because counts just inside the myocardium can smear into the space outside the wall, but there are no counts outside the wall to be smeared back into myocardium. On the other hand, the counts in the middle of the myocardial wall go down less, because some of the counts that smear away from the center of the myocardium are compensated by counts from nearby regions of the myocardium, which are blurred back to the center. Figure 7(B) plots the peak counts in the myocardium [the peak of the profile in Fig. 6(C)] as a function of wall thickness for several different imaging resolutions. The general shape of this figure is quite similar to that in Figure 7(A). In Figure 7(A), it is the mean counts in an anatomical ROI that are plotted, while in Figure 7(B) it is the maximum counts in the region (ie, in a profile). The peak of the profile determines the "brightest" counts seen in that part of the image. As seen in Figure 7(B), as the myocardium gets thicker, the peak counts increase, until after a certain thickness (approximately four times the FWHM), the peak can increase no further. At this point, just as many counts are being blurred out of the center of the myocardium as are being blurred back into the center. We can use Figure 7(B) to predict exactly how much change in image brightness will occur for a given change in thickness. Consider two diagnostically important situations: thickening of a thin myocardium, whose viability is potentially in question, and thickening of a normal or above normal thickness myocardium. From Figure 7(B) it can be seen that for very thin walls (eg, 8 mm or less), the slope of Figure 7(B) is higher for good resolution images than for poor. This means that the brightness changes more rapidly with thickening for good resolution images than for poor resolution images, implying that PET would be able to detect small changes in wall thickness in thin myocardial walls better than would SPECT. On the other hand, for thick walls (say 12 mm and thicker), good resolution images (eg, 6 mm PET) produce very little change in brightness even for large amounts of thickening; the curve in Figure 7(B) is flat. Poor resolution images, on the other hand, (eg, 14 mm FWHM SPECT) continue to get brighter with changes in thickness, even at fairly large wall thickness, although the amount of brightening for a given thickening [ie, the slope of Fig. 7(B)] gradually diminishes for larger and larger thickness. In summary, good resolution images are able to see more easily the small changes in thickening associated with thin, ischemic walls, while poor resolution images see more easily the thickening occurring in walls of normal or above normal thickness. Of course good resolution images may be "smoothed" easily into poor resolution images, but the converse is not true, and in both cases, for very thick walls, very little brightening occurs as the myocardium thickens.

The above discussion has some important clinical ramifications. For example, if brightening during systole does not appear uniform around the heart, it may be either because thickening is not uniform or because the wall is thinner in some regions than in others. Also, a region that brightens a lot may do so either because it thickens a lot or it may thicken only a little but be very thin to begin with [ie, be on the steep portion of Figure 7(B)]. Finally, very thick myocardia may experience little or no brightening even though the wall is thickening normally, because at large thickness the curve of Figure 7(B) becomes flat. This is why, in Figure 5 the thin RV wall has a larger percent increase in brightness (as seen by the peak of the profile) than do the thicker lateral or septal walls.

Yamashita[22] was one of the first to describe the clinical use of this "brightening" method for the determination of thickening. Cooke,[34] Galt,[35] Mok,[36] and Bartlett[37] further analyzed the brightening method. The nonlinear behavior of brightening versus thickening was soon realized and was characterized by Mok[36] and Bartlett[37]. In part because of the difficulty in dealing with this nonlinear relationship (ie, the nonlinearities of Figure 7), Porenta[38] described a semigeometric way of analyzing the partial volume effect to extract thickness and thickening. His method permitted absolute values of thickness to be computed at ED and ES, rather than simply a relative index, such as obtained by analysis of brightening. This absolute method, while avoiding the nonlinearities associated with the usual analysis of brightening, was shown by Porenta to be quite sensitive to noise. Bartlett[37] compared these two generic types of methods—brightening and semigeometric—and evaluated the difficulties each method has in determining thickening or percentage thickening accurately. Finally, Buvat[39] has described a "hybrid" approach to the measurement of thickening, which combines systolic brightening effects with the geometric-based method. This hybrid method appears to capitalize on the advantages of each of the two previously proposed methodologies, to produce a method that seems to behave more linearly with thickening and yet still not be too sensitive to noise. As of this writing, none of the methods have yet undergone extensive clinical testing.

Global Function From Gated Perfusion/Metabolism Scans

In addition to the brightening effect described above, one also can observe the motion of the endocardium when the perfusion or metabolism images are displayed as a gated cine. Many investigators have proposed delineating the endocardial edges at ED and ES from these gated myocardial scans to determine ejection fraction[16,18,19] and even absolute ED and ES volumes. Using such edge-based geometrical methods to determine EF and LV volumes from nuclear studies is not new. In the early days of equilibrium GBP imaging, ejection fraction measurements based on delineating the edges of the bloodpool were investigated. These methods assumed some geometric shape for the LV (eg, an ellipsoid). However, the values obtained depended very strongly on the exact definition of the edges producing high variability for EF (and very high variability for absolute volumes), and the technique was for the most part abandoned in favor of counts-based EF methods. With the advent of gated SPECT, the geometric technique has proven more robust, presumably in part because of the higher contrast obtainable from tomographic, as opposed to planar, images. Several methods have been put forth to compute EF or volumes from gated myocardial image sequences. One could draw ROIs on each short-axis image and compute the volume by adding together the areas of each ROI times its slice thickness (a method for computing volumes known as "coin stacking") or the ROIs could be drawn on the horizontal and vertical long-axis slices, at ED and ES, and techniques identical to those used with biplane contrast ventriculography. This latter approach of course requires some geometrical assumptions about the shape of the heart, but not as many as a single view (as in the case of planar imaging) would.

All the geometric methods are dependent on accurate delineation of the endocardial edge of the LV. Various methods have been proposed to delineate this surface, ranging from simple thresholding to more elaborate semiautomated methods.[16,18, 40] One difficulty is encountered when trying to delineate regions with low uptake (eg, old infarct or even regions of questionable viability). Several attempts have been made to get around this problem. In one, a count threshold based on the peak counts in the region was suggested (empirically, there are often but not always at least some counts in all regions). In another, if a region's peak counts were <50% of normal, it was suggested that one use neighboring regions to assist in the determination of the myocardial edges at that region. Of course this assumes that the walls of the region in question are similar to its neighbors. This assumption may not matter much for accurate computation of global parameters (if the region is not too large) but of course may be inadequate for regional measurements.

Despite the difficulties, much effort has been expended to begin validating the various techniques for measuring EF (and to a lesser extent absolute volumes) from manual or automatic geometric endocardial tracings. Considerable progress has been made toward confirming that the method can produce, on average, accurate values of EF.

However, more work is needed to assess the reproducibility (ie, the variability) of the technique. Although it is encouraging to know that the technique gives, on average, the correct EF, it also is necessary to know how accurate and reproducible the measurement of EF is for a single subject. This is especially important for applications in which small changes in EF over time are used to make clinical decisions. In such cases it is not sufficient that a method simply correlate well with some other "gold" standard. In addition, one must know how big a change in EF must be observed in a particular patient before one is sure that a real change, as opposed to one caused by variability in the technique, actually occurred. In addition, as of this writing, while the ability of the technique to measure absolute volumes appears promising, considerable more validation is necessary before this aspect of the technique can be used in clinical practice.

Acquisition of Gated Single Photon Emission Computer Tomography Perfusion/Metabolism Images

Gated perfusion images are acquired in a manner nearly identical to that used to acquire ungated perfusion images, but with the addition of ECG gating (see the description of GBP SPECT acquisition above). However, there are several important clinical considerations. First, which perfusion study should be gated? Ideally, all other things being equal, one would gate the study with the most counts in the myocardium, that is, the one with the best statistical quality. For Tl, this might be the stress study. Ideally, one acquires the Tl stress study soon after injection. Although the injection is at stress, the gated imaging is of course at rest and is meant to reflect resting ventricular function. However, the recent stress may well continue to affect wall motion for some time after stress, causing regions that might be viable and capable of contraction, to exhibit poor or nonexistent contraction immediately after stress.

Another difficulty with performing gated perfusion studies arises because one wishes to use the study for two purposes: assessment of perfusion and assessment of wall motion and thickening. Unfortunately, depending on how the gating is done, gating can sometimes degrade the quality of the perfusion scan. How can this happen and how can it be avoided? The problem stems from the fact that the static (ungated) perfusion image is not acquired directly but must be derived by summing together all the frames in the gated study. There are several circumstances in which summing together the gated images in this way may significantly reduce the quality of the resulting ungated perfusion image. The following are a few situations in which gating might reduce the quality of the static perfusion scan or in which the quality of the gated sequence might be compromised to ensure an adequate ungated study:

1. Use of a beat length window. Ideally, when performing a gated study, one wishes to exclude "bad" beats, that is, beats (or subsequent beats) that are exceptionally short [premature ventricular contractions (PVCs) or noise in the ECG signal] or too long. However, excluding such beats either will prolong the study or result in fewer total counts; that is, the ungated study will be of lower quality than it would have been had all the beats been used. In the near future it is hoped that manufacturers will implement acquisition schemes that avoid this problem (eg, by acquiring an ungated study simultaneously with the gated one).
2. Ignoring the beat length window. Because of the problem mentioned in situation 1 above, often one either turns off the beat length window or opens it very wide. This results in an ungated study that is uncompromised by bad beats or ECG noise. However if such beats or noise actually occurred, the gated study is compromised, perhaps making a normally contracting ventricle appear to have poor overall LV function. Unless the physician is aware that this has happened, the

study may be misread, or the ejection fraction miscomputed. In the future it is hoped that all manufacturers will at least provide the user with a histogram of number of beats versus beat length, so the user will know the composition of the beats that made up the gated study.

3. Very low heart rates. Most computer systems allow at least eight gated intervals to be acquired over the cardiac cycle. There is some evidence that this small number of gates, although causing an underestimate of EF, often may be sufficient for clinical purposes. However, in subjects with very low heart rates (perhaps 60 or less), if the eight frames are divided uniformly over the cardiac cycle, the timing of each frame may well be too coarse to give a reliable reading of wall motion or to permit accurate computation of global function. For example, at a heart rate of 60, each of the gated images would be 125 milliseconds long, more than one-third of the usual systolic interval for each image. Therefore perhaps only three images or less will sample all of systole. For still lower heart rates the situation is even worse. This is because at low heart rates, most commonly (but there are exceptions) the time for contraction stays about the same, even as the time between beats gets longer and longer [the extra time is spent either in diastasis (in normal hearts) or in slow filling]. With only eight frames then, the gated study may be compromised. One option would be to shorten the duration of the frames so as not to span the whole cardiac cycle and therefore not blur the heart as it contracts. For example, one might set each image to be 80 milliseconds, even though the heart rate was 60. This would produce a higher fidelity gated study. However, if the ungated study had to be made by adding the gated images together (as it must, as of writing this chapter), the ungated study would have only 64% of the counts that it would have had if gating had not been performed (8 frames × 80 ms/frame = 640 milliseconds total acquisition time per beat, compared with the actual time between beats of 1000 milliseconds.). Again, this problem would be solved if, for example, the manufacturers produced an ungated sequence simultaneously with the gated one.

In summary, one must thoroughly understand the gating process if one wishes to perform both a gated and an ungated perfusion study in an optimum fashion. Hopefully, in the near future, the manufacturers of computer equipment will make this process simpler, making simultaneous perfusion and function imaging easier and more reliable to perform.

References

1. Haft JI, Hammoudeh AJ, Conte PJ. Assessing myocardial viability: Correlation of myocardial wall motion abnormalities and pathologic Q waves with technetium 99m sestamibi single photon emission computed tomography. *Am Heart J* 1995;130:994–998.
2. Berman DS, Kiat H, Van Train KF, et al. Comparison of SPECT using technetium-99m agents and thallium-201 and PET for the assessment of myocardial perfusion and viability. *Am J Cardiol* 1990;66:72E–79E.
3. Chua T, Kiat H, Germano G, et al. Gated technetium-99m sestamibi for simultaneous assessment of stress myocardial perfusion, postexercise regional ventricular function and myocardial viability. Correlation with echocardiography and rest thallium-201 scintigraphy. *J Am Coll Cardiol* 1994;23:1107–1114.
4. Pace L, Cuocolo A, Marzullo P, et al. Reverse redistribution in resting thallium-201 myocardial scintigraphy in chronic coronary artery disease: An index of myocardial viability. *J Nucl Med* 1995;36:1968–1973.
5. Panza JA, Dilsizian V, Laurienzo JM, et al. Relation between thallium uptake and contractile response to dobutamine. Implications regarding myocardial viability in patients with chronic coronary artery disease and left ventricular dysfunction. *Circulation* 1995;91:990–998.

6. Parodi O, Marzullo P, Sambuceti G, et al. Non-invasive assessment of residual viability in post-myocardial infarction patients. Role of nuclear techniques. *Int J Card Imaging* 1993; 1(suppl 9):19–29.
7. Patterson RE, Pilcher WC. Assessing myocardial viability to help select patients for revascularization to improve left ventricular dysfunction due to coronary artery disease. *Semin Thorac Cardiovasc Surg* 1995;7:214–226.
8. Bartlett ML, Srinivasan G, Barker CW, et al. Left ventricular ejection fraction: Comparison of results from planar and SPECT gated bloodpool studies. *J Nucl Med* 1996;37:1795–1799.
9. Cerqueira MD, Harp GD, Ritchie JL. Quantitative gated bloodpool tomographic assessment of regional ejection fraction: Definition of normal limits. *J Am Coll Cardiol* 1992;20:934–941.
10. Dormehl IC, van Gelder AL, Hugo N, et al. Gated bloodpool SPECT and phase analysis to assess simulated Wolff-Parkinson-White syndrome in the baboon. *Nuklearmedizin* 1993;32: 222–226.
11. Indovina AG. Three-dimensional surface display in bloodpool gated SPECT. *Angiology* 1994; 45:861–866.
12. Ishino Y. Assessment of cardiac function and left ventricular regional wall motion by ^{99m}Tc multigated cardiac blood-pool emission computed tomography. *Kaku Igaku* 1992;29:1069–1081.
13. Fischman AJ, Moore RH, Gill JB, et al. Gated bloodpool tomography: A technology whose time has come. *Semin Nucl Med* 1989;19:13–21.
14. Gill JB, Moore RH, Tamaki N, et al. Multigated blood-pool tomography: New method for the assessment of left ventricular function. *J Nucl Med* 1986;27:1916–1924.
15. Underwood SR, Walton S, Ell PJ, et al. Gated blood-pool emission tomography: A new technique for the investigation of cardiac structure and function. *Eur J Nucl Med* 1985;10: 332–337.
16. DePuey EG, Nichols K, Dobrinsky C. Left ventricular ejection fraction assessed from gated technetium-99m-sestamibi SPECT. *J Nucl Med* 1993;34:1871–1876.
17. Faber TL, Akers MS, Peshock RM, et al. Three-dimensional motion and perfusion quantification in gated single-photon emission computed tomograms. *J Nucl Med* 1991;32:2311–2317.
18. Germano G, Kiat H, Kavanagh PB, et al. Automatic quantification of ejection fraction from gated myocardial perfusion SPECT. *J Nucl Med* 1995;36:2138–2147.
19. Kouris K, Abdel-Dayem HM, Taha B, et al. Left ventricular ejection fraction and volumes calculated from dual gated SPECT myocardial imaging with ^{99m}Tc-MIBI. *Nucl Med Commun* 1992;13:648–655.
20. Mannting F, Morgan-Mannting MG. Gated SPECT with technetium-99m-sestamibi for assessment of myocardial perfusion abnormalities. *J Nucl Med* 1993;34:601–608.
21. Mochizuki T, Murase K, Fujiwara Y, et al. Assessment of systolic thickening with thallium-201 ECG-gated single-photon emission computed tomography: A parameter for local left ventricular function. *J Nucl Med* 1991;32:1496–1500.
22. Yamashita K, Tamaki N, Yonekura Y, et al. Quantitative analysis of regional wall motion by gated myocardial positron emission tomography: Validation and comparison with left ventriculography. *J Nucl Med* 1989;30:1775–1786.
23. Barker WC, Bacharach SL, Freedman NMT, et al. Exercise gated bloodpool SPECT for simultaneous multi-view wall motion studies: Feasibility. *J Nucl Med* 1994;35:90P.
24. Cross SJ, Lee HS, Metcalfe MJ, et al. Assessment of left ventricular regional wall motion with bloodpool tomography: Comparison of 11CO PET with ^{99m}Tc SPECT. *Nucl Med Commun* 1994;15:283–238.
25. Freedman NMT, Bacharach SL, Cuocolo A, et al. ECG gated PET C-11 monoxide studies. An answer to the "background" question in planar Tc-99m gated bloodpool imaging. *J Nucl Med* 1992;33:938.
26. Garcia EV. Imaging guidelines for nuclear cardiology procedures, 1. *J Nucl Cardiol* 1996;3: G3–G46.
27. Bacharach SL, Green MV, Borer JS, et al. Left-ventricular peak ejection rate, filling rate, and ejection fraction-frame rate requirements at rest and exercise: Concise communication. *J Nucl Med* 1979;20:189–193.
28. Bacharach SL, Bonow RO, and Green MV. Comparison of fixed and variable temporal resolution methods for creating gated cardiac blood-pool image sequences. *J Nucl Med* 1990;31: 38–42.

29. de Graaf CN, van Rijk PP. High temporal and high phase resolution construction techniques for cardiac motion imaging: Theoretical and experimental comparison. *Int Symp Med Radionuclide Imaging* 1976:1;377–383.

30. Honda N, Machida K, Takishima T, et al. Cinematic three-dimensional surface display of cardiac bloodpool tomography. *Clin Nucl Med* 1991;16:87–91.

31. Underwood SR, Walton S, Laming PJ, et al. Left ventricular volume and ejection fraction determined by gated bloodpool emission tomography. *Br Heart J* 1985;53:216–222.

32. Mate E, Mester J, Csernay L, et al. Three-dimensional presentation of the Fourier amplitude and phase: A fast display method for gated cardiac blood-pool SPECT. *J Nucl Med* 1992;33:458–462.

33. Neumann DR, Go RT, Myers BA, et al. Parametric phase display for biventricular function from gated cardiac bloodpool single-photon emission tomography. *Eur J Nucl Med* 1993;20:1108–1111.

34. Cooke CD, Garcia EV, Cullom SJ, et al. Determining the accuracy of calculating systolic wall thickening using a fast Fourier transform approximation: A simulation study based on canine and patient data. *J Nucl Med* 1994;35:1185–1192.

35. Galt J, Garcia E, Robbins W. Effects of myocardial wall thickness on SPECT quantification. *IEEE Trans Med Imaging* 1990;9:144–150.

36. Mok DY, Bartlett ML, Bacharach SL, et al. Can partial volume effects be used to measure myocardial thickness and thickening? *IEEE Comput Cardiol* 1992:19;195–198.

37. Bartlett ML, Buvat I, Vaquero JJ, et al. Measurement of myocardial wall thickening from PET/SPECT images: Comparison of two methods. *J Comput Assist Tomogr* 1996;20:473–481.

38. Porenta G, Kuhle W, Sinha S, et al. Parameter estimation of cardiac geometry by ECG-gated PET imaging: Validation using magnetic resonance imaging and echocardiography. *J Nucl Med* 1995;36:1123–1129.

39. Buvat I, Bartlett ML, Kitsiou AN, et al. A "hybrid" method for measuring myocardial wall thickening from gated PET/SPECT images. *J Nucl Med* 1997;38:324–329.

39. Brigger P, Bacharach SL, Srinivasan G, et al. Segmentation og gated Tl-SPECT images and computation of ejection fraction: A different approach. *J Nucl Cardiol* 1999;6:286–297.

Myocardial Contractile Reserve

Vera H. Rigolin, MD, and Robert O. Bonow, MD

Introduction

In recent years, testing to evaluate the presence and extent of viable but dysfunctional myocardium has become an important component of the diagnostic assessment of patients with coronary artery disease and left ventricular (LV) dysfunction. Impaired LV function is not always an irreversible process related to previous myocardial infarction, as was once widely believed, because LV function may improve considerably after therapy for acute myocardial infarction[1–7] and after myocardial revascularization procedures in patients with chronic coronary artery disease.[8–14] The differentiation of viable from nonviable myocardium is a relevant diagnostic issue in patients being considered for coronary revascularization, because these procedures often are accompanied by high operative morbidity and mortality in the subset of patients with LV dysfunction. However, this is the same population that may ultimately benefit the most from revascularization.

Clinical Markers of Myocardial Viability

Several clinically reliable physiological markers can be used for assessing myocardial viability. Indexes of regional coronary blood flow, regional wall motion, and regional systolic wall thickening (WT) are accurate markers of viability if they are normal or near normal. However, these indexes have major limitations in identifying viable myocardium when they are reduced or absent because, by definition, regional perfusion and systolic function (regional wall motion and WT) will be severely reduced or absent[9–13] despite maintenance of tissue viability in the setting of hibernating myocardium. Thus, these three indexes are imprecise in distinguishing hibernating myocardium from myocardial scar.

Techniques to assess intact cellular metabolic processes or cell membrane integrity have intrinsic advantages over indexes of resting function and blood flow. During the past decade, numerous studies have demonstrated that nuclear cardiology techniques, involving single photon methods as well as positron emission tomography

From Dilsizian V (ed). *Myocardial Viability: A Clinical and Scientific Treatise.* Armonk, NY: Futura Publishing Co., Inc.; © 2000.

(PET), can be used to investigate perfusion, cell membrane integrity, and metabolic activity and thus provide critically important viability information in patients with LV dysfunction.

Another physiological marker of viable myocardium is the presence of residual inotropic reserve in stunned and/or hibernating myocardium that may be elicited through catecholamine stimulation. Echocardiographic approaches have evolved for this purpose and, in particular, dobutamine echocardiography to assess inotropic reserve in viable myocardium has shown considerable promise in recent years. This review will focus primarily on the strengths, applications, and limitations of these echocardiographic methods for the assessment of myocardial viability in patients with coronary artery disease and LV dysfunction. Other techniques to assess myocardial contractile reserve also will be discussed.

Acute Reversible Left Ventricular Dysfunction

Myocardial stunning is considered to be a process of myocardial injury following restoration of blood flow to previously ischemic myocardium.[2,7,15,16] This process has been studied extensively in excellent experimental models and is well validated in numerous animal investigations of coronary occlusion and reperfusion. Stunning in its purest sense represents blood flow–contraction mismatch, in that blood flow has been restored yet contractile dysfunction is present and may persist for several days to weeks before function returns spontaneously to normal.[2,7,15–17] Possible factors contributing, alone or in combination, to regional contractile dysfunction include abnormal energy utilization by contractile proteins with reduced myofilament responsiveness to calcium ion,[18–20] altered calcium transients,[21] production of cytotoxic oxygen-derived free radicals,[15–17,22,23] neutrophilic infiltration of previously ischemic tissue,[24] and damage to the extracellular collagen matrix.[25]

For years, myocardial stunning was a laboratory observation with limited clinical applicability. This has changed markedly in the current era of management of acute myocardial infarction. Recovery of regional dysfunction in patients after reperfusion therapy with thrombolytic agents or with coronary angioplasty for acute myocardial infarction is evidence that many asynergic myocardial regions in such patients represent viable but stunned myocardium.[1–7] In addition, there also is growing evidence that stunning may result from other, less severe, episodes of myocardial ischemia, including unstable angina pectoris,[7,26–28] variant angina,[7] and even exercise-induced ischemia in patients with chronic coronary artery disease.[29–31]

Contractile Reserve in Stunned Myocardium

It has been shown in several experimental situations[32–35] that stunned myocardium exhibits contractile reserve and that contractile dysfunction can be ameliorated or reversed if presented with adrenergic stimulation with agents such as epinephrine, dopamine, isoproterenol, and dobutamine (Fig. 1). This effect in the experimental laboratory has been the basis for the development of dobutamine echocardiography to assess regional contractile reserve in patients with persistent LV dysfunction after reperfusion therapy for acute myocardial infarction.

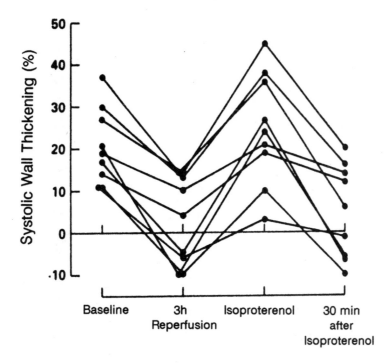

Figure 1. Contractile reserve in stunned myocardium. Contractile dysfunction after coronary occlusion and reperfusion in dogs, manifested by reduced systolic wall thickening (WT) is improved during administration of isoproterenol. After termination of isoproterenol, contractile dysfunction persists. Reproduced with permission from Reference 34.

Dobutamine Echocardiography After Acute Myocardial Infarction

Dobutamine is a synthetic catecholamine with positive inotropic effects mediated predominantly through B_1 adrenergic receptor stimulation. Direct linear correlations exist among the dose of dobutamine, the plasma concentration, and the hemodynamic effects.[36] Dobutamine has positive inotropic actions at low doses (4–8 μg/kg per minute) and increases heart rate only at doses above 10 μg/kg per minute.[37]

In a pioneering study, Pierard et al[38] evaluated 17 patients after thrombolytic therapy for acute myocardial infarction by low-dose dobutamine echocardiography and PET imaging with 13 N-ammonia and ^{18}F-2-deoxyglucose (FDG). Repeat imaging 9 ± 7 months later was performed to assess the ability of these studies to predict recovery of regional function. PET and dobutamine echocardiography were concordant regarding viability and nonviability in 62 of the 78 myocardial segments that were analyzed (79%). However, among the segments with contractile reserve on the initial dobutamine study, seven (16%) had reduced metabolic activity consistent with necrosis on the PET study, and among the segments considered nonviable (without contractile reserve) on the dobutamine study, nine (26%) had PET evidence of viability. At the follow-up examination, the regions with viability by both PET and dobutamine echocardiography improved in function, and the regions with concordance regarding nonviability by the two techniques had persistent dysfunction (Fig. 2). However, all nine of the discordant regions felt to be viable by PET but without contractile reserve did not improve in function and six had metabolic evidence of necrosis; among the seven regions predicted to be viable by echocardiography but necrotic by PET, five had improved function

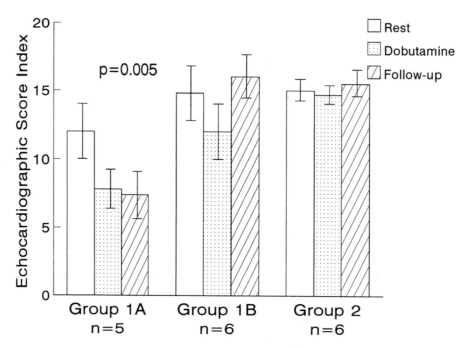

Figure 2. Changes in regional function induced by low-dose dobutamine early after thrombolytic therapy for acute myocardial infarction, in relation to resting regional function on late follow-up reevaluation at 9 ± 7 months. Patients are subdivided into three groups: Group 1A with normal perfusion and metabolism by positron emission tomography (PET), group 1B with reduced perfusion and enhanced ^{18}F-2-deoxyglucose (FDG) uptake, and group 2 with reductions in both perfusion and FDG uptake. PET and dobutamine echocardiography are concordant regarding viable myocardium in group 1A and nonviable myocardium in group 2. In group 1B, prediction of viability on the basis of FDG-blood flow mismatch does not translate into recovery of wall motion on the late follow-up evaluation. Reproduced with permission from Reference 38.

and normal metabolism on the follow-up study. Thus, although PET and dobutamine echocardiography provided concordant findings in the majority of regions, these data indicate that PET might overestimate the presence and extent of viability in the acute setting shortly after thrombolytic therapy and that dobutamine echocardiography has at least similar negative predictive value and better positive predictive value than PET for functional recovery after thrombolytic therapy.

Since the initial report of Pierard et al in 1990,[38] six other studies[39,-45] addressing the ability of low-dose dobutamine echocardiography to predict recovery of regional function after acute myocardial infarction have confirmed these findings. These seven clinical series on this subject involve a total of 291 patients studied 3–12 days after myocardial infarction with follow-up evaluations to reassess ventricular function 4 weeks to 9 months later. Overall, the sensitivity for detecting reversible regional dysfunction has ranged from 66% to 86%, with specificities ranging from 68% to 94%. The overall positive predictive accuracy of low-dose dobutamine echocardiography in these studies has averaged 71%, with a negative predictive accuracy of 87%. Similar results were found by LeClercq et al in 40 patients with acute myocardial infarction who were treated with primary angioplasty.[46] Low- and high-dose dobutamine echocardiography also has been used in the postmyocardial infarction population with similar ability to detect viability and the added benefit of the detection of ischemia.[47]

Duchak et al[40,45] compared the results of dobutamine echocardiography with resting thallium-201 single photon emission computerized tomography (SPECT) imaging in 65 consecutive patients after acute myocardial infarction. Similar to the earlier results of

Pierard et al[38] in which the echocardiographic data were compared with PET imaging, Duchak et al reported both higher sensitivity and specificity with dobutamine echocardiography (81% and 75%, respectively) compared with thallium imaging (73% and 35%, respectively) for predicting recovery of ventricular dysfunction. Elhendy et al also reported similar findings in their study of 30 patients.[48]

Although low-dose dobutamine echocardiography provides very specific information for predicting lack of improvement in regional function, the sensitivity for identifying those segments that will improve may depend on the severity of the baseline wall motion abnormality. Hypokinetic regions are more likely to manifest inotropic reserve than regions with akinesia or dyskinesia, and a greater percentage of akinetic/dyskinetic regions without evidence of inotropic reserve subsequently will improve in function during the ensuing weeks after infarction than compared with hypokinetic regions without inotropic reserve. Hence, the sensitivity for predicting recovery of function based on the presence of inotropic reserve is higher in hypokinetic than in akinetic/dyskinetic territories. The reported sensitivities in akinetic regions has ranged from 74% to as low as 35%.[40,43,45]

Myocardial Stunning Versus Acute Hibernation?

Many of the patients included in these studies underwent myocardial revascularization after the initial dobutamine echocardiogram, so that the follow-up information regarding recovery of LV function is in many cases clouded by the effect of revascularization and does not necessarily represent the ability to predict spontaneous recovery of function in patients with pure myocardial stunning who have open infarct-related arteries. In many of these patients, with a residual critical stenosis in the infarct-related artery, it is possible that persistent

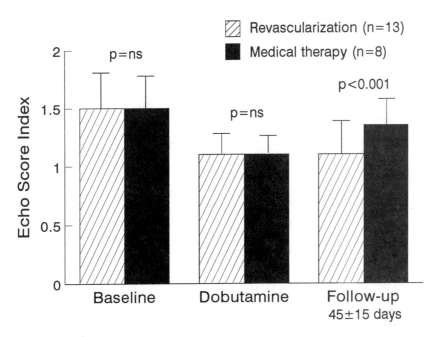

Figure 3. Myocardial contractile reserve elicited with dobutamine in patients with a recent myocardial infarction and residual stenosis in the infarct-related artery. Although dobutamine resulted in a similar reduction in echocardiographic wall motion abnormality, patients undergoing revascularization after the dobutamine test manifested a significantly greater improvement in wall motion during the follow-up period than did patients treated medically. Modified with permission from Reference 39.

myocardial hypoperfusion was present and contributed to the regional ventricular dysfunction, and that late improvement in regional wall motion was related to improvement in coronary blood flow. The data of Barilla et al[39] address this issue directly. These investigators studied 21 patients after thrombolytic therapy for acute myocardial infarction, all of whom had persistent regional dysfunction in the infarct zone and a residual stenosis in the infarct-related artery. All 21 patients manifested evidence of myocardial viability in the infarct territory, with improvement in wall motion score with low-dose dobutamine, but late improvement in wall motion during the follow-up period (mean 45 days) occurred only in patients undergoing revascularization and not in the patients treated with medical therapy alone (Fig. 3). This scenario does not fit the accepted definition of myocardial stunning. The finding that persistent myocardial hypoperfusion contributed to contractile dysfunction and that revascularization ameliorated the contractile dysfunction strongly indicate that a component of myocardial hibernation, alone or superimposed on stunned myocardium, was operative in a number of these patients.

Prognosis After Myocardial Infarction

Regardless of whether or not LV dysfunction is a result of stunning or hibernation, the detection of myocardial viability after myocardial infarction often provides prognostic information in patients treated medically and surgically, particularly when ejection fraction is reduced significantly.

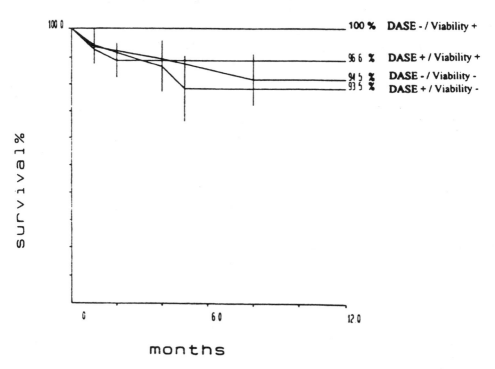

Figure 4. Kaplan-Meier survival curves in which patients are stratified according to the presence or absence of viability and ischemia detected by dobutamine stress echocardiography. Death was the only end point considered. The best survival was noted in patients with viability and without ischemia while the worst survival was seen in those without viability and with ischemia. Viability+ and viability− indicate the presence or absence of viability, respectively. DASE+ and DASE− indicate presence or absence of ischemia, respectively. (DASE = dobutamine-atropine-stress-echo). Reproduced with permission from Reference 50.

Since Barilla's study, others have been performed to address the prognostic value of dobutamine echocardiography after myocardial infarction. The largest series was the Echo Dobutamine International Cooperative (EDIC) Study in which dobutamine echocardiography was performed 12 ± 5 days after myocardial infarction in a total of 778 patients.[49] Wall motion score index at peak stress was the best predictor of cardiac death while recognition of viability was the best predictor of unstable angina. A substudy was performed utilizing the EDIC database to evaluate the impact on survival of viability detected by dobutamine echocardiography in 314 medically treated patients with severe LV dysfunction after myocardial infarction.[50] The presence of myocardial viability in these patients was associated with a higher probability of survival (Fig. 4). The higher the number of segments showing improvement in function, the better the impact of viability on survival. The presence of inducible ischemia with high dose of dobutamine was the best predictor of cardiac death.

Similarly, Previtali et al evaluated the prognostic value of dobutamine echocardiography in patients early after acute myocardial infarction treated with thrombolysis.[51] Dobutamine echocardiography was performed in 152 patients at a mean of 9 ± 5 days after the first myocardial infarction to evaluate for myocardial ischemia and viability. The patients in this study had relatively well-preserved LV function. The presence and extent of myocardial ischemia during dobutamine echocardiography was the most important predictor of both hard and spontaneous events, while myocardial viability did not have independent prognostic value. These studies suggest, therefore, that prognosis after myocardial infarction is dependent on the presence or absence of both ischemia and viability. The prognostic implications of viability seem to be most pronounced in patients with severely reduced LV function.

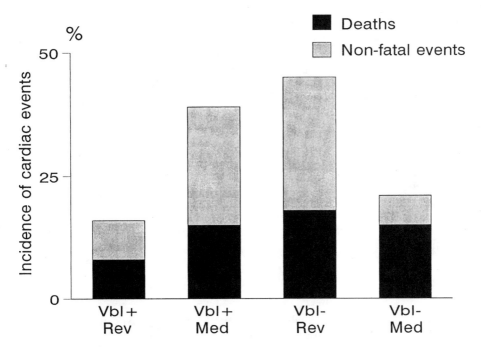

Figure 5. Bar graphs showing the frequency of cardiac death and nonfatal events in the subset of patients with left ventricular ejection fraction (LVEF) ≤33%. Patients are divided into four groups according to presence (Vbl+) or absence (Vbl−) viability determined by dobutamine stress echocardiography and treatment with revascularization (Rev) or medical therapy (Med). The incidence of cardiac events was lowest in patients with viability treated with revascularization. Modified with permission from Reference 52.

The impact of viability in patients with reduced LV function was further emphasized in a study by Anselmi et al in which 202 patients with a previous or recent myocardial infarction and regional wall motion abnormalities underwent low-dose dobutamine echocardiography.[52] In the subset of patients with severe LV dysfunction, the incidence of cardiac death was lower in patients with viability and who were revascularized (8%) than in patients with viability treated medically (15%), patients without viability and who were revascularized (18%), or patients without viability treated medically (15%) (Fig. 5).

Dobutamine stress echocardiography appears able to provide prognostic information in the myocardial infarction population. However, the assessment of both ischemia as well as viability appears to be important, suggesting that low and high doses of dobutamine are necessary for a complete evaluation.

Chronic Persistent Left Ventricular Dysfunction

Information regarding contractile reserve in normally perfused stunned myocardium cannot necessarily be extrapolated to myocardial hibernation, in which impaired function arises presumably from a functional adaptation to reduced perfusion.[13] In contrast to myocardial stunning, which represents a form of myocardial injury, the term "hibernation" connotes an adaptive, protective process to maintain myocardial viability in the setting of sustained reduction in coronary blood flow.[9–11,13] Thus, hibernation represents a form of blood flow–contraction match[13] in which there is down-regulation of contractile elements to reduce energy requirements in the face of reduced oxygen availability. In theory, hibernation may occur acutely as a result of sudden reductions in blood flow not severe enough to cause injury to myofibrillar units or to the extracellular matrix or may occur chronically in patients with chronic severe coronary artery stenoses that are flow limiting under resting conditions. Unlike myocardial stunning, in which there is a wealth of experimental validation with only recent evidence of clinical counterparts, myocardial hibernation is a concept driven by a large number of clinical observations, but one that is still waiting for an appropriate animal model with which to explore the responsible mechanism or mechanisms. Models of short-term hibernation do exist, in which reversible contractile dysfunction may be induced by reduction in coronary blood flow to levels that do not induce ischemia or necrosis, or by repeated brief episodes of ischemia that ultimately lead to decreases in both blood flow and function without further metabolic evidence of ischemia.[13,20,53–63] It is apparent from these models and from clinical studies and myocardial biopsy samples obtained from patients with chronic ischemic heart disease that contractile dysfunction may result from reduced calcium transients in early stages of the process,[20,59,60] that high-energy phosphate concentrations are not reduced,[53,56,59,63] that increased glycolytic flux may have a protective effect and prevent ischemic damage,[54,55,58] and that cellular dedifferentiation at the ultrastructural level with loss of sarcomeres and accumulation of intracellular glycogen ultimately may develop in more chronic stages of hibernation.[64,65]

Contractile Reserve in Hibernating Myocardium

Although the available models indicate that hibernating myocardium has inotropic reserve that can be elicited with catecholamine stimulation,[62,63,66] this appears to be an unstable process that can be maintained only temporarily, in keeping with the lack of normal coronary flow reserve. In acute animal models of hibernation, the response to catecholamine stimulation accurately differentiates reversible from fixed dysfunction in hypoperfused segments[67] but only low doses producing inotropy with minimal chronotropy are effective because ischemia will exacerbate dysfunction if myocardial demand increases.[62,63,68] Moreover, in the later stages of the natural history of hibernation, there may be cellular dedifferentiation and dropout of myofibrillar units[64,65] resulting in reduced or absent responsiveness to catecholamine stimulation.

Contractile Reserve in Chronic Left Ventricular Dysfunction

Data from several clinical studies reported two decades ago support the concepts derived from these experimental observations. Inotropic reserve was identified in many patients with sustained LV dysfunction using epinephrine administration or postextrasystolic potentiation during left ventriculography.[8,69–75] These methods were found to be useful in predicting the recovery of LV function after revascularization and in assessing prognosis with and without revascularization.[72,73,75]

Dobutamine Echocardiography in Chronic Left Ventricular Dysfunction

In keeping with these early reports, low-dose dobutamine echocardiography has emerged in the 1990s as a means of eliciting inotropic reserve in many patients with acute

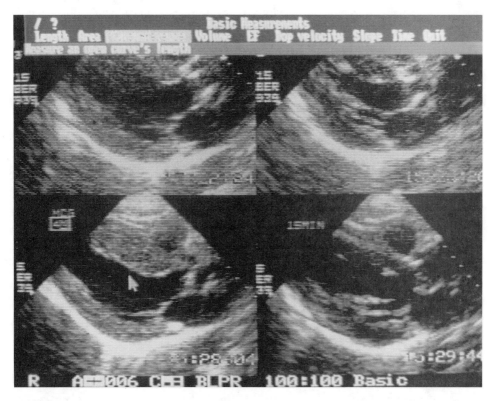

Figure 6. Evidence of contractile reserve in the anteroseptal wall as evidence of myocardial viability. Baseline echocardiography (**upper left panel**) shows severe hypokinesis with minimal to no thickening of the anteroseptal wall. During low-dose dobutamine infusion (**upper right panel**), there is marked contractile reserve with thickening of the basal and midanteroseptal wall. At peak dose of the dobutamine infusion (**lower left panel**) there is thinning and new segmental wall motion abnormalities of the basal and midposterior wall consistent with ischemia. Recovery images are shown in the bottom right panel. This study demonstrates evidence of viability in the basal and midanteroseptal wall with corresponding evidence of ischemia in the basal and midposterior walls.

and chronic LV dysfunction (Figs. 6 and 7), and there is growing awareness that such inotropic reserve identifies myocardial dysfunction that is potentially reversible. A number of investigators have examined the ability of preoperative low-dose dobutamine echocardiography to predict recovery of regional wall motion in patients with chronic coronary artery disease and LV dysfunction who are undergoing coronary artery bypass surgery (Figs. 8 and 9). A total of 402 patients have been reported in 15 studies, with excellent clinical results.[76-90] Sensitivities and specificities for predicting improvement in regional wall motion after operation have ranged from 74% to 95%. From the individual studies, the average positive predictive value of the preoperative finding of inotropic reserve was 83%, with a negative predictive value of 81%. These results are similar to those achieved using positron emission tomography or thallium reinjection imaging.[91] In addition, the viability information provided by the finding of inotropic reserve with low-dose dobutamine echocardiography in dysfunctional regions is concordant in the majority of regions with viability information examined in the same patients with thallium imaging[78,84,92] or with PET imaging with FDG.[93-95]

In the majority of investigations in this area, inotropic reserve has been classified in a binary fashion as present or absent. Afridi et al explored the more complex but commonly encountered situation of biphasic responses to dobutamine.[89] Because dobutamine causes progressive increases in oxygen demand at higher doses, it often precipitates myocardial ischemia in regions served by a critical stenosis. Hence, wall motion in some dysfunctional regions will improve at low doses of dobutamine but then deteriorate as

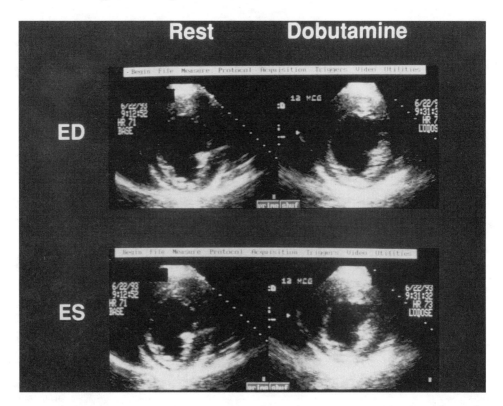

Figure 7. Parasternal short-axis views demonstrating evidence of contractile reserve by dobutamine echocardiography. Baseline end-diastolic and end-systolic frames are shown in the left panels, demonstrating no thickening or change in LV dimensions. During low-dose dobutamine infustion (**right panels**), there is a decrease in end-systolic dimensions and thickening of the myocardium, specifically the midanterior, midanteroseptum, midseptum, and midinferior wall, consistent with viability.

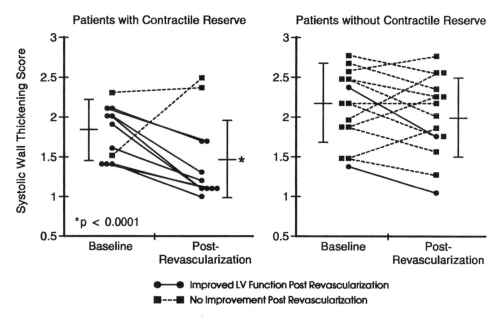

Figure 8. Changes in echocardiographic regional wall motion score before and after revascularization in patients with chronic coronary artery disease manifesting contractile reserve with low-dose dobutamine (**left panel**) and no contractile reserve (**right panel**). Circles indicate patients with improvement in LV function and squares indicate patients without improvement in ventricular function. Reproduced with permission from Reference 85.

ischemia is produced at higher doses.[89,96] Other possible contractile response patterns include recruitment of inotropic reserve only at high doses or progressive improvement in regional function at successively higher dobutamine infusion rates (ie, a normal response superimposed on abnormal baseline wall motion).

Afridi et al studied 20 patients with chronic coronary artery disease with segmental LV dysfunction before coronary angioplasty with incremental doses of 2.5–40 µg/kg per minute.[89] Follow-up echocardiograms were obtained early (<1 week) and late (≥6 weeks) after angioplasty. Of the 320 ventricular segments, 148 had abnormal wall motion at baseline, of which 114 were revascularized. Recovery of function after angioplasty occurred in 25% of the revascularized segments at the early study and in 33% at the late study. Of the 34 abnormal segments not revascularized, recovery of function occurred in only one segment. During dobutamine echocardiography, abnormal segments exhibited one of four responses: (1) a biphasic response with improvement at low dose and worsening at high dose (28% of segments), (2) sustained improvement through peak dose (18% of segments), (3) worsening at low doses (15% of segments), and (4) no change (39% of segments). A biphasic response had the highest predictive value (72%) for recovery of function followed by worsening only (35%), while the lowest predictive value was observed in segments with either no change (13%) or sustained improvement (15%) during dobutamine. Combining biphasic and worsening responses resulted in a sensitivity of 74% and specificity of 73% for detecting individual segments that would recover after angioplasty. Dobutamine responsive wall motion was detected most often at doses of 5 or 7.5 µg/kg per minute, and worsening usually was seen at doses ≥20 µg/kg per minute, although it was seen in some patients as early as 7.5 µg/kg per minute dose. These data underscore the complex nature of dobutamine responsiveness that must be considered when interpreting clinical viability studies using dobutamine echocardiography. Dobutamine should be started at a low dose with slow increments for optimal results. Impor-

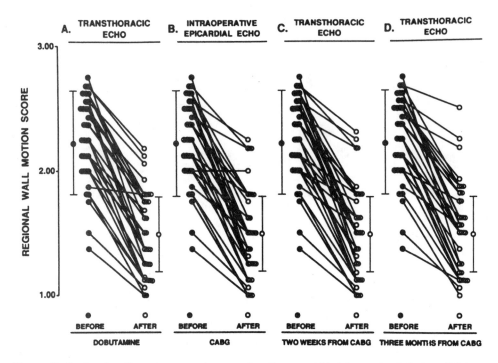

Figure 9. Regional wall motion score between baseline and (**A**) dobutamine infusion, (**B**) intra-operative epicardial echocardiography, (**C**) 2 weeks after coronary artery bypass surgery, and (**D**) 3 months after coronary artery bypass surgery. Reproduced with permission from Reference 87.

tantly, a test for viability should not be terminated after low doses of dobutamine if it is safe to continue testing at more maximal doses, because the demonstration of contractile reserve and inducible ischemia in the same segments is fairly definitive proof that the segment will improve with revascularization. This is in keeping with the wealth of previous experience with thallium-201 imaging, indicating that evidence of inducible ischemia with reversible perfusion defects is an accurate indicator of viability and potential improvement in regional dysfunction after revascularization.[97–100]

Prognostic Implications

Similar to the experience gained thus far with PET imaging[101,102] and the earlier experience with epinephrine infusions and postextrasystolic potentiation during left ventriculography,[73] the identification of viable myocardium with dobutamine echocardiography appears to provide important prognostic information in patients with LV dysfunction.[103–105] Patients with inotropic reserve appear to have an initial survival advantage compared with those patients without inotropic reserve, which cannot be explained by differences in baseline LV function, symptoms, or coronary anatomy.[103] Nonetheless, survival in patients with inotropic reserve appears to be enhanced significantly by myocardial revascularization.[103,105]

The impact of the detection of viability and the subsequent treatment modality in patients with coronary artery disease and reduced LV function was further emphasized in a recent study by Afridi et al in which 318 patients with chronic coronary artery disease and LV ejection fraction <35% were evaluated with dobutamine echocardiography.[105]

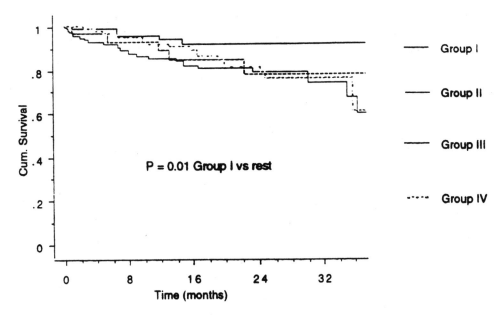

Figure 10. Kaplan-Meier survival curves in four groups of patients with coronary artery disease and severe LV dysfunction evaluated with dobutamine stress echocardiography. Group I: Presence of viability/treatment with revascularization. Group II: Presence of viability/medical treatment. Group III: Absence of viability/treatment with revascularization. Group IV: Absence of viability/medical treatment. Survival is highest in patients with viability treated with revascularization. Reproduced with permission from Reference 105.

The patients then were divided into four groups according to the presence or absence of viability and whether or not they were revascularized. Patients then were followed for 18 ± 10 months. The death rate was lowest in the group with viability who underwent revascularization (6%). The death rate was 20% in the group with viability who did not undergo revascularization, 17% in the group without viability who underwent revascularization, and 20% in the group without viability or revascularization (Fig. 10). This study not only emphasizes the prognostic implications of the presence of viability but also the benefit of revascularization in patients with viability and the lack of benefit in those without.

The major limitation of dobutamine echocardiography is the lack of quantitative methods of assessing wall motion abnormalities and WT, thus requiring visual interpretation of regional function and changes in regional function during interventions. This may be difficult in the assessment of regions with baseline contractile abnormalities.

Dobutamine Echocardiography Compared With Single Photon Emission Computerized Tomography/Positron Emission Tomography Imaging

The detection of contractile reserve during dobutamine echocardiography may identify reversible myocardial dysfunction in acute and chronic settings with reasonably high accuracy. These data are comparable with nuclear perfusion imaging and PET studies. SPECT and PET studies seem to have higher sensitivities compared with dobutamine echocardiography in identification of myocardial viability, but dobutamine echocardiography appears to be more specific. The optimal imaging technique in various subsets of patients is not defined clearly yet, and few studies have directly compared both modalities.

Panza et al compared 30 patients with transesophageal dobutamine echocardiography and stress-redistribution-reinjection thallium imaging.[92] More myocardial segments were considered viable by thallium scintigraphy than with low-dose dobutamine echocardiography (84% versus 56%, $p < 0.001$). In areas that were considered viable based on semiquantitative thallium imaging, 69% were concordant with echocardiography. The greater the amount of thallium activity, the higher the percent of myocardial segments responding to dobutamine stimulation (Fig. 11). In segments that demonstrated contractile improvement with dobutamine, only 2% did not have evidence of viability with thallium scintigraphy. No data regarding functional improvement after coronary revascularization were given in this study.

Arnese et al[78] evaluated the predictive value of stress-reinjection thallium SPECT imaging and dobutamine echocardiography in 38 patients with severe LV dysfunction. Segments that had akinesis or severe hypokinesis were examined for improvement in function 3 months after bypass surgery, as assessed by regional WT on echocardiography. Thallium criteria for viability included normal perfusion, regional thallium activity 50% of "normal" activity, or a reversible defect. Thickening of akinetic or severely dyskinetic segments with low-dose dobutamine (10 μg/kg per minute) was considered criteria for viability by echocardiography. Thallium scintigraphy detected 3 times the number of viable segments as did low-dose dobutamine echocardiography (103 versus 33 segments), with a higher sensitivity for an improvement of segmental function (89% for thallium SPECT and 74% for echocardiography). However, low-dose dobutamine echocardiography had a higher specificity and positive predictive value (95% and 85%, respectively) than did thallium reinjection imaging (48% and 33%, respectively). This study demonstrated no overall improvement in LV function following revascularization, which

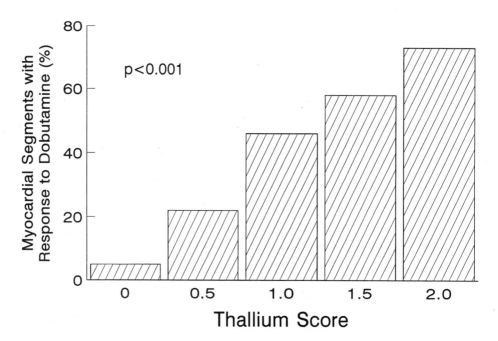

Figure 11. Relation between regional thallium activity (graded on a 5-point visual scale) and the likelihood of inotropic reserve during dobutamine echocardiography. Inotropic reserve is significantly related to regional thallium activity. Reproduced with permission from Reference 92.

may be explained by the finding that only 22% of all akinetic or severely dyskinetic segments improved following revascularization.

Rather than a binary relationship between thallium evidence of myocardial viability and contractile reserve, the likelihood that a dysfunctional segment will demonstrate contractile reserve with dobutamine is related to the extent of thallium uptake in that segment[84,92]; that is, the severity of the perfusion defect correlates with the dobutamine responsiveness.

The available data suggest that more patients and myocardial segments appear viable based on thallium imaging than with dobutamine echocardiography[77,78,83,84,92,106,107] although other investigators have found similar sensitivities.[108] Regional discordance also has been noted, with greater evidence of viability in the anterior and septal regions with thallium scintigraphy compared with dobutamine echocardiography.[107] The comparative detection of viability with sestamibi and dobutamine echocardiography is unclear[108,109] but appears to favor echocardiography.[108] The specificity and predictive value of dobutamine echocardiography and myocardial perfusion imaging have been reported to be similar in two studies[83,108] but a more recent publication revealed improved specificity for functional recovery with dobutamine echocardiography.[78]

Similar findings have been reported in the limited number of studies comparing dobutamine echocardiography and metabolic PET imaging with FDG.[93–95] A greater number of dysfunctional myocardial segments have been identified as viable by PET than by echocardiography, indicating that there are regions of viable myocardium that are metabolically active but lack inotropic reserve. The regions with discordant findings between the two techniques tend to be those that are presumably hibernating in which blood flow is reduced at rest. In contrast, there is excellent agreement between PET and dobutamine echocardiography in identifying myocardial regions that have preserved blood flow and are presumably stunned.[94,95] Discrepancies between dobutamine echocardiography and SPECT or PET imaging may reflect the underlying alterations in cellular metabolism and function. Blood flow and flow reserve may be reduced to such an extent that contractile reserve is lost while transmembrane pump activity is preserved. The dependency of contractile reserve on myocardial blood flow (MBF) was demonstrated by Lee et al.[110] In their study of 19 patients with chronic LV dysfunction, dobutamine PET and echo studies suggested that the ability to exhibit contractile reserve depends on the level of MBF at rest and during inotropic stimulation. The dependency on blood flow is supported further by the finding that nitroglycerin enhances the ability of dobutamine echocardiography to detect hibernating myocardium, presumably by increasing coronary flow to hypoperfused regions.[111]

Preserved transmembrane pump activity may be imaged directly with thallium or sestamibi or could be assessed by investigating the metabolic processes necessary to generate the high-energy processes to maintain membrane integrity. This higher degree of myocyte metabolism compared with functional integrity is suggested by several recent studies.[92,94,95]

Alternatively, more necrosis may be present when there is no significant augmentation in function with dobutamine infusion, that is, there are less viable cells within a region. This may be inferred from other investigators who have shown that the magnitude of regional tracer activity reflects the mass of viable tissue, which in turn correlates with systolic function.[78,84,92,112,113] The critical mass of viable cells necessary to allow for inotropic reserve was evaluated histologically by Baumgartner et al.[114] Twelve patients with coronary artery disease and severely impaired LV function were evaluated with dobutamine echocardiography prior to cardiac transplant. Five of these patients also underwent PET studies and seven underwent thallium-SPECT analysis. Although the number of patients in this study was small, histological evaluation of the explanted hearts after transplantation suggested that contractile reserve as evidenced by a positive response to dobutamine requires at least 50% viable myocytes in a given segment.

The "overestimation" of viability with techniques such as rest-redistribution thallium scintigraphy or PET imaging with FDG may result from the detection of small regions of viable myocardium, which are of inadequate size to permit improvement in systolic function. The distribution of viable cells also may be important, especially with regards to the recovery of ventricular function. A heterogeneous admixture of necrotic and viable cells may not manifest improved contraction after revascularization, despite the presence of adequate metabolic function in at least some of the cells. However, even without the return of cardiac function, the presence and maintenance of viability may be crucial for long-term prognosis, perhaps by the prevention of infarct expansion, ventricular remodeling, and the development of heart failure.

The potential reasons for the discordance between perfusion imaging and dobutamine echocardiography are multiple. First, and perhaps most importantly, all studies have the potential for anatomic misalignment between the perfusion study and echocardiogram, because the techniques and orientation of the heart are inherently different. This is especially problematic because the standard for functional recovery in most studies is the echocardiographic determination of wall motion. Thus, for the dobutamine echocardiographic procedures, correct registration of the segments is virtually guaranteed, while with a tomographic or planar perfusion study, substantial assumptions must be made regarding the location of perfusion abnormalities relative to echocardiographic landmarks.

Another factor that confounds the conclusions that may be drawn from comparative studies is the fact that different criteria were used to define viability for both echocardiography and scintigraphy in most studies. Additionally, the type of regional dysfunction may be important. For example, when areas of akinesis are analyzed, the concordance between the methods is reduced markedly (37%).[115] In these areas of severe dysfunction, the sensitivity of dobutamine echocardiography for improvement in function is only 26%.[116]

Additional problems include the timing of postrevascularization imaging, because many segments may have late recovery of contractile dysfunction. Also, pathophysiological differences in hibernation and stunning are likely to be present and may govern differences in radiotracer uptake and retention, as well as demonstration of contractile reserve with dobutamine. Thus, there may be substantial differences in the response to dobutamine and distribution of thallium activity in patients with stunning, as opposed to hibernation.[117]

Finally, a selection bias may be present when comparing the results of dobutamine echocardiography and myocardial perfusion imaging. Not all patients initially recruited for such trials are able to have adequate examinations. The technical quality of images is reported as only fair on average for echocardiography, compared with good for thallium-201, and poor quality echocardiograms are noted in up to 22% of patients.[106,118,119]

Suboptimal echocardiographic image quality usually is caused by body habitus or the presence of lung disease. However, the introduction of second harmonic imaging within the past few years has resulted in a significant decrease in the number of poorly visualized segments.[120–122] Compared with fundamental imaging, this technique has been shown to improve the number of visualized segments and alter wall motion scoring in dobutamine echocardiographic studies evaluated by both highly and less-experienced readers.[123]

Improvement in endocardial border definition also has been demonstrated with echocardiographic contrast agents. Within the past year, Optison[TM], an albumin-coated second-generation contrast agent containing an octafluorpropane gas, has been approved by the Food and Drug Administration (FDA) for LV cavity opacification. This agent has been shown to be safe,[124] hemodynamically inert,[125] and successful at opacifying the left ventricle after an intravenous injection.[125] Two hundred three patients with suboptimal resting echo images were evaluated with this agent in a phase 3 multicenter clinical trial.

With the contrast agent, there was a threefold improvement in endocardial border delineation in all patients, including those with varying degrees of LV dysfunction, pulmonary hypertension, and mitral and tricuspid regurgitation.[126,127]

Although prognostic data are not available for second harmonic imaging or intravenous (IV) contrast agents to enhance endocardial border detection as adjunctive agents for the detection of viability, the ability to better visualize the endocardium is likely to improve the diagnostic accuracy of dobutamine echocardiography.

Echocardiographic contrast agents have been under investigation for many years for the detection of myocardial perfusion. Early studies demonstrated adequate myocardial opacification with intracoronary, aortic root or left atrial injections. Myocardial contrast echocardiography performed in this fashion has been able to assess successfully myocardial viability.[128–131] By evaluating both function and perfusion, the combination of dobutamine echocardiography and contrast echocardiography has been shown to enhance the prediction of myocardial viability.[132–134] The detection of viability using the new IV contrast agents has not been evaluated fully. The IV technique is advantageous because of its extensive safety profile, ease of administration, and pure perfusion characteristics caused by lack of dependency on cellular metabolism. However, further validation of these new contrast agents as markers of perfusion is necessary before their use in the assessment of viability becomes universal.

Other Techniques to Assess Myocardial Contractile Reserve

Magnetic resonance imaging (MRI) recently has emerged as a valuable tool for the assessment of myocardial viability. MRI has major advantages because of markedly enhanced spatial resolution and accurate quantitative capabilities. Low-dose dobutamine has been used on conjunction with MRI to assess contractile reserve. Comparison of low-dose dobutamine transesophageal echo (TEE) and dobutamine MRI for the detection of myocardial viability has been made using PET as the gold standard.[135] In this study evaluating 43 patients with chronic myocardial infarction, the sensitivity for the detection viability by dobutamine TEE was 77% with a specificity of 94%. The comparable values for dobutamine MRI were 81% and 100%, respectively. Low-dose dobutamine MRI also has been evaluated in patients with recent myocardial infarction who underwent revascularization.[136] Using a semiquantitative method to assess wall motion, low-dose dobutamine MRI had an accuracy of 80% in predicting viability after infarction. The results of these studies suggest that low-dose dobutamine MRI is feasible and yields results comparable with standard techniques for the detection of viability.

The detection of viability by MRI appears to be enhanced further by evaluating both end-diastolic WT as well as dobutamine-induced contractile reserve. Baer et al evaluated viability in 35 patients with LV dysfunction and coronary artery disease with both PET and low-dose dobutamine MRI.[137] Viable myocardium by MRI was characterized by preserved end-diastolic WT ($\geq$5.5 mm) or the presence of dobutamine-induced contractile reserve. During dobutamine infusion, 242/299 segments graded as viable by PET had dobutamine-induced systolic WT whereas an additional 21 segments without dobutamine-induced systolic WT had normal end-diastolic WT. The combination of both parameters resulted in a sensitivity of 88% and a specificity of 87%.

In a follow-up study, Baer et al[138] evaluated the prognostic value of dobutamine MRI in patients with prior myocardial infarction who underwent revascularization. A total of 43 patients underwent low-dose dobutamine MRI followed by successful revascularization of the infarct-related artery. Resting MRI then was performed 4–6 months later. Systolic WT $\geq$2 mm in $\geq$50% of the infarct-related segments as well as diastolic WT

≥5.5 mm were evaluated as markers of viability. Dobutamine-induced systolic WT was found to be a better predictor of LV functional recovery (sensitivity 89%, specificity 94%) than was preserved diastolic WT (sensitivity 92%, specificity 56%). However, segments that remained akinetic after revascularization had significantly lower diastolic WT prior to revascularization than those with improved wall motion. The results of this study suggest that the quantitative assessment of dobutamine-induced systolic WT by MRI is a reliable indicator of myocardial viability. Although resting diastolic WT alone does not provide accurate viability data, the presence of significant wall thinning reliably suggests the presence of irreversible myocardial damage. The assessment of myocardial viability with dobutamine can therefore be restricted to those patients with preserved diastolic WT.

Recently, contrast enhanced MRI with gadolinium diethylenetriamine pentaacetic acid has been evaluated as an additional tool for the assessment of myocardial viability.[139] Compared with dobutamine stress echocardiography and thallium-SPECT imaging, delayed hyperenhancement of contrast MRI images suggests the presence of nonviable myocardium. The prognostic value of this technique in patients undergoing revascularization currently is being investigated. The incremental benefit information provided by contrast enhancement in patients undergoing functional assessment with dobutamine also has not been reported.

Dobutamine stimulation also has been evaluated in conjunction with radionuclide angiography. Increased regional but not global LV ejection fraction (LVEF) with dobutamine infusion preoperatively appears to predict improvement in LV function after revascularization.[140,141]

Conclusions

Dobutamine echocardiography has shown enormous promise for assessing viability in patients with coronary artery disease and either acute or chronic LV dysfunction. It is now clear that a number of dysfunctional myocardial regions will manifest metabolic evidence of viability, with either FDG or thallium uptake, but lack inotropic reserve during dobutamine administration. It is conceivable that some hibernating regions are balanced so delicately between the reductions in flow and function that any catecholamine stimulation to increase oxygen demands will merely result in ischemia and inability to elicit contractile reserve. Whether the PET or SPECT information is more accurate than the dobutamine echocardiographic data regarding the potential for such regions to improve in function after revascularization awaits further study. MRI and contrast echocardiography recently have emerged as additional diagnostic tools for the assessment of myocardial viability. Their precise role in the diagnostic assessment of myocardial viability currently is under investigation.

Above all, the clinical relevance of viability assessment by these and other imaging modalities requires extensive study. Over 80% of dysfunctional myocardial regions identified as viable by these various imaging techniques may improve after revascularization, but the specific patients likely to benefit clinically from this information are not delineated fully. At present, the identification of viable myocardium is only one factor that enters into the equation to recommend or not recommend revascularization in the patient with impaired LV function. As in any other patient with coronary artery disease, this decision also should be based on clinical presentation, coronary anatomy, LV function, and evidence of inducible ischemia. Increasingly, however, determination of the viability of myocardial territories to be revascularized plays a pivotal role in this decision-making process. Definitive, accurate, and cost-effective methods are essential to make this determination, and noninvasive techniques to assess myocardial function will be called on with increasing frequency in the future for this purpose.

References

1. Reduto LA, Freund GC, Baeta JM, et al. Coronary artery reperfusion in acute myocardial infarction: Beneficial effects of intracoronary streptokinase on left ventricular salvage and performance. *Am Heart J* 1981;102:1168–1177.
2. Braunwald E, Kloner RA. The stunned myocardium: Prolonged, postischemic ventricular dysfunction. *Circulation* 1982;66:1146–1149.
3. Anderson JL, Marshall HW, Bray BE, et al. A randomized trial of intracoronary streptokinase in the treatment of acute myocardial infarction. *N Engl J Med* 1983;308:1312–1318.
4. Stack RS, Phillips HR III, Grierson DS, et al. Functional improvement of jeopardized myocardium following intracoronary streptokinase infusion in acute myocardial infarction. *J Clin Invest* 1983;72:84–95.
5. Sheehan FH, Doerr R, Schmidt WG, et al. Early recovery of left ventricular function after thrombolytic therapy for acute myocardial infarction: An important determinant of survival. *J Am Coll Cardiol* 1988;12:289–300.
6. Topol EJ, Weiss JL, Brinker LA, et al. Regional wall motion improvement after coronary thrombolysis with recombinant tissue plasminogen activator: Importance of coronary angioplasty. *J Am Coll Cardiol* 1985;6:426–433.
7. Bolli R. Myocardial "stunning" in man. *Circulation* 1992;86:1671–1691.
8. Helfant RH, Pine R, Meister SG, et al. Nitroglycerin to unmask reversible asynergy: Correlation with postcoronary bypass ventriculography. *Circulation* 1974;50:103–113.
9. Rahimtoola SH. Coronary bypass surgery for chronic angina—1981: A perspective. *Circulation* 1982;65:225–241.
10. Braunwald E, Rutherford JD. Reversible ischemic left ventricular dysfunction: Evidence for "hibernating" myocardium. *J Am Coll Cardiol* 1986;8:1467–1470.
11. Rahimtoola SH. The hibernating myocardium. *Am Heart J* 1989;117:211–213.
12. Dilsizian V, Bonow RO, Cannon RO, et al. The effect of coronary artery bypass grafting on left ventricular systolic function at rest: Evidence for preoperative sublinical myocardial ischemia. *Am J Cardiol* 1988;61:1248–1254.
13. Ross J Jr. Myocardial perfusion-contraction matching: Implications for coronary artery disease and hibernation. *Circulation* 1991;83:1076–1083.
14. Elefteriades JA, Tolis G Jr, Levi E, et al. Coronary artery bypass grafting in severe left ventricular dysfunction: Excellent survival with improved ejection fraction and functional state. *J Am Coll Cardiol* 1993;22:1411–1417.
15. Bolli R, Jeroudi MO, Patel BS, et al. Marked reduction of free radical generation and contractile dysfunction by antioxidant therapy begun at the time of reperfusion: Evidence that myocardial "stunning" is a manifestation of reperfusion injury. *Circ Res* 1989;65:607–622.
16. Bolli R. Mechanism of myocardial stunning. *Circulation* 1990;82:723–738.
17. Bolli R. Oxygen-derived free radicals and postischemic myocardial dysfunction ("stunned myocardium"). *J Am Coll Cardiol* 1988;12:239–249.
18. Greenfield RA, Swain JL. Disruption of myofibrillar energy use: Dual mechanisms that may contribute to postischemic dysfunction in stunned mycocardium. *Circ Res* 1987;60:283–289.
19. Kusuoka H, Porterfield JK, Weisman HF, et al. Pathophysiology and pathogenesis of stunned myocardium: Depressed $Ca2+$ activation of contraction as a consequence of reperfusion-induced calcium overload in ferret heart. *J Clin Invest* 1987;79:950–961.
20. Marban E. Myocardial stunning and hibernation: The physiology behind the colloquialisms. *Circulation* 1991;83:681–688.
21. Kraus SM, Jacobus WE, Becker LC. Alterations in sarcoplasmic reticulum calcium transport in the postischemic "stunned" myocardium. *Circ Res* 1989;65:526–530.
22. McCord JM. Oxygen-derived free radicals in postischemic tissue. *N Engl J Med* 1985;312:159–163.
23. Przyldenk K, Kloner RA. Superoxide dismutase plus catalase improve contractile function in the canine model of "stunned myocardium." *Circ Res* 1986;58:148–156.
24. Engler R, Cowell JW. Granulocytes cause reperfusion ventricular dysfunction after 15-minute ischemia in the dog. *Circ Res* 1987;61:20–28.

25. Zhao M, Zhang H, Robinson TF, et al. Profound structural alterations of the extracellular collagen matrix in postischemic dysfunction ("stunned") but viable myocardium. *J Am Coll Cardiol* 1987;10:1322–1334.
26. Nixon JV, Brown CN, Smitherman TC. Identification of transient and persistent wall motion abnormalities in patients with unstable angina by two-dimensional echocardiography. *Circulation* 1982;65:1497–1503.
27. Renkin J, Wijns W, Ladha Z, et al. Reversal of segmental hypokinesis by coronary angioplasty in patients with unstable angina, persistent T wave inversion, and left anterior descending coronary artery stenosis: Additional evidence for myocardial stunning. *Circulation* 1990;82: 913–921.
28. Jeroudi MO, Cheirif J, Habib G, et al. Prolonged wall motion abnormalities after chest pain at rest in patients with unstable angina: A possible manifestation of myocardial stunning. *Am Heart J* 1994;127:1241–1250.
29. Homans DC, Sublett E, Dai XZ, et al. Persistence of regional left ventricular dysfunction after exercise-induced myocardial ischemia. *J Clin Invest* 1986;77:66–73.
30. Camici P, Araujo LI, Spinks T, et al. Increased uptake of 18F-fluorodeoxyglucose in post-ischemic myocardium of patients with exercise-induced angina. *Circulation* 1986;74:81–88.
31. Kloner RA, Allen J, Cox TA, et al. Stunned left ventricular myocardium after exercise treadmill testing in coronary artery disease. *Am J Cardiol* 1991;68:329–334.
32. Dyke SH, Urschel CW, Sonnenblick EH, et al. Detection of latent function in acutely ischemic myocardium in the dog: Comparison of pharmacologic stimulation and postextrasystolic potentiation. *Circ Res* 1975;36:490–497.
33. Ellis SG, Wynne J, Braunwald E, et al. Response of reperfusion-salvaged, stunned myocardium to inotropic stimulation. *Am Heart J* 1984;107:13–19.
34. Bolli R, Zhu WX, Myers ML, rt al. Beta-adrenergic stimulation reverses postischemic myocardial dysfunction without producing subsequent functional deterioration. *Am J Cardiol* 1985;56:964–968.
35. Becker LC, Levine JH, DiPaula AF, et al. Reversal of dysfunction in postischemic stunned myocardium by epinephrine and postextrasystolic potentiation. *J Am Coll Cardiol* 1986;7: 580–589.
36. Leier C, Unverferth D, Kates R. The relationship between plasma dobutamine concentrations and cardiovascular responses in cardiac failure. *Am J Med* 1979;66:238–242.
37. Tuttle R, Pollock D, Todd G. The effect of dobutamine on cardiac oxygen balance, regional blood flow and infarction severity after coronary artery narrowing in dogs. *Circ Res* 1977;41: 357–364.
38. Pierard LA, De Lansheere CM, Berthe C, et al. Identification of viable myocardium by echocardiography during dobutamine infusion in patients with myocardial infarction after thrombolytic therapy: Comparison with positron emission tomography. *J Am Coll Cardiol* 1990;15:1021–1031.
39. Barilla F, Gheorghiade M, Alam M, et al. Low-dose dobutamine in patients with acute myocardial infarction identifies viable but not contractile myocardium and predicts the magnitude of improvement in wall motion abnormalities in response to coronary revascularization. *Am Heart J* 1991;122:1522–1531.
40. Duchak J, Smart S, Wynsen J, et al. Low dose dobutamine induced infarction zone wall thickening correlates with thallium by delayed SPECT imaging. *Circulation* 1994;86(suppl I):I384. Abstract.
41. Smart SC, Sawada S, Ryan T, et al. Low-dose dobutamine echocardiography detects reversible dysfunction after thrombolytic therapy of acute myocardial infarction. *Circulation* 1993;88: 405–415.
42. Previtali M, Poli A, Lanzarini L, et al. Dobutamine stress echocardiography for assessment of myocardial viability and ischemia in acute myocardial infarction treated with thrombolysis. *Am J Cardiol* 1993;72:14G–130G.
43. Salustri A, Elhendy A, Garyfallydis P, et al. Prediction of improvement of ventricular function after acute myocardial infarction using low-dose dobutamine stress echocardiography. *Am J Cardiol* 1994;74:853–856.
44. Watada H, Ito H, Oh H, et al. Dobutamine stress echocardiography predicts reversible dysfunction and quantitates the extent of irreversibly damaged myocardium after reperfusion of anterior myocardial infarction. *J Am Coll Cardiol* 1994;24:624–630.

45. Smart SC. The clinical utility of echocardiography in the assessment of myocardial viability. *J Nucl Med* 1994;35(suppl):49S–58S.
46. Leclercq F, Messner-Pellenc P, Moragues C, et al. Myocardial viability assessed by dobutamine echocardiography in acute myocardial infarction after successful primary coronary angioplasty. *Am J Cardiol* 1997;80:6–10.
47. Previtali M, Lanzarini L, Poli A, et al. Dobutamine stress echocardiography early after myocardial infarction treated with thrombolysis. *Int J Cardiol Imaging* 1996;12:97–104.
48. Elhendy A, Trocino G, Salustri A, et al. Low dose dobutamine echocardiography and rest-redistribution thallium-201 tomography in the assessment of spontaneous recovery of left ventricular function after recent myocardial infarction. *Am Heart J* 1996;131:1088–1096.
49. Sicari R, Picano E, Landi P, et al. Prognostic value of dobutamine-atropine stress echocardiography early after acute myocardial infarction. *J Am Coll Cardiol* 1997;29:254–260.
50. Picano E, Sicari R, Landi P, et al. Prognostic value of myocardial viability in medically treated patients with global left ventricular dysfunction early after an uncomplicated myocardial infarction. *Circulation* 1998;98:1078–1084.
51. Previtali M, Fetiveau R, Lanzarini L, et al. Prognostic value of myocardial viability and ischemia detected by dobutamine stress echocardiography early after acute myocardial infarction treated with thrombolysis. *J Am Coll Cardiol* 1998;32:380–386.
52. Anselmi M, Golia G, Cicoira M, et al. Prognostic value of detection of myocardial viability using low-dose dobutamine echocardiography in infarcted patients. *Am J Cardiol* 1998;81:21G–28G.
53. Opie LH. Effects of regional ischemia on metabolism of glucose and fatty acids: Relative rates of aerobic and anaerobic energy production during myocardial infarction and comparison with effects of anoxia. *Circ Res* 1976;38(suppl I):52–74.
54. Apstein CS, Deckelbaum L, Mueller M, et al. Graded global ischemia and reperfusion: Cardiac function and lactate metabolism. *Circulation* 1977;55:864–872.
55. Apstein CS, Deckelbaum L, Hagopian L, et al. Acute cardiac ischemia and reperfusion: Contractility, relaxation, and glycolysis. *Am J Physiol* 1978;235:H637–H648.
56. Canty JM Jr, Klocke FJ. Reductions in regional myocardial function at rest in conscious dogs with chronically reduced regional coronary artery pressure. *Circ Res* 1987;61(suppl II):107–116.
57. Marshall RC, Zhang DY. Correlation of contractile dysfunction with oxidative energy production and tissue high energy phosphate stores during partial coronary flow disruption in the rabbit heart. *J Clin Invest* 1988;82:86–95.
58. Vanoverschelde JLJ, Janier MF, Bakke JE, et al. Rate of glycolysis during ischemia determines extent of ischemic injury and functional recovery after reperfusion. *Am J Physiol* 1994;267:H1785–H1794.
59. Kitakaze M, Marban E. Cellular mechanism of the modulation of contractile function by coronary perfusion pressure in ferret hearts. *J Physiol (Lond)* 1989;414:455–472.
60. Wier WG, Yue DT. Intracellular $[Ca^{2+}]$ transients underlying the short-term force-interval relationship in ferret ventricular myocardium. *J Physiol (Lond)* 1986;376:507–530.
61. Opie LH. Coronary flow rate and perfusion pressure as determinants of mechanical function and oxidative metabolism of isolated perfused rat heart. *J Physiol* 1965;180:529–541.
62. Schulz R, Guth BD, Pieper K, et al. Recruitment of an inotropic reserve in moderately ischemic myocardium at the expense of metabolic recovery: A model of short term hibernation. *Circ Res* 1992;70:1282–1295.
63. Schulz R, Rose J, Martin C, et al. Development of short-term myocardial hibernation: Its limitation by the severity of ischemia and inotropic stimulation. *Circulation* 1993;88:684–695.
64. Vanoverschelde JJ, Wijns W, Depre C, et al. Mechanisms of chronic regional postischemic dysfunction in humans: New insights from the study of noninfarcted collateral-dependent myocardium. *Circulation* 1993;87:1513–1523.
65. Maes A, Flameng W, Nuyts J, et al. Histological alterations in chronically hypoperfused myocardium: Correlation with PET findings. *Circulation* 1994;90:735–745.
66. Bolukoglu H, Liedtke JA, Nellis S, et al. An animal model of chronic coronary stenosis resulting in hibernating myocardium. *Am J Physiol* 1992;263:H20–H29.

67. Schultz R, Myazaki S, Thaulow E. Consequences of regional inotropic stimulation of ischemic myocardium on regional blood flow and function in anesthetized swine. *Circ Res* 1989;64: 1116–1126.
68. Willerson K, Hutton I, Watson J, et al. Influence of dobutamine on regional blood flow and ventricular performance during acute and chronic myocardial ischemia in dogs. *Circulation* 1976;53:828–833.
69. Horn HR, Teicholz LE, Cohn PF, et al. Augmentation of left ventricular contraction pattern in coronary artery disease by an inotropic catecholamine: The epinephrine ventriculogram. *Circulation* 1974;49:1063–1071.
70. Dyke SH, Cohn PF, Gorlin R, et al. Detection of residual myocardial function in coronary artery disease using postextrasystolic potentiation. *Circulation* 1974;50:694–699.
71. Hamby RI, Aintablian A, Wisoff BG, et al. Response of the left ventricle in coronary artery disease to postextrasystolic potentiation. *Circulation* 1975;51:428–435.
72. Cohn LH, Collins JJ, Cohn PF. Use of the augmented ejection fraction to select patients with severe left ventricular dysfunction for coronary revascularization. *J Thorac Cardiovasc Surg* 1976;72:835–840.
73. Nesto RW, Cohn LH, Collins JJ, et al. Inotropic reserve: A useful predictor of increased 5 year survival and improved postoperative left ventricular function in patients with coronary artery disease and reduced ejection fraction. *Am J Cardiol* 1982;50:39–44.
74. Bodenheimer MM, Banka VS, Hermann GA, et al. Reversible asynergy: Histopathologic and electrographic correlations in patients with coronary artery disease. *Circulation* 1976;53: 792–796.
75. Popio KA, Gorlin R, Bechtel D, et al. Postextrasystolic potentiation as a predictor of potential myocardial viability: Preoperative analysis compared with studies after coronary bypass surgery. *Am J Cardiol* 1977;39:944–953.
76. Gerber BL, Vanoverschelde JLJ, Bol A, et al. Myocardial blood flow glucose uptake, and recruitment of inotropic reserve in chronic left ventricular ischemic dysfunction: Implications for the pathophysiology of chronic myocardial hibernation. *Circulation* 1996;94:651–659.
77. Perrone-Filardi P, Pace L, Prastaro M, et al. Assessment of myocardial viability in pateints with chronic coronary artery disease: Rest-4 hour-24 hour 201Tl tomography versus dobutamine echocardiography. *Circulation* 1996;94:2712–2719.
78. Arnese M, Cornel JH, Salustri A, et al. Prediction of improvement of regional left ventricular function after surgical revascularization: A comparison of low-dose dobutamine echocardiography with 201Tl single-photon emission computed tomography. *Circulation* 1995;91: 2748–2752.
79. Haque T, Furukawa T, Takahashi M, et al. Identification of hybernating myocardium by dobutamine stress echocardiography: Comparison with thallium-201 reinjection imaging. *Am Heart J* 1995;130:553–563.
80. Skopicki HA, Weissman NJ, Rose GA, et al. Thallium imaging, dobutamine echocardiography, and positron emission tomography for the detection of myocardial viability. *J Am Coll Cardiol* 1996;27:162A. Abstract.
81. Vanoverschelde JJ, D'Hondt AM, Marwick T, et al. Head to head comparison of exercise-redistribution-reinjection thallium single-photon emission tomography and low-dose dobutamine echocardiography for prediction of reversibility of chronic left ventricular ischemic dysfunction. *J Am Coll Cardiol* 1996;28:432–442.
82. Bax JJ, Cornel JH, Vissner FC, et al. Prediction of recovery or regional left ventricular dysfunction following revascularization: Comparison of F18-fluorodeoxyglucose SPECT, thallium stress-reinjection SPECT and dobutamine echocardiography. *J Am Coll Cardiol* 1996;28:558–564.
83. Charney R, Schwinger ME, Chung J, et al. Dobutamine echocardiography and resting-redistribution thallium-201 scintigraphy predicts recovery of hibernating myocardium after coronary revascularization. *Am Heart J* 1994;128:864–869.
84. Perrone-Filardi P, Pace L, Prastaro M, et al. Dobutamine ehocardiography predicts improvement of hypoperfused dysfunctional myocardium after revascularization in patients with coronary artery disease. *Circulation* 1995;91:2556–2565.
85. Cigarroa CG, deFilippi CR, Brickner E, et al. Dobutamine stress echocardiography identifies hibernating myocardium and predicts recovery of left ventricular function after coronary revascularization. *Circulation* 1993;88:430–436.

86. Marzullo P, Parodi O, Reisenhofer B, et al. Value of rest thallium-201/technetium-99m sestamibi scans and dobutamine echocardiogrphy for detecting myocardial viability. *Am J Cardiol* 1993;71:166–172.

87. La Canna G, Alfieri O, Giubbini R, et al. Echocardiography during infusion of dobutamine for identification of reversible dysfunction in patients with chronic coronary artery disease. *J Am Coll Cardiol* 1994;23:617–626.

88. Sehgal R, Lambert KL, Saham GM, et al. Prediction of viable myocardium by dobutamine echocardiography in patients with chronic left ventricular dysfunction. *Clin Res* 1994;42: 160A. Abstract.

89. Afridi I, Kleiman NS, Raizner AE, et al. Dobutamine echocardiography in myocardial hibernation: Optimal dose and accuracy in predicting recovery of ventricular function after coronary revascularization. *Circulation* 1995;91:663–670.

90. deFellipe CR, Willet DR, Irani WN, et al. Comparison of myocardial contrast echocardiography and low-dose dobutamine stress echocardiography in predicting recovery of left ventricular function after coronary revascularization in chronic ischemic heart disease. *Circulation* 1995;91:990–998.

91. Bonow RO. The hibernating myocardium: Implications for management of congestive heart failure. *Am J Cardiol* 1995;75:17A–25A.

92. Panza JA, Dilsizian V, Laurienzo JM, et al. Relation between thallium uptake and contractile response to dobutamine: Implications regarding myocardial viability in patients with chronic coronary artery disease and left ventricular dysfunction. *Circulation* 1995;91:990–998.

93. Baer FM, Voth E, Deutsch HJ, et al. Assessment of viable myocardium by dobutamine transesophageal echocardiography and comparison with fluorine-18 fluorodeoxyglucose positron emission tomography. *J Am Coll Cardiol* 1994;24:343–353.

94. Elsner G, Sawada S, Foltz J, et al. Dobutamine stimulation detects stunned but not hibernating myocardium. *Circulation* 1994;90:I117. Abstract.

95. Hepner AM, Bach DS, Bolling SF, et al. A positive dobutamine stress echocardiogram predicts viable myocardium in ischemic cardiomyopathy: A comparison with PET. *Circulation* 1994;90:I117. Abstract.

96. Chen C, Li L, Chen LL, et al. Incremental doses of dobutamine induce a biphasic response in dysfunctional left ventricular regions subtending coronary stenoses. *Circulation* 1995;92: 756–766.

97. Berger BC, Watson DD, Burwell LR, et al. Redistribution of thallium at rest in patients with stable and unstable angina and the effect of coronary artery bypass surgery. *Circulation* 1979;60:1114–1125.

98. Iskandrian AS, Hakki A, Kane SA, et al. Rest and redistribution thallium-201 myocardial scintigraphy to predict improvement in left ventricular function after coronary artery bypass grafting. *Am J Cardiol* 1983;51:1312–1316.

99. Kiat H, Berman DS, Maddahi J, et al. Late reversibility of tomographic myocardial thallium-201 defects: An accurate marker of myocardial viability. *J Am Coll Cardiol* 1988;12:1456–1463.

100. Dilsizian V, Rocco TP, Freedman NMT, et al. Enhanced detection of ischemic but viable myocardium by the reinjection of thallium after stress-redistribution imaging. *N Engl J Med* 1990;323:141–146.

101. Eitzman D, Al-Aouar Z, Kanter HL, et al. Clinical outcome of patients with advanced coronary artery disease after viability studies with positron emission tomography. *J Am Coll Cardiol* 1992;20:559–565.

102. Di Carli MF, Davidson M, Little R, et al. Value of metabolic imaging with positron emission tomography for evaluating prognosis in patients with coronary artery disease and left ventricular dysfunction. *Am J Cardiol* 1994;73:527–533.

103. Chaudry FA, Tauke JT, Alessandrini RS, et al. Prognostic implications of myocardial contractile reserves in patients with coronary artery disease and left ventricular dysfunction. J Am Coll Cardiol 1999;34:730–738.

104. Williams MJ, Olabshian J, Lauer MS, et al. Prognostic value of dobutamine echocardiography in patients with left ventricular dysfunction. *J Am Coll Cardiol* 1996;27:132–139.

105. Afridi I, Grayburn P, Panza J, et al. Myocardial viability during dobutamine echocardiography predicts survival in patients with coronary artery disease and severe left ventricular systolic dysfunction. *J Am Coll Cardiol* 1998;32:921–926.

106. Simek CL, Watson DD, Smith WH, et al. Dipyridamole thallium-201 imaging versus dobutamine echocardiography for the evaluation of coronary artery disease in patients unable to exercise. *Am J Cardiol* 1993;72:1257–1262.

107. Hendel RC, Chaudhry FA, Parker MA, et al. Regional discordance in myocardial viability assessment with thallium-201 rest-redistribution imaging and low-dose dobutamine echocardiography. *Circulation* 1995;92:I550. Abstract.

108. Marzullo P, Parodi O, Reisenhofer B, et al. Value of rest thallium-201/technetium-99m sestamibi scans and dobutamine echocardiography for detecting myocardial viability. *Am J Cardiol* 1993;71:166–172.

109. Senior R, Raval U, Lahiri A. Technetium-88m labeled sestamibi imaging reliably identifies retained contractile reserve in dyssynergic myocardial segments. *J Nucl Cardiol* 1995;2:296–302.

110. Lee HL, Davila-Roman VG, Ludbrook PA, et al. Dependency of contractile reserve on myocardial blood flow. *Circulation* 1997;96:2884–2891.

111. Ma L, Chen L, Gillam L, et al. Nitroglycerin enhances the ability of dobutamine stress echocardiography to detect hibernating myocardium. *Circulation* 1997;96:3992–4001.

112. Perrone-Filardi P, Bacharach SL, Dilsizian V, et al. Metabolic evidence of viable myocardium in regions with reduced wall thickening and absent wall thickening in patients with chronic ischemic left ventricular dysfunction. *J Am Coll Cardiol* 1992;20:161–168.

113. Bonow RO, Dilsizian V, Cuocolo A, et al. Identification of viable myocardium in patients with chronic coronary artery disease and left ventricular dysfunction: Comparison of thallium-201 with reinjection and PET imaging with 18F-fluorodeoxyglucose. *Circulation* 1991;83:26–37.

114. Baumgartner H, Porenta G, Yuk-Kong L, et al. Assessment of myocardial viability by dobutamine echocardiography, positron emission tomography and thallium-201 SPECT: Correlation with histopathology in explanted hearts. *J Am Coll Cardiol* 1998;32:1701–1708.

115. Perrone-Filardi P, Pace L, Squame F, et al. Do rest-redistribution thallium tomography and low-dose dobutamine echocardiography yield comparable viability information in dysfunctional myocardium? *Circulation* 1994;90(suppl I):314. Abstract.

116. Pirelli S, Crivellaro W, Faletra F, et al. Dobutamine stress echocardiography and rest thallium-201 scintigraphy in patients with previous myocardial infarction and single vessel coronary artery lesion: Prediction of functional recovery after revascularization. *J Am Coll Cardiol* 1995;25:340A. Abstract.

117. Smart SC, Knickelbine T, Carlos ME, et al. Dobutamine echocardiography and rest SPECT Tl-201 scintigraphy are more concordant in detecting viability in hibernating than stunned myocardium. *J Am Coll Cardiol* 1995;25:126A. Abstract.

118. Marwick TH, Nemec JJ, Pashkow FJ, et al. Accuracy and limitations of exercise echocardiography in a routine clinical practice. *J Am Coll Cardiol* 1992;19:74–81.

119. Hoffmann R, Lethen H, Marwick T, et al. Analysis of interinstitutional observer agreement in interpretation of dobutamine stress echocardiograms. *J Am Coll Cardiol* 1996;27:330–336.

120. Kornbluth M, Liang DH, Schnittger I. Native tissue harmonic imaging improves endocardial border definition and wall motion scoring. *J Am Coll Cardiol* 1998;31(suppl A):76. Abstract.

121. Mulvagh SL, Foley DA, Gilman G, et al. Noncontrast tissue harmonic imaging markedly enhances image quality in technically difficult echocardiograms. *J Am Coll Cardiol* 1998;31(suppl A):76. Abstract.

122. Chin C, Hancock J, Brown A, et al. Improved endocardial definition and evaluation of dobutamine stress echocardiography using second harmonic imaging. *J Am Coll Cardiol* 1998;31(suppl A):76. Abstract.

123. Kancherla MK, Parker M, Greenfield S, et al. Second harmonic imaging improves interpretation of dobutamine stress echocardiography for less experienced echocardiographers. *J Am Coll Cardiol* 1999. Abstract. In press.

124. Dittrich HC, Kuvelas T, Dadd K, et al. Safety and efficacy of the ultrasound contrast agent FS069 in normal humans: Results of a phase one trial. *Circulation* 1995;92(suppl 1):I464. Abstract.

125. Skyba DM, Camarano G, Goodman NC, et al. Hemodynamic characteristics, myocardial kinetics and microvascular rheology of FS069, a second-generation echocardiographic contrast agent capable of producing myocardial opacification from a venous injection. *J Am Coll Cardiol* 1996;28:1292–1300.

126. Cohen J, Bruns D, Hausner E, et al. A multicenter trial comparing FS069 and Albunex for left ventricular endocardial border delineation. *J Am Coll Cardiol* 1997;10:519A. Abstract.
127. Cheirif J, Segar D, Hausner E, et al. FS069 greatly improves the diagnostic utility of ultrasound for left ventricular function. *J Am Soc Echocardiogr* 1997;10:390. Abstract.
128. Spotnitz WD, Matthew TL, Keller MW, et al. Intraoperative demonstration of coronary collateral flow using myocardial contrast two-dimensional echocardiography. *Am J Cardiol* 1990;65:1259–1261.
129. Sabia PJ, Powers ER, Jayaweera AR, et al. Functional significance of collateral flow in patients with recent acute myocardial infarction: A study using myocardial contrast echocardiography. *Circulation* 1992;85:2080–2089.
130. Vernon S, Camarano G, Kaul S, et al. Myocardial contrast echocardiography demonstrates that collateral flow can preserve myocardial function beyond a chronically occluded coronary artery. *Am J Cardiol* 1996;78:958–960.
131. Sabia PJ, Powers ER, Ragosta M, et al. An association between collateral blood flow and myocardial viability in patients with recent myocardial infarction. *N Eng J Med* 1992;372: 1825–1831.
132. Iliceto S, Galiuto L, Marchese A, et al. Analysis of microvascular integrity, contractile reserve, and myocardial viability after acute myocardial infarction by dobutamine echocardiography and myocardial contrast echocardiography. *Am J Cardiol* 1996;77:441–445.
133. Meza MF, Ramee S, Collins T, et al. Knowledge of perfusion and contractile reserve improves the predictive value of recovery of regional myocardial function postrevascularization. *Circulation* 1997;96:3459–3465.
134. Meza MF, Kates MA, Barbee W, et al. Combination of dobutamine and myocardial contrast echocardiography to differentiate postischemic from infarcted myocardium. *J Am Coll Cardiol* 1997;29:974–984.
135. Baer FM, Voth E, LaRosee K, et al. Comparison of dobutamine transesophageal echocardiography and dobutamine magnetic resonance imaging for detection of residual myocardial viability. *Am J Cardiol* 1996;78:415–419.
136. Dendale P, Franken PR, Holman E, et al. Validation of low-dose dobutamine magnetic resonance imaging for the assessment of myocardial viability after infarction by serial imaging. *Am J Cardiol* 1998;82:375–377.
137. Baer FM, Voth E, Schneider CA, et al. Comparison of low dose dobutamine-gradient echo magnetic resonance imaging and positron emission tomography with 18F-flourodeoxyglucose in patients with chronic coronary artery disease. *Circulation* 1995;91:1006–1015.
138. Baer FM, Theissen P, Schneider CA, et al. Dobutamine magnetic resonance imaging predicts contractile recovery of chronically dysfunctional myocardium after successful revascularization. *J Am Coll Cardiol* 1998;31:1040–1048.
139. Ramani K, Judd RM, Holly TA, et al. Contrast magnetic resonance imaging in the assessment of myocardial viability in patients with stable coronary artery disease and left ventricular dysfunction. *Circulation* 1998;98:2687–2694.
140. Coma-Canella I, del val Gomez M, Salazar L, et al. Stress radionuclide studies after acute myocardial infarction: Changes with revascularization. *J Nucl Cardiol* 1996;3:403–409.
141. Schechter D, Milgater E, Bocher M, et al. Value of dobutamine/nitrate radionuclide angiography in predicting revascularization effects on ventricular function. *J Cardiovasc Surg* 1994; 35(6suppl 1):81–84.

Chapter 11

Morphological and Echocardiographic Features of Viable and Nonviable Myocardium

Jamshid Shirani, MD, Madhulika Chandra, MD, and Edmund H. Sonnenblick, MD

Introduction

Coronary artery disease (CAD) was first identified as an etiology for congestive cardiomyopathy in 1969[1] and the term "ischemic cardiomyopathy" was proposed shortly after to refer to such an association.[2] Early necropsy studies in patients with ischemic cardiomyopathy often revealed degrees of left ventricular (LV) dysfunction and dilation disproportionate to the extent of myocardial replacement fibrosis.[3] It has since become clear that a substantial proportion of dysfunctional (asynergic) myocardial segments in patients with chronic ischemic cardiomyopathy is comprised of viable tissue with a potential for functional recovery after revascularization.[4-12] The contractile dysfunction in these viable myocardial segments results from prolonged resting hypoperfusion (hibernating myocardium) or acute, severe, ischemia-reperfusion (stunned myocardium).[13-16] Myocardial viability in asynergic LV segments now can be detected by the assessment of regional perfusion,[17-23] metabolic activity,[24-40] contractile reserve,[41-64] or microvascular patency (integrity).[62-73] The presence of large areas of viable myocardium can predict an improved outcome following revascularization in patients with chronic ischemic cardiomyopathy.[31,74-77]

Currently, the echocardiographic evaluation of myocardial viability relies primarily on the assessment of contractile response to inotropic (mainly dobutamine) stimulation.[50-64] In the last decade, a number of studies have demonstrated the accuracy of dobutamine stress echocardiographic (DSE) in predicting the outcome of asynergic myocardium following revascularization.[50-64] Meanwhile, the performance and interpretation of DSE studies have been facilitated greatly by the technical advances in the field of echocardiography. These include digital acquisition and display of images, application of new ultrasound techniques such as harmonic imaging,[78-80] power Doppler imaging,[81,82] and the use of contrast agents for endocardial border delineation.[83-89] New techniques and concepts also are developing rapidly in the field of myocardial contrast echocardiog-

From Dilsizian V (ed). *Myocardial Viability: A Clinical and Scientific Treatise.* Armonk, NY: Futura Publishing Co., Inc.; © 2000.

raphy (MCE) for assessment of regional blood flow ("microvascular patency" or "integrity").[62-73,90-100] Quantitative assessment of myocardial blood flow (MBF) also may be possible with the use of developing methods of image analysis in association with MCE.[87,90,92,99-111] In this chapter the morphological and echocardiographic features of viable and nonviable myocardium are presented.

Myocardial Asynergy in Chronic Ischemic Cardiomyopathy

Resting segmental wall motion abnormality in ischemic heart disease can result from one or a combination of several pathophysiological mechanisms (Table 1). Complete and persistent lack of myocardial perfusion results in irreversible dysfunction secondary to loss of myocytes and eventual replacement fibrosis (scar).[1,2,112] Such myocardial segments show no perfusion, metabolic activity, or contractile reserve. Following acute ischemia, if myocardial perfusion is restored adequately before myocyte necrosis has ensued, then the postischemic segment may remain asynergic for a variable period of time prior to spontaneous functional recovery (stunned myocardium).[15,16] Following timely and complete reperfusion, the stunned myocardium shows normal resting perfusion, exhibits contractile reserve, and preferentially metabolizes fatty acids, the metabolic substrate of the normal myocardium.[113-116] The hibernating myocardium is an asynergic LV segment with prolonged and persistent reduction in resting coronary blood flow, to a level that is just adequate for maintenance of tissue viability.[13,14] Such myocardial regions exhibit reduced perfusion,[13,14,17,18,35,50] active metabolism with preferential glucose utilization (perfusion-metabolism mismatch),[27,29,35] limited recruitable contractile reserve,[20,23,27,35,50-64] and a potential for recovery of function only after successful restoration of coronary blood flow.[19,35] In the absence of appropriate animal models, the exact cellular and molecular pathways leading to myocardial hibernation remain poorly understood.[117] It is proposed that myocardial hibernation is the consequence of an adaptive mechanism that allows myocyte survival in the setting of chronically reduced perfusion.[13,14] Whether or not myocardial hibernation can result from recurrent brief episodes of ischemia (repetitive stunning) in some myocardial segments with preserved resting blood flow remains controversial.[118] Chronic hypoperfusion eventually may lead to structural alterations in the myocytes ranging from mild, reversible changes in the cellular content of contractile proteins to irreversible, severe degeneration of the cells.[119-126] When extensive, functional and structural changes may lead to ischemic cardiomyopathy

Table 1

Diagnostic Features, Histopathology, and Response to Revascularization of Asynergic Myocardium in Ischemic Heart Disease

	Resting Wall Motion Abnormality	Perfusion	Contractile Reserve	Metabolism	Pathology	Recovery of Function
Scar	√	∅	∅	∅	Fibrosis	∅
Prolonged severe ischemia	√	↓↓	∅	↓*	Cellular degeneration	∅
Hibernating	√	↓	√ or ∅	√*	Loss of contractile proteins	√
Stunned	√	√	√	√†	Reperfusion injury	√

∅, Absent; ↓, reduced; ↓↓, severely reduced; √, present.

* Primarily glucose.

† Primarily fatty acid.

with global LV dysfunction and congestive heart failure, even in the absence of significant replacement fibrosis.[3,127,128] Following successful revascularization, the time course and extent of functional recovery of the hibernating myocardium primarily depends on the degree of structural changes in the myocytes.[125–127]

The aforementioned classification of asynergic myocardium has provided a useful framework for the understanding of segmental LV function in chronic CAD. It also has made possible a uniform approach to defining the predominant pathophysiological mechanism of myocardial asynergy as assessed by various diagnostic techniques. However, this oversimplified scheme may ignore the inherent heterogeneity of myocardial structure, frequently present even within small LV segments.

Structural Correlates of Reversible and Irreversible Left Ventricular Segmental Asynergy

Cardiac myocytes are believed to be terminally differentiated cells, unable to reenter the cell cycle.[129,130] Therefore, LV size and function in human disease is determined by a dynamic balance between the: (1) magnitude of irreversible cell loss, (2) structure and performance of the remaining myocytes, and (3) status of the nonmyocyte compartment (primarily the extracellular matrix) of the heart.

Irreversible Cell Loss

In ischemic cardiomyopathy, cell loss occurs through necrosis (with subsequent replacement fibrosis), apoptosis (programmed cell death), or myocytolysis (severe cellular degeneration and complete, irreversible loss of contractile proteins). Myocardial replacement fibrosis in chronic ischemic cardiomyopathy is present in the form of transmural or subendocardial scars in the infarct region and microscopic or patchy fibrosis in the noninfarct region of the LV.[131] The extent of myocardial replacement fibrosis in part determines segmental perfusion,[131–134] contractile reserve,[135] and metabolic activity,[132] as well as global LV size and systolic function. For example, the extent of postinfarct LV remodeling is influenced highly by the size of the index infarct.[136] There is an overall inverse correlation between the amount of replacement fibrosis and degree of regional thallium-201 (^{201}Tl) (thallium) uptake in ischemic cardiomyopathy.[131,133,134] Asynergic myocardial segments with enhanced ^{18}F-2-deoxyglucose (FDG) uptake show significantly less replacement fibrosis when compared with regions with low FDG uptake (24% ± 13% versus 49% ± 20%; $p = 0.002$) on positron emission tomography (PET).[125] Similarly, when both perfusion and metabolism are assessed by PET, normal segments contain lower proportions of fibrous tissue (8%) compared with areas of mismatch (11%–13%), mild to moderate matched defects (34%–35%), or severe matched defects (74%).[124,137] Following administration of nitrate[41] or dobutamine,[135] myocardial segments with lower content of fibrous tissue more often exhibit contractile reserve. Several studies have shown an overall inverse correlation between the degree of regional replacement fibrosis and the likelihood of recovery of function in asynergic myocardial segments following revascularization.[124–127]

Despite the aforementioned correlation, it is increasingly evident that factors other than the extent of myocardial fibrosis may determine the functional characteristics of the asynergic myocardium in chronic ischemic cardiomyopathy. Accordingly, some markedly enlarged hearts of patients with ischemic cardiomyopathy contain as little as 8% gross replacement fibrosis.[3] Also, as many as 50% of asynergic LV segments of patients with CAD, without prior electrographic (ECG) evidence of infarction, may appear normal on histological examination or contain <10% fibrous tissue.[138] The percentage of fibrous tissue in hypokinetic, noninfarcted myocardium may not differ from that of normokinetic segments in patients with chronic CAD (19.8% versus 20.2%; $p < 0.05$).[120] In patients with ischemic cardiomyopathy, the volume fraction of replacement collagen may range widely (4.4%–38%) in myocardial segments with similar thallium uptake.[134] Finally, asynergic myocardial segments showing a perfusion-metabolism mismatch by PET also may contain variable amounts (21%–45%) of fibrous tissue.[132] These observations indicate that factors other than the magnitude of myocardial fibrosis, such as the distribution of collagen[131] or presence of dysfunctional myocytes (see below), may affect the behavior of individual asynergic LV segments. In addition, cell loss through mechanisms other than necrosis may result in a reduced mass of functional myocytes in the absence of replacement fibrosis.

Apoptosis is a highly regulated and active process, which results in cell death in the absence of an inflammatory reaction or replacement fibrosis. Apoptosis occurs most commonly in cells that are progressing through the cell cycle.[139] Thus, it generally is believed that terminally differentiated adult cells such as myocytes do not undergo apoptosis under physiological conditions. However, several recent studies have indicated that apoptosis may be observed in myocardial infarction, end-stage ischemic cardiomyopathy, and stretched myocytes.[140–142] Apoptosis has been demonstrated in explanted hearts of patients with chronic ischemic cardiomyopathy.[141] However, data regarding the occurrence of apoptosis in earlier stages of ischemic cardiomyopathy remain inconclusive.[143,144]

In addition to necrosis and apoptosis, cell loss in chronic ischemic cardiomyopathy may result from severe and progressive loss of the cellular content of contractile proteins (myocytolysis).[119] Unlike necrosis, myocytolysis is not associated with an inflammatory response or with replacement fibrosis. In addition, in contrast to both necrosis and apoptosis, the dysfunctional cell is not cleared through phagocytosis. Aggregates of these myocytolytic cells may be present in LV regions with severe, persistent ischemia and appear as empty shells ("ghost cells"). Extensive myocytolysis may result in segmental LV dysfunction and preclude recovery of function after revascularization, even in the absence of significant replacement fibrosis.

Reversible Myocyte Dysfunction

In addition to cell loss, myocyte stunning or hibernation may contribute to segmental LV dysfunction. In stunning, the underlying histomorphological changes depend on the severity and duration of the ischemic episode, before reperfusion occurs. When coronary blood flow is restored rapidly, myocytes may appear normal histomorphologically despite abnormal contractile function. The latter is associated with reduced intracellular stores of adenosine triphosphate (ATP) and decreased sensitivity of the contractile apparatus to calcium.[145,146] However, more prolonged and severe episodes of ischemia before reperfusion may lead to contraction band necrosis, secondary to massive calcium influx. Contraction band necrosis is associated with destruction of the sarcolemma and myofibrillar apparatus, as well as agglutination of the myofibrillar proteins. Clinically, most asynergic LV segments characterized as stunned contain a mixture of cells with ischemic or reperfusion injury, as well as structurally intact myocytes.

Chronic, persistent reduction in resting coronary blood flow may alter myocyte function through a range of histomorphological and ultrastructural changes, which characterize hibernating myocardium (Table 2). The extent and duration of regional hypoperfusion[147] determine the severity of structural abnormalities in hibernating myocardium. Chronic hypoperfusion results in progressive depletion of the contractile apparatus, deposition of glycogen, and accumulation of large numbers of morphologically abnormal

Table 2

Histologic Features of Hibernating Myocardium

I. Cellular changes
  A. Light microscopy
    Depletion of contractile apparatus
    Glycogen deposition
    Tortuous nuclei with evenly distributed heterochromatin
    Increased number of small mitochondria
    Preserved cell volume
    Absence of degenerative changes, that is, acute myocyte necrosis, multilamellar
      bodies, lipid/phospholipid droplets, and gross intracellular edema
  B. Electron microscopy
    Loss of organized endoplasmic reticulum
    Loss of sarcoplasmic reticulum
    Lack of T-tubules
    Absence of degenerative ultrastructural changes, that is, cytoplasmic vascuolization,
      cytosolic edema, mitochondrial swelling, membrane disruption, accumulation of
      secondary lysosomes, membranous whorls, or lipid droplets
II. Extracellular changes
    Increased amount of types I and III collagen (perivascular and interstitial)
    Increased amount of fibronectin
    Decreased capillary density
    Well-preserved microvascular endothelium, pericytes, and interstitial mesenchymal
      cells

mitochondria, without loss of cell volume. The myocyte nucleus becomes irregular in shape, and the nuclear heterochromatin distributes uniformly rather than in clumps.[117,118,120–126,137] There often is a substantial loss of sarcoplasmic reticulum. Generally, the loss of contractile proteins begins at the perinuclear region, progresses toward the periphery of the myocyte, and eventually leads to the disappearance of all sarcomeres from the cell. However, cell membrane integrity may be preserved despite significant loss of contractile proteins. Although the histomorphological changes in hibernating myocardium are regarded as adaptive, this unstable condition eventually will progress to irreversible cellular degeneration if blood flow is not restored.[143] The likelihood and time course of functional recovery correlate directly with the severity of the ultrastructural changes in hibernating myocardium.[125,143,147] It should be emphasized that LV regions clinically characterized as hibernating may represent a variable admixture of replacement fibrosis, hibernating myocytes, and normal-appearing cells.

Nonmyocyte Compartment

Fibrous Matrix

In addition to the myocytes, the cardiac interstitium also undergoes significant alteration in response to ischemia-reperfusion and chronic, persistent hypoperfusion.[148–151] In stunned myocardium, ischemic and reperfusion injuries activate metalloproteinases resulting in dissolution of collagen matrix, which may contribute to contractile dysfunction.[149,150] A healing process that often fails to restore LV geometry then follows collagen dissolution. In hibernating myocardium, the matrix (interstitial) collagen often is expanded with increased amounts of types I and III collagen and fibronectin[151] and a reduction in the number of capillaries.[123,151,152] The extent of interstitial fibrosis in hibernating myocardium correlates with the severity and duration of hypoperfusion.[147]

Capillary Density

Extensive microvascular injury may follow ischemia-reperfusion. This may lead to intramyocardial hemorrhage and further damage to the remaining myocytes. Electron microscopic examination of the microvessels after late (60–90 minutes) reperfusion following coronary occlusion reveals loss of pinocytotic vesicles in endothelial cells, endothelial blebs, endothelial cell separation, and neutrophil infiltration.[153] Information regarding the status of microvessels in the hibernating myocardium is limited; however, preliminary results indicate that capillary density may be reduced significantly in some chronically hypoperfused segments.[151]

Echocardiographic Assessment
of Myocardial Viability

The echocardiographic evaluation of myocardial viability primarily relies on the detection of recruitable contractile reserve in asynergic LV segments. Such augmentation of contractility may occur in response to vasodilators,[41] inotropic agents,[50-64] or a properly timed premature ventricular contraction (PVC).[43-48] Currently, segmental contractile reserve is assessed most commonly by the response of the asynergic myocardium to graded dobutamine infusion.[50-64]

Dobutamine Stress Echocardiography

Dobutamine, a synthetic catecholamine (modified from isoproterenol) with a half-life of ~2 minutes, is a racemic mixture of stereoisomers with α_1-, β_1-, and β_2-adrenergic agonist activity.[154] At low doses (2.5–10 μg/kg per minute), it augments myocardial contractility without significant chronotropic effect and at higher doses, results in increased heart rate and peripheral vasodilation.[155] Systolic blood pressure increases significantly in normal individuals and modestly in those with LV dysfunction; diastolic blood pressure remains unchanged. Myocardial workload and oxygen demand are, thus, increased in a dose-related fashion in response to dobutamine. In patients with ischemic cardiomyopathy, dobutamine infusion rates of 2.5–15 μg/kg per minute (mean 10.8 ± 0.9) result in increases in heart rate, cardiac index, mean arterial pressure, and LV ejection fraction (LVEF) of 23%, 57%, 5%, and 6%, respectively.[156] These hemodynamic changes are associated with a decrease in pulmonary capillary wedge pressure and improved contractility in some segments with resting asynergy.[156] The contractile response of hibernating myocardium to dobutamine appears transient and is associated with metabolic deterioration[157,158] despite a modest increase in regional blood flow.[157]

Dobutamine increases MBF in direct correlation with the degree of epicardial coronary artery flow reserve.[155,159] In normal subjects, dobutamine infusion results in a threefold increase in MBF.[160] In patients with suspected CAD, dobutamine (at 8 μg/kg per minute) increases blood flow by an average of 137% in normal myocardium and by 47% in myocardium supplied by a severely stenotic coronary artery.[155] The degree of enhancement in MBF by dobutamine is limited in the absence of collateral flow reserve.[155] During administration of incremental doses of dobutamine (5–40 μg/kg per minute), myocardial perfusion, as assessed by ^{15}O-labeled water PET, increases by 102%

in regions without and by only 30% in regions with stress-induced asynergy.[159] The appearance and magnitude of dobutamine-induced wall motion abnormality correlates directly with the severity of coronary artery stenosis ($r = 0.68$) and inversely with myocardial fractional flow reserve ($r = -0.77$).[161] Hibernating myocardium shows a modest increase in blood flow in response to low-dose dobutamine.[157,162] A proportion of segments with inducible wall motion abnormality during dobutamine infusion will show a reduction in MBF to values below resting.[159] Dobutamine may induce myocardial ischemia at relatively low doses (2.5–15 μg/kg per minute) in some patients with ischemic cardiomyopathy.[156]

There are several patterns of contractile response to inotropic stimulation, based on the underlying myocardial pathology, resting perfusion, and blood flow reserve (Fig. 1). Infarcted/scarred tissue does not show any contractile response to inotropic stimulation. The ischemic myocardium contracts normally at rest and develops wall motion abnormality at low (5–10 μg/kg per minute) or high (20–40 μg/kg per minute) doses of dobutamine, depending on the degree of coronary flow reserve limitation. Abnormal resting wall motion with augmentation of contractility at low and high doses of dobutamine characterizes the stunned myocardium and reflects the normal blood flow reserve characteristic of these postischemic, reperfused segments. The hypokinetic or akinetic hibernating myocardium shows a "biphasic" response, with improved contractility at low doses and deterioration of wall motion at higher doses of dobutamine.[58,62,63,71] This may occur as a result of a small increase in MBF (0.20 mL/g per minute) at low doses (5–10 μg/kg per minute) of dobutamine, before the development of ischemia at higher doses.[163]

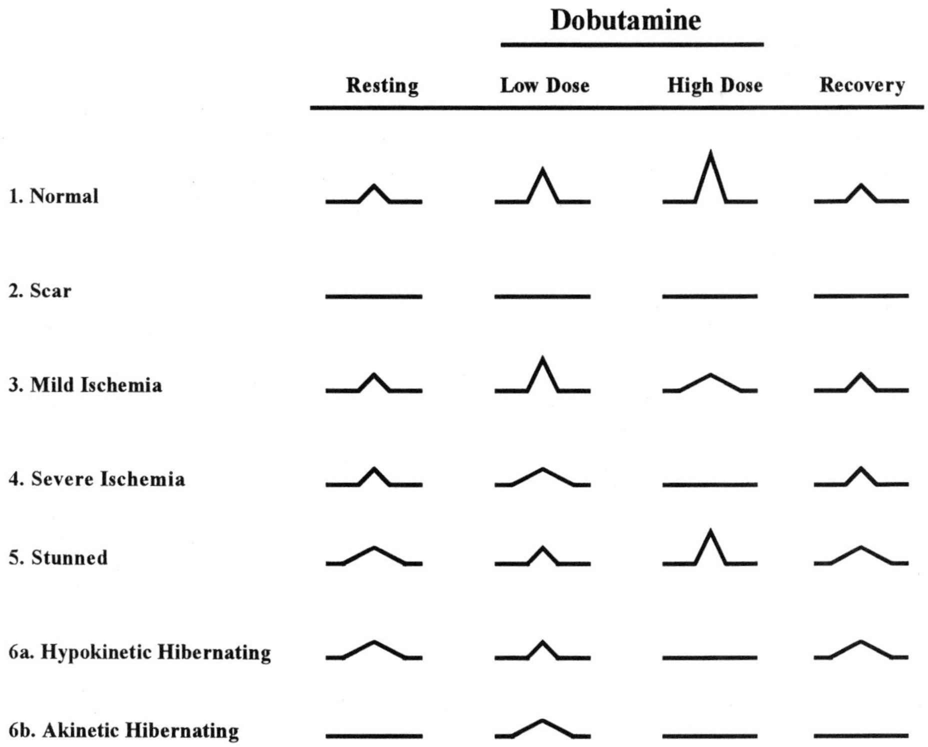

Figure 1. Diagram showing various patterns of segmental contractile response to inotropic stimulation during dobutamine stress echocardiography (DSE).

Since 1993 several studies have reported on the accuracy of DSE in predicting functional recovery of asynergic myocardium in a total of [mt]500 patients with chronic CAD (Table 3).[50-64] The overall predictive accuracy of DSE in these studies has ranged from 77% to 95%, primarily because of the differences in patient selection, DSE protocol, and other factors such as the duration of follow-up. Concerned about the safety of high-dose dobutamine in patients with severely reduced LVEF, the initial studies used relatively low doses of dobutamine (most often 5–10 μg/kg per minute).[50-57] Nevertheless, the contractile response of the asynergic myocardium to low-dose dobutamine was found to be highly predictive of postrevascularization recovery of function (positive predictive value 82%–100%).[50-57] However, functional recovery was also noted in a small (~15%) number of asynergic LV segments without contractile response to low-dose dobutamine. The latter was thought to indicate either a markedly compromised coronary flow reserve resulting in ischemia at the lowest dobutamine dose or lack of myofibrillar sensitivity to low concentrations of intracellular calcium.[51,58] Therefore, subsequent studies used lower starting and higher peak dobutamine infusion rates (2.5–40 μg/kg per minute).[58-64] This leads to an overall improvement in the sensitivity of DSE for detection of viable myocardium by identifying those segments with recruitable contractile reserve at very low (2.5 μg/kg per minute) or high (>20 μg/kg per minute) doses of dobutamine.[51, 58,164] In addition, roughly one-third of asynergic LV segments with recruitable contractile reserve at low doses of dobutamine deteriorated at higher doses. This biphasic response was found to be highly predictive of functional recovery following revascularization (overall sensitivity and specificity 69% and 87%). On the contrary, a sustained contractile response to dobutamine, observed in approximately one-fifth of the asynergic segments, appeared to indicate a low likelihood of functional recovery after revascularization. The latter is believed to either represent segments with thin subendocardial infarcts[165] or with as yet poorly characterized irreversible ischemic injury ("remodeled," "chronically stunned," or "cardiomyopathic"). It also was observed that the hypokinetic segments more often exhibited contractile reserve and had a higher likelihood of functional recovery after revascularization, compared with the akinetic segments.[50,54-56,58,62-64] However, the specificity of DSE was higher in akinetic compared with hypokinetic segments. A contractile response to dobutamine or functional recovery after revascularization was observed rarely in a dyskinetic segment.[58] These observations have influenced significantly the performance and interpretation of DSE studies for the assessment of myocardial viability.

Several studies have assessed the metabolic activity and the status of myocardial perfusion in asynergic LV segments, with and without recruitable contractile reserve by DSE.[50,55-57,61,62,157,162-164,166-168] In general, a reasonable concordance has been reported between thallium uptake and presence of contractile reserve by dobutamine.[57,164] Thus, asynergic myocardial segments with contractile reserve at low doses of dobutamine show higher uptake of thallium at rest,[50,55] late redistribution,[50] or stress-redistribution-reinjection.[61,164] A reversible thallium defect is observed more often in asynergic segments with a biphasic response, rather than other patterns of response, to dobutamine infusion.[164] However, a higher proportion of asynergic myocardial segments show viability by thallium than contractile reserve by DSE.[50,52,55-57,62,63] This has raised the possibility that a higher degree of myocyte functional integrity is required for recruitment of contractile reserve to dobutamine than for thallium uptake.[164] The latter is further supported by the observation that the presence of contractile reserve is a more potent predictor of recovery of function following revascularization than the presence of preserved membrane integrity by thallium.[169,170] A preliminary report indicates an inverse correlation between the presence of contractile reserve and percent fibrosis in transmural LV biopsies of patients with segmental wall motion abnormality.[135]

Presence of any contractile reserve by dobutamine at 5–20 μg/kg per minute has been shown to correlate well (89% concordance) with preserved metabolic activity by

Table 3

Published Reports of the Use of Dobutamine Stress Echocardiography for Assessment of Viable Myocardium

Author	Patients (number)	Age (y) Range (mean)	Dobutamine Dose (μg/kg per min/min)	Ejection Fraction (%)		Predictive Value (%)			Timing of Follow-up (mo)
				Preoperative	Postoperative	Positive	Negative	Overall	
Marzullo et al[50]	14	35–64 (54)	5–10	39	—	100	87	95	~3
Cigarroa et al[51]	49	38–73 (59)	5–20	32	—	82	86	84	≥1
Charney et al[52]	17	(63)	5–10	—	—	92	74	81	0.25
La Canna et al[53]	33	31–68 (56)	5–10	34	47	86	86	86	3
deFilippi et al[54]	23	42–75 (63)	5–20	38	47	87	93	89	2–3
Perrone-Filardi et al[55]	18	45–70 (59)	5–10	36*	42*	91	82	87	1
Arnese et al[56]	38	36–73 (59)	5–10	<40	—	85	93	91	3
Senior et al[57]	22	35–81 (61)	5–10	26	38	92	73	86	~2
Afridi et al[58]	27	(60)	2.5–40	32	—	72†	87‡	84	1.5–2
Afridi, Muin, and Grayburn[59]	41	(60)	5–20	32	—	83–100	86–100	92–93	1
Vanoverschelde et al[60]	73	35–74 (59)	5–40	36	49	73*	87*	83	5.5
Elhendy et al[61]	40	(59)	5–40	—	—	68	92	86	3
Qureshi et al[62]	34	(61)	2.5–40	39	43	72†	92‡	89†	≥1.5
Naqueh et al[63]	18	(57)	2.5–40	38	—	70†	93‡	77†	≥1.5
Cornel et al[64]	61	43–77 (61)	5–40	32	37	63	95	84	3
Cornel et al[64]	61	43–77 (61)	5–40	32	42	75	92	86	14

	Range	Total	Mean Age Range	Dose Range	Increase in Mean EF	Range of Predictive Accuracy			Range of Mean Follow-up
						Positive	Negative	Overall	
Total	1993–1998	508	54–63	2.5–40	4–13%	63–100	73–100	77–95	0.25–14
15									

* Subgroup analysis of patients with severely reduced ejection fraction.
† Only segments with biphasic contractile response.
‡ Only segments without contractile response.

FDG PET in akinetic or dyskinetic LV segments.[166] Also, the mean FDG uptake is shown to be significantly higher in segments with than without contractile reserve (68% ± 11% versus 45% ± 9%; $p < 0.001$).[166] However, a proportion (19%) of segments considered viable by FDG PET will not show recruitable contractile reserve by low-dose dobutamine.[166] Rarely, a segment with contractile reserve by dobutamine will show <50% (mean, 46% ± 3%) FDG uptake.[166] When both blood flow and glucose uptake is assessed by PET, the presence of contractile response to dobutamine correlates best with a pattern of perfusion-metabolism mismatch.[171] In a comparative study, the diagnostic accuracy of transesophageal DSE (10 μg/kg per minute) and FDG PET for prediction of functional recovery after revascularization were similar (90% versus 86%).[167]

Certain Considerations Regarding the Use of Dobutamine Stress Echocardiogram for Assessment of Myocardial Viability

Technical Limitations

The quality of the echocardiographic images remains suboptimal in a small percentage of patients undergoing DSE for assessment of myocardial viability. However, recent technical advances in the field of echocardiography have significantly reduced the number

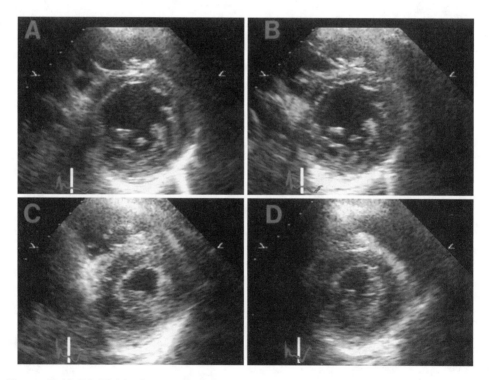

Figure 2. (**A–D**) Digitized, parasternal short-axis views at midleft ventricular (LV) cavity level shown in quad screen format at various stages of DSE. The contractile response of this normal ventricle (**A**) to dobutamine infusion is visualized easily at low (**B**) and high (**C**) doses of dobutamine and early after cessation of dobutamine infusion (**D**).

Table 4

Certain Features of Commercially Available (*) and Investigational
Echocardiographic Contrast Agents

I. First-generation (air containing) microspheres
  A. Human albumin shell
    Albunex* (Molecular Biosystems, Inc)
    Quantison (Andaris Limited)
    Quantison Depot (Andaris Limited)
  B. Cyanacrylate polymer shell
    SHU 563A (Sonovist) [Schering]
  C. Palmitic acid stabilized shell
    Levovist (Schering)
II. Second-generation (perfluorocarbon containing) microspheres
  A. Human albumin shell
    Optison (FS069)* [Molecular Biosystems, Inc]
  B. Dextrose-albumin shell
    Perfluorocarbon exposed sonicated dextrose albumin (PESDA)
  C. Phospholipid shell
    MRX-115 (ImaRx Pharmaceutical Corp.)
    Imagent (AF0150) [Alliance Pharmaceutical Corp]
  D. Surfactant stabilized shell
    Echogen (Sonus Pharmaceuticals, Inc)
    NC100100 (Nycomed Inc)

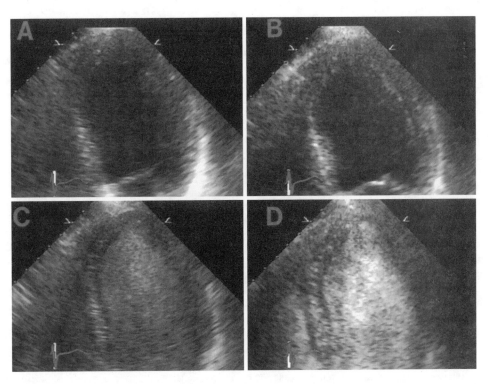

Figure 3. Apical two-dimensional (2-D) echocardiographic view of the left ventricle during (**A**) fundamental imaging, (**B**) second harmonic imaging, and (**C** and **D**) fundamental (**C**) and second harmonic (**D**) imaging following intravenous (IV) injection of contrast (Optison). Endocardial borders are better delineated during second harmonic imaging, without (**B**) and with (**D**) contrast enhancement.

of patients with technically difficult studies.[172–174] The introduction of higher frequency, broadband transducers in combination with new imaging modalities such as harmonic imaging have improved LV endocardial border delineation and assessment of wall motion abnormality.[78–80,172,173] This has been facilitated further by digital acquisition, and side-by-side display of images obtained at various stages of DSE (Fig. 2). Also, recent development of second-generation echocardiographic contrast agents, capable of consistent LV cavity opacification following intravenous (IV) administration, has improved the assessment of wall motion during DSE, especially in combination with second harmonic imaging (Table 4, Fig. 3).[86,175]

Significance of Myocyte Membrane Integrity

As mentioned above, a small proportion of asynergic LV segments without contractile response to dobutamine recover function following revascularization.[50–64] The underlying pathophysiological mechanism for lack of contractile reserve in such viable segments has not been elucidated fully. Among proposed mechanisms are: (1) severe limitation of coronary flow reserve, resulting in ischemia at the lowest dose of dobutamine,[14] and (2) significant loss of contractile elements despite preservation of cell membrane integrity.[164] Thus, some dobutamine-unresponsive segments with potential for functional recovery show uptake of perfusion tracers by radionuclide studies.[50,52,56,57,62,63] In fact, addition of perfusion to DSE data has been shown to improve the predictive accuracy of DSE.[57,63,71] In a study of 45 patients with chronic ischemic cardiomyopathy, the sensitivity of DSE for detection of recoverable myocardium was improved with addition of thallium single photon emission computed tomography (SPECT) perfusion data (87% versus 97%). The improved sensitivity of the combined data occurred in the absence of a significant change in specificity (82% versus 78%).[57]

Significance of Microvascular Integrity

Several investigators have studied the value of MCE in combination with DSE for assessment of myocardial viability.[71,72] Such studies initially were performed using intra-arterial injection of microbubbles, because the then-available air containing agents were unable to cross the pulmonary circulation in sufficient concentrations to produce myocardial enhancement following IV injection (Fig. 4).[63,71,72] This was especially true in patients with low cardiac output, pulmonary hypertension, or those with significant tricuspid valve regurgitation, conditions frequently present in chronic ischemic heart disease. An early study combining MCE and DSE included 24 patients with recent acute myocardial infarction and used intracoronary sonicated ioxaglate and low-dose (5–10 μg/kg per minute) dobutamine.[71] In this study, DSE correctly predicted the outcome of 112 of 135 asynergic segments (83%) following revascularization. Of the remaining 23 segments, 12 recovered function despite lack of contractile response to low-dose dobutamine. All 12 segments showed preserved microvascular integrity by MCE.[71] No functional recovery was noted in any of the 43 segments without contrast enhancement or contractile reserve. In another study, Nagueh et al[63] reported on 18 patients (mean age, 57 years) with ischemic cardiomyopathy (mean LVEF, 38%) who underwent preoperative DSE, intracoronary MCE with Albunex, and rest-redistribution thallium SPECT for evaluation of myocardial viability. Presence of microvascular integrity by MCE, cell membrane integrity by thallium, or any contractile reserve by DSE were all sensitive predictors of functional recovery (sensitivity, 89%–91%). However, the specificity of these methods ranged from 43% to 66% when used separately. A combination of biphasic contractile response to dobutamine and presence of microvascular integrity by MCE in asynergic

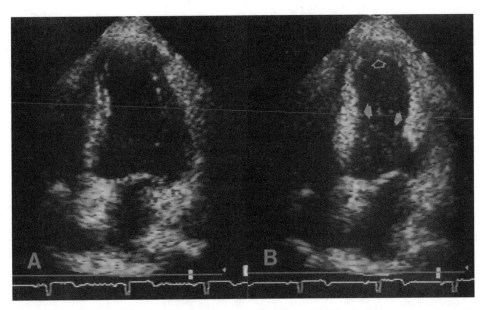

Figure 4. Second harmonic, apical 2-D echocardiographic images of the left ventricle before (**A**) and after (**B**) left main coronary injection of contrast (Albunex) in a patient with recent acute myocardial infarction. Uniform myocardial contrast enhancement is shown in ventricular septum and lateral wall (solid arrows). Minimal, patchy contrast enhancement is present in the infarct region (open arrows).

segments was the most accurate predictor of functional recovery (sensitivity, 97%; specificity, 64%).[63]

Successful myocardial contrast enhancement following IV injection of echocardiographic contrast agents has become possible with the advent of second-generation microbubbles.[93,110,175–179] Unlike their predecessors, these second-generation agents contain high-molecular-weight gases, such as perfluorocarbon, which do not diffuse out of the microbubbles as readily as air.[180] In addition, the microsphere shell is altered to allow further stabilization and maintenance of backscattering properties within the circulation (Table 4). An early attempt to assess myocardial perfusion following IV (internal jugular vein) injection of a second-generation contrast agent (FS-069) involved MCE before and after left anterior descending (LAD) coronary artery occlusion in eight anesthetized dogs.[181] Using continuous fundamental imaging, the contrast defect observed during coronary artery occlusion correlated directly ($r = 0.88$) with the area of wall motion abnormality on two-dimensional (2-D) echocardiography.[181] However, other animal studies demonstrated that the degree of myocardial enhancement following IV injection of a contrast agent often was small and obscured frequently by excessive LV cavity contrast and attenuation during continuous fundamental imaging.[180] This appeared to result, at least in part, from rapid destruction of the slow-moving microbubbles within the myocardial capillary bed by continuous exposure to ultrasonic energy. Consequently, Porter and Xie[182] used intermittent rather than continuous imaging for the assessment of myocardial perfusion following IV-injected contrast in 14 dogs. Intermittent (transient response) imaging consisted of either brief (10–60 seconds) cessation of image acquisition or ECG gated (triggered) imaging.[182] Significant improvement in the degree of myocardial contrast enhancement was noted with application of both techniques of intermittent imaging. In addition, second harmonic imaging further enhanced the myocardial contrast effect when combined with intermittent imaging. In another animal study, Firschke et al assessed the ability of MCE to define risk area and infarct area before and after LAD coronary artery occlusion in 12 dogs.[110] Direct comparison of MCE during continuous and triggered imaging in both fundamental and second harmonic imaging modalities also was made. The myocardial contrast defect during LAD occlusion was best delineated with intermittent harmonic imaging and correlated well with risk area ($r = 0.89$) and infarct area ($r = 0.96$).[110]

Intermittent harmonic imaging in conjunction with IV-injected second-generation contrast agents also has made possible the assessment of microvascular integrity in humans. An early study of 15 normal individuals showed myocardial contrast enhancement in 7/15 (47%) of patients during continuous imaging and in 14/15 (93%) of patients during intermittent harmonic imaging.[93] In another study of 30 patients, segmental MCE scores correlated well with tehnetium-99m ([99mTc]) Sestamibi (MIBI) SPECT (MIBI) perfusion scores obtained during dipyridamole stress testing.[96] Currently, there are no published reports of the simultaneous use of DSE and MCE using IV-injected contrast agents for evaluation of myocardial viability in patients with chronic CAD. However, such studies now appear feasible, especially with the developing techniques of contrast administration (continuous infusion),[178,183,184] optimization of system settings,[93,110,175,182,183,184] and new imaging modalities such as harmonic power Doppler contrast cardiography (Fig.5).[185–187] Preliminary studies of the use of harmonic power Doppler cardiography has shown good correlation with MIBI SPECT imaging at rest.[187]

Most human studies evaluating the role of MCE in assessment of myocardial viability have depended on visual estimation of the degree of myocardial contrast enhancement.[63,65,69–71] Methods of quantification of MCE data are developing rapidly and have allowed for the assessment of regional MBF, flow reserve, and blood vol-

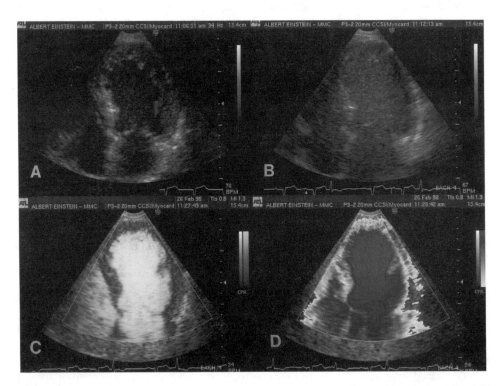

Figure 5. Apical 2-D echocardiographic views of the heart before (**A** and **B**) and after (**C** and **D**) imaging in power Doppler mode. The LV endocardial border is well visualized with power Doppler imaging (**C** and **D**). Myocardial contrast enhancement is well visualized in D, with delineation of the papillary muscle and trabeculae cornae.

ume.[92,95,97–106,178,183,184,188,189] These techniques also have provided a noninvasive tool for the diagnosis of epicardial CAD in humans that correlates well with nuclear imaging techniques.[106,189] Although significant advances have been made in understanding the pathophysiological and technical aspects of quantitative MCE, a reliable, reproducible, noninvasive method is not available yet. Further advances in this field await the development of new echocardiographic contrast agents and quantitative methods of assessment of regional blood flow during harmonic power Doppler imaging. The latter should soon allow detection of very small microvessels within the myocardium.[190,191]

Prognostic Value of Dobutamine Stress Echocardiogram in Patients with Chronic Coronary Artery Disease

The clinical utility of the methods used for detection of myocardial viability ultimately would depend on their ability to alter the therapeutic approach to and the outcome of patients with ischemic cardiomyopathy. Several studies have evaluated the prognostic significance of contractile reserve in patients with CAD.[77,192–194] The absence of contractile reserve to low-dose dobutamine in patients with CAD and severe symptomatic LV systolic dysfunction is a potent predictor of 3-year mortality.[193] However, the presence of recruitable contractile reserve and ischemia in patients with moderate to severe LV dysfunction predicts a relatively high risk of cardiac events[77,192] and mortality[77] in those treated medically. In a recent multicenter trial, the presence of viability by DSE in patients with ischemic cardiomyopathy (mean LVEF <35%) was associated with a reduced 16-month mortality in surgically treated patients compared with medically treated patients (3% versus 15%; $p < 0.01$).[194] In the absence of contractile reserve mortality was high irrespective of the therapeutic strategy (22% with medical treatment versus 28% with surgical treatment; $p =$ NS).[194]

Safety of DSE in Patients with Reduced Left Ventricular Systolic Function

Minor symptoms such as headache, anxiety, nausea, or tremor frequently occur during DSE and generally are well tolerated and of no consequence.[195] Some degree of systemic hypotension is seen in up to one-third of patients during DSE; however, symptomatic hypotension requiring discontinuation of the test is unusual.[196] Ventricular arrhythmias, mainly in the form of PVCs occur in 3.6%–6.0% of patients undergoing DSE, although life-threatening arrhythmias are extremely rare.[197–199] These arrhythmias occur more frequently in patients with recent myocardial infarction and those with frequent and repetitive ventricular arrhythmias during 24-hour Holter monitoring or during exercise stress testing.[199] Regional wall motion abnormalities induced by dobutamine may persist for as long as 25 minutes following termination of the test in some patients with severe multivessel CAD.[200] Only rare cases of acute myocardial infarction or prolonged myocardial ischemia have been reported in patients during DSE despite discontinuation of antianginal medications in most patients.[198] A recent report on 3011 studies in 2817 patients has confirmed the overall safety of DSE.[201] This is supported further by the absence of significant side effects in the studies specifically evaluating myocardial viability[50–64] or diagnosis of CAD in patients with severely reduced LVEF[202] by DSE.

Assessment of Contractile Reserve by Postextrasystolic Potentiation

Pharmacologic agents other than dobutamine (epinephrine, nitrates, dipyridimole, and nisoldipine) or nonpharmacologic stimuli such as ventricular extrasystole also have been used to assess contractile reserve in asynergic myocardium.[41–48,203,204] Normal and viable asynergic myocardium respond to appropriately timed PVCs by augmentation of contractility in the postextrasystolic beat.[42–48] However, irreversibly damaged myocardium does not show postextrasystolic potentiation (PESP) of contractility.[43,46,47] Therefore, both spontaneous and induced PVCs have been used to evaluate myocardial viability in asynergic myocardium.[42–48] In a study of 31 patients with CAD, Popio et al[46] showed recovery of function following revascularization in 11 of 12 (92%) asynergic segments with contractile reserve and 0 of 4 asynergic segments without contractile reserve as assessed by PESP. Furthermore, the degree of postoperative improvement in regional wall motion correlated directly with preoperative contractile reserve ($r = 0.66$; $p < 0.001$).[46] In another study, contractile reserve by PESP in asynergic myocardium strongly predicted improvement in global LV function after revascularization.[43] In this study, LVEF improved in 14 of 15 patients with and only 3 of 9 patients without contractile reserve.[43] Although most studies have used invasive means of PESP evaluation, a noninvasive technique of controlled PVC induction during M-mode echocardiography has been described.[205,206] In addition to premature ventricular depolarization, atrial extrasystole also has been shown to elicit PESP in patients with chronic CAD.[49] In a recent study of 60 patients, PESP induced by atrial extrasystole via a transesophageal lead was shown to be more sensitive than low-dose (5–10 μg/kg per minute) DSE (92% versus 86%; $p = 0.009$) in predicting recovery of function in asynergic myocardial segments.[49] We have observed a better concordance between microvascular integrity (using intracoronary Albunex) and PESP than contractile reserve by dobutamine (5–20 μg/kg per minute).[207,208] There is a strong correlation between the presence of PESP and microvascular integrity in asynergic myocardium.[207,208]

Summary

Now it is clear that a substantial proportion of asynergic myocardial segments in patients with chronic ischemic cardiomyopathy is comprised of viable tissue, with a potential for functional recovery following revascularization. Detection of viable myocardium in patients with chronic CAD can favorably affect the choice of therapy as well as the prognosis of such patients. DSE is a safe and reliable noninvasive method for detection of myocardial viability. Recent technological advances and development of new echocardiographic contrast agents have made significant contributions to the evaluation and understanding of myocardial viability in chronic CAD.

References

1. Raftery EB, Banks DC, Oram S. Occlusive disease of the coronary arteries presenting as primary congestive cardiomyopathy. *Lancet* 1969;29:1147.
2. Burch GE, Giles TD, Cololough HL. Ischemic cardiomyopathy. *Am Heart J* 1970;79:291.
3. Schuster EH, Bulkley BH. Ischemic cardiomyopathy: A clinicopathologic study of fourteen patients. *Am Heart J* 1980;100:506–512.
4. Rahimtoola SH. Coronary bypass surgery for chronic angina-1981. A perspective. *Circulation* 1982;65:225–241.

5. Braunwald E, Rutherford JD. Reversible ischemic left ventricular dysfunction: Evidence for the "hibernating myocardium." *J Am Coll Cardiol* 1986;8:1467–1470.

6. Shearn DL, Brent BN. Coronary artery bypass surgery in patients with left ventricular dysfunction. *Am J Med* 1986;80:405–411.

7. Kron IL, Flanagan TL, Blackbourne LH, et al. Coronary revascularization rather than cardiac transplantation for chronic ischemic cardiomyopathy. *Ann Surg* 1989;210:348–354.

8. Louie HW, Laks H, Milgalter E, et al. Ischemic cardiomyopathy: criteria for coronary revascularization and cardiac transplantation. *Circulation* 1991;84(suppl III):III290–III295.

9. Elefteriades JA, Tolis G, Levi E, et al. Coronary artery bypass grafting in severe left ventricular dysfunction: Excellent survival with improved ejection fraction and functional state. *J Am Coll Cardiol* 1993;22:1411–1417.

10. Dreyfus GD, Duboc D, Blasco A, et al. Myocardial viability assessment in ischemic cardiomyopathy: Benefits of coronary revascularization. *Ann Thorac Surg* 1994;57:1402–1408.

11. Elefteraides JA, Morales DLS, Gradel C, et al. Results of coronary artery bypass grafting by a single surgeon in patients with left ventricular ejection fractions ≤30%. *Am J Cardiol* 1997; 79:1573–1578.

12. Brundage BH, Massie BM, Botvinick EH. Improved regional ventricular function after successful surgical revascularization. *J Am Coll Cardiol* 1984;3:902–908.

13. Rahimtoola SH. The hibernating myocardium. *Am Heart J* 1989;117:211–221.

14. Rahimtoola SH. Hibernating myocardium has reduced blood flow at rest that increases with low-dose dobutamine. *Circulation* 1996;94:3055–3061.

15. Braunwald E, Kloner RA. The stunned myocardium: Prolonged, postischemic ventricular dysfunction. *Circulation* 1982;66:1146–1149.

16. Bolli R. Myocardial stunning in man. *Circulation* 1992;86:1671–1691.

17. Disizian V, Rocco TP, Freedman NMT, et al. Enhanced detection of ischemic but viable myocardium by the reinjection of thallium after stress-redistribution imaging. *N Engl J Med* 1990;323:141–146.

18. Ohtani H, Tamaki N, Yonekura Y, et al. Value of thallium-201 reinjection after delayed SPECT Imaging for predicting reversible ischemia after coronary artery bypass grafting. *Am J Cardiol* 1990;66:394–399.

19. Takeishi Y, Tono-oka I, Kubota I, et al. Functional recovery of hibernating myocardium after coronary artery bypass surgery: Does it coincide with improvement in perfusion? *Am Heart J* 1991;122:665–670.

20. Haque T, Furukawa T, Takahashi M, et al. Identification of hibernating myocardium by dobutamine stress echocardiography: Comparison with thallium-201 reinjection imaging. *Am Heart J* 1995;130:553–563.

21. Pace L, Marzullo P, Nicolai E, et al. Reverse redistribution in resting thallium-201 myocardial scintigraphy in chronic coronary artery disease: An index of myocardial viability. *J Nucl Med* 1995;36:1968–1973.

22. Scherrer-Crosbie M, Rosso J, Monin J-L, et al. Usefulness of redistribution images in viability detection after acute myocardial infarction. *Am J Cardiol* 1996;77:922–926.

23. Pagley PR, Beller GA, Watson DD, et al. Improved outcome after coronary artery bypass surgery in patients with ischemic cardiomyopathy and residual myocardial viability. *Circulation* 1997;96:793–800.

24. Tillisch J, Brunken R, Marshall R, et al. Reversibility of cardiac wall-motion abnormalities predicted by positron tomography. *N Engl J Med* 1986;314:884–888.

25. Tamaki N, Yonekura Y, Yamashita K, et al. Positron emission tomography using fluorine-18 deoxyglucose in evaluation of coronary artery bypass grafting. *Am J Cardiol* 1989;64:860–865.

26. Tamaki N, Ohtani H, Yamashita K, et al. Metabolic activity in areas of new fill-in after thallium-201 reinjection: Comparison with positron emission tomography using fluorine-18-deoxyglucose. *J Nucl Med* 1991;32:673–678.

27. Nienaber CA, Brunkren RC, Sherman CT, et al. Metabolic and functional recovery of ischemic human myocardium after coronary angioplasty. *J Am Coll Cardiol* 1991;18:966–978.

28. Gropler RJ, Geltman EM, Sampathkumaran K, et al. Functional recovery after coronary revascularization for chronic coronary artery disease is dependent on maintenance of oxidative metabolism. *J Am Coll Cardiol* 1992;20:569–577.

29. Knuuti MJ, Nuutila P, Ruotsalainen U, et al. The value of quantitative analysis of glucose utilization in detection of myocardial viability by PET. *J Nucl Med* 1993;34:2068–2075.

30. vom Dahl J, Eitzman DT, Al-Aouar ZR, et al. Relation of regional function, perfusion, and metabolism in patients with advanced coronary artery disease undergoing surgical revascularization. *Circulation* 1994;90:2356–2366.

31. Di Carli MF, Davidson M, Little R, et al. Value of metabolic imaging with positron emission tomography for evaluating prognosis in patients with coronary artery disease and left ventricular dysfunction. *Am J Cardiol* 1994;73:527–533.

32. Gewirtz H, Fischman AJ, Abraham S, et al. Positron emission tomographic measurements of absolute regional myocardial blood flow permits identification of nonviable myocardium in patients with chronic myocardial infarction. *J Am Coll Cardiol* 1994;23:851–859.

33. Soufer R, Dey HM, Ng CK, et al. Comparison of sestamibi single photon emission computed tomography with positron emission tomography for estimating left ventricular myocardial viability. *Am J Cardiol*.1995;75:1214–1219.

34. Di Carli MF, Asgaarzadie F, Schelbert HR, et al. Quantitative relation between myocardial viability and improvement in heart failure symptoms after revascularization in patients with ischemic cardiomyopathy. *Circulation* 1995;92:3436–3444.

35. Bax JJ, Cornel JH, Visser FC, et al. Prediction of recovery of myocardial dysfunction after revascularization: Comparison of fluorine-18 fluorodeoxyglucose/thallium-201 SPECT, thallium-201 stress-reinjection SPECT and dobutamine echocardiography. *J Am Coll Cardiol* 1996;28:558–564.

36. Maki M, Luotolahti M, Nuutila P, et al. Glucose uptake in the chronically dysfunctional but viable myocardium. *Circulation* 1996;93:1658–1666.

37. vom Dahl J, Altehoefer C, Sheehan FH, et al. Recovery of regional left ventricular dysfunction after coronary revascularization. Impact of myocardial viability assessed by nuclear imaging and vessel patency at follow-up angioplasty. *J Am Coll Cardiol* 1996;28:948–958.

38. Beanlands RS, DeKemp R, Scheffel A, et al. Can nitrogen-13 ammonia kinetic modeling define myocardial viability independent of fluorine-18 fluorodeoxyglucose? *J Am Coll Cardiol* 1997;29:537–543.

39. Bax JJ, Cornel JH, Visser FC, et al. Prediction of improvement of contractile function in patients with ischemic ventricular dysfunction after revascularization by fluorine-18 fluorodeoxyglucose single-photon emission tomography. *J Am Coll Cardiol* 1997;30:377–383.

40. Bax JJ, Cornel JH, Visser FC, et al. F18-fluorodeoxyglucose single-photon emission computed tomography predicts functional outcome of dyssynergic myocardium after surgical revascularization. *J Nucl Cardiol* 1997;4:302–308.

41. Helfant RH, Pine R, Meister SG, et al. Nitroglycerin to unmask reversible asynergy. Correlation with post coronary bypass ventriculography. *Circulation* 2974;50:108–113.

42. Dyke SH, Cohn PF, Gorlin R, et al. Detection of residual myocardial function in coronary artery disease using post-extra systolic potentiation. *Circulation* 1974;50:694–699.

43. Hamby RI, Aintablian A, Wisoff G, et al. Response of the left ventricle in coronary artery disease to postextrasystolic potentiation. *Circulation* 1975;51:428–435.

44. Cohn PF, Gorlin R, Herman MV, et al. Relation between contractile reserve and prognosis in patients with coronary artery disease and a depressed ejection fraction. *Circulation* 1975;51:414–420.

45. Cohn LH, Collins JJ Jr, Cohn PF. Use of the augmented ejection fraction to select patients with left ventricular dysfunction for coronary revascularization. *J Thorac Cardiovasc Surg* 1976;72:835–840.

46. Popio KA, Gorlin R, Bechtel D, et al. Postextrasystolic potentiation as a predictor of potential myocardial viability: Preoperative analyses compared with studies after coronary bypass surgery. *Am J Cardiol* 1977;39:944–953.

47. Nesto RW, Cohn LH, Collins JJ, et al. Inotropic contractile reserve: A useful predictor of increased 5 year survival and improved postoperative left ventricular function in patients with coronary artery disease and reduced ejection fraction. *Am J Cardiol* 1982;50:39–44.

48. Cooper MW, Lutherer LO, Stanton MW, et al. Postextrasystolic potentiation: Regional wall motion before and after revascularization. *Am Heart J* 1985;111:334–339.

49. Scognamiglio R, Fasoli G, Casarotto D, et al. Postextrasystolic potentiation and dobutamine echocardiography in predicting recovery of myocardial function after coronary bypass revascularization. *Circulation* 1997;96:816–820.

50. Marzullo P, Parodi O, Reisenhofer B, et al. Value of rest Thallium-201/Technetium-99m Sestamibi scans and dobutamine echocardiography for detecting myocardial viability. *Am J Cardiol* 1993;71:166–172.

51. Cigarroa CG, deFilippi CR, Brickner E, et al. Dobutamine stress echocardiography identifies hibernating myocardium and predicts recovery of left ventricular function after coronary revascularization. *Circulation* 1993;88:430–436.

52. Charney R, Schwinger ME, Chun J, et al. Dobutamine echocardiography and rest-redistribution thallium-201 scintigraphy predicts recovery of hibernating myocardium after coronary revascularization. *Am Heart J* 1994;128:864–869.

53. La Canna GL, Alfieri O, Giubbini R, et al. Echocardiography during infusion of dobutamine for identification of reversible dysfunction in patients with chronic coronary artery disease. *J Am Coll Cardiol* 1994;23:617–626.

54. deFilippi CR, Willett DL, Irani WN, et al. Comparison of myocardial contrast echocardiography and low dose dobutamine stress echocardiography in predicting recovery of left ventricular function fter coronary revascularization in chronic ischemic heart disease. *Circulation* 1995;92:2863–2868.

55. Perrone-Filardi P, Pace L, Prastaro M, et al. Dobutamine echocardiography predicts improvement of hypoperfused dysfunctional myocardium after revascularization in patients with coronary artery disease. *Circulation* 1995;91:2556–2565.

56. Arnese M, Cornel JH, Salustri A, et al. Prediction of improvement of regional left ventricular function after surgical revascularization: A comparison of low dose dobutamine with ^{201}Tl single-photon emission computed tomography. *Circulation* 1995;91:2748–2752.

57. Senior R, Glenville B, Basu S, et al. Dobutamine echocardiography and thallium-201 imaging predict functional improvement after revascularization in severe ischemic left ventricular dysfunction. *Br Heart J* 1995;74:358–364.

58. Afridi I, Kleiman NS, Raizner AE, et al. Dobutamine echocardiography in myocardial hibernation. Optimal dose and accuracy in predicting recovery of ventricular function after coronary angioplasty. *Circulation* 1995;91:663–670.

59. Afridi I, Main ML, Grayburn PA. Accuracy of dobutamine echocardiography for detection of myocardial viability in patients with an occluded left anterior descending coronary artery. *J Am Coll Cardiol* 1996;28:455–459.

60. Vanoverschelde J-LJ, D'Hondt A, Marwick T, et al. Head-to-head comparison of exercise-redistribution-reinjection thallium single-photon emission computed tomography and low dose dobutamine echocardiography for prediction of reversibility of chronic ventricular ischemic dysfunction. *J Am Coll Cardiol* 1996;28:432–442.

61. Elhendy A, Cornel JH, Roelandt JRTC, et al. Impact of severity of coronary artery stenosis and the collateral circulation on the functional outcome of dysynergic myocardium after revascularization in patients with healed myocardial infarction and chronic left ventricular dysfunction. *Am J Cardiol* 1997;79:883–888.

62. Qureshi U, Nagueh SF, Afridi I, et al. Dobutamine echocardiography and quantitative rest-redistribution ^{201}Tl tomography in myocardial hibernation: Relation of contractile reserve to ^{201}Tl uptake and comparative prediction of recovery of function. *Circulation* 1997;95:626–635.

63. Nagueh, SF, Vaduganathan P, Ali N, et al. Identification of hibernating myocardium: Comparative accuracy of myocardial contrast echocardiography, rest-redistribution Thallium-201 tomography and dobutamine echocardiography. *J Am Coll Cardiol* 1997;29:985–993.

64. Cornel JH, Bax JJ, Elhendy A, et al. Biphasic response to dobutamine predicts improvement of global left ventricular function after surgical revascularization in patients with stable coronary artery disease: Implications of time course of recovery on diagnostic accuracy. *J Am Coll Cardiol* 1998;31:1002–1010.

65. Sabia PJ, Powers ER, Ragosta M, et al. An association between collateral blood flow and myocardial viability in patients with recent myocardial infarction. *N Engl J Med* 1992;327:1825–1831.

66. Ito H, Tomooka T, Sakai N, et al. Lack of myocardial perfusion immediately after successful thrombolysis: A predictor of poor recovery of left ventricular function in anterior myocardial infarction. *Circulation* 1992;85:1699–1705.

67. Hirata N, Nakano S, Taniguchi K, et al. Assessment of regional and transmural myocardial perfusion by means of intraoperative myocardial contrast echocardiography during coronary artery bypass grafting. *J Thorac Cardiovasc Surg* 1992;104:1158–1166.

68. Hirata N, Shimazaki Y, Nakano S, et al. Evaluation of regional myocardial perfusion in areas of old myocardial infarction after revascularization by means of intraoperative myocardial contrast echocardiography. *J Thorac Cardiovasc Surg* 1994;108:1119–1124.

69. Ragosta M, Camarano G, Kaul S, et al. Microvascular integrity indicates myocellular viability in patients with recent myocardial infarction. New insights using myocardial contrast echocardiography. *Circulation* 1994;89:2562–2569.

70. Camarano G, Ragosta M, Gimple LW, et al. Identification of viable myocardium with contrast echocardiography in patients with poor left ventricular systolic function caused by recent or remote myocardial infarction. *Am J Cardiol* 1995;75:215–219.

71. Iliceto S, Galiuto L, Marchese A, et al. Analysis of microvascular integrity, contractile reserve, and myocardial viability after acute myocardial infarction by dobutamine echocardiography and myocardial contrast echocardiography. *Am J Cardiol* 1996;77:441–445.

72. Bolognese L, Antoniucci D, Rovai D, et al. Myocardial contrast echocardiography versus dobutamine echocardiography for predicting functional recovery after acute myocardial infarction treated with primary coronary angioplasty. *J Am Coll Cardiol* 1996;28:1677–1683.

73. Nanto S, Masuyama T, Lim Y-J, et al. Demonstration of functional border zone with myocardial contrast echocardiography in human hearts: Simultaneous analysis of myocardial perfusion and wall motion abnormalities. *Circulation* 1993;88:447–453.

74. Eitzman D, Al-Aouar Z, Kanter HL, et al. Clinical outcome of patients with advanced coronary artery disease after viability studies with positron emission tomography. *J Am Coll Cardiol* 1992;20:559–565.

75. Lee KS, Marwick TH, Cook SA, et al. Prognosis of patient with left ventricular dysfunction, with and without viable myocardium after myocardial infarction: Relative efficacy of medical therapy and revascularization. *Circulation* 1994;90:2687–2694.

76. Haas F, Haehnel CJ, Picker W, et al. Preoperative positron emission tomographic viability assessment and perioperative and postoperative risk in patients with advanced ischemic heart disease. *J Am Coll Cardiol* 1997;30:1693–1700.

77. Anselmi M, Golia G, Cicoira M, et al. Prognostic value of detection of myocardial viability using low-dose dobutamine echocardiography in infarcted patients. *Am J Cardiol* 1998;81:21G–28G.

78. Thomas JD, Rubin DN. Tissue harmonic imaging: Why does it work? *J Am Soc Echocardiogr* 1998;11:803–808.

79. Rubin DN, Yazbek DH, Odabashian J, et al. Why does tissue harmonic imaging improve image quality: A quantitative examination demonstrating side-lobe suppression. *J Am Coll Cardiol* 1998;31:127A. Abstract.

80. Kasprzak JD, Paellinck B, Vletter WB, et al. Tissue harmonic imaging enables improved detection of left ventricular endocardial border comparable and complementary to contrast blood pool enhancement. *J Am Coll Cardiol* 1998;31:127A. Abstract.

81. Goldman M, Dent J, Buckley S, et al. Is power motion imaging superior to standard 2 dimensional echocardiography for myocardial visualization? *J Am Soc Echocardiogr* 1997;10:397.

82. Main ML, Asher CR, Odabaashian JA, et al. A comparison of frequency conversion technology, power motion imaging, and intravenous Albunex for improved endocardial border resolution in patients with technically difficult echocardiograms. *J Am Coll Cardiol* 1998;31:127A. Abstract.

83. Ten Cate FJ, Cornel JH, Widimsky P, et al. Clinical experience with Albunex: A standard echocontrast agent for intravenous and intracoronary use. *Am J Card Imaging* 1991;5:217–223.

84. Geny B, Mettauer B, Muan B, et al. Safety and efficacy of a new transpulmonary echo contrast agent in echocardiographic studies in patients. *J Am Coll Cardiol* 1993;22:1193–1198.

85. Crouse LJ, Cheirif J, Hanly DE, et al. Opacification and border delineation improvement in patients with suboptimal endocardial border definition in routine echocardiography: Results of the phase III Albunex multicenter trial. *J Am Coll Cardiol* 1993;22:1494–1500.

86. Porter TR, Xie F, Kricsfeld A, et al. Improved endocardial border resolution during dobutamine stress echocardiography with intravenous sonicated dextrose albumin. *J Am Coll Cardiol* 1994;23:1440–1443.

87. Porter TR, Xie F, Anderson JR, et al. Multifold sonicated dilutions of albumin with fifty percent dextrose improve left ventricular contrast videointensity after intravenous injection in human beings. *J Am Soc Echocardiogr* 1994;7:465–471.

88. Skyba DM, Camarano G, Goodman NC, et al. Hemodynamic characteristics, myocardial kinetics and microvascular rheology of FS-069, a second-generation echocardiographic contrast agent capable of producing myocardial opacification from a venous injection. *J Am Coll Cardiol* 1996;28:1292–1300.

89. Lindner JR, Dent JM, Moos SP, et al. Enhancement of left ventricular cavity opacification by harmonic imaging after venous injection of Albunex. *Am J Cardiol* 1997;79:1657–1662.

90. Klein AL, Bailey AS, Moura A, et al. Reliability of echocardiographic measurements of myocardial perfusion using commercially produced sonicated serum albumin (Albunex). *J Am Coll Cardiol* 1993;22:1983–1993.

91. Agati L, Voci P, Bilotta F, et al. Influence of residual perfusion within the infarct zone on the natural history of left ventricular dysfunction after acute myocardial infarction: A myocardial contrast echocardiographic study. *J Am Coll Cardiol* 1994;24:336–342.

92. Skyba DM, Jayaweera AR, Goodman NC, et al. Quantification of myocardial perfusion with myocardial contrast echocardiography during left atrial injection of contrast. Implications for venous injection. *Circulation* 1994;90:1513–1521.

93. Porter TR, Xie F, Kricsfeld D, et al. Improved myocardial contrast with second harmonic transient ultrasound response imaging in humans using intravenous perfluorcarbon-exposed sonicated dextrose albumin. *J Am Coll Cardiol* 1996;27:1497–1501.

94. Meza MF, Mobarek S, Sonnemaker R, et al. Myocardial contrast echocardiography in human beings: Correlation of resting perfusion defects to sestamibi single photon emission computed tomography. *Am Heart J* 1996;132:528–535.

95. Firschke C, Lindner JR, Goodman NC, et al. Myocardial contrast echocardiography in acute myocardial infarction using aortic root injections of microbubbles in conjunction with harmonic imaging: Potential application in the cardiac catheterization laboratory. *J Am Coll Cardiol* 1997;29:207–216.

96. Kaul S, Senior R, Dittrich H, et al. Detection of coronary artery disease with myocardial contrast echocardiography. Comparison with ^{99m}Tc-Sestamibi single photon emission computed tomography. *Circulation* 1997;96:785–792.

97. Kaul S. A glimpse of the coronary microcirculation with myocardial contrast echocardiography. *J Invest Med* 1995;43:345–360.

98. Kaul S. Assessment of coronary microcirculation with myocardial contrast echocardiography: Current and future applications. *Br Heart J* 1995;73:490–495.

99. Kaul S. Myocardial contrast echocardiography. 15 years of research and development. *Circulation* 1997;96:3745–3760

100. Kaul S. Myocardial contrast echocardiography. *Curr Prob Cardiol* 1997;22:549–640.

101. Rovai D, Ghelardini G, Trivella MG, et al. Intracoronary air-filled albumin microsphere for myocardial blood flow measurement. *J Am Coll Cardiol* 1993;22:2014–2021.

102. Cheirif J, Narkiewitz-Jodko J, Bravenec J, et al. Myocardial contrast echocardiography: Relation between on-line and off-line assessment of myocardial perfusion. *Echocardiography* 1993;10:471–484.

103. Jayaweera AR, Edwards N, Glasheen WP, et al. In vivo myocardial kinetics of air-filled albumin microbubbles during myocardial contrast echocardiography. Comparison with radiolabelled red blood cells. *Circ Res* 1994;74:1157–1165.

104. Halmann M, Beyar R, Rinkevich D, et al. Digital subtraction myocardial contrast echocardiography: Design and application of a new analysis program for myocardial perfusion imaging. *J Am Soc Echocardiogr* 1994;7:355–362.

105. Meltzer RS, Ohad DG, Reisner S, et al. Quantitative myocardial ultrasonic integrated backscatter measurements during contrast injections. *J Am Soc Echocardiogr* 1994;7:1–8.

106. Ismail S, Jayaweera AR, Goodman NC, et al. Detection of coronary stenosis and quantification of the degree and spatial extent of blood flow mismatch during coronary hyperemia with myocardial contrast echocardiography. *Circulation* 1995;91:821–830.

107. Wei K, Skyba DM, Firschke C, et al. Interactions between microbubbles and ultrasound: In vitro and in vivo observations. *J Am Coll Cardiol* 1997;29:1081–1088.
108. Kaul S. New developments in ultrasound systems for contrast echocardiography. *Clin Cardiol* 1997;20:I27–I30.
109. Meza MF, Kates MA, Barbee RW, et al. Combination of dobutamine and myocardial contrast echocardiography to differentiate postischemic from infarcted myocardium. *J Am Coll Cardiol* 1997;29:974–984.
110. Firschke C, Lindner JR, Wei K, et al. Myocardial perfusion imaging in the setting of coronary artery stenosis and acute myocardial infarction using venous injection of a second generation echocardiographic contrast agent. *Circulation* 1997;96:959–967.
111. Schwarz KQ, Chen X, Steinmetz S. Methods for quantifying ultrasound backscatter and two-dimensional video intensity: Implications for contrast-enhanced sonography. *J Am Soc Echocardiogr* 1998;11:155–168.
112. Stinson EB, Billingham ME. Correlative study of regional left ventricular histology and contractile function. *Am J Cardiol* 1977;39:378–383.
113. Mickle DA, del Nido PJ, Wilson GJ, et al. Exogenous substrate preference of the post-ischaemic myocardium. *Cardiovasc Res* 1986;20:256–263.
114. Myears DW, Sobel BE, Bergmann SR. Substrate use in ischemic and reperfused canine myocardium: Quantitative considerations. *Am J Physio* 1987;253:H107—H114.
115. Liedtke AJ, Nelson DL, Cox MM, et al. Changes in substrate metabolism and effects of excess fatty acids in reperfused myocardium. *Circ Res* 1988;62:535–542.
116. Lopaschuk GD, Spafford MA, Davies NJ, et al. Glucose and palmitate oxidation in isolated working hearts reperfused after a period of transient global ischemia. *Circ Res* 1990;66:546–553.
117. Vanoverschelde J-LJ, Wijns W, Borgers M, et al. Chronic myocardial hibernation in humans. From bedside to bench. *Circulation* 1997;95:1961–1971.
118. Vanoverschelde J-LJ, Wijns W, Depré C, et al. Mechanisms of chronic regional postischemic dysfunction in humans. New insights from the study of noninfarcted collateral-dependent myocardium. *Circulation* 1993;87:1513–1523.
119. Zimmer G, Zimmerman R, Hess OM, et al. Decreased concentration of myofibrils and myocyte hypertrophy are structural determinants of impaired left ventricular function in patients with chronic heart disease: A multiple logistic regression analysis. *J Am Coll Cardiol* 1992;20:1135–1142.
120. Flameng W, Suy R, Schwarz F, et al. Ultrastructural correlates of left ventricular contraction abnormalities in patients with chronic ischemic heart disease: Determinants of reversible segmental asynergy postrevascularization surgery. *Am Heart J* 1981;102:846–856.
121. Flameng W, Wouters L, Sergeant P, et al. Multivariate analysis of angiographic, histologic, and electrocardiographic data in patients with coronary heart disease. *Circulation* 1984;70:7–17.
122. Flameng W, Vanhaecke J, Van Belle H, et al. Relation between coronary artery stenosis and myocardial purine metabolism, histology and regional function in humans. *J Am Coll Cardiol* 1987;9:1235–1242.
123. Borgers M, Thone F, Wouters L, et al. Structural correlates of regional myocardial dysfunction in patients with critical coronary artery stenosis: Chronic hibernation? *Cardiovasc Pathol* 1993;2:237–245.
124. Maes A, Flameng W, Nuyts J, et al. Histologic alterations in chronically hypoperfused myocardium. Correlation with PET findings. *Circulation* 1994;90:735–745.
125. Depré C, Vanoverschelde J-LJ, Melin JA, et al. Structural and metabolic correlates of the reversibility of chronic left ventricular ischemic dysfunction in humans. *Am J Physiol* 1995;268:H1265—H1275.
126. Depré C, Vanoverschelde J-LJ, Gerber B, et al. Correlation of functional recovery with myocardial blood flow, glucose uptake and morphologic features in patients with chronic left ventricular ischemic dysfunction undergoing coronary artery bypass grafting. *J Thorac Cardiovasc Surg* 1997;113:371–378.
127. Schwarz ER, Schaper J, vom Dahl J, et al. Myocyte degeneration and cell death in hibernating human myocardium. *J Am Coll Cardiol* 1996;27:1577–1585.
128. Baltrami CA, Finato N, Rocco M, et al. Structural basis of end-stage failure in ischemic cardiomyopathy in humans. *Circulation* 1994;89:151–163.

129. Li F, Wang X, Capasso JM, et al. Rapid transition of cardiac myocytes from hyperplasia to hypertrophy during postnatal development. *J Mol Cell Cardiol* 1996;28:1737–1746.

130. Soonpaa MH, Field LJ. Survey of studies examining mammalian cardiomyocyte DNA synthesis. *Circ Res* 1998;83:15–26.

131. Shirani J, Lee J, Srinivasan G, et al. Relation between the severity of reduction in thallium activity within irreversible defects and percent collagen replacement in chronic ischemic cardiomyopathy. *Circulation* 1997;96:I309. Abstract.

132. Dilsizian V, Quigg RJ, Shirani J, et al. Histomorphologic validation of thallium reinjection and fluorodeoxyglucose PET for assessment of myocardial viability. *Circulation* 1994;90:I314. Abstract.

133. Shirani J, Lee J, Kitsiou AN, et al. Histomorphologic profile of myocardial segments with normal thallium activity in chronic ischemic cardiomyopathy. *J Am Coll Cardiol* 1998;31:I84A. Abstract.

134. Shirani J, Lee J, Pick R, et al. Histomorphologic correlates of reversible and mild-moderate irreversible thallium defects in chronic ischemic cardiomyopathy. *Circulation* 1998;98:I-370. Abstract.

135. Hennessy TG, Diamond P, Holligan B, et al. Histological changes in dysfunctional myocardial segments undergoing revascularization and their correlation with dobutamine stress echocardiography. *Circulation* 1997;96:I713. Abstract.

136. Chareonthaitawee P, Christian TF, Hirose K, et al. Relation of initial infarct size to extent of left ventricular remodeling in the year after acute myocardial infarction. *J Am Coll Cardiol* 1995;25:567–573.

137. Shivalkar B, Maes A, Borgers M, et al. Only hibernating myocardium invariably shows early recovery after coronary revascularization. *Circulation* 1996;94:I308. Abstract.

138. Bodenheimer MM, Banka VS, Hermann GA, et al. Reversible asynergy. Histopathologic and electrographic correlations in patients with coronary artery disease. *Circulation* 1976;53:792–796.

139. Hetts SW. To die or not to die. An overview of apoptosis and its role in disease. *J Am Med Assoc* 1998;279:300–307.

140. Kajstura J, Cheng W, Reiss K, et al. Apoptotic and necrotic myocyte cell deaths are independent contributing variables of infarct size in rats. *Lab Invest* 1995;74:86–107.

141. Narula J, Haider N, Virmaani R, et al. Apoptosis in myocytes in end-stage heart failure. *N Engl J Med* 1996;335:1182–1189.

142. Cheng W, Li B, Kajustura J, et al. Stretch induced programmed myocyte cell death. *J Clin Invest* 1995;96:2247–2259.

143. Elsasser A, Shlepper M, Klovekorn W-P, et al. Hibernating myocardium. An incomplete adaptation to ischemia. *Circulation* 1997;96:2920–2931.

144. Ausma J, Dispersyn G, Thone F, et al. Chronic myocardial hibernation is not a prelude to apoptosis. *Circulation* 1997;96:I744. Abstract.

145. Van Bilsen M, Van der Vusse GJ, Willemsen PHM, et al. Lipid alterations in isolated, working rat hearts during ischemia and reperfusion: Its relation to myocardial damage. *Circ Res* 1989;64:304–314.

146. Soei LK, Sassen LM, Fan DS, et al. Myofibrillar Ca^{2+} sensitization predominantly enhances function and mechanical efficiency of stunned myocardium. *Circulation* 1994;90:959–969.

147. Schwarz ER, Schoendube FA, Kostin S, et al. Prolonged myocardial hibernation exacerbates cardiomyocyte degeneration and impairs recovery of function after revascularization. *J Am Coll Cardiol* 1998;31:1018–1026.

148. Swan HJC. Left ventricular dysfunction in ischemic heart disease: Fundamental importance of the fibrous matrix. *Cardiovasc Drugs Ther* 1994;8:305–312.

149. Zhao M, Zhang H, Robinson TF, et al. Profound structural alterations of the extracellular collagen matrix in postischemic dysfunctional ("stunned") but viable myocardium. *J Am Coll Cardiol* 1987;10:1322–1334.

150. Charney RH, Takahashi S, Zhao M, et al. Collagen loss in the stunned myocardium. *Circulation* 1992;85:1483–1490.

151. Elsasser A, Decker E, Muller KD, et al. Hibernating myocardium: Extracellular matrix alterations are useful predictors of the chances for functional recovery. *Circulation* 1997;96:I689. Abstract.

152. Borgers M, Ausma J. Structural aspects of the chronic hibernating myocardium in man. *Basic Res Cardiol*.1995;90:44–46.
153. Kloner RA, Rude RE, Carlson N, et al. Ultrastructural evidence of microvascular damage and myocardial cell injury after coronary artery occlusion: Which comes first? *Circulation* 1980; 62:945–952.
154. Ruffolo RR. The pharmacology of dobutamine. *Am J Med* 1987;294:244–248.
155. Meyer SL, Curry GS, Donsky MS, et al. Influence of dobutamine on hemodynamics and coronary blood flow in patients with and without coronary artery disease. *Am J Cardiol* 1976;38:103–108.
156. Pozen RG, Di Bianco R, Katz RJ, et al. Myocardial metabolic and hemodynamic effects of dobutamine in heart failure complicating coronary artery disease. *Circulation* 1981;63: 1279–1285.
157. Chen C, Li L, Chen LL, et al. Incremental doses of dobutamine induce a biphasic response in dysfunctional left ventricular regions subtending coronary stenoses. *Circulation* 1995;92: 756–766.
158. Indolfi C, Piscione F, Perrone-Filardi P, et al. Inotropic stimulation by dobutamine increases left ventricular regional function at the expense of metabolism in hibernating myocardium. *Am Heart J* 1996;132:542–549.
159. Severi S, Underwood R, Mohiaddin RH, et al. Dobutamine stress: Effect on regional myocardial blood flow and wall motion. *J Am Coll Cardiol* 1995;26:1187–1195.
160. Krivokapich J, Czernin J, Schelbert HR. Dobutamine positron emission tomography: Absolute quantitation of rest and dobutamine myocardial blood flow and correlation with cardiac work and percent diameter stenosis in patients with and without coronary artery disease. *J Am Coll Cardiol* 1996;28:565–572.
161. Bartunek J, Marwick TH, Rodrigues AC, et al. Dobutamine-induced wall motion abnormalities: Correlations with myocardial fractional flow reserve and quantitative coronary angiography. *J Am Coll Cardiol* 1996;27:1429–1436.
162. Lee HH, Davila-Roman VG, Ludbrook PA, et al. Dependency of contractile reserve on myocardial blood flow. Implications for the assessment of myocardial viability with dobutamine stress echocardiography. *Circulation* 1997;96:2884–2891.
163. Sun KT, Czernin J, Krivokapich J, et al. Effects of dobutamine stimulation on myocardial blood flow, glucose metabolism, and wall motion in normal and dysfunctional myocardium. *Circulation* 1996;94:3146–3154.
164. Panza JA, Dilsizian V, Laurienzo JM, et al. Relation between thallium uptake and contractile response to dobutamine. Implications regarding myocardial viability in patients with chronic coronary artery disease and left ventricular dysfunction. *Circulation* 1995;91:990–998.
165. Bax JJ, Cornel JH, Elhendy A, et al. The impact of subendocardial scarring on prediction of improvement of regional wall motion after revascularization by dobutamine echocardiography. *J Am Coll Cardiol* 1998;31:182A. Abstract.
166. Baer FM, Voth E, Deutsch HJ, et al. Assessment of viable myocardium by dobutamine transesophageal echocardiography and comparison with fluorine-18 fluorodeoxyglucose positron emission tomography. *J Am Coll Cardiol* 1994;24:343–353.
167. Baer FM, Voth E, Deutsch HJ, et al. Predictive value of low dose dobutamine transesophageal echocardiography and fluorine-18 fluorodeoxyglucose positron emission tomography for recovery of regional left ventricular function after successful revascularization. *J Am Coll Cardiol* 1996;28:60–69.
168. Gerber BL, Vanoverschelde J-L J, Bol A, et al. Myocardial blood flow, glucose uptake, and recruitment of inotropic reserve in chronic left ventricular ischemic dysfunction: Implications for the pathophysiology of chronic myocardial hibernation. *Circulation* 1996;94:651–659.
169. Bax JJ, Wijns W, Cornel JH, et al. Accuracy of currently available techniques for prediction of functional recovery after revascularization in patients with left ventricular dysfunction due to chronic coronary artery disease: Comparison of pooled data. *J Am Coll Cardiol* 1997;30: 1451–1460.
170. Bonow RO. Identification of viable myocardium. *Circulation* 1996;94:2674–2680.
171. Chan RKM, Lee KJ, Calafiore P, et al. Comparison of dobutamine echocardiography and positron emission tomography in patients with chronic ischemic left ventricular dysfunction. *J Am Coll Cardiol* 1996;27:1601–1607.

172. Chin D, Hancock J, Brown A, et al. Improved endocardial definition and evaluation of dobutamine stress echocardiography using second harmonic imaging. *J Am Coll Cardiol* 1998;31:76A. Abstract.

173. Spencer K, Bednarz J, Godoy I, et al. Second harmonic imaging improves endocardial visualization during dobutamine stress echocardiography without contrast. *J Am Coll Cardiol* 1998;31:437A. Abstract.

174. Falcone RA, Marcovitz PA, Perez JE, et al. Intravenous albunex during dobutamine stress echocardiography: Enhanced localization of left ventricular endocardial borders. *Am Heart J* 1995;130:254–258.

175. Porter T, Li S, Hiser W, et al. Simultaneous assessment of wall motion and myocardial perfusion using a rapid acquisition intermittent harmonic imaging pulsing interval of 5–15 Hertz following acute myocardial infarction and during stress echocardiography. *J Am Coll Cardiol* 1998;31:123A. Abstract.

176. Nanto S, Lim Y-J, Masuyama T, et al. Diagnostic performance of myocardial contrast echocardiography for detection of stunned myocardium. *J Am Soc Echocardiogr* 1996;9:314–319.

177. Galiuto L, Marchese A, Cavallari D, et al. Evaluation of postinfarction viable myocardium at jeopardy by dobutamine echocardiography and myocardial contrast echocardiography. *Echocardiography* 1994;11:337–341.

178. Porter TR, Li S, Kilzer KL, et al. Correlation between quantitative angiographic parameters of coronary stenosis severity and quantitative measurements of myocardial contrast intensity during dobutamine stress echocardiography using a continuous infusion of microbubbles. *Circulation* 1997;96:I213. Abstract.

179. Masani ND, Yao J, Cao Q, et al. Accurate infarct size estimation using NC100100 in mixed coronary territories: Increased accuracy of three-dimensional echo vs two-dimensional echo. *Circulation* 1997;96:I214. Abstract.

180. Porter TR, Xie F. Visually discernible myocardial echocardiographic contrast after intravenous injection of sonicated dextrose albumin microbubbles containing high molecular weight, less soluble gases. *J Am Coll Cardiol* 1995;25:509–515.

181. Dittrich HC, Bales GL, Kuvelas T, et al. Myocardial contrast echocardiography in experimental coronary artery occlusion with a new intravenously administered contrast agent. *J Am Soc Echocardiog.* 1995;8:465–474.

182. Porter TR, Xie F. Transient myocardial contrast after initial exposure to diagnostic ultrasound pressures with minute doses of intravenously injected microbubbles. Demonstration and potential mechanisms. *Circulation* 1995;92:2391–2395.

183. Wei K, Firoozan S, Jayaweera AR, et al. Detection of coronary stenoses from venous administration of microbubbles: Bolus injection or continuous infusion? *Circulation* 1997;96:I214. Abstract.

184. Porter TR, Li S, Oster R, et al. Correlation in humans between myocardial contrast defects observed with a continuous intravenous infusion of microbubbles during dobutamine stress and quantitative angiography. *Circulation* 1997;96:I214. Abstract.

185. Becher H, Tiemann K, Schlief R, et al. Harmonic power Doppler contrast echocardiography: Preliminary clinical results. *Echocardiography* 1997;14:637–642.

186. Agrawal DI, Malhotra S, Nanda N, et al. Harmonic power Doppler contrast edchocardiography: Preliminary experimental results. *Echocardiography* 1997;14:631–635.

187. Senior R, Kaul S, Soman P, et al. Myocardial prefusion imaging with color power Doppler contrast echocardiography and intravenous BR-1. *J Am Coll Cardiol* 1998;31:123A. Abstract.

188. Porter TR, D'Sa A, Turner C, et al. Myocardial contrast echocardiography for the assessment of coronary blood flow reserve: Validation in humans. *J Am Coll Cardiol* 1993;21:349–355.

189. Porter TR, Li S, Kricsfeld D, et al. Detection of myocardial perfusion in multiple echocardiographic windows with one intravenous injection of microbubbles using transient response second harmonic imaging. *J Am Coll Cardiol* 1997;29:791–799.

190. Burns PN, Powers JE, Hope-Simpson D, et al. Harmonic power mode Doppler using microbubble contrast agents: An improved method for small vessel flow imaging. *Proc IEEE UFFC* 1994:1547–1550.

191. Burns PN, Powers JE, Hope-Simpson D, et al. Power Doppler imaging combined with contrast enhancing harmonic Doppler: A new method for small vessel imaging. *Radiology.* 1994;193:366. Abstract.

192. Williams MJ, Odabashian J, Lauer MS, et al. Prognostic value of dobutamine echocardiography in patients with left ventricular dysfunction. *J Am Coll Cardiol* 1996;27:132–139.
193. Marmor A, Schneeweiss A. Prognostic value of noninvasively obtained left ventricular contractile reserve in patients with severe heart failure. *J Am Coll Cardiol* 1997;29:422–428.
194. Afridi I, Panza JA, Zoghbi WA, et al. Dobutamine echocardiography predicts outcome in patients with coronary artery disease and severe ventricular dysfunction. *Circulation* 1997; 96:I590. Abstract.
195. Mertes H, Sawada SG, Ryan T. Symptoms, adverse effects, and complications associated with dobutamine stress echocardiography. Experience in 1118 patients. *Circulation* 1993;88:15–19.
196. Geleijnse ML, Fioretti PM, Roelandt JRTC. Methodology, feasibility, safety and diagnostic accuracy of dobutamine stress echocardiography. *J Am Coll Cardiol* 1997;30:595–606.
197. Poldermans D, Fioretti PM, Boersma E, et al. Safety of dobutamine-atropine stress echocardiography in patients with suspected or proven coronary artery disease. *Am J Cardiol* 1994; 73:456–459.
198. Picano E, Mathias W Jr, Pingitore A, et al. Safety and tolerability of dobutamine-atropine stress echocardiography: A prospective, multicentre study. Echo Dobutamine International Cooperative Study Group. *Lancet* 1994;344:1190–1192.
199. Bigi R, Partesana R, Verzoni A, et al. Incidence and correlates of complex ventricular arrhythmias during dobutamine stress echocardiography after acute myocardial infarction. *Eur Heart J* 1995;16:1819–1824.
200. Tsoukas A, Ikonomidis I, Cokkinos P, et al. Significance of persistent left ventricular dysfunction during recovery after dobutamine stress echocardiography. *J Am Coll Cardiol* 1997;30: 621–626.
201. Secknus M, Marwick TH. Evolution of dobutamine echocardiography protocols and indications: Safety and side effects in 3011 studies over 5 years. *J Am Coll Cardiol* 1997;29:1234–1240.
202. Sharp SM, Sawada SG, Segar DS, et al. Dobutamine stress echocardiography: Detection of coronary artery disease in patients with dilated cardiomyopathy. *J Am Coll Cardiol* 1994;24: 934–939.
203. Borges A, Djorkievic-Dikic A, Mathias W, et al. The prognostic value of myocardial viability recognized by low dose dipyridamole echocardiography in ischemic chronic left ventricular dysfunction. *J Am Coll Cardiol* 1998;31:81A. Abstract.
204. Rosanio S, Sheiban I, Tonni S, et al. Nisoldipine echocardiography: A new method for assessing myocardial viability after acute myocardial infarction treated with thrombolysis. *J Am Coll Cardiol* 1998;31:82A. Abstract.
205. Cohn PF, Angoff GH, Zoll PM, et al. A new, noninvasive technique for inducing postextrasystolic potentiation during echocardiography. *Circulation* 1977;56:598–605.
206. Cohn PF, Angoff GH, Sloss LJ. Noninvasively induced postextrasystolic potentiation of ischemic and infarcted myocardium in patients with coronary artery disease. *Am Heart J* 1979;97:187–194.
207. Chandra M, Sonnenblick EH, Hla A, et al. Relation of postextrasystolic potentiation of contractility to microvascular integrity in asynergic myocardium. *Circulation* 1998;98:I-569. Abstract.
208. Chandra M, Sonnenblick EH, Strom JA, et al. Differential contractile response of asynergic myocardium to paired pacing and dobutamine. *J Am Coll Cardiol* 1999;33:412A. Abstract.

Timing and Myocardial Salvage: Lessons Learned From the Thrombolytic and Revascularization Multicenter Trials

Thomas J. Ryan, MD

Introduction

In 1977 two quite different but equally important events occurred that signaled the dawn of the reperfusion era. First was the publication of the seminal studies of Reimer et al showing irreversible ischemic myocardial cell injury develops as the duration of abrupt occlusion of a normal coronary artery is prolonged in the experimental animal.[1] After 40 minutes of ischemia, myocyte necrosis was subendocardial but with increasing duration of coronary occlusion irreversible injury progresses as a wave front toward the subendocardium. Reperfusion after 2 hours of coronary occlusion salvaged approximately 70% of the myocardium at risk; after 3 hours it salvaged approximately 30%; and after 4 hours it salvaged none. These were the earliest studies to suggest the presence of a subepicardial zone of ischemic but viable myocardium that is available for pharmacologic or surgical salvage for at least 3 or perhaps 6 hours following coronary occlusion in the dog.

The second was a series of studies undertaken at the University of Goettingen, Germany by Doctor K. Peter Rentrop that involved selective coronary angiography in patients during the early hours of acute myocardial infarction. Total occlusion of the infarct-related artery was seen in 75% (26 of 35) of the patients and >90% occlusion in the remaining patients.[2] By the following year (1978) Rentrop began to recanalize acute coronary occlusions with guide wires and small catheters using a modified Dotter technique. Injecting contrast media selectively into the infarct-related artery provided the first direct, in vivo evidence of coronary thrombosis in the genesis of acute myocardial infarction by the demonstration of mobile filling defects in the arterial lumen.[3] It was these observations that stimulated the investigators to undertake the approach used two decades earlier by Sherry and associates who pioneered the use of the thrombolytic agent streptokinase (SK) to restore flow and salvage myocardium in humans undergoing acute myocardial infarction.[4]

From Dilsizian V (ed). *Myocardial Viability: A Clinical and Scientific Treatise.* Armonk, NY: Futura Publishing Co., Inc.; © 2000.

An intracoronary infusion of SK was chosen because it would, for the first time, incorporate into the technique angiographic documentation of the result as well as achieve a high concentration of thrombolytic agent at the occlusion site.[5] In the first patients studied, cessation of chest pain and decrease of ST segment elevation accompanied restoration of coronary flow that usually was demonstrable within 30 minutes. These findings provided the strongest evidence to date for the causative role of occlusive coronary thrombosis in the pathogenesis of acute myocardial infarction. Corroboration was provided by DeWood's landmark study in 1980 that reported retrieval of thrombotic material from the infarct-related artery in patients undergoing coronary artery bypass surgery during evolving acute myocardial infarction.[6]

Intracoronary Streptokinase—Early Experience

The earliest studies that reported a benefit on mortality were carried out with the use of intracoronary SK. The first of these was the first Western Washington Study carried out in community and teaching hospitals that randomized patients following diagnostic coronary arteriography to either routine care or intracoronary SK.[7] Ultimately, 134 patients received intracoronary SK (4000 U/min begun 4.5 hours after symptom onset) and 116 randomized to routine care. At 30 days the mortality was 3.7% in the treatment arm and 11.2% for the control patients ($p = 0.02$). However, the reduction in early mortality was not sustained and by 1 year the mortality difference had narrowed to 8.2% in the intracoronary SK group and 14.7% in the controls ($p = 0.10$).[8] As the investigators point out, the greatest shortcoming of intracoronary SK therapy was the difficulty in providing rapid treatment once the patient arrived in the hospital. The mean time from the onset of symptoms to treatment was 4.6 hours. This relatively late therapy did not improve left ventricular (LV) function in the treatment group as compared with the control group.[9] Importantly, however, in patients with open infarct related-arteries with normal or near-normal flow [thrombolysis in myocardial infarction (TIMI) grade 2 or 3] following completion of the intracoronary SK infusion, 80 patients had reperfusion, 13 partial reperfusion, and 41 no reperfusion. Mortality at 1 year was low (2.5%) in those with complete reperfusion but significantly higher in those with partial reperfusion (3 of 13, 23%) and those with no reperfusion (6 of 41, 14.6%) ($p = 0.02$).[8] This improved survival with late reperfusion, unaccompanied by evidence of improved LV function or reduction in infarct size, sparked the beginning of the discussion of the open artery hypothesis that continues to the present time.

Impact of Thrombolytic Therapy on Mortality

Pooling data from the relatively small, inconclusive trials of intravenous (IV) SK infusion over variable time intervals that were performed in the early 1980s, Stampfer et al[10] found a significant mortality reduction of 18% in patients treated within 24 hours of pain onset. This meta-analysis was the basis for the first appropriately sized mortality study of thrombolytic therapy in acute myocardial infarction, the Gruppo Italiano per lo Studio Della Sopravvivenza nell' Infarcto Miocardico-I (GISSI-I) megatrial carried out by the Italian Association of Hospital Cardiologists.[11] This study randomized 11 712 patients who were admitted within 12 hours of symptom onset and randomized to conventional therapy (control) or to a modern regimen of high-dose IV SK (1.5 million units administered over 60 minutes). In addition to showing overall hospital mortality at 21 days was 10.7% in SK recipients versus 13% in control recipients, an 18% reduction [$p = 0.0002$, relative risk (RR) 0.81], it was clearly demonstrated that the extent of beneficial effect was a function of time from onset of pain to SK infusion with the RR 0.74, 0.81, 0.87, and 1.19 for the 0–3, 3–6, 6–9, and 9–12 hour subgroups. In patients who were treated within 1 hour of the onset of chest pain there was a 47% reduction in mortality.

The 1-year mortality data in the GISSI study demonstrated that the benefits of thrombolytic therapy are sustained without the use of follow-up coronary angiography and the frequent use of coronary bypass surgery or percutaneous transluminal coronary angioplast (PTCA). In the group overall, the 1-year mortality was 17.2% in the treatment group and 19.0% in the control.[12]

There have been many randomized placebo-controlled trials designed to evaluate mortality using IV thrombolytic therapy. The Second International Study of Infarct Survival (ISIS-2) was the second large trial that evaluated both SK and aspirin using a 2 × 2 factorial design.[13] This trial entered 17 187 patients with suspected myocardial infarction from 417 coronary care units and 16 countries. Patients were randomized to receive oral aspirin, IV SK in a dose of 1.5 million units given over 1 hour, both drugs, or placebos. The double-placebo group had a 35-day cumulative vascular morality of 13.2%, while the mortality was 10.7% for those receiving aspirin, a mortality reduction of 18.9%; 10.4% for those receiving IV SK, a reduction of 21.5%; and 8.0% for those receiving both drugs, a reduction of -39.4%, with each group being compared with the patients receiving double placebo.

The most striking finding in this trial was the magnitude of benefit for those patients receiving aspirin therapy and the added benefit of combined aspirin and SK therapy. As in other trials, early therapy was more effective than later treatment, with those receiving both aspirin and SK within the first 4 hours of symptom onset having a mortality of 6.4% as compared with a mortality of 13.1% (a 51% reduction) for the corresponding double-placebo group. This study also suggested that patients with symptoms for >12 hours may benefit from thrombolytic therapy. Of the 1222 patients who were randomized to either aspirin and SK or double placebo between 12 and 24 hours the mortality was 7.4% in the SK-aspirin group versus 11.5% in the double-placebo group ($p < 0.05$). As in the earlier GISSI-I trial patients with ST segment, depression not only derived no benefit but there was a trend toward showing harm.

Other Thrombolytic Agents

The Anglo-Scandinavian Study of Early Thrombolysis (ASSET) entered 5011 patients under the age of 75 years with clinically suspected acute myocardial infarction into a placebo-controlled randomized trial using 100 mg of tissue-type plasminogen activator (t-PA) over 3 hours plus heparin but neither the treatment nor the control group received aspirin. The 30-day mortality in the treatment group was 7.2% and 9.8% in the controls ($p = 0.001$). In this study the stroke rate was 1.1% in the treated patients and 1.0% in the controls. The 12-month mortality remained significantly lower in the treatment group as compared with the controls (13.2% versus 15.1%, $p < 0.05$).[14]

Anisoylated plasminogen SK activator complex (APSAC) was studied in the APSAC Intervention Mortality Study (AIMS) that enrolled 1258 patients under the age of 71 years with symptoms of acute myocardial infarction of <6 hours duration.[15] Inclusion criteria required ST elevation on the entry electrocardiogram (ECG) prior to randomization that included the IV APSAC medication as a 30-mg bolus over 5 minutes or a placebo. At 30 days the mortality was 6.4% for the treatment group and 12.1% for the control group, a significant 50% reduction in mortality ($p = 0.0006$). These striking findings were replicated in a smaller randomized trial of APSAC versus heparin.[16] This study enrolled 213 patients with symptoms in <4 hours duration. The 30-day mortality in the treated group was 5.6% compared with 12.6% in the heparin group, a 55% reduction in mortality ($p = 0.032$).

Fibrinolytic Therapy Trialists' Collaborative Group

The Fibrinolytic Therapy Trialists' (FTT) collaborative group has gathered all the data available on randomized trials of thrombolytic therapy and recently has provided recommendations for therapy in patients with suspected myocardial infarction based on the data from all published trials of >1000 patients.[17] The nine trials that comprise this database include 58 600 patients of whom 6177 (10.5%) died, 564 (1.0%) had a stroke, and 436 (0.7%) had major noncerebral bleeds. The overall benefit for the 45 000 patients with ST elevation or bundle branch block on the ECG was an absolute mortality reduction of 30 per thousand for those presenting within 6 hours of the onset of symptoms, 20 per thousand for those presenting from 7 to 12 hours, and a questionable 10 per thousand for those presenting between 13 and 18 hours. There were four additional strokes per thousand in the fibrinolytic group of whom two died. One had a moderate or severe disabling neurologic deficit and one did not. These investigators report that the benefits of thrombolytic therapy were not limited by age, sex, blood pressure, heart rate, or prior history of myocardial infarction or diabetes.

Of the various subsets identified in this meta-analysis, the ECG was an important predictor of reduced mortality (Fig. 1). For patients with bundle branch block or anterior ST segment elevation the number of lives saved per thousand were 49 and 37, respectively. Patients with inferior ST elevation benefited much less (eight lives saved per thousand) and those with ST depression, not at all. There was a marked decline in treatment benefit as a function of time from onset of symptoms to initiation of therapy with twice as many lives saved when treatment is started in the 1st hour as opposed to

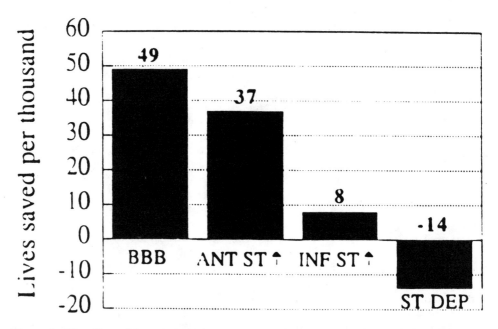

Figure 1. The effect of thrombolytic therapy on mortality according to admission electrocardiogram (ECG). Patients with bundle branch block (BBB) and anterior ST segment elevation (ANTST ↑) derived the most benefit from thrombolytic therapy. Effects in patients with inferior ST segment elevation (INFST ↑) are much less, while patients with ST segment depression (STDEP) do not benefit. Based on data from Reference 17 and reprinted with permission from Reference 22.

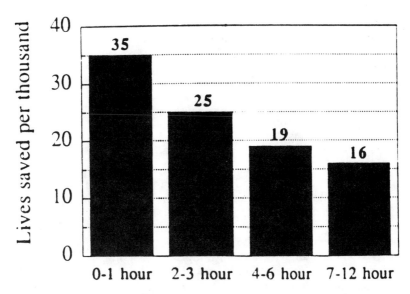

Figure 2. Effect of thrombolytic therapy on mortality according to time from symptom onset. Patients treated early derive the most benefit. Based on data from Reference 17 and reprinted with permission from Reference 22.

7–12 hours (Fig. 2). Up to age 75 years there is an increased survival benefit with age but the very elderly do not achieve an absolute increase in survival with thrombolytic therapy. Other subgroups of patients who are most likely to benefit include those with hypotension (blood pressure < 100 mm Hg), tachycardia (heart rate > 100 beats/min), and those with diabetes.

Angiographic Recanalization and Patency

Early achievement of infarct-related artery patency allows rapid coronary artery perfusion to limit infarct size, which in turn decreases LV dysfunction and improves survival. This is the paradigm that is invoked to explain the incontrovertible evidence that fibrinolytic therapy, when administered to patients within 12 hours of the onset of symptoms of acute myocardial infarction associated with ST segment elevation or presumably new bundle branch block that may obscure ST segment shifts, results in improved survival. However, there are, a number of caveats that are worthy of discussion before considering the matter established beyond all doubt.

First, it must be acknowledged that TIMI grade 3 flow (complete perfusion) is not synonymous with effective reperfusion of jeopardized myocardial tissue. A vessel may be opened successfully but too late to salvage tissue. Angiography in such cases may demonstrate TIMI grade 3 flow while nuclear imaging studies indicate a preponderance of nonviable tissue. Using intracoronary injections of technetium-99m (^{99m}Tc) microalbumin aggregates, before and after treatment, Schofer et al observed no improvement in scintigraphic defect size in 6 of 14 patients in whom the infarct-related artery was opened using intracoronary fibrinolysis.[18] Similarly, Ito and colleagues[19] reported that one in four patients with angiographically successful reperfusion fail to demonstrate myocardial flow as measured by contrast echocardiography. It has long been recognized that angiographic filling of the coronary arteries is influenced by a number of factors including the force of injection of contrast media, the administration of intracoronary nitroglycerin, the thrombolytic agent used, its dose, route, and timing of administration, to mention a few.

Second, because recanalization can occur spontaneously only those studies that have demonstrated the status of the artery prior to therapy are able to report true reperfusion rates, that is, the percentage of infarct-related arteries that are initially closed but subsequently opened by therapy. The TIMI Phase 1 Trial was such a study and one of the first trials to suggest that t-PA was a superior fibrinolytic agent to IV SK.[20] This was based on the finding of a 60% (59 of 99) recanalization rate of totally occluded infarct-related arteries at 90 minutes following the infusion of t-PA compared with a recanalization rate of 35% (40 of 115) at a similar time frame following the administration of SK. These patients underwent coronary angiography within a mean of 4.5 hours from the onset of symptoms and it was found that 58 of 316 patients (18%) had open vessels prior to either drug infusion. These findings have important implications for understanding the real meaning of "patency rates" as reported in most studies that have an angiographic measurement at some point in time following the administration of therapy but have no measurement prior to therapy. In the early studies of Rentrop and colleagues, repeat angiography 10–14 days after the administration of intracoronary SK showed an acute recanalization rate of 61% and a later patency of 77%. Acute recanalization occurred in only 8% of patients who did not receive a thrombolytic agent but after 10–14 days the patency rate had increased to 77% such that there was no difference between those patients that received thrombolytic therapy and those who had not.[21] When we consider that approximately 20% of patients with acute myocardial infarction will have patent arteries prior to therapy, patency rates overestimate true recanalization rates. For example, assuming a pretherapy patency rate of 20%, a reported posttherapy patency rate of 50% would translate to a recanalization rate of 37.5% (subtracting the 20 patients per 100 that would have open vessels prior to therapy from both numerator and denominator results in $30 \div 80 = 37.5$). Similarly, a patency of 80% would indicate a recanalization rate of 75%.[22]

Infarct Size and Left Ventricular Function

If indeed the early achievement of infarct artery patency allows rapid coronary perfusion to limit infarct size, clinical measurements of infarct size would be of key importance. It is now acknowledged that infarct size measurements from single proton emission computerized tomography (SPECT) ^{99m}Tc sestamibi correlate well with measures of LV function, LV volumes, and myocardial enzymes.[23–31] Additionally, a strong linear correlation has been found between the time to treatment and infarct size[9,32–37] (Fig. 3). Treatment 1 hour from the onset of symptoms reduces infarct size by 75%, salvaging 15% of the left ventricle. On the other hand, treatment at 3 hours reduces infarct size by only 35%, salvaging 7% of the left ventricle, and treatment at 5 hours fails to save any myocardium.

In light of these considerations it would seem predictable that the preponderance of fibrinolytic trials would show beneficial effects both on survival and on measurements of global LV function. As pointed out by Van der Werf this is not the case.[38] In the New Zealand trial[39] using SK a significant improvement in global ejection fraction as well as survival was found in the 172 patients with a first myocardial infarction but not when the entire group of 219 patients was compared with control ($p = 0.09$). In the European Cooperative Study Group Trial[40] the difference in global ejection fraction between patients treated with t-PA (Alteplase) and controls was only 2.2 percentage points ($p = 0.04$) while the reduction in mortality at 14 days was large (51%). In both the Western Washington Trial with intracoronary SK[7] and the TIMI Phase I Trial with t-PA[41] improved long-term survival was seen in the fibrinolytic group without a significant effect on

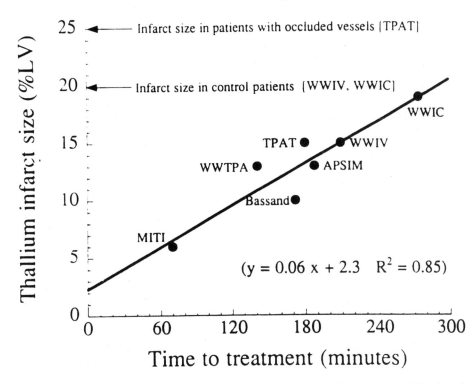

Figure 3. Linear relationship between infarct size measured by thallium-201 and the time from symptom onset to treatment. Little reduction in infarct size is achieved when treatment is started later than 4 hours from the onset of symptoms. MITI, Myocardial Infarction Triage and Intervention Trial[33,36]; WWTPA, Western Washington Myocardial Infarction Registry and Emergency Department Tissue Plasminogen Activator Treatment Trial[37]; TPAT, Tissue Plasminogen Activator, Toronto Trial[35]; APSIM, Anisoylated Plasminogen Streptokinase Activator Complex (APSAC), An Acute Myocardial Infarction Trial[32]; WWIV, Western Washington Intravenous Streptokinase Trial[34]; WWIC, Western Washington Intracoronary Streptokinase Trial.[9] Reprinted with permission from Reference 22.

LV function. Successful recanalization of the infarct-related artery was the most important predictor of late survival in both trials.[7,41,42] If preservation of LV contractile function is the most important benefit of successful coronary reperfusion one also would expect divergence of the survival curves over time. The consistent reduction in mortality observed over 4 years of follow-up in a number of controlled trials suggests that effects of reperfusion other than salvage of myocardium are involved.[43]

There also would appear to be a time-to-treatment paradox. Van der Werf has reported that in post hoc analysis of the data from the European Cooperative Study Group[38] there was an 82% reduction in mortality ($p = 0.009$) at 14 days in patients treated within 3 hours after the onset of symptoms of acute myocardial infarction, while global ejection fraction at 10–22 days was nearly identical in the surviving patients and controls. In contrast, in patients treated after 3 hours, the 14-day mortality in the fibrinolytic group was only slightly lower than that of controls and in the surviving patients treated within 3–5 hours after symptom onset, global ejection fraction was significantly higher at 4 percentage points ($p = <0.001$) in the thrombolytic group. In the Western Washington Trial with IV SK,[34] the reduction in 14-day mortality in patients treated within 3 hours was 11.3% in controls and 5.2% in the SK group (a mortality reduction of 54%), yet there was an improvement in ejection fraction of only 2 percentage points (51% versus 49%) in a subgroup of surviving patients at 2 months. In patients treated between

3 and 6 hours after the onset of symptoms the 14-day mortality was identical in both groups (7.5%) while ejection fraction at 2 months was 5 percentage points higher in the SK group compared with controls (50% versus 45%). These observations suggest that when an effective thrombolytic agent is given very early in the course of an acute myocardial infarction, some patients with extremely poor LV function will be saved. These patients would have died if no thrombolytic treatment had been given or if thrombolytic therapy had been given later. The extremely low ejection fractions in these early reperfused patients will hide the gain in ejection fraction observed in other reperfused patients and therefore confound the comparison with surviving controls.

These observations are still consistent with the findings of Mathey and colleagues[44] who studied the relationship between LV wall motion and the time to treatment in 69 patients admitted <3 hours after the onset of acute transmural myocardial infarction. There was a significant relation between time to treatment and the severity of regional hypokinesia at the infarct site. Compared with those treated later, patients treated <2 hours after symptom onset had significantly greater improvement in regional LV function and less severe hypokinesia at follow-up. Wall motion was within 2 standard deviations of the normal mean in 82% compared with only 46% in patients treated 2–5 hours after symptom onset ($p < 0.025$).

Global Utilization of Streptokinase and Tissue-Type Plasminogen Activator for Occluded Coronary Artery Trials

Although angiographic comparisons between the more clot-specific fibrinolytic agent t-PA and SK had shown t-PA to be superior in establishing coronary recanalization[20] and infarct-related artery patency,[45,46] the mortality results of 2 mega trials comparing the administration of these two agents in over 46 000 patients showed no difference.[47–49] It was suggested that the omission of IV heparin may have negated the early patency advantage of t-PA in both of these trials leading to lower than expected patency rates and resulting in suboptimal mortality reductions.[50,51]

In view of this and other considerations the now landmark trial of Global Utilization of Streptokinase and Tissue-Type Plasminogen Activator for Occluded Coronary Arteries (GUSTO) repeated the comparison of t-PA with SK using overall 30-day mortality as the primary end point.[52] However, there were two important differences. First, t-PA was administered in an accelerated fashion, over a period of 1.5 hours with two-thirds of the dose given in the first 30 minutes.[53] Second, IV heparin administration, along with aspirin, was begun with t-PA infusion and was continued at least 48 hours after completion of infusion.[52] There were four treatment groups: SK and subcutaneous heparin (30-day mortality, 7.2%), SK and IV heparin (30-day mortality, 7.4%), accelerated t-PA and IV heparin (30-day mortality, 6.3%), and the combination of both thrombolytic agents with IV heparin (30-day mortality, 7.0%). This represented a 14% reduction in mortality for accelerated t-PA as compared with the two SK-only strategies ($p = 0.001$). A significant excess of hemorrhagic strokes among the accelerated t-PA group (0.72%) and the combination therapy (0.94%) was also reported ($p = 0.03$ and 0.001, respectively).

Of greater importance than the findings of this large-scale trial that demonstrated that accelerated t-PA given with IV heparin provides a survival benefit over previous standard fibrinolytic regimens were the findings of the GUSTO angiographic substudy carried out in parallel with the main study.[54] The angiographic substudy was designed to examine whether the rate with which coronary artery patency is restored after the initiation of therapy further effects outcome. To accomplish this, the investigators carried out a second randomization of 2431 consenting patients to cardiac angiography at one of four times after the initiation of therapy: 90 minutes, 180 minutes, 24 hours, or 5–7 days. The group undergoing angiography at 90 minutes also underwent angiography at 5–7 days (see Table 1).

Among the 1210 patients randomized to angiography 90 minutes after starting therapy there was improved patency, especially TIMI grade 3 flow with accelerated t-PA over the other three regimens ($p < 0.001$). TIMI grade 3 flow at 90 minutes also was a significant predictor of 30-day survival ($p < 0.01$). To determine whether differences in mortality among the four strategies matched differences in 90-minute patency, a model was developed for predicting mortality differences in the main trial from the angiographic substudy.[55]

The model assumed that any differences in treatment effects on 30-day mortality were mediated through differences in 90-minute patency for the four treatments. The predicted rates then were compared with observed mortality rates of the remaining patients in the main trial for each treatment group. The predicted and observed 30-day mortality rates of the four treatments were SK with subcutaneous heparin, 7.46% versus 7.28%; SK with IV heparin, 7.26% versus 7.39%; accelerated t-PA, 6.31% versus 6.37%; and SK plus t-PA, 6.98% versus 6.96%. The correlation between predicted and observed results was 0.97.

The close relation between the predicted and observed 30-day mortality rates supports the concept that an important mechanism for improved survival with thrombolytic therapy is achievement of the early, complete perfusion. The close match provided in this study provides a strong biological explanation for the mortality differences seen in GUSTO-I and a sound rationale for the additional survival advantage of the accelerated t-PA regimen.

Additional important observations were made in the angiographic substudy[54] that are worthy of comment. Patency grades, regardless of treatment assignment, showed that a lack of patency at 90 minutes was associated with a mortality of 8.9%, a patency of TIMI-2 flow was associated with a mortality of 7.4%, and the rate among those with TIMI grade 3 flow was 4.4% ($p = 0.08$). There also was an effect of early patency on ventricular function. Patients with TIMI grade 3 flow at 90 minutes had a significantly higher ejection fraction, 62% ± 14% and a greater percentage of preserved regional motion, 31%, than those who had a lesser degrees of patency. This investigation also demonstrated that the rate at which the infarct-related artery becomes patent in patients given SK "catches up" to the rate in those given t-PA (see Fig. 4). By 3 hours after the start of treatment,

Table 1

Treatment Given and Infarct-Related Artery Perfusion Status

	SK + SQH	SK + IVH	Acclerated t-PA + IVH	Combined Limb
TIMI-2 or -3 (%)				
90 min	54	60	81	73
180 min	73	74	76	85
24 h	77	80	86	94
5–7 days	72	84	84	80
TIMI-3 (%)				
90 min	29	32	54	38
180 min	35	41	43	53
24 h	51	41	45	60
5–7 days	51	58	58	55

TIMI, thrombolysis in myocardial infarction; SK, streptokinase; SQH, subcutaneous heparin; IVH, intravenous heparin; t-PA, tissue-type plasminogen activator.

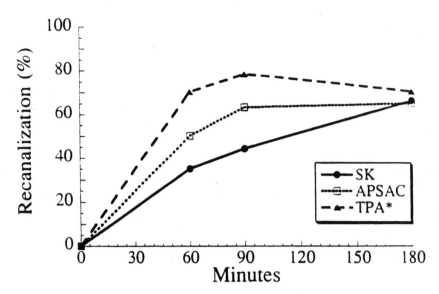

Figure 4. Time course of reperfusion for SK, APSAC, and accelerated t-PA showing that accelerated t-PA opens about two-thirds of closed vessels by 60 minutes. APSAC and SK work more slowly, taking about 90 minutes and 180 minutes, respectively, to achieve a 65% recanalization rate. Reprinted with permission from Reference 22.

patency rates were equal. This suggests that despite this catching up phenomenon, it occurs too late to result in an equally favorable clinical outcome.[54]

Implications

The importance of early reperfusion now has been well established in a prospective randomized controlled trial and should focus attention on the various measures that can accomplish this goal. One of the most important of these is the National Heart Attack Alert Program (NHAAP) established in 1991 by the National Heart, Lung and Blood Institute with the goal of reducing each component of the delay in time to treatment[53] (Table 2). The GUSTO findings also emphasize that there is considerable room for improvement in thrombolytic therapy when we consider that even with a combination of accelerated t-PA, aspirin, and IV heparin, 46% of the patients in the angiographic substudy did not have TIMI grade 3 flow at 90 minutes.[56] Third-generation thrombolytic agents such as TNK-t-PA, r-PA (retaplase), or t-PA combined with fibrin-specific mono-

Table 2

National Heart Attack Alert Program

Goal: Improve Time to Treatment of Acute Myocardial Infarction

1. Reduce door to needle time with acute myocardial infarction protocol
2. Evaluate new technologies for rapid identification of acute myocardial infarction patients
3. Improve transport time with improved Emergency-911 standards and emergency medical treatment procedures
4. Improve patient time to presentation by focusing on high-risk patients
5. Improve general public awareness via local and national media campaigns

clonal antibodies and staphylokinase are all deserving of investigation to improve early reperfusion and TIMI grade 3 flow to further reduce mortality from acute myocardial infarction.[56]

Because time to treatment is such a critical component, primary angioplasty as a means of achieving early reperfusion in acute myocardial infarction warrants careful monitoring. To employ this approach to reperfusion therapy, the cardiac catheterization team must be assembled, the patient transported to the catheterization laboratory, arterial access obtained, the diagnostic catheterization performed, the angioplasty balloon readied, and the procedure performed. In the setting of acute myocardial infarction, during the time that all these steps are being carried out, the infarct-related artery is occluded and myocardial tissue necrosis is ongoing. For these reasons the recently published American College of Cardiology/American Heart Association (ACC/AHA) *Guidelines for the Management of Patients with Acute Myocardial Infarction* expresses the concern "that a routine policy of primary PTCA for patients with acute myocardial infarction will result in unacceptable delays in achieving reperfusion in a substantial number of cases."[57] The Guidelines recommend balloon dilation within 60 minutes of the diagnosis of acute myocardial infarction.

In an effort to understand further the importance of time delay in primary angioplasty, it is helpful to examine the profile of infarct-related artery patency over time. As shown in Figures 4 and 5, the benefit of front-loaded t-PA as compared with SK is caused by more rapid early reperfusion, that is, between 60 and 180 minutes. After 180 minutes, current thrombolytic regimens appear to have equal rates of infarct-related artery patency. When one plots primary angioplasty on the same graph, one can see the importance of time in this reperfusion strategy. If the door to balloon time is rapid, for example, 60 minutes as in the First Primary Angioplasty in Myocardial Infarction Study (PAMI-I)[58] and the Netherlands Study,[59] this strategy compares favorably with thrombolytic regimens with infarct-related artery patency approaching 95%.[60] However, when the door to balloon time is over 2 hours, patency is achieved at the early time points in only a minority of patients.[61]

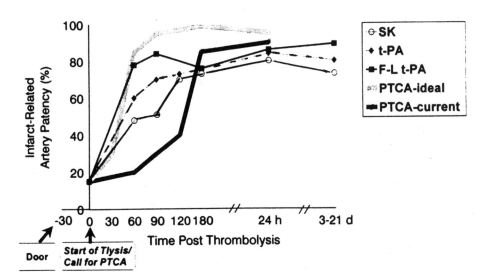

Figure 5. Patency profile of reperfusion strategies; importance of time to reperfusion. The infarct-related artery patency profile for different thrombolytic regimens, and primary angioplasty with different door to balloon times (F-L t-PA, front-loaded t-PA). Data for thrombolytic therapy are taken with permission from References 46, 54, and 61. Data for primary PTCA are taken with permission from References 58 and 62. Reprinted with permission from Reference 63.

References

1. Reimer KA, Lowe JE, Rasmussen MM, et al. The wavefront phenomenon of ischemic cell death. 1. Myocardial infarct size vs duration of coronary occlusion in dogs. *Circulation* 1977; 56:786.
2. Rentrop KP, Branke H, Karsch KR, et al. Coronary angiographic findings and left ventricular pump function in acute infarction and changes in the chronic stage infarction. *Z Kardiol* 1979;68:335–350.
3. Rentrop KP, Blanke H, Karsch KR, et al. Initial experience with transluminal recanalization of the recently occluded infarct-related coronary artery in acute myocardial infarction: Comparison with conventionally treated patients. *Clin Cardiol* 1979;2:92–105.
4. Fletcher AP, Akljaersio N, Smyrniotis FE, et al. Treatment of patients suffering from early myocardial infarction with massive and prolonged streptokinase therapy. *Trans Assoc Am Physicians* 1958;71:287–296.
5. Rentrop KP, Blanke H, Karsch KR, et al. Acute myocardial infarction: Intracoronary application of nitroglycerine and streptokinase. *Clin Cardiol* 1979;2:354–363.
6. DeWood MA, Spores J, Notske R, et al. Prevalence of total coronary occlusion during the early hours of transmural myocardial infarction. *N Engl J Med* 1980;303:897–902.
7. Kennedy JW, Ritchie JL, Davis KB, et al. Western Washington randomized trial of intracoronary streptokinase in acute myocardial infarction. *N Engl Med* 1983;309:1477–1482.
8. Kennedy JW, Ritchie JL, Davis KB, et al. Western Washington randomized trial of intracoronary streptokinase in acute myocardial infarction. A 12-month follow-up report. *N Engl Med* 1988;312:1073–1078.
9. Ritchie JL, Davis KB, Williams DL, et al. Global and regional left ventricular function and tomographic radionuclide perfusion: The Western Washington Intracoronary Streptokinase in Myocardial Infarction Trial. *Circulation* 1984;70:867–875.
10. Stampfer MJ, Goldhaber SZ, Yusuf S, et al. Effects of intravenous streptokinase on acute myocardial infarction: Results pooled from randomized trials. *N Engl J Med* 1982;307:1180–1182.
11. Gruppo Italiano per lo Studio della Streptochinase nell Infarto Miocardico (GISSI). Effectiveness of intravenous thrombolytic treatment in acute myocardial infarction. *Lancet* 1986; 1:397–402.
12. Gruppo Italiano per lo Studio della streptochi-nasi nell'Infarto Miocardico (GISSI). Long-term effects of intravenous thrombolysis in acute myocardial infarction: Final report of the GISSI study. *Lancet* 1987;ii:871–874.
13. Second International Study of Infarct Survival (ISIS-2) Collaborative Group. Randomised trial of intravenous streptokinase, oral aspirin, both, or neither among 17 187 cases of suspected acute myocardial infarction. *Lancet* 1988;ii:349–360.
14. Wilcox RG, von-der-Lippe G, Olsson CG, et al. Effects of alteplase in acute myocardial infarction: 6-month results from the ASSET study. Anglo-Scandinavian Study of the Early Thrombolysis. *Lancet* 1990;335:1175–1178.
15. AIMS Trial Study Group. Effect of intravenous APSAC on mortality after acute myocardial infarction: Preliminary report of a placebo-controlled clinical trial. *Lancet* 1988;I:545–549.
16. Meinertz T, Kasper W, Schumacher M, et al. The German multicenter trial of anisoylated plasminogen streptokinase activator complex versus heparin for acute myocardial infarction. *Am J Cardiol* 1988;62:347–351.
17. Fibrinolytic Therapy Trialists' Group. Indications for fibrinolytic therapy in suspected acute myocardial infarction: Collaborative overview of early mortality and major morbidity results from all randomised trials of more than 1000 patients. *Lancet* 1994;343:311–322.
18. Schofer J, Montz R, Mathey DG. Scintigraphic evidence of the "no reflow" phenomenon in human beings after coronary thrombolysis. *J Am Coll Cardiol* 1985;5:593–598.
19. Ito H, Tommoka T, Sakai N, et al. Lack of myocardial perfusion immediately after successful thrombolysis. A predictor of poor recovery of left ventricular function in anterior myocardial infarction. *Circulation* 1992;85:1699–1705.
20. The TIMI Study Group. The Thrombolysis in Myocardial Infarction (TIMI) Trial. Phase 1 findings. *N Engl J Med* 1985;312:932–936.

21. Rentrop KP, Feit F, Blanke H, et al. Effects of intracoronary streptokinase and intracoronary nitroglycerine infusion on coronary angiographic patterns and mortality in patients with acute myocardial infarction. *N Engl J Med* 1984;311:1457–1463.

22. Martin GV, Kennedy JW. Choice of thrombolytic agent. In: Julian DG, Bruanwald E, eds. *Management of Acute Myocardial Infarction*. Long, England: WB Saunders Co Ltd; 1994:71–105.

23. Gibbons RJ, Holmes DR, Reeder GS, et al. Immediate angioplasty compared with the administration of a thrombolytic agent followed by conservative treatment of myocardial infarction. The Mayo Coronary Care Unit and Catheterization Laboratory Groups. *N Engl J Med* 1993; 328:685–691.

24. Gibbons RJ. Perfusion imaging with ^{99m}Tc-sestamibi for the assessment of myocardial area at risk and the efficacy of acute treatment in myocardial infarction. *Circulation* 1991;84:137–142.

25. Christian TF, Behrenbeck T, Gersh BJ, et al. Relation of left ventricular volume and function over one year after acute myocardial infarction to infarct size determined by technetium-99m sestamibi. *Am J Cardiol* 1991;68:21–26.

26. Christian TF, Clements IP, Gibbons RJ. Noninvasive identification of myocardium at risk in patients with acute myocardial infarction and nondiagnostic electrocardiograms with technetium-99m-sestamibi. *Circulation* 1991;83:1615–1620.

27. Christian TF, Gibbons RJ, Gersh BJ. Effect of infarct location on myocardial salvage assessed technetium-99m isonitrile. *J Am Coll Cardiol* 1991;17:303–308.

28. Behrenbeck T, Pelikka PA, Huber KC, et al. Primary angioplasty in myocardial infarction: Assessment of improved myocardial perfusion with technetium-99m isonitrile. *J Am Coll Cardiol* 1991;17:365–372.

29. Christian TF, Behrenbeck T, Pelikka PA, et al. Mismatch of left ventricular function and infarct size demonstrated by technetium-99m isonitrile imaging after reperfusion therapy for acute myocardial infarction: Identification of myocardial stunning and hyperkinesia. *J Am Coll Cardiol* 1990;16:1632–1638.

30. Gibbons RJ, Verani MS, Behrenbeck T, et al. Feasibility of tomographic ^{99m}Tc-hexakis-2-methoxy-2-methylpropyl-isonitrile imaging for the assessment of myocardial area at risk and the effect of treatment in acute myocardial infarction. *Circulation* 1989;80:1277–1286.

31. Wackers FJ, Gibbons RJ, Verani MS, et al. Serial quantitative planar technetium-99m isonitrile imaging in acute myocardial infarction: Efficacy for noninvasive assessment of thrombolytic therapy. *J Am Coll Cardiol* 1989;14:861–873.

32. Bassand JP, Machecourt J, Cassagnes J, et al. Multicenter trial of intravenous anisoylated plasminogen streptokinase activator complex (APSAC) in acute myocardial infarction: Effects on infarct size and left ventricular function. *J Am Coll Cardiol* 1989;13:988–997.

33. Bassand JP, Cassagnes J, Machecourt J, et al. Comparative effects of APSAC and rt-PA on infarct size and left ventricular function in acute myocardial infarction. A multicenter randomized study. *Circulation* 1991;84:1107–1117.

34. Ritchie JL, Cerqueira M, Maynard C, et al. Ventricular function and infarct size: The Western Washington Intravenous Streptokinase in Myocardial Infarction Trial. *J Am Coll Cardiol* 1988;11:689–697.

35. Armstrong PW, Baigrie RS, Daly PA, et al. Tissue Plasminogen Activator: Toronto (TPAT) placebo controlled randomized trial in acute myocardial infarction. *J Am Coll Cardiol* 1989; 13:1469–1476.

36. Weaver WD, Cerqueira M, Hallstrom AP, et al. Prehospital-initiated vs hospital-initiated thrombolytic therapy. The Myocardial Infarction Triage and Intervention Trial. *JAMA* 1993; 270:1211–1216.

37. Althouse R, Maynard C, Cerqueira MD, et al. The Western Washington myocardial infarction registry and emergency department tissue plasminogen activator treatment trial. *Am J Cardiol* 1990;66:1298–1303.

38. Van-de-Werf F. Discrepancies between the effects of coronary reperfusion on survival and left ventricular function. *Lancet* 1989;i:1367–1369.

39. White HD, Norris RM, Brown MA, et al. Effect of intravenous streptokinase on left ventricular function and early survival after acute myocardial infarction. *N Engl J Med* 1987;317:850–855.

40. Van de Werf F, Arnold AER. Intravenous tissue plasminogen activator and size of infarct, left ventricular function, and survival in acute myocardial infarction. *Br Med J* 1988;297:1374–1379.

41. Dalen JE, Gore JM, Braunwald E, et al. Six- and twelve-month follow-up of the phase I thrombolysis in myocardial infarction (TIMI) trial. *Am J Cardiol* 1988;62:179–185.

42. Stadius ML, Davis K, Ritchie MC, et al. Risk stratification for 1 year survival based on characteristics identified in the early hours of acute myocardial infarction. *Circulation* 1986;74:703–711.

43. Van de Werf F. Thrombolysis for acute myocardial infarction: Why is there no extra benefit after hospital discharge? *Circulation* 1995;91:2862–2864.

44. Mathey DG, Sheehan FH, Schofer J, et al. Time from onset of symptoms to thrombolytic therapy: A major determinant of myocardial salvage in patients with acute transmural infarction. *J Am Coll Cardiol* 1985;6:518–525.

45. Verstraete M, Bernard R, Bory M, et al. Randomized trial of intravenous recombinant tissue type plasminogen activator versus intravenous streptokinase in acute myocardial infarction: Report from the European Study Group for Recombinant Tissue-type Plasminogen Activator. *Lancet* 1985;I:842–847.

46. Granger CB, Califf RM, Topol EJ. Reivew of thrombolytic therapy for acute myocardial infarction. *Drugs* 1992;44:293–325.

47. Gruppo Italiano per lo Studio della Sopravvivenza nell'Infarto Miocardico. GISSI-2: A factorial randomized trial of alteplase versus streptokinase and heparin versus no heparin among 12 490 patients with acute myocardial infarction. *Lancet* 1990;336:65–71.

48. The International Study Group. In-hospital mortality and clinical course of 20 891 patients with suspected acute myocardial infarction randomized between alteplase and streptokinase with or without heparin. *Lancet* 1990;336:71–75.

49. Third International Study of Infarct Survival (ISIS-3) Collaborative Group. ISIS-3: A randomized comparison of streptokinase vs tissue plasminogen activator vs anistreplase and of aspirin plus heparin vs aspirin alone among 41 299 cases of suspected acute myocardial infarction. *Lancet* 1993;339:753–770.

50. Prins MH, Hirsh J. Heparin as adjunctive treatment after thrombolytic therapy for acute myocardial infarction. *Am J Cardiol* 1991;67:3A–11A.

51. White HW. GISSI-2 and the heparin controversy. *Lancet* 199;336:297–298.

52. The GUSTO Investigators. An international randomized trial comparing four thrombolytic strategies for acute myocardial infarction. *N Engl J Med* 1993;329:673–682.

53. Lambrew CT. The National Heart Attack Alert Program: A review. *J Thromb* 1994;1:153–156.

54. The GUSTO Angiographic Investigators. The effects of tissue plasminogen activator, streptokinase, or both on coronary-artery patency, ventricular function, and survival after acute myocardial infarction. *N Engl J Med* 1993;329:1615–1622.

55. Simes RJ, Topol EJ, Holmes DR, et al. Link between the angiographic substudy and mortality outcomes in a large randomized trial of myocardial reperfusion. *Circulation* 1995;91:1923–1928.

56. Braunwald E. The open-artery theory is alive and well-again. *N Engl J Med* 1993;329:1630–1632.

57. Ryan TJ, Anderson JL, Antman EA, et al. ACC/AHA guidelines for the management of acute myocardial infarction. *J Am Coll Cardiol* 1996;28:1328–1428.

58. Grines CL, Browne KF, Marco J, et al. A comparison of immediate angioplasty with thrombolytic therapy for acute myocardial infarction: The Primary Angioplasty in Myocardial Infarction Study Group. *N Engl J Med* 1993;328:673–679.

59. Zijlstra F, de Boer MJ, Hoorntje JC, et al. A comparison of immediate coronary angioplasty with intravenous streptokinase in acute myocardial infarction. *N Engl J Med* 1993;328:680–684.

60. de Boer MJ, Suryapranata H, Hoorntje JCA, et al. Limitation of infarct size and preservation of left ventricular function after primary coronary angoplasty compared with intravenous streptokinase in acute myocardial infarction. *Circulation* 1994;90:753–761.

61. Cannon CP, McCabe CH, Diver DJ, et al. Comparison of front-loaded recombinant tissue-type plasminogen activator, anistreplase and combination thrombolytic therapy for acute myo-

cardial infarction: Results of the Thrombolysis in Myocardial Infarction (TIMI) 4 Trial. *J Am Coll Cardiol* 1994;24:1602–1610.

62. Cannon CP, Henry TD, Schweiger MJ, et al. Current management of ST elevation myocardial infarction and outcome of thrombolytic ineligible patients: Results of the multicenter TIMI 9 Registry. *J Am Coll Cardiol* 1995;(special issue):231A. Abstract.

63. Cannon CP, Braunwald E. Time to reperfusion: The critical modulator in thrombolysis in primary angioplasty *J Thromb Thrombolysis* 1996;3:117–125.

Part V.

Perfusion, Metabolism, and Cell Membrane Integrity

Introduction to Tracer Kinetics

Stephen L. Bacharach, PhD

Introduction

Nuclear cardiology is based on the ability to introduce a radiolabeled pharmaceutical into the body and to follow its distribution in the body with time. How the tracer distributes itself in the body with time depends first on delivery of the pharmaceutical to the tissue of interest (eg, by blood flow) and second on the physiology of that tissue, that is, on the physiological processes that are responsible for uptake or clearance of the tracer from the tissue of interest. It is these dependencies that make studying tracer kinetics so important. By following the uptake and clearance of the tracer (ie, by measuring its kinetic behavior) one hopes to determine some aspect of the physiological processes involved. The rate at which a tracer is taken up by (or cleared from) a certain volume of tissue may of course be dependent on flow, on diffusion, on relative solubilities of the tracer in blood and tissue, on a variety of active and passive cell membrane transport processes, on metabolic processes, etc. In nuclear cardiology we primarily look at static images of a distribution of radiotracer (eg, a Tl-201 scan), so we may forget that most radiopharmaceuticals have a quite complex temporal behavior, and that this behavior is related to many important physiological processes. If one can begin to understand how these physiological factors influence the kinetic behavior of the tracer, one also may begin to understand the physiological significance of even the static image. The purpose of this chapter is first to introduce, in an elementary and easy to understand way, how one can use knowledge of the underlying physiology to predict how a tracer will behave in the body with time and then, second, to show how to use this knowledge in reverse, that is, to see how one can use a measurement of the time behavior of a tracer in a tissue in order to predict what the underlying physiology must be. We will limit our discussion to a few quite simple, practical cases—cases that illustrate all the fundamental ideas and that will allow the reader to gain sufficient understanding to pursue a more detailed study on their own, using any of the large number of more advanced texts on the subject.[1-5] The principal model we will consider is that of measuring blood flow with inert, freely diffusable tracers. This model is worth understanding even if one is not interested in using such tracers, because the principles learned from this simple model are extended easily to more complicated situations.

Example of a Simple Model
(Inert and Freely Diffusable Tracers)

Some tracers undergo no metabolic reactions in the body at all; they simply arrive at the tissue and then distribute themselves and wash out according to blood flow and diffusion. Despite this simplistic behavior, these tracers can be quite valuable for making

From Dilsizian V (ed). *Myocardial Viability: A Clinical and Scientific Treatise.* Armonk, NY: Futura Publishing Co., Inc.; © 2000.

certain physiological measurements, especially for measuring blood flow. Some examples of such tracers are inert gases such as ^{133}Xe, ^{85}Krypton, and ^{15}O-labeled water. Water of course does take part in metabolic processes, but the accumulation and clearance of a bolus of injected water may be rapid enough (a few minutes), so that on this short a timescale, it too can be thought of as being inert. Obviously, because inert diffusable tracers do not take part in metabolic processes, their distribution and clearance will not be affected by metabolism, and so they cannot be used to measure metabolism. Instead, by looking at the manner in which they accumulate and clear, they can be used to measure relative or even absolute blood flow. To see how this can be done, consider Figure 1. Figure 1 illustrates an idealized model of a small volume of tissue being supplied with blood. The group of capillaries supplying this volume of tissue is, in the model of Figure 1, assumed to be supplied by a small vessel (eg, an arteriole) and the volume of tissue is in turn assumed to be drained by another small vessel (eg, a venule). A model such as the one in Figure 1, while quite simple, is probably also quite realistic for most "small" tissue volumes (we'll worry about what small means in a moment). If one were able to inject a bolus of an inert and freely diffusable tracer (eg, ^{15}O-labeled water, krypton, or xenon) directly into the small arteriole supplying this volume of tissue the sequence of events depicted in Figure 1(B)–(D) would occur. First, the bolus would travel down the arteriole, as shown in Figure 1(B). Next, the bolus would enter the small volume of tissue and distribute itself over this volume, as in Figure 1(C). Here it assumed that the volume is small enough so that the tracer diffuses throughout the volume instantaneously, where by "instantaneously" we mean simply in a time very short compared with the measurement time of the experiment (which in turn, as we will see shortly, is dictated by the flow rate we are trying to measure). Finally, as fresh blood enters the volume, it will dilute the tracer, which is distributed there, and the tracer will begin to wash out of the volume, as depicted in Figure 1(D). It seems fairly intuitive that the faster new, fresh blood enters the volume, the faster will be the rate of washout; that is, the washout rate will be faster for high flows than for low flows. It also seems fairly intuitive that for a given flow rate, if the volume of tissue were very large, it would take much longer for the tracer to wash out than

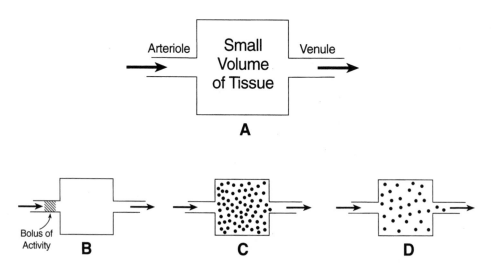

Figure 1. A: A simple model of a small volume of tissue, showing blood supplied by an incoming arteriole and removed by a venule. It is assumed that the tracer injected comes instantly into equilibrium in the tissue, hence the tissue volume is very small. **B:** A Bolus of activity has been injected into the arteriole, but has not yet arrived in the tissue. **C. And D:** The activity distributes itself in the volume, and then begins to leave the volume, and is replaced by fresh blood, diluting the remaining activity in the tissue.

if the volume of tissue were small. It is sometimes useful to restate the problem by imagining Figure 1 as a bucket with a hose attached that supplies water to the bucket and another hose that drains the bucket. The injected tracer might be a colored dye. The faster fresh water is made to flow into the bucket, the faster will any tracer (or dye) be diluted and wash out of the bucket. Similarly, if the bucket is very large, it will take a lot longer for the dye to wash out than if the bucket is small (for the same flow of water into the bucket).

The entire process described in Figure 1 can of course be stated quantitatively. Imagine that the amount of activity injected is Q_0 μCi. Assume that the volume of the tissue is V mL, and that the flow through the arteriole is F ml/min. When the Q_0 μCi enters the volume of tissue, it is assumed that it instantaneously is distributed in the tissue. If the tracer were ^{15}O-labeled water (H_2 ^{15}O), in the hose and bucket analogy, the concentration of tracer in the tissue would be Q_0 μCi distributed in a volume of V mL, or Q_0/V μCi/mL. Now in any short period of time dt, the amount of fluid carried away by the output pipe would be F times dt or $F * dt$. If the concentration in the bucket were Q/V at that time, then the amount of radioactivity removed in dt would be

$$\text{amount removed} = Q/V * F * dt \text{ microcuries.}$$

Note that the units in the above equation work out as they should (microcuries/milliliters * milliliters/minute * minute = microcuries).

Therefore the change in activity dQ in this time dt is

$$dQ = -(Q/V)Fdt. \tag{1}$$

where the minus sign simply signifies that it's a decrease in activity.

For the mathematically inclined reader, the solution to this equation can be obtained by integrating both sides (or by looking up the solution in a table) and is

$$\text{activity in bucket at time } t = Q(t) = Q_0 e^{-(F/V)t}; \tag{2}$$

that is, the activity falls exponentially as a function of time, with exponential constant F/V. Therefore if we injected an amount Q_0 into the bucket, the activity would fall exponentially.

To use this model to compute blood flow, one simply would monitor the count rate from the bucket versus time and plot on semilog paper. The slope would be F/V, that is, the flow per unit volume of tissue (well, per unit volume in the bucket in this case). Alternatively, a computer could be used to fit the plot of measured count rate from the bucket versus time, to compute the exponential constant (F/V).

One important factor needs to be considered to change this model from a model describing a bucket and hoses to one describing capillaries and tissue. In Figure 2 the model has been redrawn to emphasize that the "hoses" actually are vessels (capillaries inside the tissue) and that the volume V is composed of tissue. Although the tracer (H_2 ^{15}O in this case) is freely diffusable, water does not dissolve equally well in blood and soft tissue. Its solubility is slightly greater in blood than in soft tissue, so the concentration of activity being carried away by the capillaries is slightly higher than you might otherwise expect. If the concentration of tracer in tissue is Q/V, the concentration in the blood being removed will be $Q/\lambda V$, where λ is called the "partition coefficient" and simply is the relative solubility of the tracer in blood compared with tissue.

$$\lambda = (\text{solubility of tracer in tissue})/(\text{solubility of tracer in blood})$$

$$= {\sim}0.92 \text{ for water in myocardium compared to blood.}$$

This changes Equation (2) above to

$$Q(t) = Q_0 e^{-(F/\lambda V)t}. \tag{3}$$

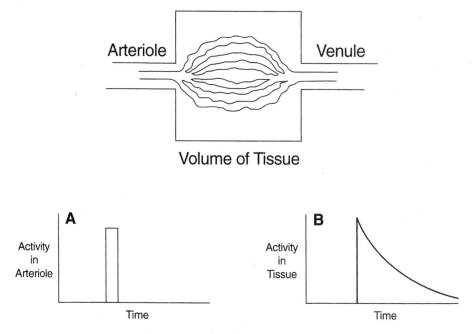

Figure 2. (**Top**) A more realistic representation of Figure 1(A). (**A**) Plot of the activity concentration seen by a detector over the arteriole, as a function of time, assuming a perfect bolus injection. (**B**) Plot of activity over the tissue as a function of time, showing the exponential washout as activity flows out the venule, and incoming fresh blood dilutes the activity remaining in the tissue.

Now lets look at the details of how the tracer concentration in the tissue behaves as time goes by. We will imagine putting a detector over the arteriole supplying the tissue and a second detector over the tissue. The detector over the arteriole will see nothing until the bolus goes by and then if the bolus is very narrow, it will for a brief instant see the counts from the Q_0-μCi bolus as it goes by and then nothing again. We are temporarily assuming that the bolus is "perfect"; that is, it's very narrow and has not spread out in time at all. Figure 2(A) shows the plot of count rate from the detector over the arteriole as a function of time [on the y axis of this plot, we have assumed that the detector could be calibrated to measure activity (eg, microcuries), instead of just counts per second]. The detector over the tissue [Figure 2(B)] will see no activity until the Q_0 μCi enters the tissue. At that time the count rate will instantly (since the bolus is assumed to be perfectly sharp) rise to a count rate corresponding to Q μCi. Thereafter, the count rate will fall exponentially with time, as described by Equation (3) above.

So far, the solution to the model shown in Figures 1 and 2 assumes a perfect bolus injection administered directly to the tissue of interest (eg, the myocardium), a situation that cannot really be attained in practice. Instead, one usually injects intravenously. Even if this intravenous injection is a sharp bolus, by the time the activity reaches the right heart, traverses the lungs, and is ejected by the left ventricle, the bolus will be quite spread out. Figure 3(A) illustrates what the detector over the arteriole in Figure 2 would show when a venous "bolus" injection is administered. This plot of activity entering the tissue versus time is called the "input function." If the input function is not a bolus, none of the above equations will be correct. New tracer will keep entering the tissue even as old tracer is washing out. This problem can be solved easily as follows. We know Equation (3) works for a bolus injection into the arteriole, that is, a bolus input function that looks like Figure 2(A). An actual input function might look like Figure 3(A). We can think of Figure 3(A) as being made up

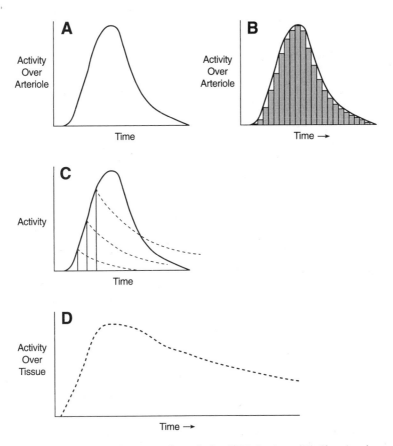

Figure 3. (**A**) A realistic input function after a bolus IV injection. (**B**) Showing how the input function in (A) can be thought of as a sum of many perfect bolus injections. (**C**) Each of the idealized bolus injections in (B) will produce an exponential decay in the tissue. (**D**) The sum of all the exponential decays in (C) will look as shown here.

of a large number of perfect bolus injections, as shown in Figure 3(B). Each of these bolus injections would produce an exponential time versus activity curve from the tissue that would look like that in Figure 2(B). Therefore, the actual tissue uptake and clearance curve would be a sum of all the exponentials produced by all the bolus injections, as shown in Figure 3(C) and (D). Just as we could use the measured tissue versus time curve to determine F/V with a perfect bolus injection, so too can we use the measured tissue versus time curve to measure flow in the case of an input function that looks like Figure 3(A). It would be tedious to do it with a paper and pencil, but it would be quite possible. One would plot the measured tissue curve and then take the measured input function and take a guess at an F/V value. Draw in the exponentials representing this value of F/V as in Figure 3(C), add them together as in Figure 3(D), and compare the result with the actual measured tissue curve. Figure 4 illustrates this process. In Figure 4(B) the data points represent actual measured tissue values (eg, as might be obtained from a region of the myocardium). The input function is assumed to be the one shown in Figure 4(A). One first takes a guess as to what F/V is (it doesn't matter if this guess is wrong; it's just a guess). Now using the measured input function of Figure 4(A), we draw, as in Figure 3(C), all the exponents with that particular value of F/V. Sum all the exponential curves together, and the result might be the solid curve in Figure 4(B). Clearly, this curve does not fit the data

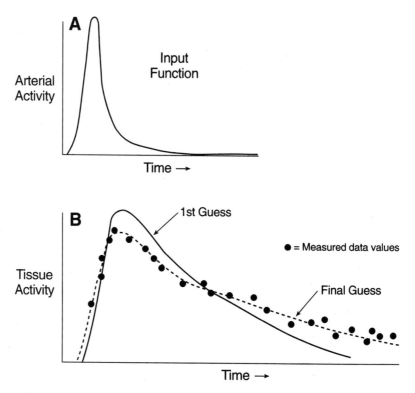

Figure 4. (**A**) A typical input function. (**B**) Solid circles represent the values of tissue activity as a function of time, as measured from a region of interest (ROI) over the actual dynamic images. The solid line represents a guess of the predicted tissue curve, based on a first guess for a flow value, which will describe the data shown by the solid circles. This guess obviously is too high a flow value, because the solid curve falls off too rapidly. After many improvements on these guesses, one would end up with the guess shown by the dashed line, resulting in a flow value that fits the measured data quite well.

very well. It drops too fast; that is, the value guessed for F/V must be too big. Another slightly smaller value then could be tried this time. By trying many guesses for F/V, the one that gave the best fit [as in the dashed line in Fig. 4(B)] of the summed exponentials to the actual measured data would be the optimum value of F/V. Clearly, although one could, with enough time, determine flow this way, the computer could do the job much faster. The computer does this computation in almost the same way as we described it being done manually, except an optimized method can be used to refine the guesses so as to converge rapidly to the best fit. The process of summing the exponential curves formed by pretending the input function is made up of many bolus injections (eg, Fig. 3) is called "convolving" the exponentials with the input function. This whole process can be expressed mathematically as follows:

$$\text{tissue curve} = Q(t) = F(A * e^{-(F/\lambda V)t}), \tag{4}$$

where $A(t)$ is the concentration of activity in the arriving blood, that is, the arterial input function; and the symbol * represents the convolution, that is, the adding together of all the exponentials weighted with the input function. Comparing Equation (3) and this Equation (4), one other difference (aside from the convolution term) stands out. How did the flow F replace the amount of injected activity, Q_0? The Q_0 term just expressed the amount of activity going into the tissue. All of it went in at once because it was a bolus. For the case of a real injection, the amount arriving at the tissue is the concentration of activity in the incoming blood $A(t)$ times the rate at which blood flows into the tissue F. Because positron emission tomography (PET) cameras [and with proper corrections, single photon emission computer tomography (SPECT) cameras] measure concentrations of activity rather than absolute amounts of activity, usually both sides of Equation (3) are divided by V. If we divide both sides of Equation (3) by V and let $q(t)$ stand for the measured concentration of activity (so $q(t) = Q(t)/V$)] then the above equation becomes

$$\text{tissue concentration curve} = q(t) = (F/V)(A(t) * e^{-(F/\lambda V)t}). \tag{5}$$

Practical Issues of Applying Kinetic Models to Cardiac Studies

We will continue to discuss the simple model of measuring flow with H_2 ^{15}O and now begin to worry about some of the real practicalities involved in making the measurement. Again, we will stick with the H_2 ^{15}O model not because it is of particular clinical importance, but rather because it illustrates very well, in a simple way, all the practical complications of kinetic modeling and how one goes about solving them.

Measuring the Arterial Input Function

To measure flow using the model of Equation (5), one must measure the tissue activity concentration as a function of time and the input function as a function of time (in fact, these two measurements are needed for the majority of kinetic models). Because the input function is the concentration of activity in the arteriole supplying the tissue, it need not be measured with a detector as shown in Figure 2. The arterial concentration is the same in all arterial vessels (apart from a small time delay) and also is equal to the concentration of activity in the left side of the heart. There are several ways to determine the arterial input function. The arterial concentration could be measured by repeatedly sampling blood from an arterial catheter. This is a somewhat invasive method, although it has been the method of choice for years in brain studies performed with PET. Alternatively, some radiotracers are taken up very slowly by tissue, and in that case, one often can give a slower injection and assume that venous samples may be substituted for arterial ones. Often, however, this assumption is not valid. For cardiac studies with PET, or more recently with fast SPECT cameras, it is possible to use the images of the left ventricular (LV) and left atrial cavities to measure the input function. Figure 5 shows a single transaxial image of the heart at various times after injection of a bolus of H_2 ^{15}O into the antecubital vein. One can see sequentially, first the right ventricle and then the left ventricle (most of the lungs are out of the field of view), and finally a more uniform distribution as the water diffuses into the tissues (especially the myocardium). By placing a region of interest (ROI) over the left atrium and basalar portion of the left ventricle, it is possible to measure the arterial input function. Only the basalar portion of the LV cavity should be used, to avoid possible contamination of the input function with activity from the myocardium itself (which may contract more vigorously at the midventricular and apical levels). Figure 6(A) and (B) shows an appropriate ROI placed on the heart and the resulting arterial input function. In practice ROIs are drawn on several adjacent slices and the data averaged together. It is the result of this process that is shown in Figure

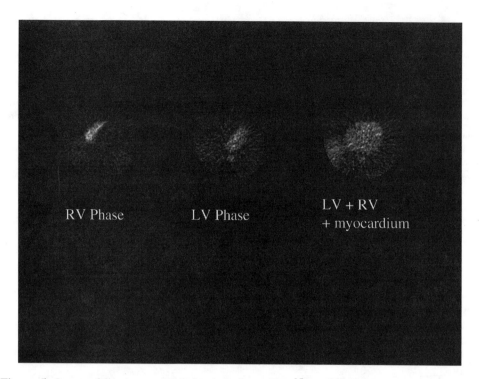

RV Phase

LV Phase

LV + RV
+ myocardium

Figure 5. Images following an IV bolus injection of $H_2\ ^{15}O$. The first image represents data accumulated during the first 10 or 15 seconds after injection. Almost all the activity is concentrated in the right ventricular (RV) phase. The second image in the sequence was made by adding all the data from time of injection to approximately 45 seconds. By the end of this time, activity also is seen clearly in the left ventricular (LV) phase. Finally, the last image in the sequence is the image made from data from 1 to 2 minutes postinjection. The water has been delivered to the myocardium and is roughly in equilibrium with the arterial concentration; so the LV, RV, and myocardium all show up as bright areas in the image, making distinguishing the myocardium nearly impossible.

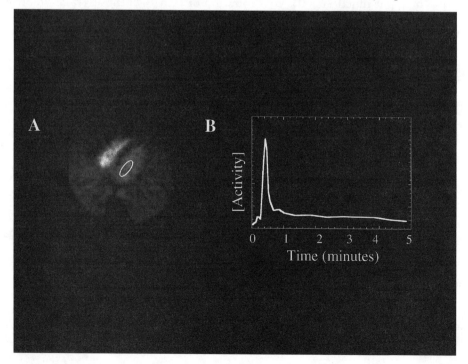

Figure 6. (**A**) Showing a small ROI drawn in the LV and left atrium. (**B**) The arterial input function obtained from the region drawn in (A) (averaged with similar regions on two other slices), following a bolus injection of $H_2\ ^{15}O$.

6(B). This noninvasive method for measuring the arterial input function has been found to agree quite well with direct arterial sampling.[6,7]

Measuring the Tissue Time Activity Curve

The measurement of the tissue time activity curve is made easily by placing an ROI over the portion of the myocardium of interest. For most tracer studies, defining the myocardial ROI is quite straightforward. One simply draws regions on the myocardial images when uptake of the tracer by the myocardium is maximal. The difficulty for H_2 ^{15}O water studies is that water doesn't produce a distinguishable image of the myocardium. By the time the tracer has diffused into the myocardium, its concentration in the myocardium is about the same as that in the blood pool (eg, as in the last panel of Fig. 5), making the myocardium indistinguishable from the LV cavity. Most other tracers [^{18}F-2-deoxyglucose (FDG), ^{201}Thallium, ^{99}Tc-MIBI, etc] don't have this problem because these tracers concentrate in the myocardium and clear from the blood. An easy way around the problem (and a way that can enhance the myocardial image for many other tracers) is to subtract a fraction of the early image (when the image is dominated by right ventricular [RV] and LV cavity activity) from the late image (when the image is a combination of LV cavity activity and myocardial activity). The resulting image is (approximately) myocardium alone. Figure 7 illustrates the procedure for our H_2 ^{15}O study. When the early phase of the water image [Fig. 7(B); containing RV and LV] is scaled appropriately and subtracted from the late phase

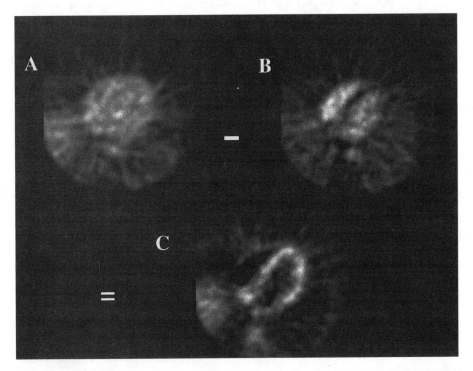

Figure 7. (**A** and **B**) Showing the early and late phases of the H_2 ^{15}O images, just as in Figure 5(B) and (C). When these two images are scaled and subtracted from each other the resultant image is as shown in (C). (**C**)This image gives an approximate representation of the myocardium, which can be used to draw myocardial ROIs to produce tissue time activity curves.

[Fig. 7(A); containing RV, LV, and myocardium], the resulting image [Fig. 7(C)] contains primarily myocardium. Although the image in Figure 7(C) is only an approximate representation of the myocardium, it often is good enough to be used to define ROIs for the purpose of measuring the tissue time activity curve. Alternatively, some researchers have used an additional blood pool scan, using labeled carbon monoxide ($C^{15}O$), an excellent red blood cell tag.[6] The blood pool image then can be used to subtract out the blood pool component from the late water image and, as discussed below, can be used to correct for a phenomenon called "spillover."

Correction for Spillover and Partial Volume Effects

No matter how good the definition of the myocardial ROI is, there almost always will be the possibility of some spillover of activity in the LV cavity to the myocardial ROI. This is true for two reasons. First, because no matter what the tracer, the entire injected dose must pass through the cavity, while only a small fraction of the dose ultimately makes its way into the myocardium (remember that only approximately 3%–5% of the cardiac output goes to the myocardium). Second, the resolution of even the best nuclear scanner is only approximately 5 mm or so, while the myocardial wall usually is approximately 10 mm (and can be much thinner in pathological situations). Thus partial volume effects, caused by the finite resolution of the scanner compared with the size of the object (10 mm), cause counts from the LV cavity to blur or spillover into the myocardial ROI.[8,9] This effect is illustrated in Figure 8, in which the early images of the heart are shown for a perfect scanner on the top and for a scanner with a more realistic resolution on the bottom. The result of this spillover is that the

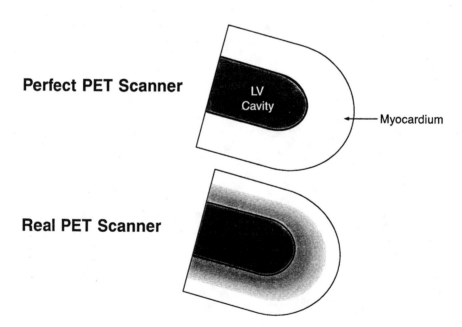

Figure 8. (**Top**) An image of the heart from an ideal scanner, with perfect resolution, showing activity primarily in the LV cavity. (**Bottom**) The same image, but imaged using a scanner with more realistic resolution. Now intensity (ie, counts) from the LV cavity will "blur" into the myocardium, causing myocardial tissue time activity curves to be contaminated with arterial activity.

myocardial tissue curve is "contaminated" by containing some counts from the LV cavity. The tissue curve will appear not as in Figure 4(B) but instead as a sum of the curves in Figure 4(B) plus a fraction of the curve in Figure 4(A). The larger the contamination, the larger the fraction of the arterial curve [Fig. 4(A)] will be added to the underlying tissue curve. There are several solutions to this problem. The solution we shall explore here is to try to use the model itself to compensate for this contamination.[10,11] This is easy to do and illustrates a useful general principle in kinetic modeling, namely, inclusion not only of physiology in the model, but inclusion also of imperfections in the scanner (ie, its finite resolution) and imperfections in our ability to draw perfect ROIs.

The usual way to measure flow with Equation (5) is to use a computer to fit the measured myocardial tissue activity curve [Fig. 4(B)] to Equation (5). However, we now recognize that the measured myocardial tissue curve actually is the sum of the true myocardial tissue curve plus some unknown fraction of the input function. That is, some unknown fraction S of the counts in the LV cavity will spill over into the myocardial ROI. Therefore we must modify Equation (5) to include this spillover.

measured myocardial activity = true myocardial activity + spillover

$$M(t) = q(t) + S * (\text{input function}),$$

where S is the (unknown) fraction of counts from the LV cavity, which spill over into the myocardial ROI. Therefore Equation (5) becomes

$$M(t) = (F/V)(A(t) * e^{-(F/\lambda V)t}) + (S)A(t). \tag{6}$$

The computer now has a slightly more complicated equation to fit, with one additional unknown term, the fraction of counts S, spilling over from the LV cavity into the myocardial ROI. In general, the more unknowns the computer is asked to determine, the larger will be the standard deviations in the estimates of these unknowns. However, for this particular case, this is not completely true, because not only are there more unknowns to compute, there also are more data, that is, the extra counts from the counts that have spilled over and the knowledge of $A(t)$. It has even been suggested that one might intentionally draw the ROI so as to overlap partially into the LV cavity,[12] thereby enhancing that part of the data that permits computation of S.

One final addition to our kinetic model might be considered—a modification that again would be valuable no matter what the tracer or model. Even if there were no activity in the LV cavity to spill over into the myocardial ROI, how the myocardial ROI was drawn could affect the results. This is because what is measured in an ROI is the tissue activity concentration. Therefore if one draws the ROI too large, the mean value in the ROI will be too low.[9] Usually, this is thought of as being caused by the finite resolution of the scanner, that is, to the so-called "partial volume" effect.[8,9] That is, even if one drew an ROI that exactly matched the true myocardial anatomical borders, the finite resolution of the scanner would cause some of the counts within those borders to be blurred outside of the ROI, reducing the value within the ROI. The result of this partial volume effect is that the myocardial portion of the measured tissue time activity curve is reduced by an unknown fraction that we'll call P (for the partial volume effect). The equation that the computer must fit then becomes

$$M(t) = P(F/V)(A(t) * e^{-(F/\lambda V)t}) + (S)A(t). \tag{7}$$

Now our computer program must solve not only for flow per unit volume (F/V), but also for the spillover fraction S and for the partial volume correction factor P.

We have seen then that kinetic models can permit us to predict not just how physiology will influence our measurement of tissue uptake and clearance, but also how some of the physical limitations of our measurement device (the PET or SPECT scanner) can affect the measurements. By suitable inclusion of both physiology and technical factors in the model, one can use kinetic data to make accurate measurements of physiological parameters even in the presence of technical limitations.

More Complicated Models

The model described in detail above often is referred to as a "one-compartment" model, because, as can be seen from Figure 1, there only was one tissue compartment (ie, the box in Fig. 1). We will not dwell on more complex models in this chapter, except to note briefly that they are relatively straightforward (albeit mathematically messy) extensions of the simple one-compartment model. Instead of just one input pipe and one output pipe, as in Figure 1, the box in Figure 1 may be connected to a second box, which may in turn be connected to a third box, etc. Each of the boxes (or compartments) is included only if one can ascribe some physiological significance to it and each compartment usually is connected bidirectionally to its adjacent compartment (unless some physiological restriction is known to prevent transport in one of the directions). For example, Figure 9 shows a model containing three compartments. This model has been used for many different tracers, with each of the three compartments representing different physiological components depending on the tracer and the organ being studied. The model in Figure 9 has been used to described the uptake and washout of ^{201}Tl, in which case compartment A represented the arterial blood, compartment B the interstitial space, and compartment C the myocardial cells. All the arrows shown in Figure 9 were allowable in this model, indicating bidirectional exchange between the arterial supply and the interstitial space and both sequestration and release from the myocardial cells. Alternatively, Figure 9 is used widely to represent the uptake of FDG. In this case, box A might represent FDG in the plasma of the extracellular space, box B the FDG in the myocardial cells, and box C the phosphorylated FDG in the cells. Once FDG has been phosphorylated it usually is assumed that it can no longer be dephosphorylated back to FDG, so the arrow representing k4 (the arrow going from box C to box B in Fig. 9) would not need to be present. Exactly how these more complicated models are solved (and how one determines how to use the known physiology to create the model) is left for more advanced texts.[1–3,5,13] Basically, however, the equations are just extensions of those in Equations (1)–(7). Just as with our simple water blood flow model, the solution to the equations often are based on sums of exponentials.

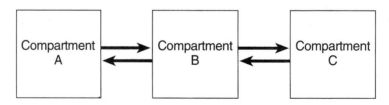

Figure 9. A three-compartment model, showing possible exchange of radiotracer bidirectionally between all three compartments.

Quantitating Myocardial Uptake

Some tracers, like Tc-MIBI or even (for times short compared with redistribution) Tl-201, can be thought of as nearly like microspheres. To a first approximation, their uptake is independent of how much tracer already might be in the myocardium, and once there a large fraction of the delivered dose "sticks" to the myocardium; that is, once taken up by the myocardium, they are not released (or released only slowly compared with the imaging time). In such cases it often is useful to be able to quantify the amount of tracer taken up in a manner so as to be able to compare the tracer uptake in one region of the heart with the uptake in the same region under different physiological conditions. For example, one might wish to compare Tl or MIBI uptake when the compound is injected at stress with the uptake of the same region when the compound is injected at rest. This is not the comparison that usually is made between regions at stress and rest. The usual comparison is performed by normalizing all the regions in the stress image, for example, to one particular region (eg, one thought to be "normal"). Then the rest image is normalized similarly and the comparisons are made between these normalized values. Such a comparison completely masks any absolute differences in uptake that may occur between stress and rest. For example, if the total amount of MIBI in a particular region is twice as great at stress than at rest, this fact is not evident from the usual normalization. At first one might think such a computation would be impossible without being able to quantify absolute myocardial uptake. This is not so. Even if the data are from "nonquantitative" SPECT imaging (eg, no attenuation correction, no correction for scatter, etc), it is possible to make such comparisons (at least approximately) if one can measure the input function. The corrections for attenuation, etc, to a first approximation can be ignored, because in general, whatever their effects are at rest, they are the same at stress (or during any other pair of physiological conditions). Why is the input function needed to make this comparison? Because without it, the result would depend not just on the differences in function of the myocardium between the two physiological conditions, but also on the function of all other organs in the body between these two conditions. Imagine that one had injected the same activity at rest as at stress. If at rest the liver (or any other organ) took up much more activity than at stress, then far less of the activity would be available to the myocardium at rest. That is, the amount of tracer available to the myocardial tissue depends on the concentration of tracer in the arterial blood supplying the myocardium. If that concentration falls rapidly with time because of uptake by the liver or clearance by the kidneys, then less activity will be available to the myocardium itself. The total amount of tracer available to the myocardium is not determined solely by the injected dose. Instead it is determined by the concentration of the tracer in the arterial supplying the myocardium. This is what determines how much tracer each cell perfused by that blood "sees." Because the arterial concentration changes with time (and presumably the flow does not, at least not during the uptake period), we must normalize our Tl or MIBI images by dividing by the area under the arterial curve, that is by the integral of the arterial input function. This concept is illustrated in Figure 10. As yet, this procedure is used only in PET studies. However, in the future, it may well be possible to quantitate the arterial input function from SPECT studies. Note again that absolute quantitation of the arterial input function is not required; only relative quantitation is required. That is, whatever errors are made (because of no attenuation correction, etc) are assumed to exist equally for both injections (eg, rest and stress). In this way the ratio of stress-to-rest uptake can be preserved.

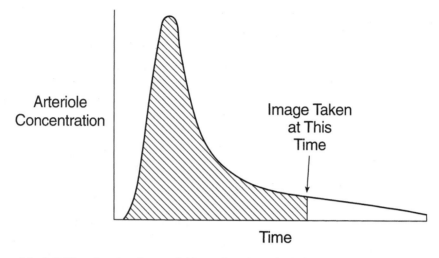

Figure 10. Solid line showing the arterial input function. Shaded area represents the integral (ie, area under the curve) from time 0 up to the imaging time. If stress injection images and rest injection images were normalized to this area, it would be possible to compare rest and stress uptake.

References

1. Bassingthwaighte JB, Holloway GA. Estimation of blood flow with radioactive tracers. *Semin Nucl Med* 1976;6:141–161.
2. Carson RE. The development and application of mathematical models in nuclear medicine. *J Nucl Med* 1991;32:2206–2208.
3. Carson RE. Mathematical modeling, and compartmental analysis. In: Harbert WCEJC , Neumann RD, eds. *Nuclear Medicine Diagnosis, and Therapy.* New York: Thieme; 1996:167–193.
4. Huang S-C, Phelps ME. Principles of tracer kinetic modeling in positron emission tomography and autoradiography. In: *Positron Emission Tomography and Autoradiography.* Phelps ME, Mazziotta JC, Schelbert HR, eds. New York: Raven Press; 1986:237–286.
5. Lassen NA, Perl W. *Tracer Kinetic Methods in Medical Physiology.* New York: Raven Press; 1979.
6. Bergmann SR. Noninvasive quantitation of myocardial blood-flow in human-subjects with oxygen-15-labeled water and positron emission tomography. *J Am Coll Cardiol* 1989;14:639–652.
7. Iida H. Use of the left-ventricular time-activity curve as a noninvasive input function in dynamic oxygen-15-water positron emission tomography. *J Nucl Med* 1992;33:1669–1677.
8. Hoffman EJ, Huang S-C, Phelps ME. Quantitation in positron emission computed tomography, 1. Effect of object size. *J Comput Assist Tomogr* 1979;3:299–308.
9. Bacharach SL. Image analysis. In: Henry J, Wagner N, eds. *Principles of Nuclear Medicine.* Philadelphia, Pa: W.B. Saunders; 1995:393–404.
10. Herrero P, Markham J, Bergmann SR. Quantitation of myocardial blood-flow with (H$_2$O)–O-15 and positron emission tomography—Assessment and error analysis of a mathematical approach. *J Comput Assis Tomogr* 1989;13:862- 873.
11. Iida H. Measurement of absolute myocardial blood-flow with (H$_2$O)–O-15 and dynamic positron-emission tomography—Strategy for quantification in relation to the partial-volume effect. *Circulation* 1988;78:104–115.
12. Hutchins GD, Caraher JM, Raylman RR. A region of interest strategy for minimizing resolution distortions in quantitative myocardial pet studies. *J Nucl Med* 1992;33:1243–1250.
13. Jacquez JA. *Compartmental Analysis in Biology, and Medicine.* Holland, Amsterdam: Elsevier/ North; 1972.

Thallium-201 Scintigraphy:

Experience of Two Decades

Vasken Dilsizian, MD

Introduction

The application of radioactive tracers for cardiac evaluation offers the unique opportunity of measuring physiological parameters, noninvasively, as an adjunct to anatomical information. Numerous advances in radiopharmaceuticals and instrumentation over the last decades has improved our understanding of myocardial perfusion, contraction, and metabolism in various cardiovascular diseases.

Historical Background

The first application of radioactive tracers dates back to 1927, when Blumgart and Weiss examined the pulmonary circulation time in normal subjects with radon, using a cloud chamber as the radiation detection device.[1] In 1957, Love and Burch were able to measure tracer concentration in the heart, lungs, and blood, after intravenous administration of ionic rubidium using a single probe placed over the chest.[2] In 1964, Ross and colleagues examined coronary blood flow by injecting xenon directly in the coronary arteries and measuring precordial activity of xenon.[3] This approach minimized the potential of background activity from the lungs, chest wall, and intracavity blood pool interfering with the measurements of coronary blood flow. However, despite advances in the application of tracer technique, the spatial resolution of the instruments was inadequate for identifying patients with significant coronary artery narrowing. In 1972, using a multicrystal scintillation camera and intracoronary injection of xenon, Cannon and coworkers were able to demonstrate alterations in regional blood flow under basal condition in patients with coronary artery disease.[4] While some investigators were applying regional inert gas clearance method with xenon and kryton for making measurement of coronary perfusion, others were injecting macroaggregated albumin or microsphere into the coronary arteries for evaluation of regional perfusion.[5,6] Extensive studies using macroaggregated particulates in human subjects was shown to be safe, without hemodynamic sequelae, as long as the size of particles was kept below 50 μm and less than 50 000 particles were injected into the coronary arteries.[7] In 1974, Gould and coworkers intro-

From Dilsizian V (ed). *Myocardial Viability: A Clinical and Scientific Treatise.* Armonk, NY: Futura Publishing Co., Inc.; © 2000.

duced the concept that by studying alterations in regional blood flow in the basal state as well as during coronary vasodilation, hemodynamic significance of a coronary artery narrowing can be determined.[8]

Intravenously Injected Ionic Tracers

Myocardial perfusion can be assessed by several monovalent cations that may have similar biological properties, such as potassium, rubidium, and thallium, but diverse physical properties in terms of physical half-life and the number and energies of photons emitted. Myocardial uptake of potassium and rubidium was first demonstrated by Love and coworkers in 1954 with subsequent development of improved collimator by the same authors to image the myocardial distribution of potassium-42 in 1966.[9,10]

Because potassium is the major intracellular cation in muscle and is virtually absent in scar tissue, it is a particularly well-suited radionuclide for differentiating normal and ischemic but viable myocardium from fibrotic or scarred myocardium. Earlier studies had shown an association between abnormalities in regional potassium metabolism and acute myocardial injury. In animals studied under conditions of (1) normal flow, (2) ischemia

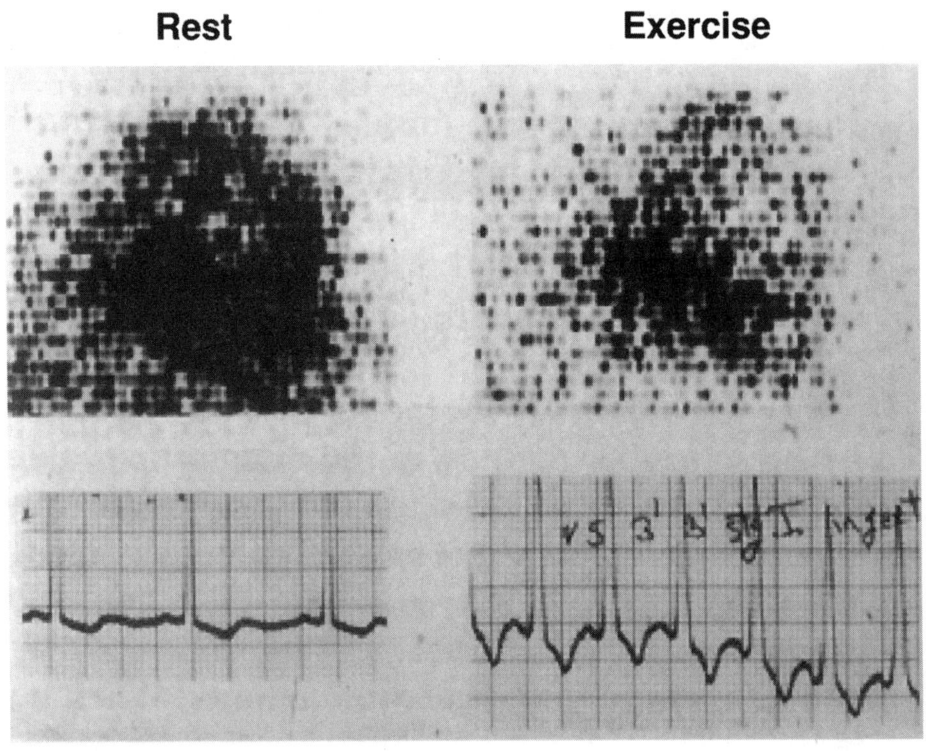

Rest   **Exercise**

Figure 1. Potassium-43 myocardial images obtained in the anterior view at rest (**left**) and with exercise (**right**) to point of angina pectoris using planar imaging. The electrocardiogram (ECG) at the time of administration of potassium-43 is below each image. There is decreased radionuclide accumulation in the anterior wall during stress but not present at rest. Coronary arteriography showed proximal narrowing of the left anterior descending and left circumflex coronary arteries. Modified and reprinted with permission from Reference 12.

(partial occlusion of coronary artery and pacing), and (3) infarction (total occlusion of a coronary artery), a linear relationship was demonstrated between the distribution of potassium-43 and microspheres.[11] These studies in animals spurred the application of potassium in humans to detect coronary artery disease and myocardial injury. In clinical studies, the combination of exercise treadmill testing with potassium-43 imaging was able to identify patients with angina pectoris and myocardial territories supplied by significantly narrowed coronary arteries[12,13] (Fig. 1). However, the relatively high-energy γ-spectrum of potassium-43 (373–619 keV) created image degradation and resolution problems in terms of routine clinical application of potassium-43 with Anger-type scintillation cameras for detection of coronary artery disease. At the present time, Anger-type scintigraphic cameras, which are used widely in most nuclear medicine laboratories, have a 1.25-cm-thick sodium iodide crystal as the photon detector. Because of the nature of the crystal, the optimum combination of efficiency and resolution is obtained with tracers emitting 100 to 200-keV energies. Furthermore, the collimators most commonly used in nuclear laboratories provide the optimum combination of resolution and sensitivity with lower-energy photons.

Thallium-201 has biological properties similar to potassium-43 but with lower photon energy (80 keV mercury X-ray emission) and shorter physical half-life (74 hours). Although the energy spectrum of thallium is somewhat lower than optimal for conventional scintillation cameras [ideal photopeak in the range of 140 keV, like technetium-99m (^{99m}Tc)], it overcomes some of the limitations of potassium-43[14–16] (Fig. 2). The photon energies of thallium are low enough to be well collimated and to allow high-efficiency detection with the 1.25-cm-thick sodium iodide crystal of most Anger-type scintillation cameras. These favorable physical and biological properties of

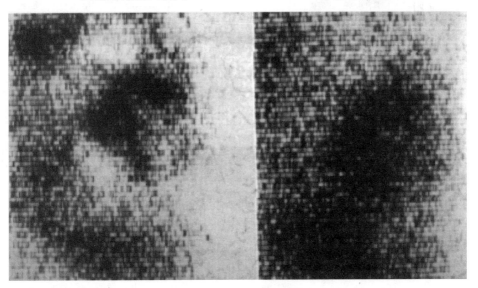

Thallium-201   **Potassium-43**

Figure 2. Myocardial perfusion image with thallium-201 (**left**) and potassium-43 (**right**) in a dog with ligation of the left anterior descending coronary artery. The apical defect can be seen with both tracers, but is better defined on the thallium image. Modified and reprinted with permission from Reference 13.

thallium-201 propelled the clinical application of myocardial imaging in many hospitals.

Physiology of Myocardial Thallium Uptake

For the last two decades, thallium has been a clinically important tracer with which to assess both regional blood flow and myocardial viability. Support for the application of thallium for the evaluation of myocardial perfusion and viability comes from observations in animal models of acute myocardial ischemia in which abnormalities in transmyocardial potassium flux have been observed. Experimental studies have shown progressive decrease of potassium/sodium ratio after coronary artery occlusion.[17] These findings in animals also were described in man, in association with angina pectoris produced by atrial pacing. Furthermore, because the uptake and retention of thallium by myocardial cells is an active process, thallium scintigraphy has the unique potential for distinguishing viable from nonviable myocardium with greater precision than can be achieved by the assessment of regional anatomy or function alone.

Initial Thallium Uptake

Myocardial uptake early after intravenous injection of thallium is proportional to regional blood flow with a high first-pass extraction fraction in the range of 85% with rapid clearance from the intravascular compartment by peripheral tissue extraction.[18] Myocardial extraction of thallium is dependent on energy utilization, membrane adenosine triphosphatase (ATPase), and active transport. Thallium-201 is a monovalent cation that is transported across the myocyte sarcolemmal membrane via the Na-K ATPase transport system and by facilitative diffusion.[19,20] Peak myocardial concentration of thallium generally is within 5 minutes of intravenous injection. Thallium extraction is linearly proportional at normal or low levels of myocardial blood flow (MBF),[21] whereas thallium extraction rises proportionally less at higher blood flow values.[22] Experimental studies with thallium have demonstrated that the cellular extraction of thallium across the cell membrane is unaffected by hypoxia unless irreversible injury is present.[23,24] Similarly, pathophysiological conditions of chronic hypoperfusion (hibernating myocardium) and postischemic dysfunction (stunned myocardium), in which regional contractile function is impaired in the presence of myocardial viability, do not adversely alter extraction of thallium.[25–27] Thus, intracellular uptake of thallium across the sarcolemmal membrane is maintained for as long as sufficient blood flow is present to deliver thallium to the myocardial cell. Thallium does not actively concentrate in regions of infarcted or scarred myocardium. Therefore, decreased myocardial uptake early after thallium injection could be caused either by reduced regional blood flow or infarction.

Thallium Redistribution

Although the initial distribution of thallium primarily is a function of blood flow, the later distribution (redistribution) of thallium over a 3- to 4-hour period is a function of regional blood volume and is unrelated to flow.[28] Redistribution of thallium begins within 10–15 minutes after injection[29] and is prolonged in regions of hypoperfusion[30] and is related to the rate of thallium clearance from the blood.[31] The rate of thallium clearance from myocardial segments is linked to the concentration gradient across the myocytes and the blood such that thallium clearance is more rapid from normal myocardial segments with high-thallium activity when compared with myocardial segments with reduced thallium activity (Fig. 3). This phenomenon is known as differential washout. In animal studies, redistribution on a delayed image was shown to represent reduced thallium concentration in normal segments along with increased thallium concentration in ischemic segments.[28,32,33] Clearance of thallium from the normal myocardium mirrored the thallium clearance from the blood while in ischemic segments there was slow accumulation of the tracer from the recirculating thallium within the blood.[32,33] Thus, myocardial concentration of thallium changes over time. During the redistribution phase, there is a continuous exchange of thallium between the myocardium and the extracardiac compartments, driven by the concentration gradient of the radiotracer and myocyte viability. Thus, the extent of defect resolution, from the initial to delayed redistribution images over time, termed reversible defect, reflects one index of myocardial viability. When only scarred myocardium is present, the degree of the initial thallium defect persists over time without redistribution, termed irreversible defect. When both viable and scarred myocardium are present, thallium redistribution is incomplete, giving the appearance of partial reversibility on delayed images.

Myocardial imaging with thallium offers information that is different from coronary angiography and perhaps complementary information to the structural abnormalities of

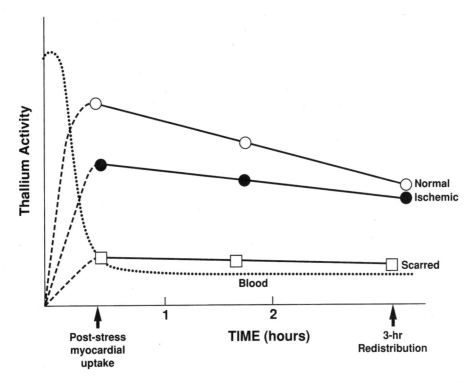

Figure 3. Schematic diagram of thallium clearance from normal and ischemic myocardium. Thallium clearance is more rapid from the normal myocardium with high thallium activity when compared with the ischemic myocardium with reduced thallium activity (differential washout).

the coronary arteries. Because myocardial imaging with thallium provides information regarding perfusion at the level of the myocytes, the thallium scan can appear to be normal in the setting of a totally occluded coronary artery with ample collaterals. Conversely, because retention of thallium several hours after the administration of the tracer (redistribution image) reflects myocardial mass that is viable, the scan may appear abnormal in the setting of a patent coronary artery if recanalization of the vessel has occurred following an acute myocardial infarction.

Clinical Applications of Thallium Scintigraphy

Imaging After Acute Myocardial Infarction

After the acute phase of myocardial infarction, the two most important factors that affect short- and long-term survival are the state of left ventricular function and the amount of viable myocardium perfused by stenotic coronary arteries.[34,35] Thus, an assessment of global left ventricular function at rest and the extent of myocardium in jeopardy relative to infarct size, may have important prognostic implications.

Because infarct size relative to the total myocardial risk area is highly variable,[36,37] the differentiation between viable and scarred or necrotic myocardium early after myocardial infarction is important, particularly in those patients who are being considered for revascularization. Parameters such as coronary artery patency,[38-41] electrocardiographic (ECG) Q-waves,[42,43] or regional left ventricular contraction at rest[44-46] do not predict accurately myocardial viability. Thus, a variety of methods have been developed to differentiate more reliably viable from nonviable myocardium. In general, these methods involve the measurement of myocardial perfusion and/or metabolism or functional response of the myocardium to inotropic stimulation such as dobutamine.

Imaging Patients With Chronic Coronary Artery Disease

Unlike acute myocardial syndromes (unstable angina or myocardial infarction) where impairment of coronary blood flow is caused by abrupt plaque rupture, thrombus formation, and vascular occlusion,[47-50] chronic coronary artery syndromes result from a slower progression of atherosclerosis in response to chronic endothelial injury.[48] Clinical manifestations of such slow progression of atherosclerosis include chronic stable angina, silent ischemia/infarction, and chronic hibernation.

Myocardial Ischemia

Imbalance between oxygen supply, usually caused by reduced myocardial perfusion, and oxygen demand, determined primarily by the rate and force of myocardial contraction, is termed ischemic myocardium. Clinical presentation of such imbalance may be symptomatic (angina pectoris) or asymptomatic (silent ischemia). If the oxygen supply-demand imbalance is transient (ie, triggered by exertion) it represents reversible ischemia. In the absence of myocardial necrosis, the degree of regional contractile dysfunction has been shown to be proportional to the extent of myocardial ischemia (Fig. 4).[51-54] On the

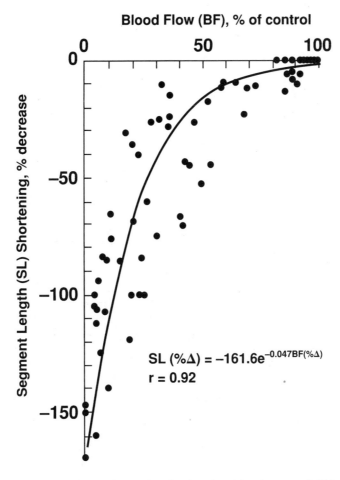

Figure 4. The exponential relation between reductions in regional myocardial blood flow (MBF; radioactive microsphere technique) and segmental shortening (ultrasonic dimension technique) in conscious dogs with acute graded levels of coronary artery stenosis. Modified and reprinted with permission from Reference 53.

other hand, if regional oxygen supply-demand imbalance is prolonged (ie, during myocardial infarction), high-energy phosphates will be depleted, regional contractile function will deteriorate progressively,[55] and cell membrane rupture with cell death will follow (myocardial infarction).

Thallium Protocols

There are a number of thallium protocols that currently are used for assessing myocardial perfusion and viability (Fig. 5). Advantages and disadvantages of these various protocols (stress-3- to-4-hour redistribution, late (24-hour) redistribution, thallium reinjection, and rest redistribution) are reviewed below.

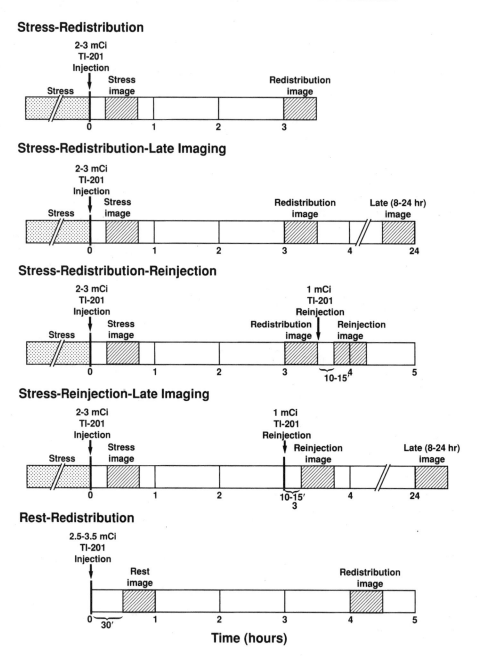

Figure 5. Thallium protocols for assessing myocardial viability. Reprinted with permission from Reference 158.

Stress-3- to-4-Hour-Redistribution Imaging

Stress and Coronary Flow Reserve

Regional MBF is critically dependent on the driving pressure gradient and the resistance of the vascular bed. Advanced degrees of coronary artery disease may exist at rest without myocardial ischemia because of compensatory dilatation of the resistance vessels.[56] In a canine model, over 80% occlusion of the coronary artery was necessary before ischemia was observed under basal state.[57] Because the pressure drop across a stenosis varies directly with the length of the stenosis and inversely with the fourth power of the radius (Bernoulli's theorem), resistance almost triples as the severity of coronary artery stenosis increases from 80% to 90%.[58] Consequently, during exercise or pharmacologic stress testing, when the resistance to the distal bed and the pressure distending the stenotic coronary artery declines, myocardial ischemia ensues.

Coronary blood flow in myocardial regions without coronary artery stenosis may increase to approximately four- to five-fold during vigorous aerobic exercise.[59,60] However, in the setting of moderate-to-severe coronary artery stenosis, the degree of coronary flow increase may be attenuated when compared with myocardial regions without coronary artery stenosis. The insufficient coronary blood flow increase during stress results in impaired subendocardial perfusion and myocardial ischemia.[61] In patients with coronary artery disease, an inverse relationship has been shown between the increase in MBF and the percentage of coronary artery stenosis once the lumen is narrowed by approximately 40%–50%.[62] Thus, when a radiotracer such as thallium is injected at peak exercise, the relative differences in regional MBF will be reflected in disproportionate concentrations of

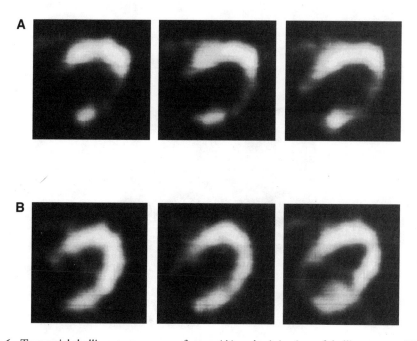

Figure 6. Transaxial thallium tomograms of stress (A) and reinjection of thallium at rest (B) from a patient with coronary artery disease. Myocardial perfusion abnormality is seen in the lateral region on the stress images but not on the reinjection images.

regional thallium activity on the stress images. Myocardial perfusion imaging, therefore, identifies subcritical coronary artery stenosis when performed in conjunction with exercise or pharmacologic stress but not at rest (Fig. 6).

Three- to-Four-Hour Redistribution

In 1977, Dr. Pohost made the observation that thallium defects on immediate postexercise images may normalize or redistribute if images were repeated several hours after the initial stress study.[28] The presence of thallium redistribution subsequently was described after the injection of thallium at rest as well as in patients undergoing pharmacologic stress studies. Consequently, the acquisition of redistribution images 3–4 hours after the administration of intravenous thallium at peak stress or at rest became the standard for thallium scintigraphic studies. However, further experience indicated that there are limitations of stress-3- to-4-hour-redistribution imaging in differentiating viable from nonviable myocardium.

Stress-induced thallium defects that redistribute on 3- to-4-hour delayed images are accurate indicators of ischemic myocardium. However, the converse, abnormal thallium defects during stress that persist on delayed images, does not necessarily indicate scarred myocardium. Ischemic but viable regions as well as regions with mixed viable and scarred myocardium may appear irreversible on stress-redistribution studies (Fig. 7). Many patients with irreversible thallium defects on stress-redistribution imaging have no evidence of prior myocardial infarction and will have normal thallium uptake after revascularization.[63–68] Using thallium quantification, Gibson and coworkers demonstrated that 45% of segments with irreversible defects had improved thallium uptake after coronary artery bypass surgery.[64] Segments that were likely to improve had thallium activity that was >50% of the activity in normal regions (Fig. 8). Similar results were obtained after successful percutaneous coronary artery angioplasty.[65,68] Thus, stress-3- to-4-hour-redistribution thallium studies may under-

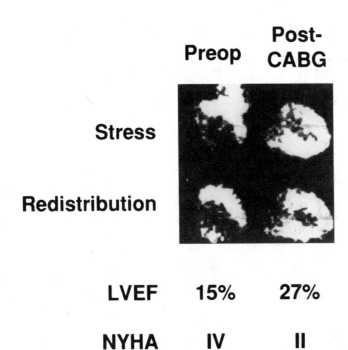

Figure 7. Evidence for viable myocardium in a region with irreversible thallium defect. Pre- and postoperative anterior planar thallium images demonstrate partially reversible inferior and fixed apical thallium defects preoperatively that normalizes after coronary artery bypass surgery. The left ventricular ejection fraction (LVEF) increased from 15% before to 27% after surgery. Modified and reprinted with permission from Reference 63.

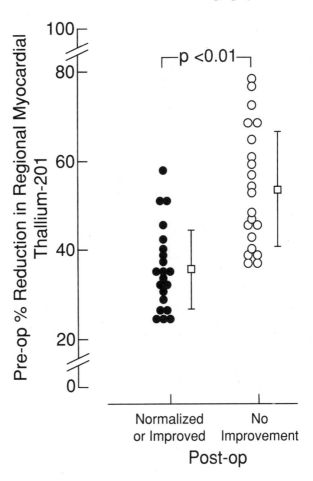

Figure 8. Percentage of reduction in regional thallium uptake for irreversible defects that normalized or improved after revascularization (solid circles) as compared with irreversible defects that did not improve after revascularization (open circles). Note that the irreversible defects that normalized or improved after surgery had a significantly smaller reduction in regional myocardial thallium activity preoperatively (preop). Reprinted with permission from Reference 64.

estimate the presence of ischemic but viable myocardium in many patients with coronary artery disease.

Late (24-Hour) Redistribution Imaging

Among patients demonstrating irreversible thallium defects on conventional stress-redistribution studies, the identification of viable myocardium may be improved by allowing a longer period for thallium redistribution (Fig. 9). A possible explanation for late redistribution is that in certain ischemic myocardial regions supplied by critically stenosed coronary arteries, the initial uptake of thallium is low (because delivery is impaired) and the rate of thallium clearance (from the myocardium to the blood) and accumulation (from the recirculating tracer within the blood over the 3- to-4-hour-redistribution period) is very slow. Thus, ischemic but viable myocardium may mimic the appearance of scarred myocardium. However, if a greater time is allowed for redistribution, then a greater number of viable myocardial regions may be differentiated from scarred myocardium.

In patients with coronary artery disease, 21% of the segments with irreversible thallium defects on the 3- to-4-hour delayed images showed redistribution when late images were obtained 18–24 hours after exercise.[69] Myocardial segments demonstrating such late thallium redistribution usually were perfused by critically stenosed coronary arteries.[66-70] Thus, regional thallium activity on redistribution images, acquired either early (2–4 hour) or late

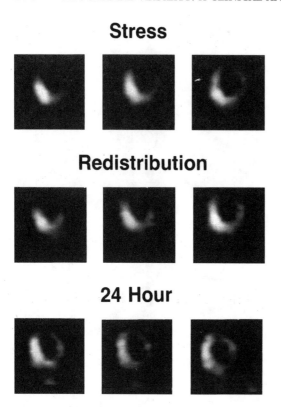

Figure 9. Short-axis thallium tomograms during stress, redistribution, and 24-hour imaging from a patient with coronary artery disease. There are extensive anterior and lateral thallium abnormalities during stress, which persist on redistribution images but that improve at 24 hours. Modified and reprinted with permission from Reference 92.

(8–72 hour) after stress, demonstrates the distribution of viable myocytes and the extent of scarred myocardium. In a subsequent prospective study,[70] late redistribution was observed in 53% of the patients and in 22% of the segments with 4-hour irreversible defects (Fig. 10). In patients undergoing revascularization, 95% of segments that demonstrated late redistribution at 18–24 hours showed improved thallium uptake after revascularization.[67] However, as with early (2–4 hour) redistribution imaging, the absence of late (8–72 hour) redistribution underestimated the presence of viable myocardium. Up to 37% of segments that remained irreversible on both 3- to-4-hour and 24-hour studies showed improvement in function after revascularization.[67] In addition, despite implementing 50% longer imaging time, a number of late redistribution studies had suboptimal count statistics at 24 hours. These data suggest that although late thallium imaging improves the identification of viable myocardium, it continues to underestimate segmental improvement after revascularization.

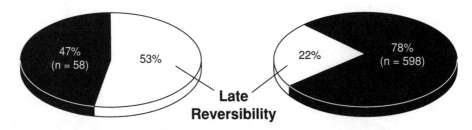

Figure 10. Pie chart showing the frequency of late reversibility and nonreversibility in 118 consecutive patients. In this prospective study, late redistribution was observed in 53% of the patients (**left**) and in 22% of the segments with 4-hour irreversible defects (**right**). Modified and reprinted with permission from Reference 70.

Thallium Reinjection

Although standard stress-3- to-4-hour-redistribution thallium scintigraphy may underestimate the presence of ischemic but viable myocardium in many patients with coronary artery disease, reinjection of thallium at rest after stress-3- to-4-hour-redistribution imaging substantially improves the assessment of myocardial ischemia and viability.[71] Among patients with coronary artery disease studied using thallium single photon emission tomography (SPECT), 33% of abnormal myocardial regions on stress appeared to be irreversible on 3- to-4-hour-redistribution images. However, after reinjecting a second dose of 1 mCi (37 MBq) of thallium at rest immediately after redistribution images and followed by image acquisition 10–15 minutes later, 49% of the apparently irreversible defects on 3- to-4-hour-redistribution images demonstrated improved or normal thallium uptake.[71] Moreover, in the subgroup of patients who underwent coronary angioplasty, 87% of myocardial regions identified as viable by reinjection studies had normal thallium uptake and improved regional wall motion after coronary angioplasty. In contrast, all regions with irreversible defects on reinjection imaging before angioplasty had abnormal regional wall motion after coronary angioplasty. Improved identification of viable myocardium with thallium reinjection has been confirmed by other medical centers both with exercise and after pharmacologic stress.[72–80] A patient example demonstrating the effect of thallium reinjection is shown in Figure 11.

Figure 11. Short-axis thallium tomograms during stress, redistribution, and reinjection imaging in a patient with coronary artery disease. There are extensive thallium abnormalities in the anterior and septal regions during stress that persist on redistribution images but improve markedly on reinjection images. Reprinted with permission from Reference 71.

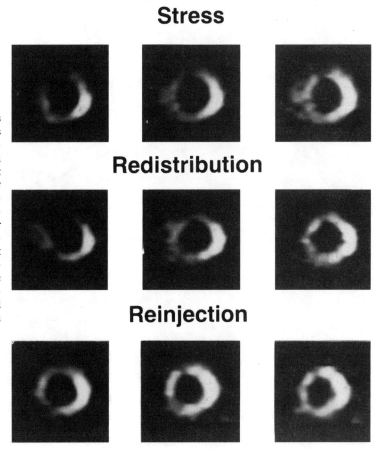

Scientific Basis for the Ability of Thallium-201 Reinjection to Assess Viability

That myocardial regions identified by thallium uptake following thallium reinjection represent viable myocardium is supported by improved regional function after revascularization[71–80] and preserved metabolic activity by fluorodeoxyglucose (FDG) positron emission tomography (PET).[75,81] In addition, a significant inverse correlation between the magnitude of thallium activity after reinjection and regional volume fraction of interstitial fibrosis has been demonstrated in comparative clinicopathological studies (Fig. 12).[82] The available data

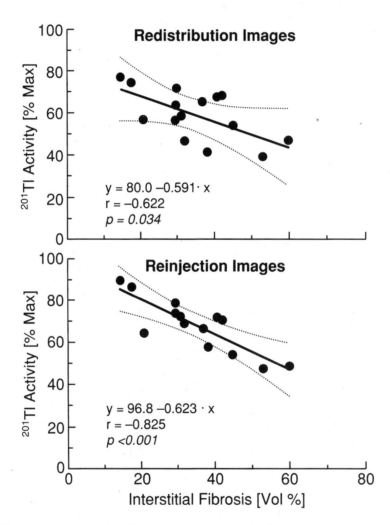

Figure 12. Graphs showing the relation between regional thallium activity on redistribution (**top panel**) and reinjection (**bottom panel**) images and regional volume fraction of interstitial fibrosis in patients with chronic stable coronary artery disease undergoing coronary artery bypass surgery. Two transmural biopsy specimens were taken during surgery and volume fraction of interstitial fibrosis was assessed by use of light microscopic morphometry. Dotted lines indicate 95% confidence limits for the regression line. The %Max indicates percentage of maximum normal activity. When compared with redistribution images, regression analysis reveals a significantly improved correlation ($p < 0.01$) between thallium reinjection and regional volume fraction of interstitial fibrosis. Modified and reprinted with permission from Reference 82.

Table 1

Thallium-201 Stress-Redistribution-Reinjection Imaging for Predicting Recovery of Regional Function: Pre- and Postrevascularization Studies

Author	Pts	LVEF (%)	Sens (%)	Spec (%)	PPV (%)	NPV (%)
I. When success of revascularization (either repeat thallium imaging or coronary angiography postoperatively) was taken into consideration in the analysis of regional data						
Dilsizian et al.[71]	20	44 ± 12	100 (13/13)	80 (8/10)	87 (13/15)	100 (8/8)
Bartenstein et al.[76]	19	—	83 (10/12)	86 (6/7)	91 (10/11)	75 (6/8)
II. When success of revascularization was not taken into consideration in the analysis of regional data						
Ohtani et al.[73]	24	—	89 (33/37)	50 (12/24)	73 (33/45)	75 (12/16)
Tamaki et al.[75]	11	—	95 (38/40)	38 (6/16)	79 (38/48)	75 (6/8)
Haque et al.[77]	26	43 ± 14	88 (29/33)	50 (5/10)	85 (29/34)	56 (5/9)
Vanoverschelde et al.[78]	73	36 ± 12	77 (129/167)	56 (155/277)	51 (129/251)	80 (155/193)
Gursurer et al.[80]	12	32 ± 3	99 (80/81)	47 (14/30)	83 (80/96)	93 (14/15)

Pts = patients; LVEF = left ventricular ejection fraction; Sens = sensitivity; Spec = specificity; PPV = positive predictive value; NPV = negative predictive value.

suggest that enhanced thallium uptake after reinjection in otherwise irreversible stress-redistribution defects accurately predicts improvement in regional function at rest after revascularization for as long as the outcome of revascularization is successful (Table 1).

The following is a possible explanation for the salutary results of thallium reinjection technique clinically. The initial myocardial uptake of thallium (postinjection) reflects regional

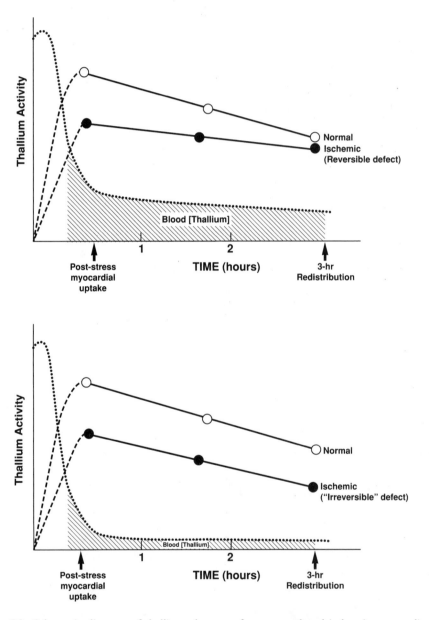

Figure 13. Schematic diagram of thallium clearance from normal and ischemic myocardium in relation to blood activity of thallium. If the blood thallium level remains the same (or increases) during the period between stress and 3-hour-redistribution imaging (**top panel**), then an apparent defect in a region with viable myocytes should improve over time. On the other hand, if the blood thallium concentration is low (or decreases) during the period between stress and 3-hour-redistribution imaging (**lower panel**), the delivery of thallium may be insufficient, and the thallium defect may remain irreversible even though the underlying myocardium is viable.

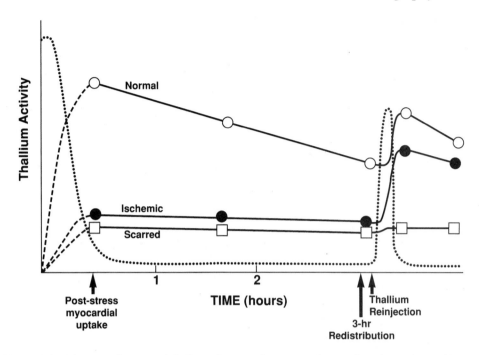

Figure 14. Schematic diagram of thallium clearance from normal, severely ischemic but viable, and scarred myocardium. In view of insufficient thallium delivery from the blood, ischemic but viable regions with severely reduced thallium defect on stress may appear irreversible on 3-hour redistribution (even with 24-hour imaging), unless blood levels of thallium are increased with thallium reinjection.

blood flow while redistribution of thallium in a given defect depends not only on the severity of the initial defects but also on the presence of viable myocytes,[83] the concentration of the tracer in the blood,[84,85] and the rate of decline of thallium levels in the blood.[30,31,86,87] Thus, the heterogeneity of regional blood flow observed on the initial stress-induced thallium defects may be independent of the subsequent extent of thallium redistribution.[88,89] If the blood thallium level remains the same (or increases) during the period between stress and 3-to-4-hour-redistribution imaging, then an apparent defect in a region with viable myocytes that can retain thallium should improve. On the other hand, if the blood thallium concentration is low (or decreases) during the imaging interval, the delivery of thallium may be insufficient and the thallium defect may remain irreversible even though the underlying myocardium is viable[90] (Fig. 13). This suggests that some ischemic but viable regions may never

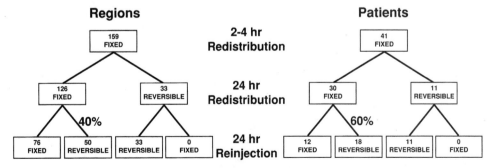

Figure 15. Flow diagram displaying the fate of "fixed" thallium defects on the 2-to-4-hour-standard-redistribution studies, 24-hour redistribution, and after reinjection of thallium at 24 hours. Modified and reprinted with permission from Reference 91.

redistribute, even with late (24 hour) imaging, unless blood levels of thallium are increased (Fig. 14). This hypothesis is supported by a study where thallium reinjection was performed immediately after 24-hour-redistribution images were obtained.[91] Improved thallium uptake after reinjection occurred in 40% of regions (involving 60% of patients) that appeared fixed on late (24 hour) redistribution images (Fig. 15). This percentage is remarkably similar to the 37% of irreversible defects at 24 hours that improve after revascularization, as previously reported.[67]

Late Redistribution Imaging After Thallium Reinjection. If thallium reinjection after stress-3- to-4-hour redistribution improves detection of ischemic and viable myocardium, it is possible that delaying the redistribution period between reinjection and repeat imaging from 10 minutes to 24 hours may identify additional viable regions. In patients with chronic coronary artery disease who underwent four sets of images (stress, 3-

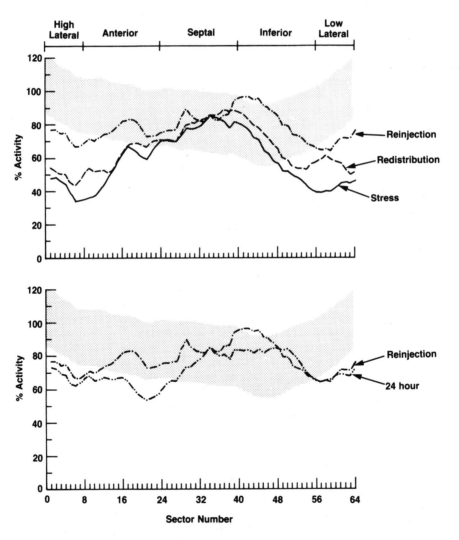

Figure 16. Quantitative regional thallium activity. The myocardial sectors in the anterior and inferior regions remain irreversible on the redistribution study but improve after reinjection and do not change at 24 hours. In addition, the anterolateral and inferolateral regions demonstrate partial reversibility on the redistribution study, improve further after reinjection, but show no further improvement after 24 hours. Reprinted with permission from Reference 92.

to-4-hour redistribution, reinjection, and 24-hour-redistribution images), only 11% of myocardial regions (involving 6% of patients) that remained irreversible after both 3-to-4-hour redistribution and reinjection showed evidence of late redistribution. Thus, most of the clinically relevant information pertaining to viability was obtained by a stress-redistribution-reinjection protocol.[92] These observations have been confirmed by other medical centers,[93,94] and therefore, late imaging after stress-redistribution-reinjection studies seems unnecessary (Fig. 16).

Issues Regarding Interpretation of Thallium Reinjection Studies

Pre- and Postrevascularization Studies

Adequacy of Revascularization and Functional Outcome

Most studies utilizing thallium reinjection technique do not reexamine regional perfusion or vessel patency after revascularization. Although functional studies are acquired before and after the revascularization, repeat thallium studies or coronary angiography are not performed postoperatively.[73,75,77,78,80] For an asynergic region to improve function after revascularization, it must not only retain viable myocardium but also be revascularized adequately[71,76] (Fig. 17). As illustrated in Table 1, summarizing pre- and postrevascularization studies utilizing thallium stress-redistribution-reinjection technique, the reported specificities and negative predictive accuracies vary greatly among

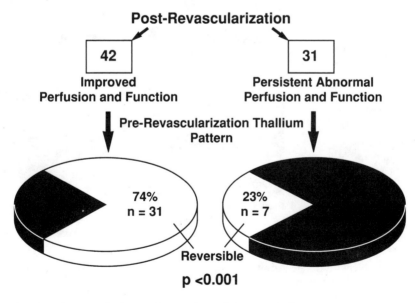

Figure 17. Flow diagram displaying the prerevascularization thallium pattern in asynergic regions with improved perfusion and function (**left**) and those with persistent abnormal perfusion and function (**right**) after revascularization. A larger proportion of asynergic regions with improved perfusion and function after revascularization demonstrated reversible thallium defects on their prerevascularization thallium study compared with those with lack of improvement in regional perfusion and function. Reprinted with permission from Reference 95.

studies. Lack of postoperative assessment of success of revascularization adversely effects the specificity and the negative predictive accuracy of the thallium reinjection technique.

Stress-Induced Reversible and Mild-to-Moderate Irreversible Defects: Are They Equally Accurate for Predicting Recovery of Regional Function After Revascularization?

A potential limitation inherent in many comparative studies of thallium reinjection before and after revascularization is in the grouping of stress-induced reversible and mild-to-moderately reduced irreversible thallium defects. Although regions with mild-to-moderately reduced irreversible thallium defects indeed retain viable myocardium, the mere presence of viable myocardium does not necessarily indicate ischemic myocardium (Table 2).

When performing rest-redistribution studies, mild-to-moderately reduced irreversible thallium defects represent viable myocardium with the potential of recovery after revascularization. However, the same concept may not apply when performing stress studies. Most mild-to-moderate irreversible thallium defects on stress studies represent an admixture of viable (nonischemic) and scarred myocardium, and there-

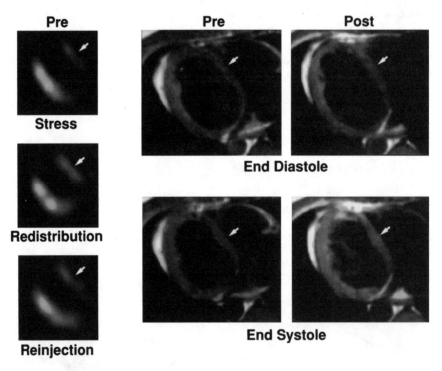

Figure 18. Persistent postrevascularization regional asynergy is shown in a patient with prerevascularization mild-to-moderate irreversible thallium defect. Matched transaxial tomograms are displayed for thallium stress, redistribution, and reinjection (**left**), with corresponding end-diastolic and end-systolic magnetic resonance imaging (MRI) tomograms pre- and postrevascularization (**right**). Mild-to-moderate septal thallium abnormality is seen during stress (shown by the arrowhead) that persists on redistribution and reinjection images (irreversible defect). Corresponding MRI tomograms demonstrate abnormal systolic wall thickening (WT) in the septal region prerevascularization, which remains abnormal postrevascularization. Reprinted with permission from Reference 95.

_____**Table 2**_____

Assessment of Myocardial Viability With Thallium Stress Protocols

Scintigraphic Interpretation	Clinical Interpretation	Probability of Functional Recovery After Revascularization
I. Reversible defects		
Complete	Ischemic, viable myocardium	High
Partial	Ischemic, mixed viable/scarred myocardium	Likely
II. Irreversible defects		
Mild-Moderate	Nonischemic, mixed viable/scarred myocardium	Low
Severe	Nonischemic, scarred myocardium	Unlikely

fore, may not improve after revascularization (Figure 18). In a recent study, asynergic regions with reversible thallium defects on the prerevascularization thallium studies were shown more likely to improve after revascularization when compared with asynergic regions with mild-to-moderate irreversible defects (79% versus 30%, respectively, $p < 0.001$).[95] Even at a similar mass of viable myocardial tissue (as reflected by the final thallium content), the presence of inducible ischemia (a reversible defect) was associated with an increased likelihood of functional recovery (Fig. 19). Thus, a more accurate noninvasive determination of myocardial viability requires the demonstra-

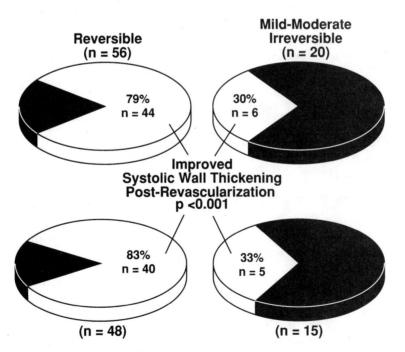

Figure 19. Recovery of asynergic regions after revascularization regardless of the final thallium content (**top panel**), and at the same final thallium content of 60% threshold value (**lower panel**). Pie charts comparing the proportion of asynergic myocardial regions that improved after revascularization in reversible (**left**) and mild-to-moderate irreversible (**right**) thallium defects. Reprinted with permission from Reference 95.

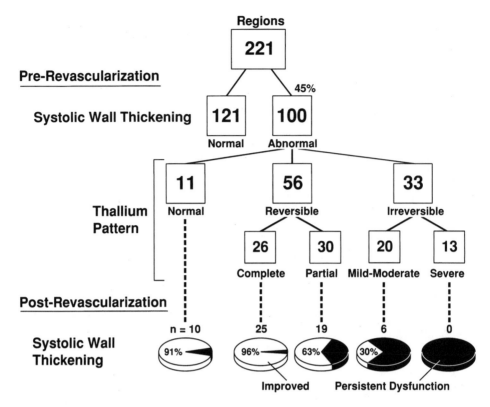

Figure 20. Flow diagram of prerevascularization systolic WT and thallium pattern and postrevascularization functional outcome of the 221 revascularized regions. Reprinted with permission from Reference 95.

tion of myocardial ischemia, which may explain the apparent lower specificity of thallium reported in the literature (Fig. 20).

Issues Regarding Modification of the Thallium Reinjection Protocol

Elimination of 3- to-4-Hour-Redistribution Image

There are a number of other pre- and postrevascularization studies (not listed in the table) in which the authors acquired only two sets of images, stress and reinjection, and eliminated the 3- to-4-hour-redistribution image. In view of the clinical success of thallium reinjection, many nuclear laboratories have adopted the practice of eliminating 3-to-4-hour-redistribution imaging. This approach assumes that a stress-reinjection protocol (without the 3- to-4-hour-redistribution image) provides the same information regarding stress-induced ischemia and viability as a stress-redistribution-reinjection protocol. Reinjection of thallium without acquiring 3- to-4-hour-redistribution images could be confounded by underperfusion at rest (Fig. 21). Because apparent washout of thallium may occur between redistribution and reinjection studies, reliance on reinjection images alone would underestimate defect reversibility and hence viability in up to 25% of ischemic regions.[71,96] Reversible stress-redistribution defects that appear to washout after reinjection and thus appear "fixed" on stress-reinjection images result from a dispropor-

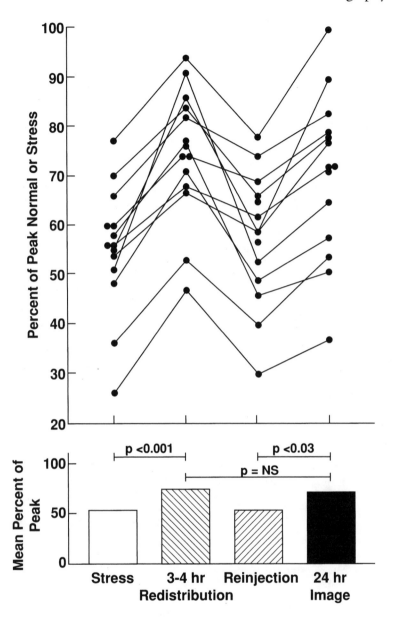

Figure 21. Relative regional thallium activity (presented as a percent of normal activity) in 14 regions demonstrating the phenomenon of apparent thallium washout caused by low differential uptake. **Top panel**: Individual data points are displayed for stress, 3- to-4-hour redistribution, reinjection, and 24-hour images. **Bottom panel**: Mean thallium activity in relation to each of the four corresponding images. If the 3- to-4-hour-redistribution images were eliminated and the reinjection images were acquired alone, these regions would be assigned incorrectly to be irreversible. On the 24-hour images, redistribution again is apparent, indicating reversibility of the defect, and the relative thallium activity is similar to that observed on the 3- to-4-hour-redistribution studies. Reprinted with permission from Reference 96.

tionately smaller increment in regional thallium activity after reinjection in some ischemic regions that are underperfused at rest compared with the uptake in normal regions, a phenomenon termed "differential uptake."[71,96] Thus, to capture ischemic but viable myocardium accurately, all three images (stress, redistribution, and reinjection) should be acquired and the maximum final thallium content on either redistribution or reinjection should be used for viability assessment. Alternatively, a stress-reinjection protocol appears to be a reasonable alternative to stress-redistribution-reinjection imaging, as long as late (24 hour) imaging is performed in those patients with irreversible defects.[96] Thus, high predictive accuracy for ischemic and viable myocardium can be achieved with thallium imaging with either a stress-redistribution-reinjection or stress-3- to-4-hour-reinjection–late redistribution imaging. For either of these protocols, the third set of images is only necessary if an irreversible defect exists on the stress-redistribution or the stress-reinjection images.

Early Thallium Reinjection After Stress

An alternative approach to stress-redistribution-reinjection imaging would be to reinject thallium immediately after the stress images are completed and acquire a "redistribution" image 3–4 hours later. This modified redistribution image would represent redistribution of both the stress and the reinjected thallium doses and thereby avoid the acquisition of three sets of images.

When Kiat and coworkers applied such an early thallium reinjection protocol, 24% of irreversible thallium defects on stress-modified-redistribution images became reversible when a third set of images was acquired 24 hours later.[97] Although other investigators have reported good agreement between 1-hour after early reinjection and 3-hour-modified-redistribution images, an independent validation of the accuracy of the early reinjection technique was not provided.[98] In a subsequent publication, stress-early reinjection imaging was compared with conventional stress-redistribution-reinjection thallium imaging among two groups of patients with similar clinical parameters.[99] Consistent with previous observations, the frequency of reversible defects was significantly less with early reinjection compared with the standard stress-redistribution-reinjection protocol. Recently, in addition to acquiring stress-early reinjection images, a second 1-mCi (37 MBq) dose of thallium was reinjected after modified redistribution images were completed and a third set of images was acquired.[100] When modified redistribution images after early reinjection were compared with the delayed (postredistribution) reinjection images, early thallium reinjection underestimated myocardial viability in approximately 25% of irreversible defects. These preliminary data suggest that a delay period after exercise is necessary to determine accurately myocardial ischemia and viability among patients with chronic left ventricular dysfunction.

Rest-Redistribution Imaging

The stress-redistribution-reinjection thallium protocol provides important diagnostic and prognostic information regarding both inducible ischemia and myocardial viability. However, if the clinical question to be addressed is one of the presence and extent of viable myocardium within dysfunctional regions and not inducible ischemia, it is reasonable to perform only rest-redistribution thallium imaging.

Thallium defects on resting images have been reported during angina-free periods in patients with unstable angina and without myocardial infarction as well as in patients with severe coronary artery disease in the absence of an acute ischemic process or previous myocardial infarction.[101,102] Furthermore, it has been recognized that many of these defects on the initial rest images may redistribute over the next 2–4 hours (Fig. 22). Since

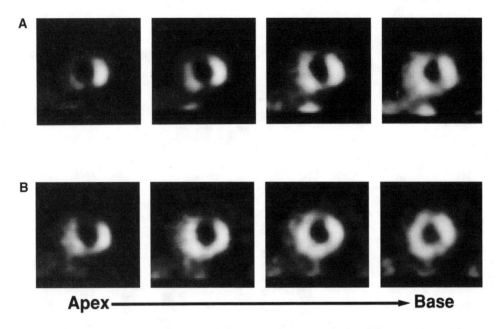

Figure 22. Rest-redistribution short-axis thallium tomograms are displayed from a patient with coronary artery disease. There are extensive thallium abnormalities in the anteroapical, anteroseptal, and inferior regions on the initial rest images (A). On 3- to-4-hour-redistribution images (B), the inferior region remains fixed (scarred myocardium), while the anteroapical and anteroseptal regions show significant reversibility, suggestive of viable myocardium. Reprinted with permission from Reference 159.

these initial reports, several studies have evaluated the efficacy of rest-redistribution thallium imaging in predicting the outcome of myocardial regions after revascularization.[103–105] Among regions with reversible rest-redistribution thallium defects preoperatively, 77%–86% had normal thallium uptake and/or improved left ventricular function after revascularization. However, 22%–38% of regions with irreversible rest-redistribution defects preoperatively also showed improved left ventricular contraction postoperatively. Thallium defects in each of these studies were classified as being reversible, partially reversible, or irreversible. However, the severity of the irreversible thallium defects was not assessed. Recently, improved results were obtained using quantitative analysis in which the severity of reduction in thallium activity was assessed within irreversible rest-redistribution thallium defects.[106–108]

Which Thallium Protocol for Identifying Chronic Coronary Artery Disease (Hibernating Myocardium)?

In most cases, the identification of presence and extent of myocardial ischemia is much more important clinically in terms of patient management and risk stratification than knowledge of myocardial viability. Regional left ventricular dysfunction arising from a transient period of myocardial ischemia (repetitive stunning) and/or a prolonged period of myocardial hypoperfusion at rest (hibernation) may be reversible, while regional dysfunction arising from transmural myocardial infarction or mixed scarred and viable myocardium may be irreversible after revascularization. The distinction between reversible and irreversible asynergic regions may be accomplished by demonstrating stress-induced

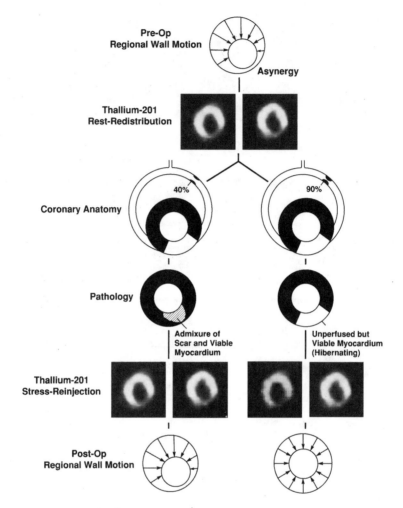

Figure 23. A schematic diagram of how exercise stress may produce greater regional MBF heterogeneity when compared with rest-redistribution imaging and thereby differentiate an asynergic region with mixed scarred and viable myocardium from a region with underperfused but viable (hibernating) myocardium. A preoperative asynergic myocardial region that exhibits reduced thallium uptake at rest and remains irreversible on the redistribution study may represent a region with patent (40% stenosis) coronary artery after thrombolytic therapy (**left**) or a region with critically narrowed (90% stenosis) coronary artery without myocardial infarction (**right**). In the case of the patient with 40% coronary artery stenosis and prior myocardial infarction, the dysfunctional myocardium (assessed several months after the acute infarction) represents mixed scarred and viable myocardium that will not recover after revascularization. In contrast, in the patient with 90% coronary artery stenosis without prior myocardial infarction the dysfunctional myocardium perfused by this artery represents underperfused but viable myocardium that will recover completely after revascularization. These two situations can be differentiated by performing a stress-redistribution-reinjection study (demonstrating ischemia) but not by a rest-redistribution study. The apparent reduced thallium activity at rest and lack of subsequent redistribution probably relates to partial volume and recovery coefficient effects in the presence of thinned or nonthickening myocardium. Reprinted with permission from Reference 130.

ischemia (reversible thallium defect) in regions that are asynergic on the basis of repetitive stunning and/or hibernation and scar or lack of ischemia (irreversible thallium defect) in regions that are asynergic as a result of transmural infarction or mixed scarred and viable myocardium. Such a distinction, prospectively, has important clinical implications, especially in patients who are being considered for interventional therapy.

The impact of a stress study in differentiating an asynergic region with mixed scarred and viable myocardium from a region with underperfused but viable (hibernating) myocardium is outlined in Figure 23. It has been well recognized that regional contraction itself could influence the appearance of myocardial perfusion images.[109–113] A region with minimal or absent systolic wall thickening may appear to have reduced thallium activity on a rest-redistribution study as a result of partial volume and recovery coefficient effects in the presence of thinned or nonthickening myocardium. Hence, an asynergic region with a mild-to-moderately reduced rest-redistribution thallium pattern may represent either a mixed scarred and viable (nonischemic) myocardium or a region with predominantly viable myocardium. These two asynergic regions may be distinguished by demonstrating stress-induced ischemia (a reversible thallium defect) in the case of viable myocardium and absence of ischemia (an irreversible thallium defect) in the case of mixed scarred and viable (nonischemic) myocardium.[95]

If the clinical question is one of myocardial viability within asynergic regions, then a rest-redistribution thallium protocol along with quantitative analysis of the severity of the thallium defect may suffice. On the other hand, if the clinical question is one of ischemia and viability, then stress-redistribution-reinjection or stress-reinjection-late redistribution imaging provides the most comprehensive information.

Which Thallium Protocol for Identifying Stunned Myocardium?

The process of thallium accumulation early after myocardial infarction is complex, a time during which alterations in the two primary determinants of thallium uptake, blood flow and tissue viability, may be occurring over relatively brief periods of time. In experimental models of myocardial stunning, the extraction of thallium remained essentially unaltered as long as myocardial necrosis was absent. There are a number of experimental data to show that thallium does not localize in nonviable, necrotic myocardium and thus may be useful to assess myocardial infarct size.[83,114,115] The observations in the experimental laboratory were confirmed in patients studied before and after thrombolytic therapy.[116,117] In patients who were reperfused within 2.5 hours from onset of symptoms, thallium images showed normal or improved uptake after thrombolysis, which correlated to later improvement in regional wall motion. In contrast, patients who were reperfused 5 hours after the onset of acute symptoms displayed no such improvement in regional thallium uptake or in regional wall motion abnormality.[116]

Although thallium uptake after reperfusion appears to correlate well with myocardial infarct size, early postreperfusion thallium uptake may overestimate myocardial viability. When thallium is injected immediately after reperfusion, the initial uptake of thallium may reflect hyperemic flow and, therefore, overestimate salvaged, viable myocardium.[117] However, necrotic myocardium cannot retain thallium and, despite its initial uptake, thallium washout is accelerated in necrotic tissue.[28,118] Consequently, rapid early thallium washout might be used to indicate nonviability. The ambiguity of initial postreperfusion resting studies may be lessened with redistribution imaging, which allows time for thallium washout in necrotic myocardium and for thallium "wash-in" in viable tissue. In theory, it is possible to utilize this knowledge of thallium kinetics both to assess infarct size and to estimate myocardial salvage after infarction. Thus early imaging, which reflects

MBF, and delayed imaging, which reflects infarct size, can be applied clinically for this purpose.[119–121] In fact, the evaluation of myocardial infarct size with thallium performed approximately 8 weeks after myocardial infarction has been associated with worse survival.[121] However, it should be noted that there may be practical limitations to imaging a patient within the first few hours after myocardial infarction.

There are only a few studies in which rest-redistribution thallium imaging was performed early, within 1–3 days, after myocardial infarction.[122,123] Among patients demonstrating viability in the infarct zone by rest-redistribution thallium, the infarct-related artery was patent in all patients and left ventricular function improved significantly during follow-up. In contrast, in patients demonstrating lack of myocardial viability in the infarct zone by thallium, one-third of infarct-related arteries remained occluded and left ventricular function declined in this group over time (Fig. 24). Additional studies in a larger number of patients are needed to assess the role of thallium imaging early after infarction.

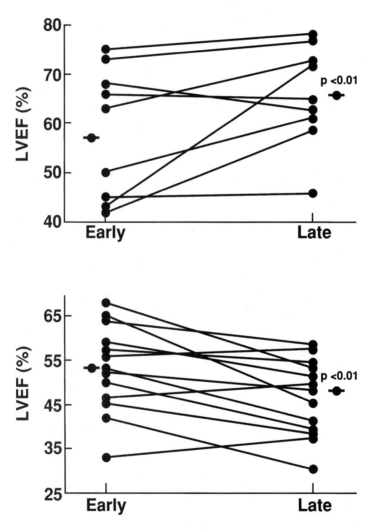

Figure 24. Early and late LVEF in patients with presence of infarct zone viability by thallium (**upper panel**) and lack of infarct zone viability by thallium (**lower panel**). Late left ventricular function improved in patients exhibiting infarct zone viability by thallium but not in patients without infarct zone viability ($p < 0.001$). Modified and reprinted with permission from Reference 122.

No-Reflow Phenomenon

The "no-reflow" phenomenon refers to a lack of tissue perfusion despite restoration of blood flow in the epicardial artery. It may be possible theoretically to take clinical advantage of the no-reflow phenomenon in assessing myocardial salvage with thallium. Such identification of patients who exhibit the no-reflow phenomenon may have prognostic implications.

Because significant hyperemia may occur acutely during reperfusion, early injection of thallium will reflect neither myocardial risk area nor infarct size. Furthermore, given the kinetics of thallium uptake, it is not possible to inject the radiotracer prior to reperfusion therapies, because the imaging phase would delay such therapy. However, by delaying thallium imaging to approximately 24 hours after infarction, initial images may reflect myocardial risk area caused by persistence of flow abnormalities in the risk zone (no-reflow) while avoiding the initial hyperemia. Delayed images then could be used to estimate the degree of salvage. This approach, while potentially feasible, has not been investigated in clinical trials.

The complexity of the interaction of myocardial perfusion, ischemia, and viability is highlighted by investigations that have indicated possible deleterious effects of reperfusion.[124,125] In patients with acute myocardial infarction who were treated with thrombolysis and/or angioplasty, capillary perfusion to the vascular bed served by the culprit artery was assessed by intracoronary injection of echocardiographic contrast material.[126] The results showed that patients who exhibited the no-reflow phenomenon had significantly more congestive heart failure and lack of improvement in left ventricular function compared with those in whom blood flow was reestablished after reperfusion (Fig. 25).

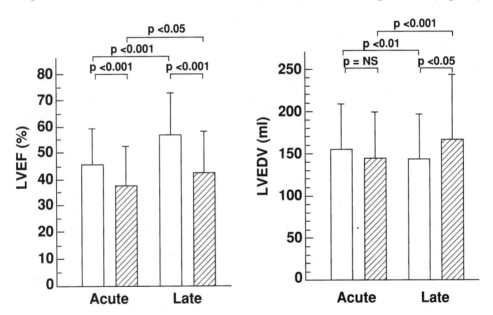

Figure 25. No-reflow phenomenon. Bar graphs showing the temporal changes in mean ± SD LVEF (**left**: LVEF[%]) and end-diastolic volume (**right**: LVEDV [mL]) from the early to late stage in patients with and without the no-reflow phenomenon assessed by myocardial contrast echocardiography (MCE). Patients with MCE no-reflow (crossed bar) showed a little functional improvement, while patients with MCE reflow (open bar) showed significant temporal improvement in ventricular function. Ventricular function was significantly better in patients with MCE reflow than those with MCE no-reflow. LVEDV increased in the late stage in patients with MCE no-reflow and decreased in patients with MCE reflow. Therefore, late-stage LVEDV was significantly greater in patients with MCE no-reflow than those with MCE reflow. Modified and reprinted with permission from Reference 126.

Thallium and ¹⁸F-fluoro-deoxyglucose (FDG) Imaging

Because delayed thallium images reflect cation flux and sarcolemmal membrane integrity, it is possible that thallium may yield comparable viability information as metabolic imaging with FDG. Preserved or enhanced FDG uptake in asynergic myocardial regions identifies viable myocardium that has been shown to predict not only improved regional and global left ventricular function after revascularization but also improved survival when compared with patients treated with medical therapy alone. In a canine model of 2 hours of coronary occlusion followed by 4 hours of reperfusion, thallium was injected before reperfusion and FDG was administered 3 hours after reflow.[127] Both thallium redistribution and preserved FDG uptake accurately identified viable myocardium after reperfusion. On the other hand, lack of thallium redistribution and reduced FDG uptake identified irreversibly injured, necrotic myocardium.

Comparison With Stress-Redistribution-Reinjection Imaging

In patients with chronic coronary artery disease, the similar predictive accuracies of FDG PET imaging and thallium reinjection for differentiating viable from nonviable myocardium have prompted comparative studies of the two imaging techniques in the same patients.[75,81] In the first study, 94% of regions demonstrating either complete or

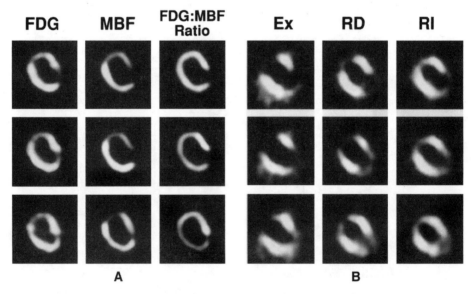

Figure 26. Concordance of positron emission tomography (PET) (A) and thallium reinjection data (B). Tomographic ¹⁸F-2-deoxyglucose (FDG), myocardial blood flow (MBF), and FDG-to-blood flow ratio (FDG:MBF), generated from the quantitative ¹⁵O-water data with partial volume and spillover correction are shown on the left panel. The corresponding thallium data for exercise (Ex), 3- to-4-hour redistribution (RD), and reinjection (RI) are shown on the right panel. Standard exercise-redistribution thallium studies demonstrate an apparently irreversible anteroapical defect. MBF is reduced in this region and in the septum according to PET. However, FDG images demonstrate uptake and, hence, viability in all regions, most notably the anteroapical region. Functional images of FDG-to-blood flow ratio demonstrate enhanced FDG uptake relative to blood flow (mismatch) involving the apex and septum. Thallium reinjection images mirror the FDG images, with evidence of enhanced thallium uptake and, hence, viability in the anteroapical region. Reprinted with permission from Reference 81.

partial reversibility on stress-redistribution thallium studies were viable by FDG PET.[81] FDG uptake was preserved in 91% of mildly reduced (60%–84% of peak activity) and 84% of moderately reduced (50%–59% of peak activity) irreversible thallium regions. Hence, the level of thallium activity itself in mild-to-moderate defects might be a clinically reliable marker of myocardial viability. Furthermore, among regions considered irreversible on 3-to-4-hour-redistribution images, the severity of reduction in thallium activity correlated with the likelihood of metabolic activity as assessed by FDG uptake. In regions with severe irreversible thallium defects (≤50% of peak activity) on redistribution imaging, the results of thallium reinjection were comparable with PET, with a concordance between the two techniques of 88% for viable or nonviable myocardium.[81] An example of this concordance is demonstrated in Figure 26. These initial observations at the National Institutes of Health were confirmed by other investigators.[75,128] In a subsequent study, the increase in regional thallium activity from redistribution to reinjection was computed, normalized to the increase observed in a normal region, and termed differential uptake.[129] The magnitude of increase in thallium activity (differential uptake) was significantly greater in mild-to-moderate defects than in severe irreversible defects, suggesting that these regions represent viable myocardium as confirmed by the corresponding PET data (Fig. 27).

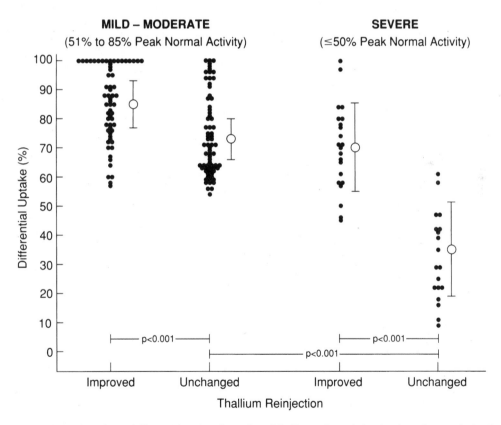

Figure 27. Plots show differential regional uptake of thallium after reinjection based on analysis of changes in the magnitude of regional thallium activity in regions with irreversible thallium defects on redistribution imaging. **Left panel**: Regions with mild-to-moderate reduction in thallium activity on redistribution images (ranging from 51% to 85% of peak normal activity). **Right panel**: Regions with severe reduction in thallium activity (≤50% of peak activity). Within each panel, regions are further subdivided on the basis of improved or unchanged relative thallium activity after reinjection. Mild-to-moderate defects in which relative thallium activity was unchanged after reinjection had significantly greater increase in absolute thallium activity than similar regions that represented severe irreversible defects. Reprinted with permission from Reference 129.

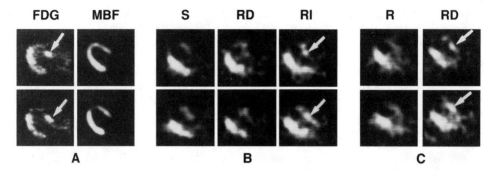

Figure 28. Concordance between PET (A), stress-redistribution-reinjection (B) and rest-redistribution (C) imaging is demonstrated in this patient example. Two consecutive transaxial tomograms are displayed for FDG and MBF by PET, with corresponding thallium tomograms of stress (S), redistribution (RD), reinjection (RI), and rest (R)-redistribution. On the PET study, MBF is reduced in the anteroapical, anteroseptal, and posteroseptal regions. FDG uptake in the corresponding regions demonstrates a mismatch in the posteroseptal region (arrowhead) and a match between FDG uptake and blood flow in the anteroapical and anteroseptal regions. Corresponding single photon emission tomography (SPECT) thallium images reveal extensive perfusion abnormalities involving the apical and septal regions during stress, which persist on redistribution images. However, thallium reinjection images show improved thallium uptake in the posteroseptal region (arrowhead), while the apical region remains fixed. On rest-redistribution images, the apical region has severely reduced thallium activity, which remains fixed, while the posteroseptal region that was abnormal on the initial rest study shows significant improvement in the 3- to-4-hour-redistribution study, suggesting viable myocardium. Reprinted with permission from Reference 130.

Comparison With Rest-Redistribution Imaging

There are only limited data comparing rest-redistribution thallium imaging with PET.[130,131] In a study in which quantitative thallium scintigraphic findings obtained from patients undergoing both stress-redistribution-reinjection and rest-redistribution SPECT imaging were compared with PET (Fig. 28), it was concluded that either thallium protocol might yield clinically satisfactory information as long as the severity of thallium defects are quantified within rest-redistribution images.[130] However, in the absence of contraindications to stress testing, stress-redistribution-reinjection imaging provides a more comprehensive assessment of the extent and severity of myocardial ischemia, without loss of information on myocardial viability.

Comparison With Thallium Uptake After Reinjection in Regions With Reverse Redistribution

On conventional stress-redistribution imaging, reverse redistribution indicates either the appearance of a new defect on the redistribution images or the worsening of a defect apparent on stress images. However, it remains unclear whether regions demonstrating the phenomenon of reverse redistribution represent scarred or viable myocardium. Hence, the clinical significance of reverse redistribution in chronic coronary artery disease is uncertain.

Because thallium reinjection is a valuable technique for detecting myocardial viability, its effect was examined among patients with chronic coronary artery disease, all of whom demonstrated reverse redistribution on standard stress-redistribution studies.[132] Enhanced thallium uptake after reinjection occurred in 82% of regions with reverse redistribution (Fig. 29). Regions with improved thallium uptake after reinjection were associated with absence of ECG

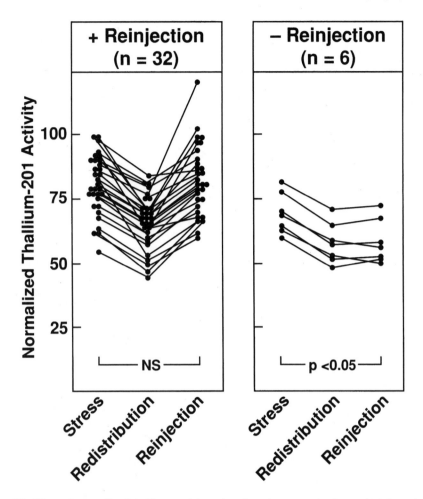

Figure 29. Plots of normalized thallium activity values based on quantitative analysis in each region with reverse redistribution during stress, redistribution, and reinjection. The plots show regions with (+ reinjection, **right panel**) and without (− reinjection, **left panel**) enhanced thallium uptake after reinjection, respectively. Reprinted with permission from Reference 132.

and functional indices of myocardial necrosis and were supplied by severely stenosed coronary arteries with good collaterals. Furthermore, metabolic activity as assessed by FDG was preserved by PET imaging in such regions. In contrast, regions with reverse redistribution in which thallium activity failed to increase after reinjection were associated with ECG Q-waves, severely impaired regional contraction, and severely reduced FDG and blood flow (FDG/blood flow match) by PET. These observations indicate that thallium reinjection may be helpful in differentiating scarred from viable myocardium in regions with reverse redistribution.[132] Similar results were obtained by other investigators.[133]

Thallium and FDG Single Photon Emission Tomography (SPECT) Imaging

The clinical application of FDG has been hampered by the limited availability and high cost of PET and cyclotron technology. Recently, because of the relatively long

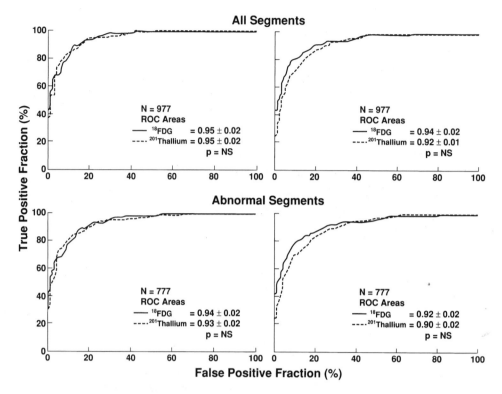

Figure 30. Plots of receiver operating characteristic (ROC) curves for thallium and FDG SPECT to predict myocardial viability as defined by 50% (**left**) and 60% (**right**) FDG PET threshold values for all segments (**top panel**) and abnormal thallium segments (**lower panel**) are shown. Area under the ROC curve for FDG SPECT and thallium SPECT are displayed for each panel. There are no significant differences between thallium and FDG SPECT for detecting myocardial viability. In all 977 segments, 877 were viable at 50% threshold (**upper left panel**) and 818 were viable at 60% threshold (**upper right panel**). Among the 777 abnormal segments, 677 were viable at 50% threshold (**lower left panel**) and 618 were viable at 60% threshold (**lower right panel**). Reprinted with permission from Reference 134.

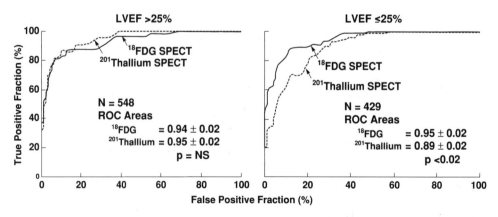

Figure 31. Plots of ROC curves for thallium and FDG SPECT to predict myocardial viability as defined by 60% FDG PET threshold value for patients with LVEF > 25% (**left**) and for patients with LVEF ≤ 25% (**right**) are shown. Area under the ROC curve for FDG SPECT and thallium SPECT are displayed for each panel. Thallium tended to underestimate myocardial viability in patients with LVEF ≤ 25% but not in patients with LVEF > 25%. For patients with LVEF > 25% (**left**), 471 of 548 segments were viable, and for patients with LVEF ≤ 25% (**right**), 347 of 429 segments were viable. Reprinted with permission from Reference 134.

physical half-life of ^{18}F (110 minutes), offsite production of FDG and subsequent transport to satellite nuclear cardiology laboratories has been proposed. This, combined with the advent of high-energy γ-camera collimators for SPECT, has made possible the use of FDG SPECT for detection of myocardial viability. In patients with chronic coronary artery disease undergoing evaluation for myocardial viability receiver operating characteristic (ROC) analysis was applied to examine regional differences in FDG uptake by SPECT and PET technologies as well as the relationship between thallium and FDG tracers.[134] Because assessment of viability is of particular concern in patients with left ventricular dysfunction, differences between the technologies and tracers in subjects with left ventricular ejection fraction (LVEF) of ≤25% compared with those with LVEF of >25% also were determined. The results showed that the overall concordance between the two technologies (SPECT and PET) and the two tracers (FDG and thallium) was

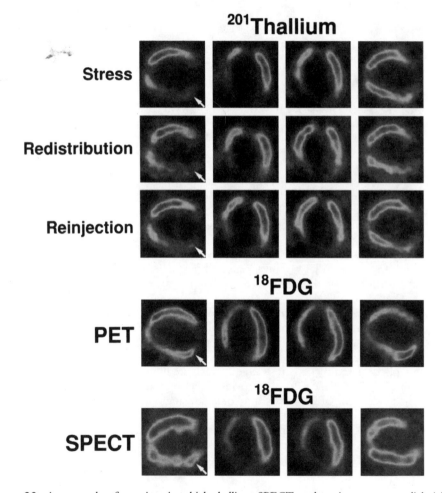

Figure 32. An example of a patient in which thallium SPECT underestimates myocardial viability when compared to FDG SPECT and FDG PET in the inferior region. Four radial long-axis tomograms are displayed for FDG SPECT, FDG PET, with corresponding thallium tomograms of stress, redistribution, and reinjection. On the FDG SPECT and PET studies, FDG uptake is preserved in the inferoseptal and inferobasal regions (shown by the arrowhead), suggestive of viable myocardium. However, thallium images show an extensive perfusion defect in the inferobasal region during stress, which persists on redistribution and reinjection images (severe irreversible thallium defect), suggestive of scarred myocardium by thallium. Reprinted with permission from Reference 134.

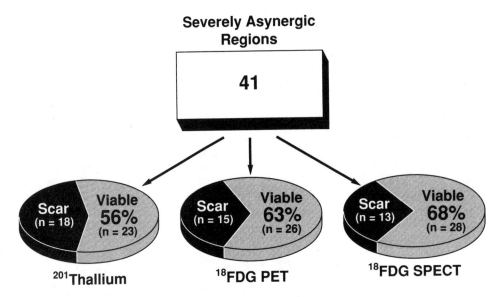

Figure 33. Flow diagram displaying the results of FDG SPECT, FDG PET, and thallium SPECT in severely asynergic regions (scarred by regional contractile function alone). There are no significant differences between FDG SPECT, FDG PET, and thallium SPECT. Reprinted with permission from Reference 134.

excellent for differentiating viable from nonviable myocardium regardless of the level of FDG PET threshold value applied (Fig. 30). However, in segments with severe irreversible thallium defects, FDG SPECT provides incremental information regarding myocardial viability in the inferior segment, especially in patients with severely impaired left ventricular function (Fig. 31). Thus, in regions judged scarred by thallium (severe irreversible defects), metabolic imaging with FDG SPECT may provide incremental information regarding myocardial viability, especially in patients with severely impaired left ventricular function in whom the effects of thallium attenuation would be particularly prominent (Fig. 32).

To correlate regional function with perfusion and/or metabolism, gated tomographic radionuclide angiography was applied, which allowed direct and accurate comparison of tomographic regional function with the assessment of myocardial viability by FDG SPECT, thallium SPECT, and FDG PET.[134] In previous studies, functional assessment of the heart has been by planar gated blood pool studies, which are limited by overlap between cardiac structures or by ECGs, which do not provide direct regional alignment. In the subset of patients who underwent SPECT gated radionuclide angiography, the agreement between SPECT and PET technologies for identifying myocardial viability with FDG in severely asynergic regions was 80%; thallium provided concordant information with FDG SPECT in 73% of these regions. In normal or mildly hypokinetic regions, thallium and FDG SPECT provided concordant information in 94% of the regions (Fig. 33).

Prognostic Value of Thallium-201

Stress-Redistribution

Beyond its value as a perfusion and viability tracer, thallium provides useful information regarding patient outcome and prognosis. In patients with chronic coronary artery disease, the presence of abnormally increased lung-to-heart ratio after stress,[135,136] transient left ventricular cavity dilatation,[137,138] and extensive reversible and irreversible thallium defects[139,140] have been shown to be important predictors of adverse outcome. These scintigraphic variables provide incremental prognostic information to those obtained from clinical evaluation, exercise treadmill testing, and coronary angiography.[141,142] When thallium imaging variables were assessed following acute myocardial infarction,[143] the combination of reversible defects and increased lung-to-heart ratio had a significantly greater sensitivity for predicting future cardiac death, recurrent myocardial infarction, or unstable angina than submaximal exercise testing or coronary angiography (Fig. 34). Thallium identified the low-risk subgroup much better than submaximal exercise testing or coronary angiography.[143]

Large irreversible defects provide a scintigraphic corollary of resting left ventricular dysfunction, while stress-induced reversible defects reflect the extent of ischemic myocar-

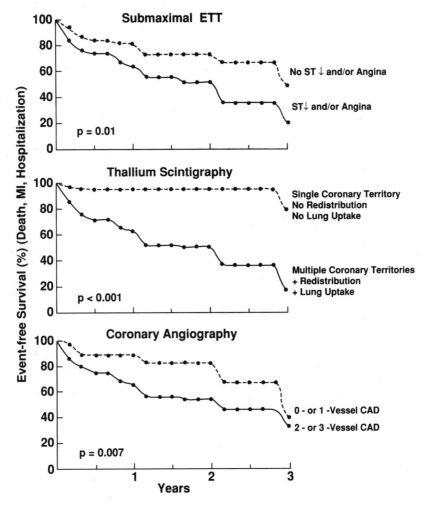

Figure 34. Cumulative event-free survival as a function of time for different subgroups formed by the submaximal exercise test response (**top**), thallium scintigraphic findings (**middle**), or coronary angiographic findings (**bottom**) before hospital discharge. The solid and dashed lines represent the high-risk and low-risk cumulative probability, respectively. Modified and reprinted with permission from Reference 143.

dium. Among patients undergoing preoperative thallium studies prior to a major elective vascular (noncardiac) surgery, reversible thallium defect was the most important predictor of perioperative cardiac events, dominated by nonfatal myocardial infarction. On the other hand, the presence of irreversible thallium defect was the most important predictor of cardiac events, dominated by fatal events.[144]

Thallium Reinjection

Whether thallium reinjection provides additional prognostic information over variable derived from stress-redistribution imaging seems to depend on the patient population studied and quantitation of defect severity. In patients with prior myocardial infarction and left ventricular dysfunction (LVEF $\leq$ 40%), thallium reinjection imaging provided incremental prognostic information to clinical, exercise, and thallium stress-redistribution data when reversible and moderately irreversible defects were combined for both redistribution and reinjection using quantitative analysis (Fig. 35).[145] In a similar patient population of chronic coronary artery disease and prior myocardial infarction, when thallium data were classified qualitatively as normal, reversible, or irreversible (without taking into consideration defect severity; mild-to-moderate, or severe), the scintigraphic variable that was the strongest predictor of hard events (cardiac death or myocardial infarction) was the presence of more than three irreversible defects that remained

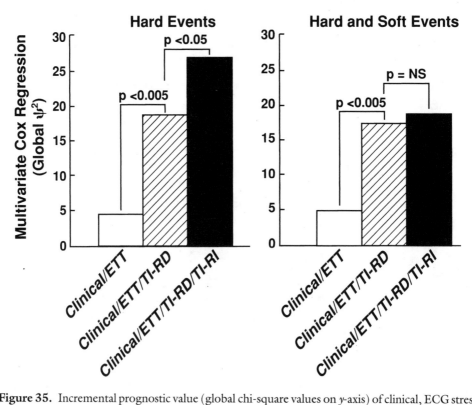

Figure 35. Incremental prognostic value (global chi-square values on y-axis) of clinical, ECG stress test (ETT), thallium stress-redistribution (Tl-RD), and reinjection (Tl-RI) data for hard events (**left**) and for hard and soft events combined (**right**). Modified and reprinted with permission from Reference 145.

fixed after thallium reinjection.[146] However, when the prognostic value of thallium reinjection was assessed retrospectively, among patients who were referred for thallium stressredistribution imaging (not selected for prior myocardial infarction or left ventricular dysfunction), the number of reversible defects was not predictive of future events on either the redistribution or the reinjection images.[147] In all three studies, planar imaging was utilized. Whether the application of SPECT imaging with quantitation of defect severity will enhance the prognostic value of thallium reinjection is a subject of ongoing investigation.

Early After Myocardial Infarction

Because of the potential profound impact on survival and left ventricular function of early reperfusion strategies in acute myocardial infarction, it is useful to assess studies performed in the prethrombolytic era separately from those performed in the current thrombolytic era. However, it should be noted that even in the current era, many patients with acute myocardial infarction do not undergo early reperfusion therapy for a number of reasons.

Risk Assessment in the Prethrombolytic Era

Many clinical variables have been identified that are associated with high clinical risk in survivors of myocardial infarction. In the presence of such high-risk indicators as recurrent angina, cardiogenic shock, malignant arrhythmias, and congestive heart failure, the patient usually undergoes early invasive evaluation. Thus, the focus of noninvasive assessment in the prethrombolytic era was the risk stratification of patients with uncomplicated myocardial infarction.

A number of studies have shown that thallium scintigraphy can identify high-risk postinfarction patients with multivessel coronary disease.[143,148,149] Gibson and coworkers investigated the prognostic value of submaximal exercise testing with thallium imaging in 140 patients with uncomplicated myocardial infarction.[143] In this study, the presence of ischemia defined by thallium scintigraphy was the most important predictor of subsequent cardiac events and was more important than any other clinical or angiographic variable (Fig. 34). Furthermore, in another study, the identification of ischemia by early thallium imaging was a better predictor of mortality than the assessment of left ventricular function alone.[150]

Risk Assessment in the Thrombolytic Era

Although the identification of viable, ischemic myocardium after infarction by thallium scintigraphy is known to provide important prognostic information, it is not clear whether these results can be extrapolated to patients receiving acute reperfusion therapy with thrombolytics or primary angioplasty. In a study of postthrombolytic patients studied with thallium SPECT imaging 3 days after infarction, a negative thallium study was associated with a favorable prognosis over a 7-month follow-up period.[151] Patients with positive scans were managed aggressively, and thus it is impossible to determine the natural history of such patients. However, recent studies have found lower prognostic value of predischarge low-level exercise thallium testing in such patients.

Tilkemeier and colleagues followed 64 patients who underwent early thrombolysis for acute myocardial infarction and 107 patients without an intervention.[152] After a mean follow-up of approximately 1 year, cardiac events (death, recurrent myocardial infarction, or revascularization) occurred in 25% of the thrombolytic group versus 32% in those without thrombolytic therapy. The sensitivity of predischarge low-level exercise thallium scintigraphy was 55% in the thrombolytic group and 81% in the group without intervention ($p < 0.05$). Others have found that multivessel coronary disease was just as likely in patients with high-grade residual stenosis of the infarct-related artery who had negative early, submaximal exercise thallium scintigraphy as in those who had positive tests.[153]

The apparent discrepant results of thallium for risk stratification after acute myocardial infarction in the pre- and postthrombolytic era may relate to the selection bias and the potential beneficial effects of reperfusion therapy on prognosis. Patients in most thrombolytic trials tend to have a lower prevalence of multivessel coronary disease and a more favorable prognosis. For example, in the substudy of Global Utilization of Streptokinase and Tissue-Type Plasminogen Activator for Occluded Coronary Arteries Study (GUSTO) Trial,[154] 62% of the patients had one-vessel disease, 24% had two-vessel coronary artery disease, and only 14% of patients had three-vessel coronary artery disease. In fact, approximately 40% of the patients had entirely normal regional wall motion in the infarct zone. The mortality rates at 30 days (early prognosis) were 3.5% in the one-vessel group, 6.5% in the two-vessel group, and 11.2% in the three-vessel group. Thus, most patients were in a relatively low-risk group, in which the positive predictive value (PPV) of any test result to identify this small percentage of patients with an adverse outcome is low. However, a negative test result, during hospitalization in postinfarction patients, has an excellent negative predictive value (NPV) for a good outcome. The favorable effects of thrombolytic therapy on prognosis likewise may limit the positive predictive accuracy of noninvasive strategies further. Thus, the results of any prognostic test must be interpreted with appropriate consideration of the pretest likelihood of risk.

Recent Advances in SPECT Technology and Instrumentation

Gated Thallium SPECT

To understand fully the pathophysiology of myocardial ischemia and viability, an assessment of both myocardial perfusion and function usually is required. In the past, this has required two separate diagnostic tests, with functional assessment performed noninvasively with radionuclide ventriculography or echocardiography. Recently, by gating the acquisition of the perfusion imaged to the ECG, a composite series of images are created that represent different phases of the cardiac cycle, which then can be displayed dynamically, analogous to an equilibrium radionuclide angiography (Fig. 36). The feasibility of this approach is now well established both with thallium[155] and ^{99m}Tc-labeled myocardial perfusion tracers,[156] and most modern SPECT cameras have the capability for ECG gating and image analysis.

The simultaneous assessment of myocardial perfusion and function may be helpful in distinguishing viable from scarred or fibrotic myocardium in patients with chronic or acute coronary artery disease. Patients with myocardial stunning would be identified by relatively normal perfusion but impaired contraction. Patients with hibernation may be identified with impaired perfusion and contraction but with preserved thallium uptake on redistribution/reinjection images or by using another tracer such as FDG. Optimal methods for the analysis of gated SPECT images have not been developed, and additional studies will be needed to determine the clinical utility of this approach.

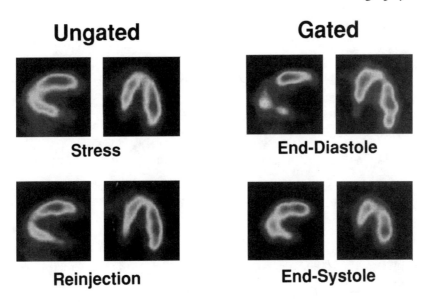

Figure 36. Left: Vertical and horizontal long-axis ungated stress-reinjection thallium SPECT images. **Right**: End-diastolic and end-systolic images corresponding to the gated stress thallium images.

Attenuation Correction

Breast attenuation artifacts in women and diaphragmatic attenuation in men are the two most commonly cited artifacts with thallium scintigraphy. When applying quantitative analysis, breast and diaphragmatic attenuation may reduce myocardial counts beyond the threshold criteria for viability thereby underestimating the extent and presence of myocardial tissue.

During SPECT imaging, as the detector moves about the patient, the projection data acquired at each incremental angle will vary depending on the differences in tissues along the projection ray, the depth of tissue, and the distance to the detector caused by the geometry of the collimator.[157] These factors influence the linear relation between thallium counts intensity in the SPECT image and the actual thallium concentration in the myocardium. Attenuation refers to the combined effects of scatter (detected photons but misregistered or undetected photons) and photon absorption by the photoelectric effect (undetected). Because the probability of attenuation by photon absorption decreases as photon energy of the radiotracer increases, this may explain, in part, the reported less severe attenuation artifacts with ^{99m}Tc-labeled perfusion tracers compared with thallium-201. Although attenuation correction is more difficult with SPECT compared with PET, a number of methods have been proposed to measure attenuation values with SPECT.[157] New instrumentation and reconstruction algorithms (attenuation maps and software) that address the attenuation problem for cardiac SPECT also have been made available commercially. Whether attenuation correction of thallium will further enhance assessment of viable myocardium is a subject of ongoing investigation.

References

1. Blumgart HC, Weiss S. Studies on the velocity of blood flow. VII. The pulmnonary circulation time in normal resting individuals. *J Clin Invest* 1927;4:399–425.

2. Love WD, Burch GE. A study in dogs of methods notable for estimating the rate of myocardial uptake of ^{86}Rb in man and the effect of L-norepinephrine and pitressin on ^{86}Rb uptake. *J Clin Invest* 1957;36:468–478.

3. Ross RS, Ueda K, Lichtlen PR, et al. Measurement of myocardial blood flow in animals and man by selective injection of radio-active inert gas into the coronary arteries. *Circ Res* 1964; 15:28–41.

4. Cannon PJ, Dell RB, Dwyer EM. Regional myocardial perfusion rates in patients with coronary artery disease. *J Clin Invest* 1972;51:978–994.

5. Quinn JL, Seratto M, Kezdi P. Coronary artery bed photo scanning using radioiodine albumin macroaggregates (RAMA). *J Nucl Med* 1966;7:107–113.

6. Ashburn WL, Braunwald E, Simon AL, et al. Myocardial perfusion imaging in man using ^{99m}Tc-MAA. *J Nucl Med* 1970;11:618–619. Abstract.

7. Grames GM, Jansen C, Gander MP, et al. The safety of the direct coronary injection of radiolabeled particles in 800 patients undergoing coronary angiography. *J Nucl Med* 1974; 15:2–6.

8. Gould KL, Lipscomb K, Hamilton G. Physiologic basis for assessing critical coronary stenosis: Instantaneous flow response and regional distribution during coronary hyperemia as measures of coronary flow reserve. *Am J Cardiol* 1974;33:87–94.

9. Love WD, Smith RO. Focusing collimator for use with the hard gamma emitters rubidium-86 and potassium-42. *J Nucl Med* 1966;7:781–786.

10. Love WD, Romney RB, Burch GE. A comparison of the distribution of potassium and exchangeable rubidium in the organs of the dog, using rubidium-86. *Circ Res* 1954;2:112–122.

11. Prokop EK, Strauss HW, Shaw J, et al. Comparison of regional myocardial perfusion determined by ionic potassium-43 to that determined by microspheres. *Circulation* 1974;50:978–984.

12. Zaret BL, Strauss HW, Martin ND, et al. Noninvasive regional myocardial perfusion with radioactive potassium: Study of patients at rest with exercise and during angina pectoris. *N Engl J Med* 1973;288:809–812.

13. Strauss HW, Harrison K, Langan JK, et al. Thallium-201 for myocardial imaging: Relation of thallium-201 to regional myocardial perfusion. *Circulation* 1975;51:641–645.

14. Lebowitz E, Greene MW, Fairchild R, et al. Thallium-201 for medical use, I. *J Nucl Med* 1975;16:151–155.

15. Bradley-Moore PR, Lebowitz E, Greene MW, et al. Thallium-201 for medical use, II: Biological behavior. *J Nucl Med* 1975;16:156–160.

16. Atkins HL, Budinger TF, Lebowitz E, et al. Thallium-201 for medical use, III: Human distribution and physical imaging properties. *J Nucl Med* 1977;18:133–140.

17. Lie JT, Pairolero PC, Holley KE, et al. Time course and zonal variations of ischemia-induced myocardial cationic electrolyte derangements. *Circulation* 1975;51:860–866.

18. Weich HF, Strauss HW, Pitt B. The extraction of thallium-201 by the myocardium. *Circulation* 1977;56:188–191.

19. Mullins LJ, Moore RD. The movement of thallium ions in muscle. *J Gen Physiol* 1960;43: 759–773.

20. Gehring PJ, Hammond PB. The interrelationship between thallium and potassium in animals. *J Pharmacol Exp Ther* 1967;155:187–201.

21. Mueller TM, Marcus ML, Ehrhardt JC, et al. Limitations of thallium-201 myocardial perfusion scintigrams. *Circulation* 1976;54:640–646.

22. Gould KL. Noninvasive assessment of coronary stenoses by myocardial perfusion imaging during pharmacologic coronary vasodilatation. *Am J Cardiol* 1978;41:279–287.

23. Leppo JA, Macneil PB, Moring AF, et al. Separate effects of ischemia, hypoxia, and contractility on thallium-201 kinetics in rabbit myocardium. *J Nucl Med* 1986;27:66–74.

24. Leppo JA. Myocardial uptake of thallium and rubidium during alterations in perfusion and oxygenation in isolated rabbit hearts. *J Nucl Med* 1987;28:878–885.

25. Moore CA, Cannon J, Watson DD, et al. Thallium-201 kinetics in stunned myocardium characterized by severe postischemic systolic dysfunction. *Circulation* 1990;81:1622–1632.

26. Sinusas AJ, Watson DD, Cannon JM, et al. Effect of ischemia and postischemic dysfunction on myocardial uptake of technetium-99m-labeled methoxyisobutyl isonitrile and thallium-201. *J Am Coll Cardiol* 1989;14:1785–1793.

27. Granato JE, Watson DD, Flanagan TL, et al. Myocardial thallium-201 kinetics and regional flow alterations with 3 hours of coronary occlusion and either rapid reperfusion through a totally patent vessel or slow reperfusion through a critical stenosis. *J Am Coll Cardiol* 1987; 9:109–118.

28. Pohost GM, Zir LM, Moore RH, et al. Differentiation of transiently ischemic from infarcted myocardium by serial imaging after a single dose of thallium-201. *Circulation* 1977;55:294–302.

29. Schwartz JS, Ponto R, Carlyle P, et al. Early redistribution of thallium-201 after temporary ischemia. *Circulation* 1978;57:332–335.

30. Grunwald A, Watson D, Holzgrefe H, et al. Myocardial thallium-201 kinetics in normal and ischemic myocardium. *Circulation* 1981;64:610–618.

31. Okada R, Jacobs M, Daggett W, et al. Thallium-201 kinetics in nonischemic canine myocardium. *Circulation* 1982;65:70–77.

32. Beller GA, Watson DD, Ackell P, et al. Time course of thallium-201 redistribution after transient myocardial ischemia. *Circulation* 1980;61:791–797.

33. Okada RD, Pohost GM. Effect of decreased blood flow and ischemia on myocardial thallium clearance. *J Am Coll Cardiol* 1984;3:744–750.

34. DeBusk RF. For the Health and Public Policy Committee of the Clinical Efficacy Assessment Subcommittee, American College of Physicians: Evaluation of patients after recent acute myocardial infarction. *Ann Intern Med* 1989;110:485–488.

35. Norris RM, Barnaby PF, Brandt PWT, et al. Prognosis after recovery from first acute myocardial infarction: Determinants of reinfarction and sudden death. *Am J Cardiol* 1984;53: 408–413.

36. Lowe JE, Reimer KA, Jennings RB. Experimental infarct size as a function of the amount of myocardium at risk. *Am J Pathol* 1978;90:363–377.

37. Topol EJ, Ellis SG. Coronary collaterals revisited: Accessory pathway to myocardial preservation during infarction. *Circulation* 1991;83:1084–1086.

38. Knoebel SB, Henry PL, Phillips JF, et al. Coronary collateral circulation and myocardial blood flow reserve. *Circulation* 1972;46:84–94.

39. Levin DC. Pathways and functional significance of coronary collateral circulation. *Circulation* 1974;50:831–837.

40. Dilsizian V, Cannon RO, Tracy CM, et al. Enhanced regional left ventricular function after distant coronary bypass via improved collateral blood flow. *J Am Coll Cardiol* 1989;14:312–318.

41. DeWood MA, Spores J, Notske R, et al. Prevalence of total coronary occlusion during the early hours of transmural myocardial infarction. *N Engl J Med* 1980;303:897–902.

42. Rozanski A, Berman D, Gray R, et al. Preoperative prediction of reversible myocardial asynergy by postexercise radionuclide ventriculography. *N Engl J Med* 1982;307:212–216.

43. Tillisch JH, Brunken R, Marshall R, et al. Reversibility of cardiac wall-motion abnormalities predicted by positron tomography. *N Engl J Med* 1986;314:884–888.

44. Heyndrickx GR, Baig H, Nelkins P, et al. Depression of regional blood flow and wall thickening after brief coronary occlusions. *Am J Physiol* 1978;234:H653–H659.

45. Rahimtoola SH. Coronary bypass surgery for chronic angina—1981: A perspective. *Circulation* 1982;65:225–241.

46. Matsuzaki M, Gallagher KP, Kemper WS, et al. Sustained regional dysfunction, produced by prolonged coronary stenosis: Gradual recovery after reperfusion. *Circulation* 1983;68:170–182.

47. Fuster V, Stein B, Ambrose J, et al. Atherosclerotic plaque rupture and thrombosis: Evolving concepts. *Circulation* 1990;82:II47–II59.

48. Fuster V, Badimon L, Badimon JJ, et al. Mechanisms of disease: The pathogenesis of coronary artery disease and the acute coronary syndromes. Parts I and II. *N Engl J Med* 1992;326:242–250, 310–318.

49. Ambrose J, Winters S, Arora R, et al. Angiographic evolution of coronary artery morphology in unstable angina. *J Am Coll Cardiol* 1986;7:472–478.

50. Ambrose J, Tannenbaum M, Alexopoulos D, et al. Angiographic progression of coronary artery disease and the development of myocardial infarction. *J Am Coll Cardiol* 1988;12:56–62.

51. Tennant R, Wiggers C. The effect of coronary occlusion on myocardial contraction. *Am J Physiol* 1935;112:351–361.

52. Downey JM. Mycoardial contractile force as a function of coronary blood flow. *Am J Physiol* 1976;230:1–6.

53. Vatner S. Correlation between acute reduction in myocardial blood flow and function in conscious dogs. *Circ Res* 1980;47:201–207.

54. Lee JD, Tajimi T, Guth B, et al. Exercise induced regional dysfunction with subcritical coronary stenosis. *Circulation* 1986;73:596–605.

55. Herman MV, Heinle RA, Klein MD, et al. Localized disorders of myocardial contraction. *N Engl J Med* 1967;277:222–232.

56. Johnson PC. Autoregulation of blood flow. *Circ Res* 1986;59:483–495.

57. Gould KL, Hamilton GW, Lipscomb K, et al. Method of assessing stress-induced regional malperfusion during coronary arteriography. Experimental validation and clinical application. *Am J Cardiol* 1974;34:557–564.

58. Klocke FJ. Measurements of coronary blood flow and degree of stenosis: Current clinical implications and continuing uncertainties. *J Am Coll Cardiol* 1983;1:31–41.

59. Cannon PJ, Weiss MB, Sciacca RR. Myocardial blood flow in coronary artery disease: Studies at rest and during stress with inert gas washout techniques. *Prog Cardiovasc Dis* 1977;20:95–120.

60. Coffman JD, Gregg DE. Reactive hyperemia characteristics of the myocardium. *Am J Physiol* 1960;199:1143–1149.

61. Gewirtz H, Williams DO, Ohley WH, et al. Influence of coronary vasodilation on the transmural distribution of myocardial blood flow distal to a severe fixed coronary stenosis. *Am Heart J* 1983;106:674–680.

62. Holman BL, Cohn PF, Adams DF, et al. Regional myocardial blood flow during hyperemia induced by contrast agent in patients with coronary artery disease. *Am J Cardiol* 1976;38:416–421.

63. Akins CW, Pohost GM, Desanctis RW, et al. Selection of angina-free patients with severe left ventricular dysfunction for myocardial revascularization. *Am J Cardiol* 1980;46:695–700.

64. Gibson RS, Watson DD, Taylor GJ, et al. Prospective assessment of regional myocardial perfusion before and after coronary revascularization surgery by quantitative thallium-201 scintigraphy. *J Am Coll Cardiol* 1983;1:804–815.

65. Liu P, Kiess MC, Okada RD, et al. The persistent defect on exercise thallium imaging and its fate after myocardial revascularization: Does it represent scar or ischemia? *Am Heart J* 1985;110:996–1001.

66. Cloninger KG, DePuey EG, Garcia EV, et al. Incomplete redistribution in delayed thallium-201 single photon emission computed tomographic images: An overestimation of myocardial scarring. *J Am Coll Cardiol* 1988;12:955–963.

67. Kiat H, Berman DS, Maddahi J, et al. Late reversibility of tomographic myocardial thallium-201 defects: An accurate marker of myocardial viability. *J Am Coll Cardiol* 1988;12:1456–1463.

68. Manyari DE, Knudtson M, Kloiber R, et al. Sequential thallium-201 myocardial perfusion studies after successful percutaneous transluminal coronary artery angioplasty: Delayed resolution of exercise-induced scintigraphic abnormalities. *Circulation* 1988;77:86–95.

69. Gutman J, Berman DS, Freeman M, et al. Time to completed redistribution of thallium-201 in exercise myocardial scintigraphy: Relationship to the degree of coronary artery stenosis. *Am Heart J* 1983;106:989–995.

70. Yang LD, Berman DS, Kiat H, et al. The frequency of late reversibility in SPECT thallium-201 stress-redistribution studies. *J Am Coll Cardiol* 1989;15:334–340.

71. Dilsizian V, Rocco TP, Freedman NM, et al. Enhanced detection of ischemic but viable myocardium by the reinjection of thallium after stress-redistribution imaging. *N Engl J Med* 1990;323:141–146.

72. Rocco TP, Dilsizian V, McKusick KA, et al. Comparison of thallium redistribution with rest "reinjection" imaging for the detection of viable myocardium. *Am J Cardiol* 1990;66:158–163.

73. Ohtani H, Tamaki N, Yonekura Y, et al. Value of thallium-201 reinjection after delayed SPECT imaging for predicting reversible ischemia after coronary artery bypass grafting. *Am J Cardiol* 1990;66:394–399.

74. Lekakis J, Vassilopoulos N, Germanidis J, et al. Detection of viable tissue in healed infarcted myocardium by dipyridamole thallium-201 reinjection and regional wall motion studies. *Am J Cardiol* 1993;71:401–404.

75. Tamaki N, Ohtani H, Yamashita K, et al. Metabolic activity in the areas of new fill-in after thallium-201 reinjection: Comparison with positron emission tomography using fluorine-18-deoxyglucose. *J Nucl Med* 1991;32:673–678.

76. Bartenstein P, Hasfeld M, Schober O, et al. Tl-201 reinjection predicts improvement of left ventricular function following revascularization. *Nucl Med* 1993;32:87–90.

77. Haque T, Furukawa T, Takahashi M, et al. Identification of hibernating myocardium by dobutamine stress echocardiography: Comparison with thallium-201 reinjection imaging. *Am Heart J* 1995;130:553–563.

78. Vanoverschelde JJ, D'Hondt AM, Gerber BL, et al. Head-to-head comparison of exercise-redistribution-reinjection thallium SPECT and low-dose dobutamine echocardiography for prediction of the reversibility of chronic left ventricular dysfunction. *J Am Coll Cardiol* 1996;28:432–442.

79. Inglese E, Brambilla M, Dondi M, et al. Assessment of myocardial viability after thallium-201 reinjection or rest-redistribution imaging: A multicenter study. *J Nucl Med* 1995;36:555–563.

80. Gursurer M, Pinarli AE, Aksoy M, et al. Assessment of viable myocardium and prediction of postoperative improvement in left ventricular function in patients with severe left ventricular dysfunction by quantitative planar stress-redistribution-reinjection Tl-201 imaging. *Int J Cardiol* 1997;58:179–184.

81. Bonow RO, Dilsizian V, Cuocolo A, et al. Identification of viable myocardium in patients with coronary artery disease and left ventricular dysfunction: Comparison of thallium scintigraphy with reinjection and PET imaging with ^{18}F-fluorodeoxyglucose. *Circulation* 1991;83:26–37.

82. Zimmermann R, Mall G, Rauch B, et al. Residual Tl-201 activity in irreversible defects as a marker of myocardial viability: Clinicopathological study. *Circulation* 1995;91:1016–1021.

83. Goldhaber SZ, Newell JB, Alpert NM, et al. Effects of ischemic-like insult on myocardial thallium-201 accumulation. *Circulation* 1983;67:778.

84. Budinger TF, Pohost GM. Indication for thallium reinjection by 3 hour plasma levels. *Circulation* 1993;88:I534. Abstract.

85. Budinger TF, Pohost GM. Thallium "redistribution": An explanation. *J Nucl Med* 1986;27:996. Abstract.

86. Gewirtz H, Sullivan MJ, Shearer DR, et al. Analysis of proposed mechanisms of thallium redistribution: Comparison of a computer model of myocardial thallium kinetics with quantitative analysis of clinical scans. *IEEE Comput Cardiol* 1981;75–80.

87. Nelson CW, Wilson RA, Angello DA, et al. Effect of thallium-201 blood levels on reversible thallium defects. *J Nucl Med* 1989;30:1172–1175.

88. Okada RD, Leppo JA, Boucher CA, et al. Myocardial kinetics of thallium-201 after dipyridamole infusion in normal canine myocardium and in myocardium distal to a stenosis. *J Clin Invest* 1982;69:199–209.

89. Leppo JA, Okada RD, Strauss HW, et al. Effect of hyperaemia on thallium-201 redistribution in normal canine myocardium. *Cardiovasc Res* 1985;19:679–685.

90. Budinger TF, Knittel BL. Cardiac thallium redistribution and model. *J Nucl Med* 1987;28:588. Abstract.

91. Kayden DS, Sigal S, Soufer R, et al. Thallium-201 for assessment of myocardial viability: Quantitative comparison of 24-hour redistribution imaging with imaging after reinjection at rest. *J Am Coll Cardiol* 1991;18:1480–1486.

92. Dilsizian V, Smeltzer WR, Freedman NMT, et al. Thallium reinjection after stress-redistribution imaging: Does 24 hour delayed imaging following reinjection enhance detection of viable myocardium? *Circulation* 1991;83:1247–1255.

93. Dae MW, Botvinick EH, Starksen NF, et al. Do 4-hour reinjection thallium images and 24-hour thallium images provide equivalent information? *J Am Coll Cardiol* 1991;17:29. Abstract.

94. McCallister BD, Clemments IP, Hauser MF, et al. The limited value of 24-hour images following 4-hour reinjection thallium imaging. *Circulation*. 1991;84:II533. Abstract.

95. Kitsiou AN, Srinivasan G, Quyyumi AA, et al. Stress-induced reversible and mild-to-moderate irreversible thallium defects: Are they equally accurate for predicting recovery of regional left ventricular function after revascularization? *Circulation*. 1998;98:501–508.

96. Dilsizian V, Bonow RO. Differential uptake and apparent thallium-201 "washout" after thallium reinjection: Options regarding early redistribution imaging before reinjection or late redistribution imaging after reinjection. *Circulation*. 1992;85:1032–1038.

97. Kiat H, Friedman JD, Wang FP, et al. Frequency of late reversibility in stress-redistribution thallium-201 SPECT using an early reinjection protocol. *Am Heart J* 1991;122:613–619.

98. van Eck-Smit BLF, van der Wall EE, Kuijper AFM, et al. Immediate thallium-201 reinjection following stress imaging: A time-saving approach for detection of myocardial viability. *J Nucl Med* 1993;34:737–743.

99. Klingensmith WC III, Sutherland JD. Detection of jeopardized myocardium with Tl-201 myocardial perfusion imaging: Comparison of early and late reinjection protocols. *Clin Nuc Med* 1993;18:487–490.

100. Dilsizian V, Bonow RO, Quyyumi AA, et al. Is early thallium reinjection after post-exercise imaging a satisfactory method to detect defect reversibility? *Circulation* 1993;88:I199. Abstract.

101. Wackers FJ, Lie KI, Liem KL, et al. Thallium-201 scintigraphy in unstable angina pectoris. *Circulation* 1978;57:738–742.

102. Gewirtz H, Beller GA, Strauss HW, et al. Transient defects of resting thallium scans in patients with coronary artery disease. *Circulation* 1979;59:707–713.

103. Berger BC, Watson DD, Burwell LR, et al. Redistribution of thallium at rest in patients with stable and unstable angina and the effect of coronary artery bypass surgery. *Circulation* 1979;60:1114–1125.

104. Iskandrian AS, Hakki A, Kane SA, et al. Rest and redistribution thallium-201 myocardial scintigraphy to predict improvement in left ventricular function after coronary artery bypass grafting. *Am J Cardiol* 1983;51:1312–1316.

105. Mori T, Minamiji K, Kurogane H, et al. Rest-injected thallium-201 imaging for assessing viability of severe asynergic regions. *J Nucl Med* 1991;32:1718–1724.

106. Ragosta M, Beller GA, Watson DD, et al. Quantitative planar rest-redistribution ^{201}Tl imaging in detection of myocardial viability and prediction of improvement in left ventricular function after coronary artery bypass surgery in patients with severely depressed left ventricular function. *Circulation* 1993;87:1630–1641.

107. Udelson JE, Coleman PS, Metherall JA, et al. Predicting recovery of severe regional ventricular dysfunction: Comparison of resting scintigraphy with ^{201}Tl and ^{99m}Tc-sestamibi. *Circulation* 1994;89:2552–2561.

108. Perrone-Filardi P, Pace L, Prastaro M, et al. Assessment of myocardial viability in patients with chronic coronary artery disease: Rest-4-hour-24-hour ^{201}Tl tomography versus dobutamine echocardiography. *Circulation* 1996;94:2712–2719.

109. Hoffman EJ, Huang SC, Phelps ME. Quantitation in positron emission tomography, 1: Effect of object size. *J Comput Assist Tomogr* 1979;3:299–308.

110. Gewirtz H, Grotte GJ, Strauss HW, et al. The influence of left ventricular volume and wall motion on myocardial images. *Circulation* 1979;59:1172–1179.

111. Parodi AV, Schelbert HR, Schwaiger M, et al. Cardiac emission computed tomography: Estimation of regional tracer concentrations due to wall motion abnormality. *J Comput Assist Tomogr* 1984;8:1083–1092.

112. Sinusas AJ, Shi QX, Vitols PJ, et al. Impact of regional ventricular function, geometry and dobutamine stress on quantitative 99mTc-sestamibi defect size. *Circulation* 1993;88:2224–2234.

113. Eisner RL, Schmarkey S, Martin SE, et al. Defects on SPECT "perfusion" images can occur due to abnormal segmental contraction. *J Nucl Med* 1994;35:638–643.

114. Granato JE, Watson DD, Flanagan TL, et al. Myocardial thallium-201 kinetics and regional flow alterations within 3 hours of coronary occlusion and either rapid reperfusion through a totally patent vessel or slow reperfusion through a critical stenosis. *J Am Coll Cardiol* 1987;9:109–118.

115. Maddahi J, Ganz W, Ninomiya K, et al. Myocardial salvage by intracoronary thrombolysis in evolving acute myocardial infarction: Evaluation using intracoronary injection of thallium-201. *Am Heart J* 1981;102:664–674.

116. Markis JE, Malagold M, Parker JA, et al. Myocardial salvage after intracoronary thrombolysis with streptokinase in acute myocardial infarction. *N Eng J Med* 1981;305:777–782.

117. Beller GA. Role of myocardial perfusion imaging in evaluating thrombolytic therapy for acute myocardial infarction. *J Am Coll Cardiol* 1987;9:661–668.

118. Granato JE, Watson DD, Flanagan TL, et al. Myocardial thallium-201 kinetics during coronary occlusion and reperfusion: Influence of methods of reflow and timing of thallium-201 administration. *Circulation* 1986;73:150–160.

119. Stewart RE, Kander N, Juni JE, et al. Submaximal exercise thallium-201 SPECT for assessment of interventional therapy in patients with acute myocardial infarction. *Am Heart J* 1991;121:1033–1041.

120. Lew AS, Maddahi J, Shah PK, et al. Critically ischemic myocardium in clinically stable patients following thrombolytic therapy for acute myocardial infarction: Potential implications for early coronary angioplasty in selected patients. *Am Heart J* 1990;120:1015–1025.

121. Cerqueira MD, Maynard C, Ritchie JL, et al. Long-term survival in 618 patients from the Western Washington Streptokinase in Myocardial Infarction Trials. *J Am Coll Cardiol* 1992; 20:1452–1459.

122. Lomboy CT, Schulman DS, Griill HP, et al. Rest-redistribution thallium-201 scintigraphy to determine myocardial viability early after myocardial infarction. *J Am Coll Cardiol* 1995;25: 201–207.

123. Komamura K, Kitakaze M, Nishida K, et al. Progressive decreases in coronary vein flow during reperfusion in acute myocardial infarction: Clinical documentation of the no reflow phenomenon after successful thrombolysis. *J Am Coll Cardiol* 1994;24:370–377.

124. Canby RC, Silber S, Pohost GM. Relations of the myocardial imaging agents 99mTc-myocardial ischemiaBI and 201-Tl to myocardial blood flow in a canine model of ischemic insult. *Circulation* 1990;81:286–296.

125. Glover DK, Okada RD. Myocardial kinetics of Tc-myocardial ischemiaBI in canine myocardium after dipyridamole. *Circulation* 1990;81:628–637.

126. Ito H, Maruyama A, Iwakura K, et al. Clinical implications of the "no reflow" phenomenon: A predictor of complications and left ventricular remodeling in reperfused anterior wall myocardial infarction. *Circulation* 1996;93:223–228.

127. Melin JA, Wijns W, Keyeux A, et al. Assessment of thallium-201 redistribution versus glucose uptake as predictors of viability after coronary occlusion and reperfusion. *Circulation* 1988; 77:927–934.

128. Ogiu N, Nakai K, Hiramori K. Thallium-201 reinjection images can identify the viable and necrotic myocardium similarly to metabolic imaging with glucose loading F-18 fluorodeoxyglucose (FDG)-PET. *Annals of Nucl Med* 1994;8:171–176.

129. Dilsizian V, Freedman NMT, Bacharach SL, et al. Regional thallium uptake in irreversible defects: Magnitude of change in thallium activity after reinjection distinguishes viable from nonviable myocardium. *Circulation* 1992;85:627–634.

130. Dilsizian V, Perrone-Filardi P, Arrighi JA, et al. Concordance and discordance between stress-redistribution-reinjection and rest-redistribution thallium imaging for assessing viable myocardium: Comparison with metabolic activity by PET. *Circulation* 1993;88: 941–952.

131. Brunken RC, Kottou S, Nienaber CA, et al. PET detection of viable tissue in myocardial segments with persistent defects at Tl-201 SPECT. *Radiology* 1989;65:65–73.

132. Marin-Neto JA, Dilsizian V, Arrighi JA, et al. Thallium reinjection demonstrates viable myocardium in regions with reverse redistribution. *Circulation* 1993;88:1736–1745.

133. Dey HM, Soufer R. Reverse redistribution on planar thallium scintigraphy: Relationship to resting thallium uptake and long-term outcome. *Eur J Nucl Med* 1995;22:237–242.

134. Srinivasan G, Kitsiou AN, Bacharach SL, et al. ^{18}F-fluorodeoxyglucose single photon emission computed tomography: Can it replace PET and thallium SPECT for the assessment of myocardial viability? *Circulation* 1998;97:843–850.

135. Boucher CA, Zir LM, Beller GA, et al. Increased lung uptake of thallium-201 during exercise myocardial imaging: Clinical, hemodynamic and angiographic implications in patients with coronary artery disease. *Am J Cardiol* 1980;46:189–196.

136. Gill JB, Ruddy TD, Newell JB, et al. Prognostic importance of thallium uptake by the lungs during exercise coronary artery disease. *N Engl J Med* 1987;317:1485–1489.

137. Stolzenberg J. Dilatation of left ventricular cavity on stress thallium scan as an indicator of ischemic disease. *Clin Nucl Med* 1980;5:289–291.
138. Krawczynska EG, Weintraub WS, Garcia EV, et al. Left ventricular dilatation and multivessel coronary artery disease on thallium-201 SPECT are important prognostic indicators in patients with large defects in the left anterior descending distribution. *Am J Cardiol* 1994;74: 1233–1239.
139. Brown KA, Boucher CA, Okada RD, et al. Prognostic value of exercise thallium-201 imaging in patients presenting for evaluation of chest pain. *J Am Coll Cardiol* 1983;1:994–1001.
140. Ladenheim ML, Pollack BH, Rozanski A, et al. Extent and severity of myocardial reperfusion as predictors of prognosis in patients with suspected coronary artery disease. *J Am Coll Cardiol* 1986;7:464–471.
141. Pollock SG, Abbott RD, Boucher CA, et al. Independent and incremental prognostic value of test performed in hierarchical order to evaluate patients with suspected coronary artery disease. *Circulation* 1992;85:237–248.
142. Iskandrian AS, Chae SC, Heo J, et al. Independent and incremental prognostic value of exercise single photon emission computed tomography (SPECT) thallium imaging in coronary artery disease. *J Am Coll Cardiol* 1993;22:665–670.
143. Gibson RS, Watson DD, Craddock GB, et al. Predication of cardiac events after uncomplicated myocardial infarction: A prospective study comparing predischarge exercise thallium-201 scintigraphy and coronary angiography. *Circulation* 1983;68:321–336.
144. Hendel RC, Whitfield SS, Villegas BJ, et al. Prediction of late cardiac events by dipyridamole thallium imaging in patients undergoing elective vascular surgery. *Am J Cardiol* 1992;70: 1243–1249.
145. Petretta M, Cuocolo A, Bonaduce D, et al. Incremental prognostic value of thallium reinjection after stress-redistribution imaging in patients with previous myocardial infarction and left ventricular dysfunction. *J Nucl Med* 1997;38:195–200.
146. Tisselli A, Pieri P, Moscatelli G, et al. Prognostic value of persistent thallium-201 defects that become reversible after reinjection in patients with chronic myocardial infarction. *J Nucl Cardiol* 1997;4:195–201.
147. Zafrir N, Leppo JA, Reinhardt CP, et al. Thallium reinjection versus standard stress/delay redistribution imaging for prediction of cardiac events. *J Am Coll Cardiol* 1998;31:1280–1285.
148. Abraham RD, Freedman SB, Dunn RF, et al. Prediction of multivessel coronary artery disease and prognosis early after acute myocardial infarction by exercise electrocardiography and thallium-201 myocardial perfusion scanning. *Am J Cardiol* 1986;58:423–427.
149. Brown KA, Weiss RM, Clements JP, et al. Usefulness of residual ischemic myocardium within prior infarct zone for identifying patients at high risk late after myocardial infarction. *Am J Cardiol* 1987;60:15–19.
150. Becker LC, Silverman KJ, Bulkley BH, et al. Comparison of early thallium-201 scintigraphy and gated blood pool imaging for predicting mortality in patients with acute myocardial infarction. *Circulation* 1983;67:1272–1282.
151. Topol EJ, Burek K, O'Neill WW, et al. A randomized controlled trial of hospital discharge three days after myocardial infarction in the era of reperfusion. *N Eng J Med* 1988;318:1083–1088.
152. Tilkemeier PL, Guiney TE, LaRaia PJ, et al. Prognostic value of predischarge low-level exercise thallium testing after thrombolytic treatment of acute myocardial infarction. *Am J Cardiol* 1990;66:1203–1207.
153. Sutton JM, Topol EJ. Significance of a negative exercise thallium test in the presence of a critical residual stenosis after thrombolysis for acute myocardial infarction. *Circulation* 1991; 83:1278–1286.
154. The GUSTO Angiographic Investigators. The effects of tissue plasminogen activator, streptokinase or both on coronary-artery patency, ventricular function and survival after acute myocardial infarction. *N Eng J Med* 1993;329:1615–1622.
155. Srinivasan G, Nour KA, Davis CM, et al. Gated thallium imaging with multiheaded SPECT differentiates attenuation from myocardial injury in routine clinical studies. *Circulation* 1996; 94:I240. Abstract.
156. DePuey EG, Rozanski A. Using gated technetium-99m sestamibi SPECT to characterize fixed myocardial defects as infarct or artifact. *J Nucl Med* 1995;36:952–955.

157. Bacharach SL, Buvat I. Attenuation correction in cardiac positron emission tomography and single-photon emission computed tomography. *J Nucl Cardiol* 1995;2:246–255.
158. Dilsizian V, Arrighi JA: Myocardial viability in chronic coronary artery disease: Perfusion, metabolism, and contractile reserve. In: Gerson MC, ed. *Cardiac Nuclear Medicine*, 3rd ed. New York: McGraw-Hill; 1997;143–191.
159. Arrighi JA, Dilsizian V. Identification of viable, nonfunctioning myocardium. In: Brown DL, ed. *Cardiac Intensive Care*, 1st ed. Philadelphia, PA: Saunders; 1998;307–327.

Technetium-99m–Labeled Myocardial Perfusion Tracers: Blood Flow or Viability Agents?

Vasken Dilsizian, MD

Introduction

To reflect regional perfusion, an ideal tracer must have high extraction by the organ of interest and rapid clearance from the blood.[1] The radiotracer that most closely parallels myocardial blood flow (MBF) would be expected to most accurately identify coronary artery narrowing. There are several classes of radiopharmaceuticals that meet these criteria, such as microspheres, thallium-201, and technetium-99m (^{99m}Tc)–labeled perfusion tracers. Radiotracers that are not highly extracted (<50%) or if the residence time in the blood is prolonged (clearance half-time of >5 minutes) cannot be used to assess regional perfusion.

Despite the excellent myocardial extraction and flow kinetics properties of thallium for evaluating myocardial perfusion and ischemia (redistribution) for evaluating viability, the energy spectrum of thallium is somewhat lower (69–80 keV mercury X-ray emission) than what is considered optimum for conventional scintillation cameras (ideal photopeak in the range of 140 keV). Consequently, attenuation of photons as a function of tissue depth is a potential limitation for thallium in patients with large body habitus. In addition, because of its long physical half-life (73 hours), the amount of thallium administered to a patient is confined by its radiation burden.

[99m]Tc–labeled compounds improve on these two limitations of thallium. The short 6-hour half-life of ^{99m}Tc permits the administration of doses 10 times higher than thallium thereby improving the resolution of the images (higher photon flux and count statistics) while maintaining a relatively low-radiation burden to the patient. Furthermore, the 140-keV energy spectrum of ^{99m}Tc result in less scatter and soft tissue attenuation with improved spatial resolution when compared with thallium. Several new classes of ^{99m}Tc-labeled complexes have been developed since 1981[2] for myocardial perfusion imaging (Table 1): (1) isonitriles (^{99m}Tc-sestamibi), (2) boronic acid adducts of technetium dioxime (BATO) (^{99m}Tc-teboroxime), (3) diphosphines (^{99m}Tc-tetrofosmin), (4) mixed ligand complexes (^{99m}Tc-furifosmin, Q12), and (5) nitrido dithiocarbamates [[99m]TcN-[bis(*N*-etoxy, *N*-ethyl dithiocarbamato) nitrido technetium(V)] (NOET). These technetium-labeled perfusion tracers are taken up by the myocardium in proportion to regional blood flow. Despite the recognized metabolic or transmembrane trap-

From Dilsizian V (ed). *Myocardial Viability: A Clinical and Scientific Treatise.* Armonk, NY: Futura Publishing Co., Inc.; © 2000.

_____**Table 1**_____

Myocardial Perfusion Tracers

Thallium-201
Isonitriles
  Technetium-99m (^{99m}Tc)–sestamibi
Boronic acid adducts of technetium dioxime (BATO) compounds
  ^{99m}Tc-teboroxime
Diphosphines
  ^{99m}Tc-tetrofosmin
Mixed ligand complexes
  ^{99m}Tc-furifosmin (Q12)
Nitrido dithiocarbamates
  ^{99m}Tc N-[bis(N-etoxy,N-ethyl dithiocarbamato) nitrido technetium(V)] NOET

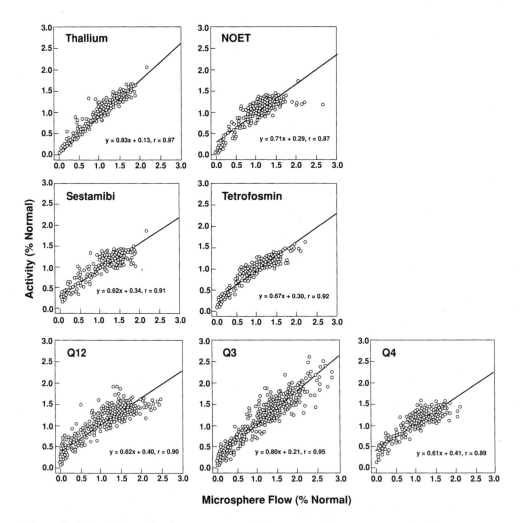

Figure 1. Plots of normalized average myocardial tracer activity versus normalized average myocardial blood flow (MBF) assessed by radioactive microspheres. Thallium shows a more ideal linear relationship with microsphere blood flow when compared with six technetium-99m (^{99m}Tc)–labeled myocardial perfusion agents. Modified and reprinted with permission from Reference 3.

ping of these ^{99m}Tc tracers, the relationship between myocardial tracer uptake and blood flow is not altered significantly except during acute myocardial ischemia, conditions of extremely low pH, or hyperemic flow.

During stress (exercise or pharmacologic), coronary blood flow in myocardial regions without coronary artery narrowing may increase to approximately four- to fivefolds above the baseline levels. However, in the setting of mild-to-moderate coronary artery narrowing, the degree of coronary flow increase may be attenuated when compared with regions without coronary artery disease. A linear relationship between tracer uptake and MBF would, therefore, differentiate between regions with normal or high blood flow (supplied by normal coronary arteries) and abnormal or low blood flow (supplied by narrowed coronary arteries). In an open-chest canine model of regional myocardial ischemia with dipyridamole-induced hyperemia, thallium showed a more ideal linear relationship between tracer uptake and MBF assessed by microspheres when compared with six ^{99m}Tc-labeled myocardial perfusion agents[3] (Fig. 1).

Clinical studies in patients have indicated that the accuracy of sestamibi, teboroxime, and tetrofosmin (three tracers that have received US Food and Drug Administration approval) for detection of coronary artery disease is similar to that of thallium.[4-6] Whether ^{99m}Tc-labeled perfusion tracers provide similar information to thallium with regards to myocardial perfusion defect size, defect reversibility, and viability remains controversial.

Technetium-99m Sestamibi

Mechanism of Sestamibi Uptake

Sestamibi is a lipophilic cationic complex that is taken up across sarcolemmal and mitochondrial membranes of myocytes by passive distribution, but at equilibrium it is retained within the mitochondria because of a large negative transmembrane potential.[7,8] Unlike thallium, which is predominantly dependent on sufficient membrane adenosine triphosphate (ATP) stores and active sodium potassium adenosine triphosphatase (ATPase) transport mechanism, sestamibi uptake does not appear to be active (Table 2). Experimental studies have demonstrated that sestamibi uptake continues as long as the cell membrane and mitochondrial processes remain intact,[9] and its clearance is related directly to the mitochondrial transmembrane potential and does not differ in ischemic from nonischemic regions.[10] Thus, while the uptake of sestamibi appears related primarily to its lipophilicity, the accumulation and retention of the tracer is related to energy-dependent processes that maintain membrane polarization. The concept that the myocardial retention of sestamibi is energy dependent suggests that this agent may be a marker of cellular viability. This has fueled substantial interest and optimism in the use of sestamibi clinically for assessing myocardial viability. Experimental models of myocardial infarction with and without reperfusion support this concept.[11-13]

Table 2
Technetium-99m Sestamibi

Lipid-soluble
Cationic perfusion tracer
Uptake is passive across mitochondrial membranes
At equilibrium, it is retained within the mitochondria because of a large negative
    transmembrane potential
Minimal redistribution compared with thallium

Sestamibi and Thallium Uptake: Similarities and Differences

Myocardial Perfusion

Like thallium, initial uptake of sestamibi reflects both regional blood flow and myocardial extraction; these vary depending on the retention mechanism involved for each individual tracer. Sestamibi is taken up by the myocardium in proportion to blood flow at normal or moderately elevated flow rates.[10,14,15] Similar to other myocardial perfusion tracers, its uptake plateaus at high flow rates, as may occur during pharmacologic vasodilatation. Thus, at flow rates above 2.0 mL/min per gram, sestamibi underestimates coronary blood flow and at very low flow rates (0.2 mL/min per gram) sestamibi overestimates coronary blood flow.[15] However, during intermediate flow rates, myocardial sestamibi activity increases linearly with coronary blood flow. Transcapillary transport and myocardial retention of both ^{99m}Tc-sestamibi and thallium are affected by the perfusion rate, capillary permeability, and by the binding characteristics within the myocardium.[9,16] Using a blood-perfused, isolated rabbit heart model, Leppo and Meerdink have shown that the average extraction fraction of sestamibi (39% ± 9%) is significantly less than that of thallium (73% ± 10%, $p < 0.001$), and that sestamibi has a higher parenchymal cell permeability and higher volume of distribution than thallium.[16]

Adenosine Stress

In canines with either critical or mild coronary artery stenosis, when thallium, sestamibi, and microspheres were injected simultaneously during adenosine infusion, the magnitude of flow heterogeneity between stenotic and normal perfusion beds was underestimated significantly when compared with thallium and microspheres[17] (Fig. 2). Al-

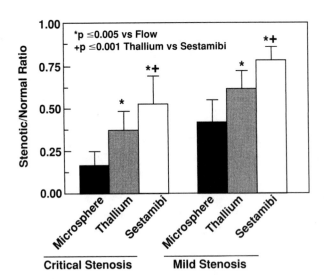

Figure 2. Bar graphs showing mean microsphere flow, thallium, and sestamibi activities expressed as the stenotic-to-normal thallium and sestamibi ratios for both critical and mild stenosis groups. Both thallium and sestamibi significantly underestimated blood flow when compared with microsphere flow. However, the degree of underestimation was significantly greater for sestamibi when compared with both microsphere flow and thallium. Modified and reprinted with permission from Reference 17.

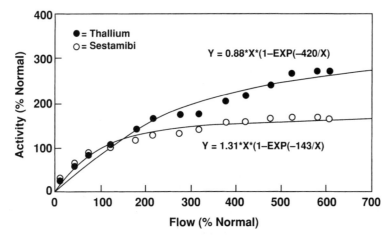

Figure 3. Graph showing myocardial sestamibi and thallium activities versus microsphere blood flow from a representative dog with a critical left anterior descending coronary artery stenosis that received intravenous adenosine. Data points represent transmural activities expressed as a percentage of activity at normal flow (1 mL/min per gram). Modified and reprinted with permission from Reference 17.

though myocardial uptake of thallium seemed to plateau at high coronary flow rates, the extent of underestimation of coronary blood flow was statistically greater with sestamibi (leveling off approximately two times normal flow) resulting in limited contrast between normal and stenotic myocardium (Fig. 3).

Dobutamine Stress

Unlike vasodilator stressors such as adenosine and dipyridamole, dobutamine stress tends to produce modest increases in blood flow. In canine models of coronary artery

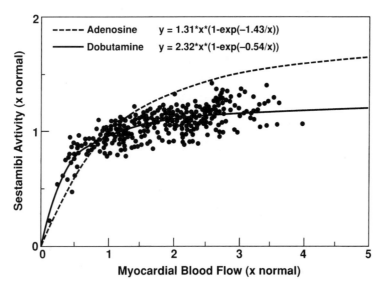

Figure 4. Normalized myocardial sestamibi activity versus microsphere flow at time of sestamibi injection during dobutamine and adenosine stress in same canine models. Sestamibi uptake plateaus earlier during dobutamine stress (at flows of just 1–1.5 mL/min per gram), and the relationship between flow and sestamibi uptake is less favorable for perfusion imaging during dobutamine stress than during adenosine stress. Modified and reprinted with permission from Reference 18.

stenoses, sestamibi activity ratios significantly underestimated dobutamine-induced flow disparity at time of sestamibi injection and therefore underestimated the physiological severity of the coronary stenoses.[18,19] Furthermore, the underestimation of the dobutamine-induced hyperemia at peak doses (30 μg/kg per minute) was greater than had been described previously with adenosine stress (Fig. 4). Dobutamine increased blood flow in normal myocardium by a factor of 2.5–3 times baseline flow, which is smaller than the fourfold increase described with vasodilator stressors, such as adenosine. Sestamibi activity ratios by γ-well counting were more favorable for adenosine stress in the groups with reduced (0.79 ± 0.03) and absent flow reserve (0.53 ± 0.06) than for dobutamine stress in the groups with reduced (0.80 ± 0.03) and absent flow reserve (0.78 ± 0.02). The reduced myocardial sestamibi uptake with dobutamine may relate to dobutamine-induced mitochondrial calcium influx thereby attenuating the negative mitochondrial membrane driving potential caused by mitochondrial calcium sequestration. This postulate is supported by preliminary data in which infusion of ruthenium red (a selective inhibitor of mitochondrial calcium influx) resulted in increased sestamibi first-pass extraction fraction during dobutamine-induced hyperemia.[20]

Myocardial Viability

In cultured chick embryo cardiac myocytes, Piwnica-Worms and colleagues studied cellular kinetics of thallium and sestamibi during metabolic inhibition, independent of perfusion.[21] Oxidative phophorylation and glycolysis were inhibited simultaneously by rotenone (10 μm) and iodoacetate (1 mmol/L), respectively, producing a decline in myocellular ATP content. Under these conditions, initial uptake rates of thallium and sestamibi responded in divergent ways to ATP depletion (Fig. 5). Initial uptake rates (extraction efficiency) of thallium declined within 20 minutes of metabolic inhibition by

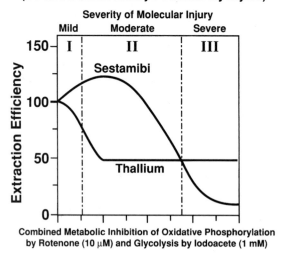

Figure 5. Schematic of the effect of severity of metabolic injury on initial uptake rates of sestamibi and thallium into cardiac myocytes, independent of perfusion. Modified and reprinted with permission from Reference 21.

A

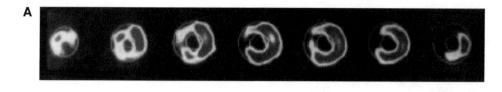

B

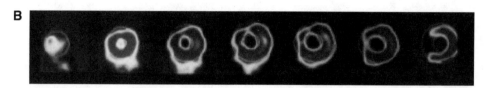

Figure 6. An example of a patient with smaller sestamibi defect size on stress (A) when compared with thallium (B). The patient performed the same level of exercise with both sestamibi and thallium. The left ventricular mass algorithm provided similar measures of total mass (197 g for thallium and 189 g for sestamibi). However, the stress-induced defect mass derived from thallium imaging (41 g) is significantly larger than that detected by sestamibi (3 g). No transmural defects are present on the sestamibi images. Modified and reprinted with permission from Reference 24.

50%–70% while initial uptake rates of sestamibi increased significantly by 10–20 minutes and remained elevated for the first 40–60 minutes of metabolic inhibition. The observed increase or near-normal uptake rates of sestamibi during mild-to-moderate metabolic injury (thallium/sestamibi mismatch) may indicate a mean plasma membrane hyperpolarization possibly resulting from opening of ATP-sensitive and arachidonic acid-activated potassium channels, before declining to low values with more severe cell injury. Similar distinctions between thallium and sestamibi uptake have been reported by other investigators.[22,23] These findings suggest that both thallium and sestamibi uptake by myocytes are affected by metabolic disturbances; however, sestamibi uptake is insensitive to mild metabolic impairment. These experimental data could explain on a metabolic basis alone the clinical observation that sestamibi defects are consistently smaller than those assessed by thallium[24] (Fig. 6).

Myocardial Perfusion Defect Size

The observed differences in extraction efficiencies of thallium and sestamibi in cultured chick embryo may have implications regarding perfusion defect size and reversibility (extent of myocardial ischemia and infarction) in the clinical setting. In a canine model of coronary artery occlusion and pharmacologic vasodilation, Leon and coworkers compared the extent of myocardial perfusion defect size with thallium and sestamibi using postmortem staining to define the extent of the hypoperfused region.[25] When coronary artery occlusion was near total (severe), sestamibi and thallium showed similar defect contrast and areas (Fig. 7). However, when coronary artery occlusion was moderate, counts in the defects were 39% higher for sestamibi compared with the thallium defects, and the area of the sestamibi defects occupied only 37% of the area of the defect on the thallium images of the same dog (Fig. 8). The extent of hypoperfused myocardium

Thallium Sestamibi
(5-10 min) (74-152 min)

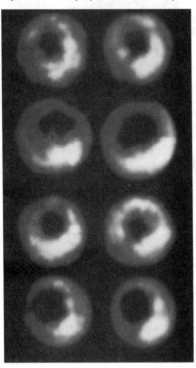

Figure 7. Bull's-eye displays from four severe or total occlusion coronary artery experiments in canines during pharmacological vasodilation. The single photon emission tomography (SPECT) thallium bull's-eye displays are on the left, and the SPECT sestamibi displays are on the right. In animals with severe or total coronary artery occlusion, thallium and sestamibi defect extent and severity are similar. Modified and reprinted with permission from Reference 25.

determined pathologically (polar display of pathological left ventricular short-axis slices) was closer to the thallium defect size than the sestamibi defect size. These observations in canines are similar to the observations made in the cultured myocytes by Piwnica-Worms and colleagues.[21] In patients with coronary artery disease undergoing thallium and sestamibi studies, sestamibi myocardial perfusion defects were consistently smaller than thallium regardless of whether the sestamibi images were acquired 120 minutes[24] or 60 minutes poststress.[26] Similar results were obtained by other investigators with another technetium-labeled perfusion tracer, tetrofosmin.[27]

Both in experimental animal and in human studies, thallium images were acquired 5–10 minutes after injection while sestamibi images were acquired 60–152 minutes after injection. The 1-to-2-hour delay between sestamibi injection and imaging was based on the best compromise between a high myocardial count rate and low background activity. A possible explanation, therefore, for the observed differences in sestamibi and thallium defect size may relate to differences in tracer redistribution, resolution, and/or response to altered metabolic states. Depending on the blood activity of the tracer after stress, continued uptake by the myocardium after the first pass may reduce the defect severity and area in the underperfused region. In view of these reports, it is recommended that sestamibi images be acquired earlier, approximately 30 minutes after injection during stress.

Despite differences in cellular kinetics between sestamibi and thallium uptake, in the clinical setting, both tracers have similar accuracy for detection of coronary artery disease.[28-32] However, beyond detection of disease, whether differences in myocardial perfusion defect size and reversibility (extent of myocardial ischemia and infarction) between

Thallium Sestamibi
(5-10 min) (74-152 min) Pathology

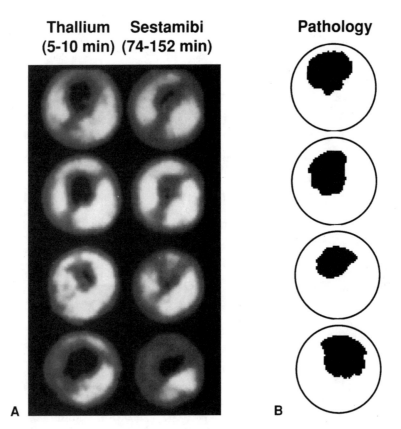

A   B

Figure 8. Bull's-eye displays from four representative experiments of moderate coronary artery stenoses during pharmacological vasodilation. (**A**) SPECT thallium bull's-eye displays are on the left, and the SPECT sestamibi displays are on the right. In every case, thallium defects are more severe and larger than sestamibi defects. (**B**) Pathological polar displays from the same four experiments are shown. The defect area in the thallium but not sestamibi displays approaches the underperfused area on the corresponding pathological display. Modified and reprinted with permission from Reference 25.

sestamibi and thallium impact assessment of myocardial viability has not been addressed clearly in the literature.

Sestamibi Redistribution

Redistribution of sestamibi has been shown both in animal models[33-36] and in patients with chronic coronary artery disease.[37-41] However, the extent of redistribution with sestamibi is significantly less than that observed with thallium. Following transient ischemia and reperfusion in a canine model, Li and coworkers[34] have demonstrated that sestamibi undergoes myocardial redistribution, albeit more slowly and less completely when compared with thallium (Fig. 9). Sestamibi redistribution over 2.5 hours also was observed in an animal model of sustained low-flow ischemia[35] (Fig. 10). In clinical studies of patients undergoing exercise studies, minimal but clinically relevant redistribution has been observed in ischemic myocardium.[37,38,40] In patients with angiographic or scintigraphic evidence of coronary artery disease, significant differences between clearance rates from normal and ischemic myocardium were found 6 hours after sestamibi injection at

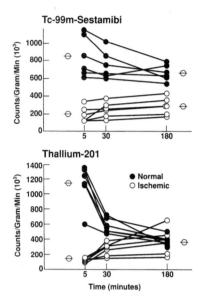

Figure 9. Sestamibi and thallium activities in myocardial biopsies from the normal (closed circles) and ischemic zones (open circles) in six dogs 5, 30, and 180 minutes after injection of the tracers. The dogs were reperfused just after the 5-min biopsies. The bisected circles represent mean activity values in each zone. For both sestamibi and thallium, note the consistent fall in normal zone activity and rise in ischemic zone activity consistent with redistribution. However by 180 min, redistribution is complete for thallium but not for sestamibi. Reprinted with permission from Reference 34.

peak stress.[37] The ratio between the activity in ischemic and normal myocardium increased in regions with mild defects from 0.70 ± 0.08 to 0.84 ± 0.13 at 6 hours after sestamibi injection (Fig. 11). Similar findings were reported by others in patients with angiographically documented coronary artery disease.[40] Significant sestamibi redistribution was observed in 31% of single photon emission tomography (SPECT) myocardial regions, from $69.9\% \pm 22.5\%$ at 5 minutes poststress to $74.5\% \pm 20.8\%$ at 120 minutes after injection of sestamibi at peak stress ($p < 0.01$). Although interpretation of data should be viewed cautiously when sestamibi imaging is delayed by 2 hours or more after

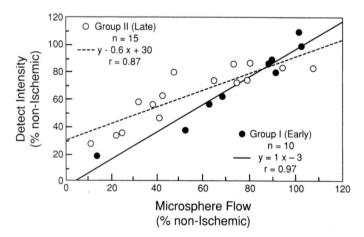

Figure 10. Scatterplot of transmural defect intensity (percent nonischemic) from γ-camera images of ex vivo myocardial slices. Ten slices from five group I dogs and 15 slices from eight group II dogs were analyzed. The relative defect intensity correlates well with the relative transmural microsphere flow deficit in identical regions early after sestamibi injection (group I). In group II, there also was good correlation between relative defect intensity and the flow deficit in the corresponding region. However, the defect was less pronounced than the flow deficit at the time of injection, suggesting that redistribution of sestamibi was detectable by quantitative analysis of high-resolution ex vivo images. Reprinted with permission from Reference 35.

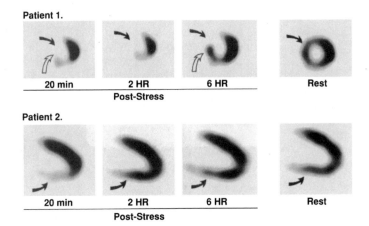

Figure 11. Clinically relevant redistribution in patients undergoing exercise sestamibi studies. Myocardial SPECT images obtained from two different patients are presented in the short-axis plane (**upper panel**) and in the vertical long-axis plane (**lower panel**) at 20 minutes, 2 hours, and 6 hours after exercise and at rest. **Upper panel:** There is sestamibi redistribution in the inferoseptal region (open arrow) but not in the anteroseptal region (closed arrow) by 6 hours. On the rest-injected image, complete normalization of all perfusion defects are seen. **Lower panel:** There is sestamibi redistribution in the inferior region (closed arrow) on both 2- and 6-hour images and complete normalization on rest-injected sestamibi image. Modified and reprinted with permission from Reference 37.

stress (underestimation of defect size and ischemia), the same concept does not apply for rest-injected studies. Contrarily, delaying sestamibi images by 2 hours or more after rest injection actually may improve viability assessment.

Indeed, redistribution of sestamibi has been observed following rest studies.[39,41] When an additional redistribution image was obtained 4 hours after injecting the tracer at rest, sestamibi redistribution occurred in 38% of regions with perfusion defects on the initial rest image that were identified as viable by thallium and positron emission tomography (PET) studies (Fig. 12). Such redistribution was observed in 22% of patients, and increased the overall concordance between thallium and sestamibi imaging regarding

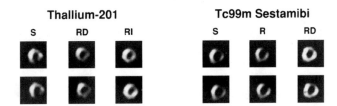

Figure 12. An example of a patient with reversible thallium defects and irreversible defects on rest-stress sestamibi imaging. Two consecutive short-axis tomograms are displayed for thallium stress (S), redistribution (RD), and reinjection (RI) with corresponding sestamibi tomograms of stress, rest (R), and redistribution. Thallium stress-redistribution images reveal partially reversible inferior and fixed anterolateral defects that improve after reinjection of thallium at rest. Same-day rest-stress sestamibi images incorrectly identified the anterolateral region as being irreversibly impaired and nonviable and the inferolateral region to be only partially reversible when compared with the thallium redistribution-reinjection study. However, sestamibi redistribution images acquired 4 hours following injection of the tracer at rest show partial reversibility in the anterolateral region and complete reversibility of the inferolateral region comparable with the thallium reinjection image. Reprinted with permission from Reference 39.

defect reversibility.[39] Using a rest-redistribution sestamibi protocol, Maurea and cowork-ers[41] reported that among regions with severe sestamibi defects at rest (mean 43% ± 8%) that were identified as viable by thallium, 24% showed improved sestamibi uptake (mean 60% ± 8%) when redistribution images were acquired approximately 5 hours later ($p <$ 0.001). Such delayed uptake of sestamibi (redistribution) was observed in 65% of the patients studied with coronary artery disease and left ventricular dysfunction. Thus, the clinical relevance of rest sestamibi redistribution has been confirmed by other investigators.

Chronic Coronary Artery Disease

As in the case for thallium, most of our knowledge with regard to the perfor-mance of sestamibi imaging for the assessment of myocardial viability is from studies in patients with chronic coronary artery disease. However, unlike the thallium data, there are a growing number of studies to suggest that sestamibi underestimates defect reversibility (ischemia) and myocardial viability in patients with chronic coronary artery disease.[39–58] Reports from several groups indicate that resting sestamibi imag-ing may significantly underestimate viability in approximately one-quarter to one-third of regions in comparison with thallium reinjection or dobutamine echocardiog-raphy.[39,43,45] The potential underestimation of viability may be evident particularly in regions with severe dysfunction or regions supplied by severely stenosed arteries. However, the concordance of sestamibi imaging to more accepted methods for via-bility assessment, such as thallium SPECT or PET metabolism, may be improved with quantitation of regional radiotracer uptake and/or acquisition of delayed redistribu-tion images.[39] However, despite the application of quantitative techniques, other studies have reported that rest sestamibi imaging underestimates myocardial viability

2-Day Sestamibi

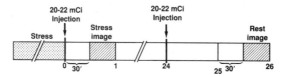

1-Day Sestamibi

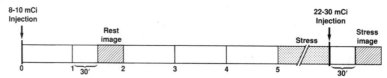

Rest-Redistribution-Stress Sestamibi

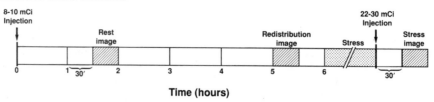

Time (hours)

Figure 13. ^{99m}Tc-sestamibi protocols for assessing myocardial ischemia and viability. Reprinted with permission from reference 136.

when compared with PET.[47,51,53,55–58] Various sestamibi protocols that currently are used for assessing myocardial ischemia and viability are shown in Figure 13.

Clinical Studies

Using conventional planar imaging and qualitative analysis among patients with chronic coronary artery disease, Cuocolo and coworkers reported that 29% of reversible myocardial regions by thallium reinjection appeared irreversible when a 2-day stress-rest sestamibi protocol was performed.[43] In our laboratory,[39] using SPECT imaging and quantitative analysis, 36% of myocardial regions that were classified as ischemic but viable by the thallium stress-redistribution-reinjection protocol was misclassified as irreversible defects on the sestamibi rest-stress protocol (Fig. 14). PET imaging was used as the gold standard to confirm viability of these regions.[39] These initial observations, both with planar and SPECT imaging, have been confirmed by subsequent studies.[40,41,44–58] Similarly, in cardiac transplant patients who were being evaluated for allograft vasculopathy, sestamibi significantly underestimated myocardial ischemic territories (reversible defects) when compared with thallium scintigraphy.[59]

If the mechanism of the thallium reinjection effect is merely that the reinjected thallium dose provides a better assessment of resting myocardial perfusion than redistribution images, then thallium reinjection results should be equivalent to results obtained when sestamibi is injected at rest. It is likely that the period of thallium redistribution after exercise may be the key factor, with the images after reinjection incorporating resting blood flow along with the metabolic information inherent in the redistribution data. These observations imply that perfusion agents that measure coronary blood flow alone may not assess myocardial viability as well as an agent that redistributes, such as thallium.

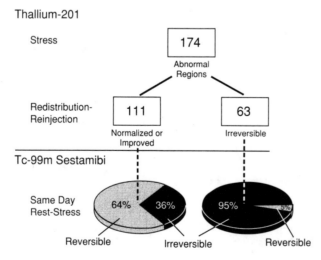

Figure 14. Flow diagram displaying the prevalence of reversible and irreversible thallium perfusion defects by stress-redistribution-reinjection and same-day rest-stress sestamibi studies in 54 patients with chronic coronary artery disease with a mean left ventricular ejection fraction (LVEF) of 34% ± 14%. Reprinted with permission from Reference 39.

Severity of Regional Sestamibi Defect

One approach that may overcome, in part, the limitations of sestamibi in assessing myocardial viability is to quantify the severity of regional sestamibi activity. Such quantitative methods have been useful in thallium imaging for identifying viable myocardium within apparently irreversible thallium defects.[60-62] In one study, among regions with irreversible sestamibi defects that were considered to be viable by thallium imaging and PET, 78% had only mild-to-moderately reduced sestamibi activity.[39] If such mild-to-moderate sestamibi defects are considered to represent nonischemic but viable myocardium, and only severe reduction in activity ($\leq$50% of normal) is considered evidence of nonviability, then the overall concordance between thallium and sestamibi studies was increased to 93% (Fig. 15). However, despite the application of quantitative techniques, other studies have reported that rest sestamibi imaging underestimates myocardial viability when compared with PET.[47,51,53,55-58] In patients with chronic coronary artery disease undergoing both rest sestamibi SPECT and ^{18}F-fluoro-deoxyglucose (FDG) PET studies, Altehoefer et al[47,53] found discordance between the severity of sestamibi defects and FDG uptake (Fig. 16). Using the same threshold quantitative values for viability, Sawada et al[51] found that the sestamibi defect size at rest was larger than[13]N-ammonia images assessed by PET. Furthermore, 47% of segments with severe sestamibi defects (<50% of peak activity) had preserved metabolic activity as assessed by FDG PET.

However, it is important to point out that the mere presence of viable myocardium (severity of regional sestamibi defect) does not necessarily indicate ischemic myocardium (stress-induced reversible defect). It is more likely for an ischemic region to improve after revascularization than nonischemic but viable myocardium (mild-to-moderate reduction in tracer activity).[63] In the study by Marzullo et al, 32% of segments exhibiting sestamibi activity of >55% of peak normal (viable at rest) showed

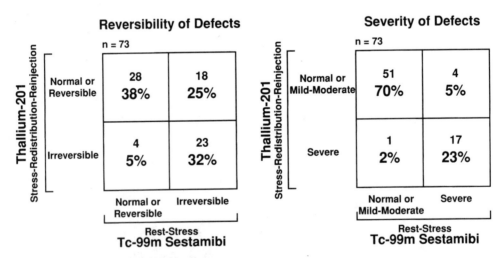

Figure 15. Diagram showing concordance and discordance between thallium stress-redistribution-reinjection and sestamibi rest-stress images in 25 patients who also underwent positron emission tomography (PET) studies. Data on reversibility of defects (normal/reversible or irreversible) are shown on the left, and severity of defects (normal/mild-to-moderate or severe) is shown on the right. Eighteen of 22 discordant regions between thallium and sestamibi studies are reversible by thallium redistribution-reinjection studies. Myocardial viability was confirmed in 17 of 18 regions by PET. Reprinted with permission from Reference 39.

Rest Images

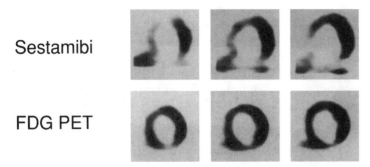

Sestamibi

FDG PET

Figure 16. Discordance between PET and rest sestamibi SPECT imaging is demonstrated in this patient with three-vessel coronary artery disease. Three consecutive short-axis tomograms are displayed for ^{99m}Tc-sestamibi (**top**), with corresponding ^{18}F-2-deoxyglucose (FDG) PET tomograms (**bottom**). Rest sestamibi images reveal extensive perfusion abnormalities involving the anteroapical, septal, and inferior regions with preserved viability in the posterolateral region and mixed viable and scarred myocardium in the septal region. FDG uptake in the corresponding regions demonstrates preserved metabolic activity and viability in all three coronary artery vascular territories. The patient had totally occluded but collateralized left anterior descending and right coronary arteries and severe stenosis of the left circumflex artery. Modified and reprinted with permission from Reference 53.

no improvement in regional contraction after revascularization.[54] Conversely, 25% of segments with normal wall motion had severely reduced ($\leq$55% of peak) sestamibi activity at rest (nonviable). Therefore, the distinction between ischemic myocardium (stress-induced reversible defect) and viable myocardium (severity of defect at rest) has important clinical implications.

Nitrate Administration

Considering the kinetics of sestamibi, in myocardial regions with decreased blood flow and partially impaired viability, uptake of sestamibi appears to be influenced by regional perfusion rather than myocyte viability.[64] In view of the limitations of rest-injected sestamibi for assessing myocardial viability some investigators have proposed injection of sestamibi during nitrate infusion. In addition to lowering preload and after-load, it has been reported that nitrates may vasodilate flow limiting epicardial coronary arteries[65] as well as collateral vessels.[66] When sestamibi was injected during nitrate infusion (10 mg of isosorbide dinitrate in 100 ml of isotonic saline solution), both defect reversibility and final sestamibi content were shown to improve the accuracy of sestamibi for predicting recovery of regional[67,68] and global[69] left ventricular function after revascularization.

Revascularization Studies

There are a growing number of studies in the literature that have evaluated ^{99m}Tc-sestamibi uptake before and after revascularization.[41,45,46,54,70] Pre- and postrevascularization studies have suggested that sestamibi may underestimate myocardial viability and functional recovery after revascularization when compared with thallium.

In 1992, Lucignani et al reported that among 54 asynergic regions studied before surgery, 42 had normal or reduced perfusion at rest and developed stress-induced ischemia, while 11 had markedly reduced or absent perfusion at rest.[46] After revascularization, although recovery of wall motion was observed in 79% of regions with stress-induced ischemia, 72% of regions with markedly reduced or absent perfusion at rest also showed improved wall motion after surgery. Among 18 patients with coronary artery disease undergoing revascularization, more favorable positive (80%) and negative (96%) predictive accuracies were attained by Udelson et al when the severity of sestamibi defect was quantified at rest[70] (Fig. 17). However, a recent publication by Maurea and coworkers suggest that such high positive and negative predictive accuracies for recovery of function after revascularization can be attained only if a rest-redistribution sestamibi protocol is utilized.[41] In their study, 83% of regions with a combination of severely reduced sestamibi uptake at rest and redistribution on 5-hour delayed images showed improvement in regional contractile function after revascularization. Global left ventricular ejection fraction (LVEF) increased in these patients from 42% ± 7%, before surgery, to 47% ± 7%, after revascularization ($p < 0.01$). In contrast, 96% of segments with severely reduced sestamibi uptake at rest that remained irreversible on 5-hour redistribution images had persistent left ventricular dysfunction after revascularization (Fig. 18). In subsequent publications, when sestamibi uptake at rest was compared with thallium uptake after rest-redistribution using quantitative analysis, one study found comparable tracer activity[71] while the

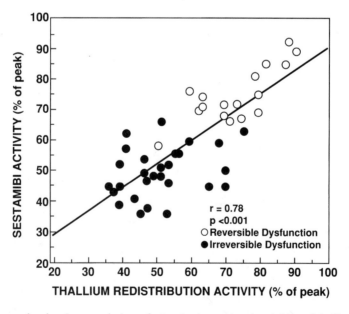

Figure 17. Scatterplot showing correlation of quantitative regional activities of thallium (at redistribution imaging after rest injection) on the abscissa and regional activities of sestamibi (at rest) on the ordinate among segments with signficant regional dysfunction in patients undergoing revascularization. Modified and reprinted with permission from Reference 70.

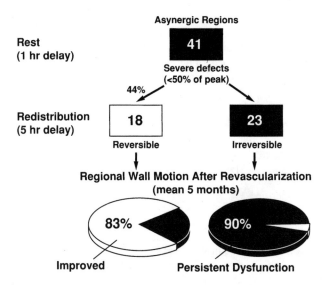

Figure 18. Flow diagram displaying the prevalence of sestamibi redistribution and recovery of function after revascularization in asynergic regions with severe reduction in resting sestamibi images. Modified and reprinted with permission from Reference 41.

other found significantly lower sestamibi uptake in regions with reversible rest-redistribution thallium defects.[72]

Summary

With the exception of few studies, sestamibi appears to underestimate myocardial ischemia (defect reversibility) and viability in patients with chronic coronary artery disease and left ventricular dysfunction compared with thallium scintigraphy and FDG PET. The factors contributing to impaired sestamibi uptake and defect reversibility when compared with thallium include differences in (1) extraction fraction, (2) blood clearance, (3) redistribution, and (4) response to altered metabolic states. To overcome the limitation of sestamibi for underestimating myocardial ischemia and viability, Berman et al have proposed dual-isotope imaging, which combines rest-redistribution thallium with stress sestamibi (Fig. 19), thereby taking advantage of the favorable properties of each of the two tracers.[73] Whether measuring redistribution of

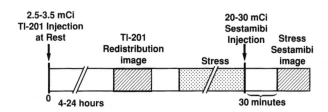

Figure 19. Dual-isotope (thallium-sestamibi) myocardial viability protocol. Reprinted with permission from Reference 136.

sestamibi after rest injections will enhance assessment of viable myocardium is a subject of ongoing investigation. Perhaps a more likely improvement could be achieved through (1) combined sestamibi perfusion and functional imaging or electrocardiogram (ECG) gated myocardial perfusion studies, (2) quantitation of regional radiotracer uptake, and (3) nitrate administration before rest sestamibi injection.

Acute Coronary Artery Disease

Myocardial Risk Area and Infarct Size Assessment

Unlike thallium, the minimal redistribution of sestamibi makes it a potentially useful tracer for application in the acute or subacute phases of myocardial infarction. The minimal redistribution over time allows greater temporal separation between the time of isotope injection and that of imaging. Specifically, the injection of sestamibi during the acute phase of myocardial infarction before reperfusion therapy may represent a true estimate of risk area and can be used to assess the degree of myocardial salvage after thrombolytic therapy or direct angioplasty. After injection of sestamibi, imaging can be delayed for several hours during which therapy is administered and the patient is stabilized. The initial sestamibi images, which can be acquired several hours after its administration, reflects the perfusion pattern at the time of sestamibi injection and vessel occlusion (myocardial risk area assessment). Approximately 24 hours after reperfusion therapy, a second injection of sestamibi can be performed at rest. The second set of sestamibi images reflects the extent of myocardial "salvage" in the infarct-related artery. Such assessment of myocardial risk area and myocardial salvage has been shown in experimental animal models and confirmed in human subjects.

Experimental Studies

In an animal model of acute myocardial infarction, DeCoster and coworkers injected sestamibi during coronary occlusion and obtained tissue biopsies from the risk area during the 90- to120-minute occlusion and 2–3 hours after reperfusion.[74] Sestamibi count profiles were nearly identical in the images obtained during occlusion and after reperfusion. In another animal model of acute coronary artery occlusion and reperfusion in which the relationship between sestamibi uptake and blood flow was assessed, sestamibi uptake correlated closely with blood flow assessed by microspheres and the autoradiographic risk area correlated to the postmortem angiographic risk area.[11] However, when the radiotracer was injected after reperfusion, its uptake tracked infarct size but no longer tracked MBF (reflecting myocardial viability; Fig. 20). Such good correlation between scintigraphic infarct size (assessed by ex vivo tomographic sestamibi images) and pathological infarct size (assessed histochemically) has been demonstrated by other investigators.[75]

These experimental data suggest that sestamibi may be a useful tracer for determining myocardial risk area and final infarct size. Optimal determination of myocardial risk area requires injection of the radiotracer prior to reperfusion, that is, during coronary occlusion. A second set of images, acquired after reinjection of the radiotracer several hours after reperfusion, may reflect final infarct size and, at least early after infarction, may be more indicative of myocardial viability than of perfusion.

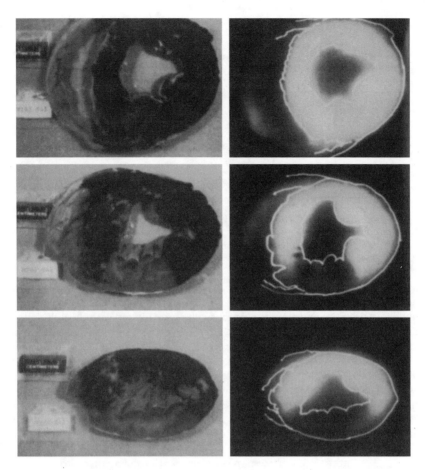

Figure 20. Postmortem dual perfusion maps (**left**) and sestamibi autoradiographs (**right**) from a representative dog injected with sestamibi after reperfusion. Shown, on the left, are three slices oriented with the right ventricle on the left and the anterior wall of the left ventricle on the bottom. Risk area is stained brick red with triphenyltetrazolium chloride (TTC). Infarct area is the pale unstained region within the risk area. Defects seen on unenhanced autoradiographs with superimposed overlay (**right**) correlate closely with the area of infarction defined by TTC staining. No significant sestamibi activity is seen in the central necrotic region, while some activity is seen in the perinecrotic area. The figure is reduced 15%. Modified and reprinted with permission from Reference 11.

Clinical Studies

In stunned but viable myocardium, in which regional contractility is impaired despite restoration of coronary blood flow, sestamibi uptake should be an accurate marker of cellular viability, and this has been confirmed in several studies.[75–82] In patients studied within the first week of thrombolytic therapy for acute myocardial infarction, sestamibi images may be used to estimate final infarct size. Sestamibi defect size has been shown to correlate well with regional wall motion at the time of discharge,[80] with late ejection fraction measurements,[80] and with peak release of creatine kinase.[81] Christian and colleagues demonstrated close correlations between final defect size and several functional parameters including end-diastolic volume index, end-systolic volume index, and ejection fraction at 1-year follow-up.[83] In a

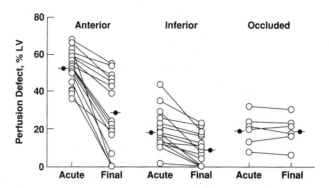

Figure 21. Sestamibi perfusion defect size by infarct location and arterial patency, as determined before reperfusion (Acute) and at discharge (Final). Both anterior and inferior infarct locations show a significant decrease in perfusion defect size after reperfusion ($p < 0.001$ for both); however, there was no significant change in patients with an occluded infarct-related artery. Modified and reprinted with permission of from Reference 85.

subsequent study in which the feasibility of serial tomographic sestamibi imaging was assessed to measure myocardial salvage, a significant decrease in sestamibi defect size was observed, from acute to discharge imaging, among patients who were treated with thrombolytic therapy compared with those who were not (Fig. 21).[84,85] These findings were confirmed by other investigators.[86,87] Santoro and colleagues reported a good correlation between final defect size and enzymatic infarct size as well as between improvement in perfusion defect and decrease in regional left ventricular dysfunction from acute to predischarge imaging.[86] In patients undergoing direct angioplasty for acute myocardial infarction,[87] although a significant decrease in sestamibi defect size was observed between acute and late imaging, this effect was highly variable. Because the area of myocardial risk varies widely even for similar anatomical location of coronary artery occlusion, it underscores the role for radionuclide imaging in such patients.

The measurement of both early sestamibi defect size (localizing myocardial risk area) and predischarge defect size (reflecting the extent of irreversible injury) may provide an assessment of the effects of treatment (myocardial salvage). Therefore, such an approach may be useful for risk stratification, especially when combined with pharmacological stress testing. For example, when myocardial infarct size exceeds 40% of the left ventricle, the incidence of cardiogenic shock is high. In addition, assessment of myocardial risk area and salvage would provide a noninvasive method for evaluating the efficacy of new pharmaceutical agents or revascularization techniques in the setting of acute myocardial infarction.

Clinical studies concerning viability assessment with sestamibi early after myocardial infarction have focused on the approach of determination of degree of myocardial salvage and final infarct size. However, to date, there are no conclusive studies examining the assessment of sestamibi as a viability tracer specifically in a population of patients early after myocardial infarction. A recent report comparing resting sestamibi SPECT with low-dose dobutamine echocardiography showed that estimates of myocardial infarct size were larger with sestamibi imaging than with echocardiography.[88] However, this study did not include follow-up assessment of ventricular function or another independent marker of myocardial viability.

Prognostic Assessment Early After Myocardial Infarction

The ultimate goal of evaluating patients early after myocardial infarction for risk area, final infarct size, amount of salvage, or residual viability is to improve their prognosis and

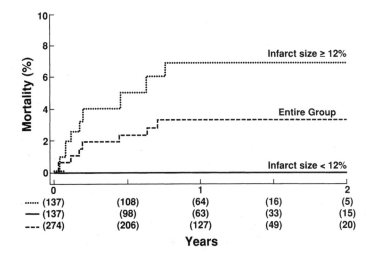

Figure 22. Plot of mortality curves for the entire study population and for the subgroups divided on the basis of median infarct size. Patients with infarct size <12% of the left ventricle had significantly better outcomes than those with infarcts involving ≥12% of the ventricle. Numbers in parentheses at the bottom of the figure indicate the patients from each group available for analysis at the given points in time. Modified and reprinted with permission from Reference 90.

to target interventional procedures to those individuals who have the most to gain prognostically. Depending on the clinical situation, such risk assessment usually involves the assessment of myocardial viability alone or in combination with stress perfusion imaging to identify additional areas at risk.

The value of stress sestamibi imaging for prognostic assessment early after myocardial infarction has not been established definitively. Among a population of patients referred for various indications for stress perfusion imaging, sestamibi imaging compares favorably with thallium imaging for prognostic evaluation.[89] Recent data suggest that assessment of infarct size with sestamibi imaging has important prognostic implications. Miller and colleagues studied 274 patients with acute myocardial infarction with acute (on presentation) and predischarge quantitative sestamibi SPECT imaging.[90] Patients were followed for a median of 12 months. These investigators demonstrated a significant association between final infarct size and overall mortality, as well as an association between myocardium at risk and subsequent cardiac mortality. Patients with infarct size <12% of the left ventricle had significantly better outcomes than those with infarcts involving ≥12% of the ventricle (Fig. 22). However, there are no large studies specifically addressing patients early after myocardial infarction. Preliminary data from several groups using dipyridamole stress imaging within several days of infarction suggest that reversible sestamibi defects have prognostic significance, which is incremental to that of clinical variables alone.[91] Additional studies are needed in this population of patients to confirm these findings.

Assessment of Acute Coronary Syndromes in the Emergency Room

The use of radionuclide perfusion imaging for early diagnostic and prognostic assessment of patients with suspected acute myocardial syndromes is an emerging area of investigation. Early risk stratification of such patients may lead to more cost-effective decision-making strategies, eliminating hospitalization costs for patients who are deter-

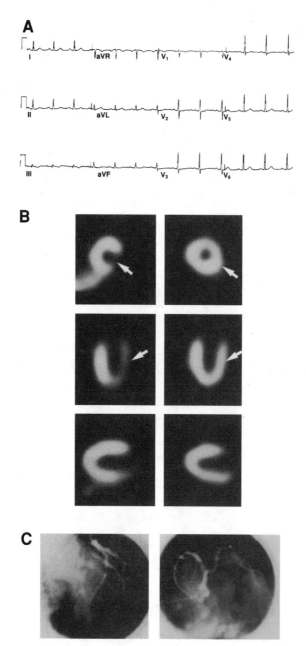

Figure 23. Assessment of acute myocardial infarction in the emergency room. The electrocardiogram (ECG) of this 60-year-old man with typical angina (**A**) shows nonspecific ST-T–wave changes but is not diagnostic for myocardial ischemia or infarction. However, sestamibi scan performed in the emergency room (**B, left column**) shows a severe perfusion defect in the lateral region, which corresponds to the 80% narrowing in the first obtuse marginal artery and a filling defect suggestive of thrombus in the left circumflex coronary artery (**C**). The patient underwent immediate administration of intracoronary urokinase and subsequent successful coronary angioplasty. Repeat sestamibi scan performed before hospital discharge (**B, right column**) shows reperfusion of the left circumflex vascular territory. Modified and reprinted with permission from Reference 94

mined to be low risk within 12–24 hours of presentation to the emergency department. Presently, even low- and intermediate-risk patients are admitted at most centers to rule out myocardial infarction, with stress testing performed 48–72 hours afterward in most patients. Acute myocardial perfusion imaging may provide early risk assessment and thus aid in the triage of emergency department patients who present with chest pain and nondiagnostic ECGs. The characteristics of sestamibi, particularly its minimal redistribution, make it the most suitable radiotracer for this indication.

There are two approaches to risk stratification in the setting of a potential acute coronary syndrome. First, perfusion imaging may be performed after the injection of radiotracer during chest pain at rest. Several clinical studies have demonstrated the feasibility of this approach.[92–96] Bilodeau and colleagues examined 45 patients who were injected with sestamibi during spontaneous episodes of chest pain, 26 of whom had significant coronary artery stenosis.[92] The specificity and negative predictive accuracies of a normal perfusion scan were 88% and 94%, respectively. Such high specificity of a normal perfusion scan for noncoronary heart disease was confirmed by others.[93] Hilton and colleagues studied 102 patients with chest pain and nondiagnostic ECGs using rest sestamibi SPECT and followed these patients for subsequent cardiac events.[94] Multivariate regression analysis showed that an abnormal perfusion study was the only independent predictor for adverse cardiac events. Among 70 patients with a normal perfusion scan, only one had a cardiac event. In contrast, the cardiac event rate in those patients with equivocal or abnormal scans was 13% and 71%, respectively[94] (Fig. 23).

There are preliminary studies to suggest that triaging patients with unexplained chest pain in the emergency department with radionuclide perfusion studies also may be cost-effective.[95] However, the time window for radiotracer injection in these patients remains unclear. Some studies have included patients whose chest pain had resolved before their arrival to the emergency room[93] and yet abnormal perfusion studies were attained in a subset of such patients. Nevertheless, the sensitivity of these perfusion studies is higher among patients injected with the radiotracer during symptoms compared with those injected following the resolution of their symptoms.[96]

A second approach for risk stratification in the emergency department involves early exercise testing with or without radionuclide imaging. Although early stress testing in this population has been proven to be safe, data from the Duke Treadmill Study indicate that approximately half of patients studied with treadmill exercise tests without perfusion imaging remained in the intermediate-risk subgroup.[97] In another study, where patients were studied with sestamibi SPECT during an episode of spontaneous chest pain or within 5 hours of such pain (acute imaging) and again during exercise or pharmacological stress within 1 week of the chest pain, there was a 91% concordance between early, acute perfusion images and late, stress perfusion images.[98] The use of radionuclide stress imaging in the emergency department remains an area of active investigation.

Technetium-99m–Teboroxime

^{99m}Tc-teboroxime is a neutral, lipophilic compound that is extracted by the myocardium in proportion to regional blood flow and its extraction remains linear even at high-flow conditions.[99,100] The first-pass extraction fraction of teboroxime is reported to be 88% at rest and 91% under hyperemic conditions.[101] In cultured myocardial cells, the accumulation of teboroxime has been shown to be 4–7.5 times greater than that of sestamibi but the differences were not as pronounced for thallium.[102,103] In human subjects, teboroxime permits accurate assessment of coronary blood flow even during pharmacological hyperemia.[104–107] Unlike sestamibi, which is retained within the mitochondria, teboroxime washes out rapidly from the myocardium at a rate proportional to regional blood flow. Approximately two-thirds of the teboroxime activity has been shown to clear from the heart with a half-time of 3.6 minutes in canines.[108] Therefore, both uptake and washout of teboroxime depend predominantly on regional MBF and are not confounded by tissue metabolism or other binding characteristics within the myocardium.[23,101,109–114] Unlike thallium and sestamibi, teboroxime uptake in cultured myocardial cells was shown to be independent of the metabolic status of the cells.[23] This makes teboroxime particularly more suitable as a blood flow tracer rather than a viability tracer.

Teboroxime has been shown to demonstrate apparent redistribution by poststenotic differential clearance at rest[101,109] and with stress.[101,110,111] However, the rapid clearance of teboroxime from myocardial cells makes imaging technically difficult. Moreover, despite its rapid clearance, some reports have suggested that teboroxime underestimates reversibility of defects (myocardial ischemia) when compared with thallium.[5,104,115–117] Larger series of studies clearly are needed to further define the role of teboroxime (if any) for the assessment of myocardial viability.

Technetium-99m–Tetrofosmin

[99m]Tc-tetrofosmin is a lipophilic phosphine dioxocation that is distributed within the myocardium in proportion to regional blood flow.[118,119] Myocardial uptake and blood clearance kinetics of tetrofosmin are similar to sestamibi. However, the clearance of tetrofosmin from lungs and liver is faster than sestamibi, which may improve the resolution of early cardiac images and reduce the overall radiation burden.[120] Unlike thallium, tetrofosmin does not redistribute significantly over time, thereby necessitating two injections of the tracer at peak exercise and at rest.[121,122]

In a canine model of adenosine-induced vasodilation with various degrees of coronary artery stenosis, tetrofosmin uptake underestimated the flow disparity when compared with thallium and microspheres.[123] When the stenosis was severe, the stenotic-to-normal circumflex artery flow ratios with adenosine were 0.22 ± 0.02 for microsphere,

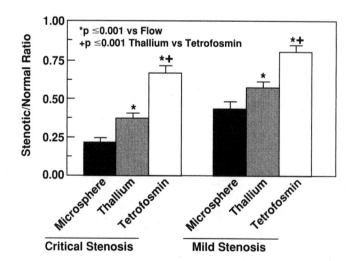

Figure 24. Bar graphs showing mean microsphere flow, thallium, and tetrofosmin activities expressed as the stenotic-to-normal thallium and tetrofosmin ratios for both critical and mild stenosis groups. Both thallium and tetrofosmin significantly underestimated blood flow when compared with microsphere flow. However, the degree of underestimation was significantly greater for tetrofosmin when compared with both microsphere flow and thallium. Modified and reprinted with permission from Reference 123.

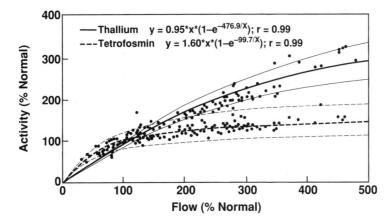

Figure 25. Normalized thallium and tetrofosmin activities plotted as a function of microsphere flow from endocardial, midwall, and epicardial samples of critically stenotic group of dogs. Heavy solid and dashed lines are mathematically modeled curve fits with 95% confidence intervals (CIs). Modified and reprinted with permission from Reference 123.

0.37 ± 0.04 for thallium, and 0.67 ± 0.05 for tetrofosmin ($p < 0.01$), and when the stenosis was mild, the flow ratios were 0.44 ± 0.05 for microsphere, 0.58 ± 0.04 for thallium, and 0.81 ± 0.04 for tetrofosmin ($p < 0.01$) (Fig. 24). Similarly, the magnitude of ex vivo image defects was significantly greater for thallium than for tetrofosmin in both groups[123] (Fig. 25). In a recent multicenter trial, when the efficacy of tetrofosmin was compared with thallium stress-redistribution scintigraphy, the overall concordance between the two tracers for defining normal or abnormal regions was approximately 80%.[6] However, when patients were categorized as showing normal, ischemia, infarction, or mixed (infarction and viable) myocardium, the concordance between tetrofosmin and thallium decreased to only 59%. Furthermore, when the 2-day stress-rest tetrofosmin protocol was compared with stress-redistribution-reinjection thallium among patients

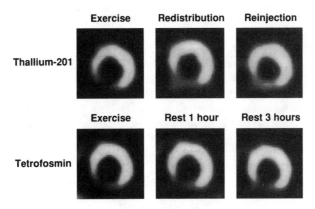

Figure 26. An example of a patient with reversible thallium and irreversible tetrofosmin defects. Short-axis tomograms are displayed for thallium stress, redistribution, and reinjection with corresponding tetrofosmin stress, 1-hour delayed rest, and 3-hour delayed rest-injected tomograms. Thallium tomograms reveal a severe inferior perfusion defect during stress with partial reversibility on redistribution and further improvement on reinjection images. Stress, 1-hour delayed rest, and 3-hour delayed rest tetrofosmin images show a severe irreversible defect in the inferior region. Modified and reprinted with permission from Reference 124.

with coronary artery disease and left ventricular dysfunction, thallium and tetrofosmin provided discordant information in 40% of segments; 88% appearing irreversible on tetrofosmin images but reversible (ischemic and viable) on thallium reinjection images.[124] A patient with discordant thallium stress-redistribution-reinjection and 2-day stress-rest as well as 3-hour delayed rest tetrofosmin imaging is shown in Figure 26. These data suggest that, similar to sestamibi, tetrofosmin underestimates myocardial ischemia and viability in patients with chronic coronary artery disease and left ventricular dysfunction.

Technetium-99m–Furifosmin (Q12)

[99m]Tc-furifosmin (Q12) is a mixed-ligand cationic complex that is taken up avidly by the myocardium in relation to regional blood flow, as measured by the radioactive microsphere technique, for flows up to 2 mL/g per minute.[125] However, with pharmacological stress (blood flow above 2 mL/g per minute), Q12 activity does not increase proportionately. Q12 is cleared primarily by the hepatobiliary system and approximately 30% by the kidneys. Similar to tetrofosmin, Q12 does not redistribute significantly from the time of injection.[125] In a pilot study, in which Q12 and thallium imaging were compared with coronary angiography for detection of 50% or greater coronary artery stenosis, the respective diagnostic sensitivities and specificities were 90% and 90% for thallium and 85% and 80% for Q12 [p = not significant (NS)].[126] Although there was good overall concordance of Q12 with thallium in normal and irreversible regions, agreement between thallium stress-redistribution-reinjection and rest-stress Q12 for detecting myocardial ischemia and viability (defect reversibility) was poor. Multicenter clinical trials currently are underway comparing Q12 with thallium in the same patients to better define Q12's role in assessing myocardial viability.

Technetium-99m N[bis(N-etoxy, N-ethyl dithiocarbamato) Nitrido Technetium(V)] NOET

[99m]TcN-NOET is a neutral lipophilic myocardial imaging agent characterized by the presence of a Tc-N triple bond group. Its electrically neutral property is similar to the BATO compounds such as teboroxime. After passive diffusion, the mechanism of NOET uptake is thought to be through linkage of the radiotracer to proteins bound in the lipid membrane of isolated myocytes.[127] In cell fractionation studies, no NOET activity was found in the cytosol or mitochondria.[128] Unlike teboroxime, NOET exhibits slow myocardial clearance and longer retention in normal myocardium. Differences in tracer clearance and retention between teboroxime and NOET are thought to be related to differences in the strength of protein binding and protein-binding profile. Unlike sestamibi and tetrofosmin (monocationic compounds), NOET appears to redistribute over time predominantly by differential clearance, in which clearance from the normal zone is more rapid than clearance from the ischemic zone.[129,130]

The first-pass extraction fraction of NOET is 75% at rest and 85% under hyperemic conditions.[131] In a canine model of partial coronary artery occlusion and vasodilation, there was a linear relation between NOET activity and radiolabeled microspheres (r = 0.94) except in low-flow zones where NOET overestimates blood flow and in high-flow zones where NOET underestimates blood flow.[131] After reflow, there was almost complete redistribution of NOET within 90 minutes. Similar findings regarding NOET and thallium uptake and kinetics were observed in canine models of sustained low flow (2 hours) and transient coronary artery occlusion (20 minutes) followed by 2 hours of reflow.[129] Data regarding the efficacy of NOET in the clinical setting is sparse. In 25 patients who underwent stress-redistribution-reinjection thallium SPECT and stress-delayed rest NOET SPECT, the diagnostic accuracy of thallium and NOET for detecting the presence and extent of coronary artery disease assessed by coronary angiography was comparable.[132]

Regarding the utility of NOET as a myocardial viability marker, recent studies have shown that uptake and retention of NOET is dependent on the structural integrity of cell membrane.[133] In an isolated perfused heart model, retention of NOET was not significantly different in the ischemic-reperfused myocardium (mild-to-moderate injury) from that of the control hearts (no cellular injury). This suggests that NOET may not be a sensitive marker of cell injury.[133,134] However, in myocardium exposed to severe irreversible cell membrane disruption with Triton X-100 (sarcolemmal membrane detergent) or sodium cyanide (cytochrome c oxidase inhibitor), clearance of NOET was accelerated significantly. The dissociation between NOET and microspheres in the low-flow zones and the lack of differentiation between mild-to-moderately injured and normal myocardium may be explained by the availability of NOET from recirculating red blood cells and redistribution. A recent study has shown that red blood cells avidly extract and retain NOET from aqueous media.[135] This suggests that myocardial uptake of NOET may continue with recirculation as long as concentration gradients between myocardial tissue and blood exist. After multiple circulatory passes, the equilibrium achieved between myocardial tissue and blood NOET activity may explain, in part, the defect resolution and redistribution kinetics of NOET over time.

Summary

The advent of ^{99m}Tc-labeled perfusion tracers has broadened the application of myocardial perfusion imaging from detection of coronary artery disease to evaluation of acute and subacute phases of myocardial infarction and in triaging patients in the emergency room. In addition, simultaneous assessment of myocardial perfusion and function with gated SPECT studies now is a clinical reality. Because of their slow myocardial clearance and redistribution, tracers such as sestamibi and tetrofosmin allow greater temporal separation between the time of isotope injection and that of imaging, which is a clinically valuable attribute when assessing patients in the emergerncy room with chest pain and/or acute infarction. On the other hand, lack of significant redistribution makes these tracers less effective in identifying viable myocardium in patients with chronic coronary artery disease and impaired blood flow at rest. Continued development of radiotracers with differing cellular extraction, retention, and clearance properties may further refine our understanding of agents that are more suitable for assessment of myocardial viability rather than blood flow.

References

1. Saperstein LA, Moses JE. Cerebral and cephalic blood flow in man: Basic consideration of the indicator fractionation technique. In: Knisely RE, ed. *Dynamic Clinical Studies with Radio-isotopes.* Washington, DC: United States Atomic Energy Commission, Division of Technical Information, No. 3; 1964:135–152.

2. Deutsch E, Bushong W, Glavan KA, et al. Heart imaging with cationic complexes of technetium. *Science* 1981;214:85–86.

3. Meleca MJ, McGoron AJ, Gerson MC, et al. Flow versus uptake comparisons of thallium-201 with technetium-99m perfusion tracers in a canine model of mycoardial ischemia. *J Nucl Med* 1997;38:1847–1856.

4. Wackers FJTh, Berman D, Maddahi J, et al. Technetium-99m hexakis 2-methoxy-isobutyl isonitirile: Human biodistribution, dosimetry, safety and preliminary comparison to thallium-201 for myocardial perfusion imaging. *J Nucl Med* 1989;30:301–311.

5. Johnson LL, Seldin DW. Clinical experience with technetium-99m teboroxime, a neutral, lipophilic myocardial perfusion imaging agent. *Am J Cardiol* 1990;66:63E–67E.

6. Zaret BL, Rigo P, Wackers FJT, et al. Myocardial perfusion imaging with Tc-99m tetrofosmin: Comparison to thallium imaging and coronary angiography in a phase III multicenter trial. *Circulation* 1995;91:313–319.

7. Piwnica-Worms D, Kronauge JF, Chiu ML. Uptake and retention of hexakis (2-methoxy-isobutyl isonitrile) technetium (I) in cultured chick myocardial cells: Mitochondrial and plasma membrane potential dependence. *Circulation* 1990;82:1826–1838.

8. Delmon-Moingeon LI, Piwnica-Worms D, Van den Abbeele AD, et al. Uptake of the cation hexakis (2-methoxyisobutylisonitrile)-technetium-99m by human carcinoma cell lines in vitro. *Cancer Res* 1990;50:2198–2202.

9. Meerdink DJ, Leppo JA. Comparison of hypoxia and ouabain effects on the myocardial uptake kinetics of technetium-99m haxakis 2-methoxy-isobutyl isonitrile and thallium-201. *J Nucl Med* 1989;30:1500–1506.

10. Okada RD, Glover D, Gaffney T, et al. Myocardial kinetics of technetium-99m-hexakis-2-methoxy-2-methylpropyl isonitrile. *Circulation* 1988;77:491–498.

11. Sinusas AJ, Trautman KA, Bergin JD, et al. Quantification of area at risk during coronary occlusion and degree of myocardial salvage after reperfusion with technetium-99m methoxy-isobutyl isonitrile. *Circulation* 1990;82:1424–1437.

12. Freeman I, Grunwald AM, Hoory S, et al. Effect of coronary occlusion and myocardial viability on myocardial activity of technetium-99m-sestamibi. *J Nucl Med* 1991;32:292–299.

13. Beanlands R, Dawood F, Wen WH, et al. Are the kinetics of technetium-99m methoxyisobutyl isonitrile affected by cell membrane metabolism and viability? *Circulation* 1990;82:1802–1814.

14. Canby RC, Silber S, Pohost GM. Relations of the myocardial imaging agents 99mTc-MIBI and 201-Tl to myocardial blood flow in a canine model of ischemic insult. *Circulation* 1990;81:286–296.

15. Glover DK, Okada RD. Myocardial kinetics of Tc-MIBI in canine myocardium after dipyridamole. *Circulation* 1990;81:628–637.

16. Leppo JA, Meerdink DJ. Comparison of the myocardial uptake of a technetium-labeled isonitrile analogue and thallium. *Circ Res* 1989;65:632–639.

17. Glover DK, Ruiz M, Edwards NC, et al. Comparison between ^{201}Tl and ^{99m}Tc sestamibi uptake during adenosine-induced vasodilation as a function of coronary stenosis severity. *Circulation* 1995;91:813–820.

18. Calnon DA, Glover DK, Beller GA, et al. Effects of dobutamine stress on myocardial blood flow, ^{99m}Tc sestamibi uptake, and systolic wall thickening in the presence of coronary artery stenoses: Implications for dobutamine stress testing. *Circulation* 1997;96:2353–2360.

19. Wu JC, Yun JJ, Heller EN, et al. Limitations of dobutamine for enhancing flow heterogeneity in the presence of single coronary stenosis: Implications for technetium-99m-sestamibi imaging. *J Nucl Med* 1998;39:417–425.

20. Calnon DA, Ruiz M, Vanzetto G, et al. Myocardial uptake of Tc-99m sestamibi during dobutamine stress is enhanced by ruthenium red, an inhibitor of mitochondrial calcium influx. *Circulation* 1997;96:I687. Abstract.

21. Piwnica-Worms D, Chiu ML, Kronauge JF, Divergent kinetics of ^{201}Tl and ^{99m}Tc-sestamibi in cultured chick ventricular myocytes during ATP depletion. *Circulation* 1992;85:1531–1541.

22. Maublant JC, Gachon P, Moins N. Hexakis (2-methoxyisobutyl isonitrile)technetium-99m and thallium-201 chloride: Uptake and release in cultured myocardial cells. *J Nucl Med* 1988;29:48–54.

23. Maublant JC, Moins N, Gachon P, et al. Uptake of technetium-99m teboroxime in cultured myocardial cells: Comparison with thallium-201 and technetium-99m sestamibi. *J Nucl Med* 1993;34:255–259.

24. Narahara KA, Vilaneuva-Meyer J, Thompson CJ, et al. Comparison of thallium-201 and technetium-99m hexakis 2-methoxyisobutyl isonitrile single-photon emission computed to-

mography for estimating the extent of myocardial ischemia and infarction in coronary artery disease. *Am J Cardiol* 1990;66:1438–1444.

25. Leon AR, Eisner RL, Martin SE, et al. Comparison of single-photon emission computed tomographic (SPECT) myocardial perfusion imaging with thallium-201 and technetium-99m sestamibi in dogs. *J Am Coll Cardiol* 1992;20:1612–1625.

26. Maublant JC, Marcaggi X, Lusson JR, et al. Comparison between thallium-201 and technetium-99m methoxyisobutyl isonitrile defect size in single-photon emission computed tomography at rest, exercise and redistribution in coronary artery disease. *Am J Cardiol* 1992;69: 183–187.

27. Matsunari I, Fujino S, Taki J, et al. Comparison of defect size between thallium-201 and technetium-99m tetrofosmin myocardial single-photon emission computed tomography in patients with single-vessel coronary artery disease. *Am J Cardiol* 1996;77:350–354.

28. Wackers FJ, Berman DS, Maddahi J, et al. Technetium-99m hexakis 2-methoxyisobutyl isonitrile: Human biodistribution, dosimetry, safety, and preliminary comparison to thallium-201 for myocardial perfusion imaging. *J Nucl Med* 1989;30:301–311.

29. Kiat H, Maddahi J, Roy LT, et al. Comparison of technetium-99m methoxy isobutyl isonitrile and thallium 201 for evaluation of coronary artery disease by planar and tomographic methods. *Am Heart J* 1989;117:1–11.

30. Kahn JK, McGhie I, Akers MS, et al. Quantitative rotational tomography with Tl-201 and Tc-99m 2-methoxy-isobutyl-isonitrile: A direct comparison in normal individuals and patients with coronary artery disease. *Circulation* 1989;79:1282–1293.

31. Iskandrian AS, Heo J, Kong B, et al. Use of technetium-99m isonitrile (RP-30A) in assessing left ventricular perfusion and function at rest and during exercise in coronary artery disease, and comparison with coronary arteriography and exercise thallium-201 SPECT imaging. *Am J Cardiol* 1989;64:270–275.

32. Dilsizian V, Rocco TP, Strauss HW, et al. Technetium-99m isonitrile myocardial uptake at rest: I. Relation to severity of coronary artery stenosis. *J Am Coll Cardiol* 1989;14:1673–1677.

33. Canby RC, Silber S, Pohost GM. Relations of the myocardial imaging agents 99mTc-MIBI and 201-Tl to myocardial blood flow in a canine model of ischemic insult. *Circulation* 1990;81:286–296.

34. Li QS, Solot G, Frank TL, et al. Myocardial redistribution of technetium-99m-methoxyisobutyl isonitrile (Sestamibi). *J Nucl Med* 1990;31:1069–1076.

35. Sinusas AJ, Bergin JD, Edwards NC, et al. Redistribution of 99mTc-sestamibi and 201Tl in the presence of a severe coronary artery stenosis. *Circulation* 1994;89:2332–2341.

36. Sansoy V, Glover DK, Watson DD, et al. Comparison of thallium-201 resting redistribution with technetium-99m-sestamibi uptake and functional response to dobutamine for assessment of myocardial viability. *Circulation* 1995;92:994–1004.

37. Franceschi M, Guimond J, Zimmerman RE, et al. Myocardial clearance of Tc-99m hexakis-2-methoxy-2-methylpropyl isonitrile (MIBI) in patients with coronary artery disease. *Clin Nucl Med* 1990;15:307–312.

38. Taillefer R, Primeau M, Costi P, et al. Technetium-99m-sestamibi myocardial perfusion imaging in detection of coronary artery disease: Comparison between initial (1-hour) and delayed (3-hour) postexercise images. *J Nucl Med* 1991;32:1961–1965.

39. Dilsizian V, Arrighi JA, Diodati JG, et al. Myocardial viability in patients with chronic coronary artery disease: Comparison of ^{99m}Tc-sestamibi with thallium reinjection and ^{18}F-fluorodeoxyglucose. *Circulation* 1994;89:578–587.

40. Richter WS, Cordes M, Calder D, et al. Washout and redistribution between immediate and two-hour myocardial images using technetium-99m sestamibi. *Eur J Nucl Med* 1995;22:49–55.

41. Maurea S, Cuocolo A, Soricelli A, et al. Myocardial viability index in chronic coronary artery disease: Technetium-99m-methoxy isobutyl isonitrile redistribution. *J Nucl Med* 1995;36: 1953–1960.

42. Rocco TP, Dilsizian V, Strauss HW, et al. Technetium-99m isonitrile myocardial uptake at rest: II. Relation to clinical markers of potential viability. *J Am Coll Cardiol* 1989;14:1678–1684.

43. Cuocolo A, Pace L, Ricciardelli B, et al. Identification of viable myocardium in patients with chronic coronary artery disease: Comparison of thallium-201 scintigraphy with reinjection and technetium-99m methoxyisobutyl isonitrile. *J Nucl Med* 1992;33:505–511.

44. Bonow RO, Dilsizian V. Thallium-201 and technetium-99m-sestamibi for assessing viable myocardium. *J Nucl Med* 1992;33:815–818.

45. Marzullo P, Sambuceti G, Parodi O. The role of sestamibi scintigraphy in the radioisotopic assessment of myocardial viability. *J Nucl Med* 1992;33:1925–1930.

46. Lucignani G, Paolini G, Landoni C, et al. Presurgical identification of hibernating myocardium by combined use of technetium-99m-hexakis-2-methoxyisobutylisonitrile single photon emission tomography and fluorine-18-fluoro-2-deoxy-D-glucose positron emission tomography in patients with coronary artery disease. *Eur J Nucl Med* 1992;19:874–881.

47. Altehoefer C, Kaiser HJ, Dorr R, et al. Fluorine-18 deoxyglucose PET for assessment of viable myocardium in perfusion defects in 99mTc-MIBI SPET: A comparative study in patients with coronary artery disease. *Eur J Nucl Med* 1992;19:334–342.

48. Ferreira J, Gil VM, Ventosa A, et al. Reversibility in myocardial perfusion scintigraphy after myocardial infarction: Comparison of SPECT 99mTc-sestamibi rest-stress single day protocol and thallium-201 reinjection. *Rev Port Cardiol* 1993;12:1013–1021.

49. Marzullo P, Parodi O, Reisenhofer B, et al. Value of rest thallium-201/technetium-99m sestamibi scans and dobutamine echocardiography for detecting myocardial viability. *Am J Cardiol* 1993;71:166–172.

50. Maurea S, Cuocolo A, Pace L, et al. Left ventricular dysfunction in coronary artery disease: Comparison between rest-redistribution thallium-201 and resting technetium-99m methoxyisobutyl isonitrile cardiac imaging. *J Nucl Cardiol* 1994;1:65–71.

51. Sawada SG, Allman KC, Muzik O, et al. Positron emission tomography detects evidence of viability in rest technetium-99m sestamibi defects. *J Am Coll Cardiol* 1994;23:92–98.

52. Maurea S, Cuocolo A, Nicolai E, et al. Improved detection of viable myocardium with thallium-201 reinjection in chronic coronary artery disease: Comparison with technetium-99m-MIBI imaging. *J Nucl Med* 1994;35:621–624.

53. Altehoefer C, vom Dahl J, Biedermann M, et al. Significance of defect severity is technetium-99m-MIBI SPECT at rest to assess myocardial viability: Comparison with fluorine-18-FDG PET. *J Nucl Med* 1994;35:569–574.

54. Marzullo P, Sambucetti G, Parodi O, et al. Regional concordance and discordance between rest thallium-201 and sestamibi imaging for assessing tissue viability: Comparison with postrevascularization functional recovery. *J Nucl Cardiol* 1995;2:309–316.

55. Delbeke D, Videlefsky S, Patton JA, et al. Rest myocardial perfusion/metabolism imaging using simultaneous dual-isotope acquisition SPECT with technetium-99m-MIBI/fluorine-18-FDG. *J Nucl Med* 1995;36:2110–2119.

56. Soufer R, Dey HM, Ng CK, et al. Comparison of sestamibi single-photon emission tomography with positron emission tomography for estimating left ventricular myocardial viability. *Am J Cardiol* 1995;75:1214–1219.

57. Rossetti C, Landoni C, Lucignani G, et al. Assessment of myocardial perfusion and viability with technetium-99m methoxybutylisonitrile and thallium-201 rest redistribution in chronic coronary artery disease. *Eur J Nucl Med* 1995;22:1306–1312.

58. Arrighi JA, Ng CK, Dey HM, Wackers FJT, Soufer R. Effect of left ventricular function on the assessment of myocardial viability by 99mTc-sestamibi and correlation with positron emission tomography in patients with healed myocardial infarcts or stable angina pectoris or both. *Am J Cardiol* 1997;80:1007–1013.

59. Rodney RA, Johnson LL. Myocardial perfusion scintigraphy to assess cardiac transplant vasculopathy. *J Heart Lung Transplant* 1992;11:S74–S78.

60. Dilsizian V, Perrone-Filardi P, Arrighi JA, et al. Concordance and discordance between stress-redistribution-reinjection and rest-redistribution thallium imaging for assessing viable myocardium: Comparison with metabolic activity by PET. *Circulation* 1993;88:941–952.

61. Bonow RO, Dilsizian V, Cuocolo A, et al. Identification of viable myocardium in patients with coronary artery disease and left ventricular dysfunction: Comparison of thallium scintigraphy with reinjection and PET imaging with ^{18}F-fluorodeoxyglucose. *Circulation* 1991;83:26–37.

62. Dilsizian V, Freedman NMT, Bacharach SL, et al. Regional thallium uptake in irreversible defects: Magnitude of change in thallium activity after reinjection distinguishes viable from nonviable myocardium. *Circulation* 1992;85:627–634.

63. Kitsiou AN, Srinivasan G, Quyyumi AA, et al. Stress-induced reversible and mild-to-moderate irreversible thallium defects: Are they equally accurate for predicting recovery of regional left ventricular function after revascularization? *Circulation* 1998;98:501–508.

64. Mehry Y, Latour JG, Arsenault A, et al. Effect of coronary reperfusion on technetium-99m methoxyisobutylisonitrile uptake by viable and necrotic myocardium in the dog. *Eur J Nucl Med* 1992;19:503–510.

65. Brown BG, Bolson EL, Petersen RB, et al. The mechanism of nitroglycerin action: Stenosis vasodilation as a major component of the drug response. *Circulation* 1981;64:1089–1097.

66. Cohen MV, Sonnenblick EH, Kirk ES. Comparative effects of nitroglycerin and isosorbide dinitrate on coronary collateral vessels and ischemic myocardium in dogs. *Am J Cardiol* 1976;37:244–249.

67. Bisi G, Sciagra R, Santoro GM, et al. Technetium-99m-sestamibi imaging with nitrate infusion to detect viable hibernating myocardium and predict postrevascularization recovery. *J Nucl Med* 1995;36:1994–2000.

68. Sciagra R, Bisi G, Santoro GM, et al. Comparison of baseline-nitrate technetium-99m sestamibi with rest-redistribution thallium-201 tomography in detecting viable hibernating myocardium and predicting postrevascularization recovery. *J Am Coll Cardiol* 1997;30:384–391.

69. Sciagra R, Bisi G, Santoro GM, et al. Influence of the assessment of defect severity and intravenous nitrate administration during tracer injection on the detection of viable hibernating myocardium with data-based quantitative techentium 99m-labeled sestamibi single-photon emission computed tomography. *J Nucl Cardiol* 1996;3:221–230.

70. Udelson JE, Coleman PS, Metherall JA, et al. Predicting recovery of severe regional ventricular dysfunction: Comparison of resting scintigraphy with ^{201}Tl and ^{99m}Tc-sestamibi. *Circulation* 1994;89:2552–2561.

71. Kauffman GJ, Boyne TS, Watson DD, et al. Comparison of rest thallium-201 imaging and rest technetium-99m sestamibi imaging for assessment of myocardial viability in patients with coronary artery disease and severe left ventricular dysfunction. *J Am Coll Cardiol* 1996;27:1592–1597.

72. Marcassa C, Galli M, Cuocolo A, et al. Rest-redistribution thallium-201 and rest technetium-99m-sestamibi SPECT in patients with stable coronary artery disease and ventricular dysfunction. *J Nucl Med* 1997;38:419–424.

73. Berman DS, Kiat H, Friedman JD, et al. Separate acquisition rest thallium-201/stress technetium-99m sestamibi dual-isotope myocardial perfusion single-photon emission computed tomography: A clinical validation study. *J Am Coll Cardiol* 1993;22:1455–1464.

74. DeCoster PM. Area-at-risk determination by technetium-99m-hexakis-2-methoxyisobutyl isonitrile in experimantal reperfused myocardial infarction. *Circulation* 1990;82:2152–2162.

75. Verani MS, Jeroudi MO, Mahmarian JJ, et al. Quantification of myocardial infarction during coronary occlusion and myocardial salvage after reperfusion using cardiac imaging with technetium-99m hexakis 2-methoxybutyl isonitrile. *J Am Coll Cardiol* 1988;12:1573–1581.

76. Sinusas AJ, Watson DD, Cannon JM, et al. Effect of ischemia and postischemic dysfunction on myocardial uptake of technetium-99m-labeled methoxyisobutyl isonitrile and thallium-201. *J Am Coll Cardiol* 1989;14:1785.

77. Beanlands RSB, Dawood F, Wen WH, et al. Are the kinetics of technetium-99m methoxyisobutyl isonitrile affected by cell metabolism and viability? *Circulation* 1990;82:1802–1814.

78. Li QS, Matsumura K, Dannals R, et al. Radionuclide markers of viability in reperfused myocaridum: Comparison between ^{18}F-2-deoxyglucose, ^{201}Tl, and. ^{99m}Tc-sestamibi. *Circulation* 1990;82:III542. Abstract.

79. Sinusas AJ, Trautman KA, Bergin JD, et al. Quantification of "area at risk" during coronary occlusion and degree of myocardial salvage after reperfusion with technetium-99m-methoxyisobutyl-isonitrile. *Circulation* 1990;82:1424–1437.

80. Gibbons RJ, Verani MS, Behrenbeck T, et al. Feasibility of tomographic technetium-99m-hexakis-2-methoxy-2-methylpropyl-isonitrile imaging for the assessment of myocardial area at risk and the effect of acute treatment in myocardial infarction. *Circulation* 1989;80:1277–1286.

81. Behrenbeck T, Pellikka PA, Huber KC, et al. Primary angioplasty in myocardial infarction: Assessment of improved myocardial perfusion with technetium-99m isonitrile. *J Am Coll Cardiol* 1991;17:365–372.

82. Beller GA, Glover DK, Edwards NC, et al. ^{99m}Tc-sestamibi uptake and retention during myocardial ischemia and reperfusion. *Circulation* 1993;87:2033–2042.

83. Christian TF, Behrenbeck T, Pellikka PA, et al. Mismatch of left ventricular function and infarct size demonstrated by technetium-99m isonitrile imaging after reperfusion therapy for acute myocardial infarction: Identification of myocardial stunning and hyperkinesis. *J Am Coll Cardiol* 1990;16:1632–1638.

84. Gibbons RJ, Verani MS, Behrenbeck T, et al. Feasibility of tomographic 99mTc-hexakis-2-methoxy-2-methylpropyl-isonitrile imaging for the assessment of myocardial area at risk and the effect of acute treatment in myocardial infarction. *Circulation* 1989;80:1277–1286.

85. Christian TF, Gibbons RJ, Gersh BJ. Effect of infarct location on myocardial salvage assessed by technetium-99m isonitrile. *J Am Coll Cardiol* 1991;17:1303–1308.

86. Santoro GM, Bisi G, Sciagra R, et al. Single photon emission computed tomography with technetium-99m hexakis 2-methoxyisobutyl isonitrile in acute myocardial infarction before and after thrombolytic treatment: Of salvaged myocardium and predictiion of late functional recovery. *J Am Coll Cardiol* 1990;15:301–314.

87. Behrenbeck T, Pellikka PA, Huber KC, et al. Primary angioplasty in myocardial infraction: Assessment of improved myocardial perfusion with technetium-99m isonitrile. *J Am Coll Cardiol* 1990;17:365–372.

88. Claeys MJ, Rademakers FE, Vrints CJ, et al. Comparative study of rest technetium-99m sestamibi SPET and low-dose dobutamine stress echocardiography for the early assessment of myocardial viability after acute myocardial infarction: Importance of the severity of the infarct-related stenosis. *Eur J Nucl Med* 1996;23:748–755.

89. Berman DS, Hachamovitch R, Kiat H, et al. Incremental value of prognostic testing in patients with known or suspected ischemic heart disease: A basis for optimal utilization of exercise technetium-99m sestamibi myocardial perfusion single-photon emission computed tomography. *J Am Coll Cardiol* 1995;26:639–647.

90. Miller TD, Christian TF, Hopfenspirger MR, et al. Infarct size after acute myocardial infarction measured by quantitative tomographic 99mTc sestamibi imaging predicts subsequent mortality. *Circulation* 1995;92:334–341.

91. Brown KA, Heller GV, Landin RJ, et al. Prognostic value of IV dipyridamol Tc99m sestamibi SPECT imaging early post myocardial infarction for prediction of in-hospital cardiac events. *Circulation* 1995;92:I-522.

92. Bilodeau L, Theroux P, Gregoire J, et al. Technetium-99m sestamibi tomography in patients with spontaneous chest pain: Correlations with clinical, electrocardiographic, and angiographic findings. *J Am Coll Cardiol* 1991;18:1684–1691.

93. Varetto T, Cantalupi D, Altieri A, et al. Emergency room technetium-99m sestamibi imaging to rule out acute myocardial ischemic events in patients with nondiagnostic electrocardiograms. *J Am Coll Cardiol* 1993;22:1804–1808.

94. Hilton TC, Thompson RC, Williams HJ, et al. Technetium-99m sestamibi myocardial perfusion imaging in the emergency room evaluation of chest pain. *J Am Coll Cardiol* 1994;23:1016–1022.

95. Radensky PW, Stowers SA, Hilton TC, et al. Cost-effectiveness of acute myocardial perfusion imaging with Tc-99m sestamibi for risk stratification of emergency room patients with acute chest pain. *Circulation* 1994;90:I528. Abstract.

96. Stowers SA, Abuan THE, Szymanski TJ, et al. Technetium-99m sestamibi SPECT and techetium-99m tetrofosmin SPECT in prediction of cardiac events in patients injected during chest pain and following resolution of pain. *J Nucl Med* 1995;36:88P. Abstract.

97. Mark DB, Hlatky MA, Harrell FE, et al. Exercise treadmill score for predicting prognosis in coronary artery disease. *Ann Intern Med* 1987;106:793–800.

98. Morris S, Mascitelli VA, Lawrence DS, et al. Acute Tc-99m SPECT myocardial perfusion imaging during spontaneous angina and stress imaging: The same defect, same location? *Circulation* 1995;92:I677. Abstract.

99. Weinstein H, Reinhardt CP, Leppo JA. Teboroxime, sestamibi and thallium-201 as markers of myocardial hypoperfusion: Comparison by quantitative dual-isotope autoradiography in rabbits. *J Nucl Med* 1993;34:1510–1517.

100. DiRocco RJ, Rumsey WL, Kuczynski BL, et al. Measurement of myocardial blood flow using a coinjection technique for technetium-99m teboroxime, technetium-99m sestamibi and thallium-201. *J Nucl Med* 1992;33:1152–1159.
101. Stewart RE, Schwaiger M, Hutchins GD, et al. Myocardial clearance kinetics of technetium-99m SQ30217: A marker of regional myocardial blood flow. *J Nucl Med* 1990;31:1183–1190.
102. Maublant JC, Moins N, Gachon P. Uptake and release of two new Tc-99m labeled myocardial blood flow imaging agents in cultured cardiac cells. *Eur J Nucl Med* 1989;15:180–182.
103. Kronauge JF, Chiu ML, Cone JS, et al. Comparison of neutral and cationic myocardial perfusion agents: Characteristics of accumulation in cultured cells. *Nucl Med Biol* 1992;19:141–148.
104. Seldin DW, Johnson L, Blood DK, et al. Myocardial perfusion imaging with technetium-99m SQ30217: Comparison with thallium-201 and coronary anatomy. *J Nucl Med* 1989;30:312–319.
105. Iskandrian AS, Heo J, Nguyen T, et al. Myocardial imaging with Tc-99m teboroxime: Technique and initial results. *Am Heart J* 1991;121:889–894.
106. Iskandrian AS, Heo J, Nguyen T. Tomographic myocardial perfusion imaging with technetium-99m teboroxime during adenosine-induced coronary hyperemia: Correlation with thallium-201 imaging. *J Am Coll Cardiol* 1992;19:307–312.
107. Henzlova MJ, Machac J. Clinical utility of technetium-99m teboroxime myocardial washout imaging. *J Nucl Med* 1994;35:575–579.
108. Narra RK, Nunn AD, Kuczynski BL, et al. A neutral technetium-99m complex for myocardial imaging. *J Nucl Med* 1989;30:1830–1837.
109. Johnson G III, Glover D, Hebert C, et al. Early myocardial clearance kinetics of technetium-99-teboroxime differentiate normal and flow-restricted canine myocardium at rest. *J Nucl Med* 1993;34:630–636.
110. Gray WA, Gewirtz H. Comparison of ^{99m}Tc-teboroxime with thallium for myocardial imaging in the presence of a coronary artery stenosis. *Circulation* 1991;84:1796–1807.
111. Johnson G III, Glover DK, Hebert CB, et al. Myocardial clearance kinetics of tc-99m-teboroxime following dipyridamole: Differentiation of stenosis severity in canine myocardium. *J Nucl Med* 1995;36:111–119.
112. Weinstein H, Dahlberg ST, McSherry BA, et al. Rapid redistribution of teboroxime. *Am J Cardiol* 1993;71:848–852.
113. Beanlands R, Muzik O, Nguyen N, et al. The relationship between myocardial retention of technetium-99m teboroxime and myocardial blood flow. *J Am Coll Cardiol* 1992;20:712–719.
114. Smith AM, Gullberg GT, Christian PE, et al. Kinetic modeling of teboroxime using dynamic SPECT imaging of a canine model. *J Nucl Med* 1994;35:484–495.
115. Fleming RM, Kirkeeide RL, Taegtmeyer H, et al. Comparison of technetium-99m teboroxime tomography with automated quantitative coronary arteriography and thallium-201 tomographic imaging. *J Am Coll Cardiol* 1991;17:1297–1302.
116. Hendel RC, Dahlberg ST, Weinstein H, et al. Comparison of teboroxime and thallium for the reversibility of exercise-induced myocardial perfusion defects. *Am Heart J* 1993;126:856–862.
117. Bisi G, Sciagra R, Santoro GM, et al. Evaluation of 99mTc-teboroxime scintigraphy for the differentiation of reversible from fixed defects: Comparison with 201Tl redistribution and reinjection imaging. *Nucl Med Commun* 1993;14:520–528.
118. Kelly JD, Forester AM, Higley B, et al. Technetium-99m Tetrofosmin as a new radiopharmaceutical for myocardial perfusion imaging. *J Nucl Med* 1993;34:222–227.
119. Sinusas AJ, Shi QX, Saltzberg MT, et al. Technetium-99m tetrofosmin to assess myocardial blood flow: Experimental validation in an intact canine model of ischemia. *J Nucl Med* 1994;35:664–671.
120. Higley B, Smith FW, Smith T, et al. Technetium-99m-1,2-bis[bis(2-ethoxyethyl)phosphino]ethane: Human biodistribution, dosimetry and safety of a new myocardial perfusion imaging agent. *J Nucl Med* 1993;34:30–38.
121. Koplan BA, Beller GA, Ruiz M, et al. Comparison between thallium-201 and technetium-99m-tetrofosmin uptake with sustained low flow and profound systolic dysfunction. *J Nucl Med* 1996;37:1398–1402.

122. Jain D, Wackers FJ, Mattera J, et al. Biokinetics of 99m Tc-tetrofosmin, a new myocardial perfusion imaging agent: Implications for a one day imaging protocol. *J Nucl Med* 1993;34: 1254–1259.

123. Glover DK, Ruiz M, Yand JY, et al. Myocardial 99mTc-tetrofosmin uptake during adenosine-induced vasodilation with either a critical or mild coronary stenosis: Comparison with 201Tl and regional myocardial blood flow. *Circulation* 1997;96:2332–2338.

124. Matsunari I, Fujino S, Taki J, et al. Myocardial viability assessment with technetium-99m-tetrofosmin and thallium-201 reinjection in coronary artery disease. *J Nucl Med* 1995;36: 1961–1967.

125. Gerson MC, Millard RW, Roszell NJ, et al. Kinetic properties of 99mTc-Q12 in canine myocardium. *Circulation* 1994;89:1291–1300.

126. Gerson MC, Lukes J, Deutsch E, et al. Comparison of technetium-99m Q12 and thallium-201 for detection of angiographically documented coronary artery disease in humans. *J Nucl Cardiol* 1994;1:499–508.

127. Uccelli L, Giganti M, Duatti A, et al. Subcellular distribution of technetium-99m-N-NOET in rat myocardium. *J Nucl Med* 1995;36:2075–2079.

128. Uccelli L, Pasqualini R, Duatti A, et al. Uptake mechanism of the neutral myocardial imaging agents. *J Nucl Med* 1993;34:18p. Abstract.

129. Vanzetto G, Calnon DA, Ruiz M, et al. Myocardial uptake and redistribution of 99m-Tc-N-NOET in dogs with either sustained coronary low flow or transient coronary occlusion: Comparison with ^{201}Tl and myocardial blood flow. *Circulation* 1997;96:2325–2331.

130. Johnson G III, Nguyen KN, Liu Z, et al. Planar imaging of ^{99m}Tc-labeled (bis(N-ethoxy, N-ethyl dithiocarbamato) nitrido technetium(V) can detect resting ischemia. *J Nucl Cardiol* 1997;4:217–225.

131. Ghezzi C, Fagret D, Arvieux CC, et al. Myocardial kinetics of TcN-NOET: A neutral lipophilic complex tracer of regional myocardial blood flow. *J Nucl Med* 1995;36:1069–1077.

132. Fagret D, Marie PY, Brunotte F, et al. Myocardial perfusion imaging with technetium-99m-Tc-NOET: Comparison with thallium-201 and coronary angiography. *J Nucl Med* 1995;36: 936–943.

133. Johnson G III, Allton IL, Nguyen KN, et al. Clearance of technetium 99m N-NOET in normal, ischemic-reperfused, and membrane-disrupted myocardium. *J Nucl Cardiol* 1996; 3:42–54.

134. Maublant J, Zhang Z, Ollier M, et al. Uptake and release of bis(N-ethoxy, N-ethyl dithiocarbamato) nitrido 99m-Tc(V) in cultured mycardial cells: Comparison with Tl-201, MIBI, and teboroxime. *Eur J Nucl Med* 1992;19:597. Abstract.

135. Johnson G III, Nguyen KN, Pasqualini R, et al. Interaction of technetium-99m-N-NOET with blood elements: Potential mechanism of myocardial redistribution. *J Nucl Med* 1997; 38:138–143.

136. Dilsizian V, Arrighi JA. Myocardial viability in chronic coronary artery disease: Perfusion, metabolism, and contractile reserve. In: Gerson MC, ed. *Cardiac Nuclear Medicine*, 3rd ed. New York: McGraw-Hill; 1997;143–191.

Myocardial Imaging of Lipid Metabolism with Labeled Fatty Acids

Ludwig E. Feinendegen, MD

Introduction

Because fatty acids are major energy supplying substrates for myocardial metabolism,[1-3] oleic acid was initially used by Evans et al in 1965[4] for the purpose of in vivo scanning of the myocardium in dogs and in human patients. It was labeled with ^{131}I by double-bond saturation. After intravenous (IV) injection, this fatty acid served as a precursor of myocardial lipids and allowed the external imaging of the myocardium. The degree of uptake depended on the nutritional state of the examined subject, and the distribution of uptake conformed to myocardial perfusion.

This led to the search for improving myocardial scintigraphy with labeled fatty acids. The γ-camera had become the instrument for studying local myocardial perfusion with ionic radionuclides such as [43]K and [129]Cs.[5] Subsequently, hexadecanoic acid was selected and labeled with ^{123}I so that it replaced the terminal methyl group.[6] It was shown to be incorporated more efficiently into the myocardial tissue than oleic acid that was iodinated by double-bond saturation. Moreover, ^{123}I with its near pure γ-energy peak of 159 keV and its half-life of 13.3 hours is well suited for clinical work with the γ-camera. This tracer allowed excellent images of the left ventricular (LV) myocardium in humans with various heart diseases. The pattern of tracer uptake coincided with myocardial mass and perfusion[7] and led to the suggestion that this labeled fatty acid eventually also may be applied to imaging of local myocardial metabolism. Similar initial data were reported for positron emission tomography (PET) using ^{11}C-labeled palmitic acid.[8] In parallel to these studies, different, variously labeled long-chain fatty acids were synthesized and tested in rodents for the purpose of developing metabolic imaging of the myocardium.[9] This work independently confirmed the particular usefulness of the terminal (ω) positioning of the radioiodine on heptadecanoic acid (ω-I-HDA) that behaved kinetically like ^{11}C-labeled palmitic acid. In fact, ^{123}I-labeled fatty acids were used for studying myocardial lipid turnover with dynamic planar imaging before dynamic PET became available confirming the findings.[10,11]

For measuring fatty acid metabolism in the myocardium in clinical practice and in view of budgetary concerns, the ^{123}I-labeled fatty acids are preferred for use with γ-camera scintigraphy either in the planar or tomographic mode. Fatty acids labeled with

From Dilsizian V (ed). *Myocardial Viability: A Clinical and Scientific Treatise*. Armonk, NY: Futura Publishing Co., Inc.; © 2000.

positron emitters such as ^{11}C or ^{18}F usually are used with PET. The latter is relatively expensive and remains confined to a limited number of appropriately equipped institutions. Attempts at labeling fatty acids with ^{99m}Tc for easy use with the γ-camera thus far have not resulted in metabolically useful substrates. This is likely caused by severe structural alterations of the fatty acid when it is linked to a technetium-containing ligand.[12]

The introduction of diagnostic imaging with labeled fatty acids in cardiology significantly contributed to the development of the medical subspeciality nuclear cardiology.[13] This chapter discusses the role of various labeled fatty acids in the diagnostic repertoire of cardiology, both for assessing local myocardial perfusion and metabolism. A single direct image of uptake and distribution of a labeled fatty acid alone is hardly satisfactory for clinical diagnosis; consideration of the influences of metabolism on the image avoids serious misinterpretations of the data.

Constraints of Measuring Metabolism in the Living Organism

To image in vivo the metabolic fate of a labeled substrate, various potential problems arise. These need to be considered, understood, and overcome before reliable data can be meaningfully analyzed.[10]

- Imaging of a labeled substrate in the stationary or dynamic mode only registers the relative amount or rate of uptake and/or release of the radionuclide and not necessarily of the labeled substrate within the chosen region of interest (ROI) in the body.
- The radionuclide must remain bound to the labeled substrate during the time of observation if the labeled substrate should truly serve as an indicator.
- Local blood supply needs to be considered; it influences the path of the labeled substrate in the body to its site of metabolism in the ROI. A diminished local perfusion, for example, may cause a reduced local uptake or release of the labeled substrate and may mimic a reduced rate of metabolism.
- Within the ROI, local diffusion and transport from the capillary vessels into the extracellular space and cells determine the rate of supply of the labeled substrate for cellular metabolism.
- The labeled substrate within the cell may be transported or may diffuse back into the extracellular space and capillary vessels. This leads to loss of the nonmetabolized tracer from the site of observation. In such an instance, loss of that tracer from the ROI is indistinguishable from loss of radionuclide from the ROI because of metabolism. If the labeled substrate or the radionuclide becomes detached from the substrate in consequence of metabolism and should recirculate in the ROI, the metabolic reaction only can be assessed when the recirculation in the ROI is accounted for separately.

To overcome these principal challenges of directly observing metabolic reactions within selected ROIs, the following requirements arise:

1. Knowledge of the metabolic reaction under study in terms of the biochemical steps involving the substrate
2. Proper choice of the radionuclide for labeling the substrate to be measured and for the type of imaging instrument
3. Optimal and usually stable positioning of the radionuclide on the substrate so that it becomes a useful metabolic indicator

4. Measurement techniques in the dynamic mode and data analysis with the help of models in compliance with the local physiology and biochemistry of the metabolic reaction

5. Proof of applicability of the method

The above requirements 1, 2, and 3 presently are the main challenges of expert radiopharmaceutical chemistry. Requirements 4 and 5 demand various applications of what one may summarily call dynamic dual parameter analysis, as discussed later.[14]

Dynamic Dual Parameter Analysis for Noninvasively Measuring Metabolism

The dynamic dual parameter analysis in measuring metabolic reactions comprises, today, a set of standard procedures for metabolic imaging. Most common and successful is the simultaneous and frequent measurement of a single labeled substrate at two different sites: peripheral arterial blood supplying the tissue and tissue site of the metabolic reaction. The resulting time-activity curve obtained from the blood describes the input of the substrate to the site of the metabolic reaction, and that obtained from the tissue relates to the rate of reaction. Appropriate models are chosen for two or three compartments giving the labeled substrate in the peripheral blood, the reaction site and the reaction. They usually allow the analysis of the time-activity curves that are obtained from blood and tissue for calculating the rates and rate constants of substrate transfer between the peripheral blood and the extracellular compartment of free substrate to the reaction site in the cell, and, depending on the protocol, also of the reaction.[14,15,16]

Other modes of dual parameter analysis apply two different radionuclides on one substrate to describe the metabolic alteration of the substrate; also, separate radioactive indicators such as two isomers are used that have similar biokinetics data exclusive of that caused by the metabolic reaction.

For example, the initial development of the external imaging of fatty acid metabolism in the human myocardium relied on the experience with the dynamic dual parameter analysis using two different radionuclides on one substrate. Thus, the fate of IV-injected DNA and its catabolite in normal mice[17] and the site and rate of catabolism of insulin in various tissues of the human body were described.[18] The success of the investigation on insulin depended on double labeling of insulin with ^{131}I and ^{51}Cr, without destroying its biological function. The frequent, that is, dynamic, registration of the two different radionuclides is easy in separate energy windows of the imaging device. These radionuclides remained together as long as the labeled insulin was intact, wherever it moved or resided. Catabolism caused the two radionuclides to separate rapidly in such a way that one of the two, namely, ^{51}Cr, by its chemical nature, remained at the cellular site of catabolism while the other, ^{131}I, readily moved away from the site to enter the free-iodine pool in the body. The change in the ratio of the two radionuclides thus signaled the fate of the insulin molecule; wherever the ratio changed, catabolism occurred, and the rate of change gave the rate of catabolism. Local organ perfusion, or diffusion and transport of the insulin did not influence the measurement.

This principal approach to observing in vivo the catabolism of insulin was crucial in preparing for the measurement of the metabolic fate of iodine labeled fatty acids in the intact living body. This will be discussed later in the context of the various labeled fatty acids.

Fatty Acid Labeling and Imaging Instruments

Planar imaging and single photon emission computed tomography (SPECT) with radioiodine-labeled fatty acids currently are both widely available and diagnostically used in investigational and clinical cardiology. Fatty acids labeled with positron emitters such as ^{11}C or ^{18}F are the substrates of choice for PET.

The expense and infrastructural complexity of running PET in a clinical setting is partly offset by three advantages:

- PET, in contrast to SPECT, allows the noninvasive quantification of substrate concentration in tissue.
- PET images today have a relatively high resolution within the millimeter range and, thus, may observe three-dimensionally metabolic reactions within tissue masses of fractions of a gram.
- A main advantage is imaging a large number of small molecular substrates. These usually cannot be labeled with a foreign nuclide without changing their metabolic specificity. The replacement of a natural carbon or nitrogen atom in a small molecular substrate by radioactive ^{11}C or ^{13}N has no biochemical effect. Similarly, a hydrogen atom may at times be replaced in small molecules by ^{18}F without interfering with a biochemical reaction to be studied. However, these positron emitting radionuclides have short half-lives: 20 minutes for ^{11}C, 10 minutes for ^{13}N, and 110 minutes for ^{18}F. This requires not only radionuclide production by cyclotrons close to the site of PET, but often also sophisticated radiopharmaceutical chemistry. For the purpose of routine work, the latter is presently often provided by automatically operating equipment.

Planar imaging or SPECT has the advantage of wide availability and relative ease of operation. Thus, it is less costly and less labor-intensive. Substrates that are labeled with single photon emitters have a relatively long half-life and usually are supplied commercially. An additional advantage is the potential for dynamic imaging in a PET equivalent manner, so that time-activity curves may be constructed for applying compartmental analyses of tracer kinetics.

Among the single photon emitters that are suitable for γ-camera imaging, so far only radioiodine has been used widely for labeling fatty acids. Iodine has an atomic radius that is similar to that of the methyl group and, thus, may replace a molecular methyl group without destroying metabolic substrate specificity. Also, iodine is linked relatively easily to organic molecules by halogen exchange reactions. Of the various isotopes of radioiodine, ^{123}I with its γ-emission of 159 keV is optimal for γ-cameras of the Anger type. Its physical half-life of 13.3 hours, nevertheless, poses a logistical problem of timely production, supply, and use of ^{123}I-labeled compounds.

On the other hand, ^{99m}Tc is obtained most easily by using the appropriate radionuclide generator, and it is used widely for γ-camera scintigraphy. However, technetium does not covalently bind to carbon, nitrogen, and oxygen, but requires sophisticated linker chemistry for substrate labeling. However, this, alters the molecular structure and usually eliminates metabolic specificity.[12]

Types of Labeled Fatty Acids
for Myocardial Scintigraphy

Various long-chain fatty acids are used as diagnostic tools in clinical practice and investigations. Several categories of different chemical structures, as shown in Figure 1, provide special applications that are discussed in this chapter.

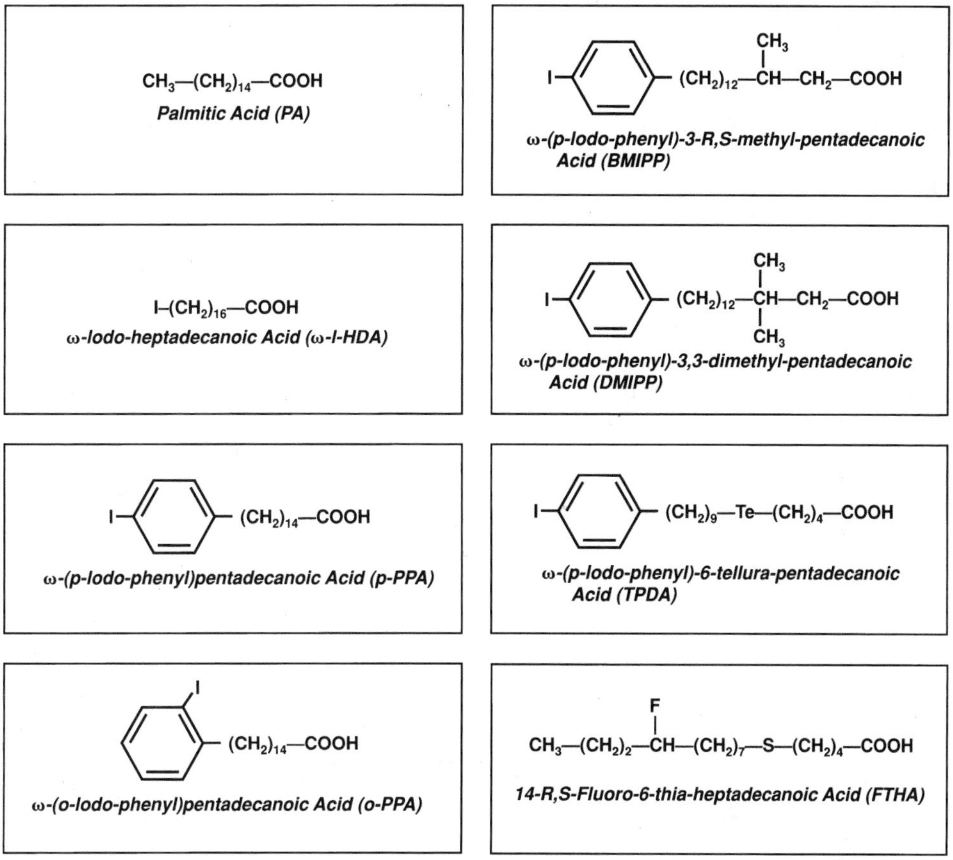

CH₃—(CH₂)₁₄—COOH

Palmitic Acid (PA)

ω-(p-Iodo-phenyl)-3-R,S-methyl-pentadecanoic Acid (BMIPP)

I—(CH₂)₁₆—COOH

ω-Iodo-heptadecanoic Acid (ω-I-HDA)

ω-(p-Iodo-phenyl)-3,3-dimethyl-pentadecanoic Acid (DMIPP)

ω-(p-Iodo-phenyl)pentadecanoic Acid (p-PPA)

ω-(p-Iodo-phenyl)-6-tellura-pentadecanoic Acid (TPDA)

ω-(o-Iodo-phenyl)pentadecanoic Acid (o-PPA)

14-R,S-Fluoro-6-thia-heptadecanoic Acid (FTHA)

Figure 1.

One category traces the fate of labeled physiological fatty acids by imaging the tracer uptake, distribution into, and release from the myocardium; the latter usually indicates the completion of catabolism via physiological β-oxidation; however, a nonmetabolized tracer also may be lost from cells in the diseased myocardium through retrograde diffusion and transport back into the capillaries. External dynamic imaging does not distinguish between these two routes of tracer loss. Into this group of tracers belong the ^{11}C-labeled palmitic acid, the ^{123}I-labeled ω-I-hexadecanoic and ω-I-HDA, and the ^{123}I-labeled ω-(p-^{123}I-phenyl)pentadecanoic acid (p-PPA).

Another category of fatty acids is chemically tailored so that the rate of their catabolism and the release of labeled catabolites from the myocardial cells is prolonged greatly without change in the rate of myocardial uptake. The advantage here is, on the one hand, technical. A prolonged retention of tracer helps to improve image quality especially by SPECT; a prolonged data collection diminishes contribution of background counts and advances image contrast. Of equal importance are biochemical differences between these tailored tracers that may help in distinguishing between specific biochemical steps in myocardial lipid metabolism without direct interference from local blood flow, as is discussed later.

Thus, one type of this category of fatty acids is preferentially trapped within the mitochondria, where β-oxidation physiologically catabolizes the fatty acids. The rate of accumulation of the tracer within the mitochondria indicates the rate of fatty acid supply for energy metabolism through β-oxidation. Into this group of tracers belong the fatty acids carrying, within their carbon chain, a foreign nuclide such as tellurium or sulfur.

A second type of analog carries one or two methyl groups on the carbon chain, in the 3 or β-position. This leads to a reduction or even blocking of the release of the tracer from the complex lipids into which these analogs are readily incorporated. If they reach the mitochondria for β-oxidation, again, a reduced rate of tracer release from the mitochondria is seen with monomethylated analogs.

A third fatty acid analog mainly remains in the fatty acid pool in the cytoplasm outside the mitochondria. Because this analog is hardly or not at all transported into mitochondria for β-oxidation, release of the tracer from the myocardium indicates predominantly retrograde diffusion and transport into the capillaries. So far, only ^{123}I labeled ω-(o-^{123}I-phenyl)pentadecanoic acid (o-PPA) behaves in this fashion.

Any of these fatty acid analogs in the same patient may be compared kinetically with each other or with a labeled physiologically behaving fatty acid or a suitable tracer of local blood flow. The differences between the kinetics of two or three of these tracers in the same patient allow the calculation of various specific aspects of myocardial lipid metabolism. Thus, the fractions of tracer entering lipid synthesis in various myocardial regions, the tracer release due to β-oxidation on the one hand and due to back-diffusion and transport on the other, may be assessed separately. This type of multiparameter analysis was diagnostically helpful in various myocardial diseases and will be discussed later.

Myocardial Fatty Acid Metabolism

The mammalian myocardium utilizes, besides oxygen, various substrates such as amino acids, long-chain fatty acids, glucose, ketone bodies, lactate, and pyruvate. Of these, long-chain fatty acids are preferred in aerobic physiological metabolism; they supply between 65% and 70% of energy for the working heart, and some 15%–20% of total energy supply comes from glucose.[19–21] A simplified scheme of fatty acid metabolism is shown in Figure 2.

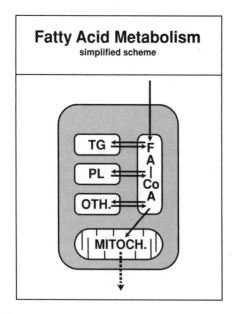

Figure 2. Simplified scheme of fatty acid metabolism. TG = tryglycerides, PL = phospholipids, OTH = other lipids, FA-CoA = fatty acid Coenzyme-A, mitoch = mitochondria. Reproduced with permission from reference 13.

Physiologically, fatty acids circulate in the peripheral blood in bondage to plasma protein, albumin and lipoproteins, and also in triglycerides from where they are set free by lipases, pass through the capillary wall, and are transported actively into the myocardial cells.[22,23,24] Approximately 40% of the long-chain fatty acids that pass through the myocardial capillaries thus are extracted normally into cells. However, this extraction fraction depends on coronary blood flow.[25–29] As flow decreases, fatty acid extraction eventually decreases too; however, extraction also may diminish with the flow rising far above the normal resting flow. This situation may occur at high values of coronary reserve,[30] which gives the ratio between flows at the conditions of maximally induced vasodilation and predilation.

The transporter protein in myocardial cells has been identified to have a molecular weight of approximately 40 kd; and within the cells, fatty acids are bound to storage protein weighing approximately 12 kd.[19,22,23] Fatty acids that are synthesized within the cell also are bound this way.

In the normal human myocardium, free fatty acids are activated metabolically or accepted in the cell by binding to coenzyme A (CoA) by the enzyme acyl-CoA-transferase.[19] The activated fatty acids then may take various metabolic routes according to their chemistry and chain length. Up to approximately 10% of the extracted fatty acids may be transported back into the capillary vessels.[31] A major pathway leads to myocardial lipids such as phospholipids and triglycerides. These lipids also constitute a reservoir for fatty acids to be returned into the free fatty pool. Depending on demand, some 80% of the extracted fatty acids, shown for palmitic and oleic acid, eventually are activated for transport from the pool of lipids via the carnitine shuttle into the mitochondria for catabolism by β-oxidation. The rate of fatty acid transfer from the pool of lipids into mitochondria in human myocardium is at least an order of magnitude slower than the rate of release of catabolites from the mitochondria.[32]

The main catabolite of fatty acid β-oxidation is carbon dioxide, which appears in the venous effluent of the coronary circulation in less than a minute after fatty acid transfer into the mitochondria.[33–35] Fatty acid catabolism by α-oxidation also may occur and is discussed with the fatty acids later, as it applies.

The metabolism of fatty acids and lipids in the mammalian myocardium reacts homeostatically to changes of physiological balances between different normal metabolites in the peripheral blood and the myocardial tissue.[36–39] Such changes are influenced by the chain length of the fatty acid; by the number of double bonds in the carbon chain of the fatty acids; by the plasma concentration of fatty acids, insulin, glucose, and various amino acids in arterial blood; and, of course, by energy consumption in response to mechanical demand on the myocardium. For example, food intake stimulates insulin secretion. This reduces the serum concentration of glucose, which again increases fatty acid utilization. On the other hand, increased plasma concentration of fatty acids in the peripheral circulation leads to enhanced fatty acid oxidation in the myocardium, which again raises the levels of intracellular adenosine triphosphate (ATP) and acetyl-CoA with the consequence of inhibition of pyruvate dehydrogenase.[40] This way, the entry of lactate into the citric acid cycle and eventually glucose utilization in the myocardium are reduced. Changes in energy consumption and even psychological stress influence fatty acid and lipid turnover in the myocardium.[41]

Imaging of labeled fatty acids in the myocardium, of course, only allows the observation of the tracer uptake rates and distribution into and release from the myocardium. This is presented schematically in Figure 3. The rate of release is determined by the rate of lipid turnover and not by β-oxidation, which, in principle, is a rapid process. Radioiodine either in the free or bound form may, on completion of β-oxidation of the labeled long-chain fatty acid, be released rapidly from the myocardium into the circulating blood or even the interstitial space in the case of free iodine.[34] In this case, recirculating radio-

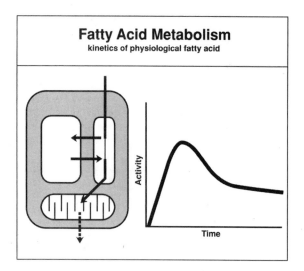

Fatty Acid Metabolism
kinetics of physiological fatty acid

Activity

Time

Figure 3. External measurement by dynamic imaging principally registers tracer inflow, peak accumulation, and release within the chosen region of interest in the myocardium, as shown on the right.

iodine in the myocardium needs to be subtracted from the myocardial image to observe specifically the kinetics of the lipid-bound tracer.[42,43]

Applying imaging with labeled fatty acids for the diagnosis in clinical cardiology demands attention to the physiological adaptations to various diurnal, alimentary, physical, and psychological influences with their concomitant alterations in local substrate concentrations and reactions. Hence, investigational protocols must be designed carefully. Individual adaptive responses of lipid metabolism should be avoided or specifically planned as part of the protocol, so that external imaging gives useful information.

Myocardial pathology is accompanied or caused by severe derangements of the homoeostasis of myocardial metabolism, and fatty acids and lipids are involved accordingly.[44] This offers diagnostic advantages of tracer techniques with labeled fatty acids. For example, during ischemia long-chain fatty acids are oxidized less readily, and glucose becomes the preferred substrate for energy supply.[1,2,20,21,45,46] Hypoxia severely disturbs cellular metabolism, impairs the carnitine shuttle, and eventually causes a cellular accumulation of inhibitory metabolites. These amplify the reduction in fatty acid oxidation and shift metabolism toward glycolysis and use of lactate.[47] If supplied in excess of metabolic capacity in the ischemic tissue, fatty acids form esters, which may become toxic to membranous structures of the cells.[40] Thus, fatty acids also tend to be lost by retrograde diffusion through disrupted membranes of the hypoxic cells into the capillary vessels.[24,48,49]

Myocardial imaging of labeled fatty acids and imaging of local myocardial blood flow (MBF) in conjunction with quantification of cardiac function and wall motion in the individual patient enhances, of course, the diagnostic relevance of an alteration of either one of them. After initiation of ischemia,[50,51] the sequence of events primarily leads to a reduced supply of metabolic substrates, followed by disturbed metabolism that eventually leads to impairment of cardiac function.[52,53]

The duration of a given degree of ischemia appears to determine the extent of damage. This is indicated partially by the time it takes for the myocardium to recover fully its function after myocardial perfusion is restored.[54,55] Two minutes of ischemia cause wall motion abnormality to last less than approximately 45 minutes; a limited time of 5 minutes of ischemia causes abnormal wall motion for approximately 3 hours; after 15 minutes of ischemia wall motion is disturbed for some 6 hours.[40] Consequences of ischemic injury in terms of myocardial stunning and hibernation may be discernable. The former appears characterized by reduced cardiac function and restored MBF, while, hibernation exhibits both reduced local blood flow and cardiac function for a various length of time. Stunning appears to be caused by membranous damage in the mitochondria from attacks by metabolic oxygen radicals resulting in uncoupling of mitochondrial metabolism and energy production.[53] ATP is reduced. Yet, stunning allows for a relatively fast recovery whereas hibernating myocardium, still being viable, recovers comparatively slowly. The metabolic causes of these specific adaptations or mixtures of those in the myocardium in response to ischemia are not understood fully.

Different forms of nonischemic cardiomyopathies often are not diagnosed easily at an early stage of disease.[30,56] The particular metabolic disturbances in this disease group, even if they are still far from being understood, are increasingly recognized by metabolic imaging, also using labeled fatty acids. It may be predicted that metabolic imaging of the myocardium will become a major tool for the early diagnosis of different pathological entities underlying the various clinical representations in this group of diseases.

More detailed findings with different types of labeled fatty acids as tracers for myocardial imaging in the mode of single or multiple parameter analysis are given in the subsequent sections. They will show the potential power of the various approaches in the clinical diagnosis of heart diseases, when more conventional tests and structural imaging are less revealing.

^{11}C-Palmitic Acid

Normal Myocardium

The labeling of palmitic acid with ^{11}C usually in the carboxyl group permits the observation of the biokinetics of the physiological substrate in the myocardium using dynamic PET (Fig. 4). In this way, a standard is set for assessing noninvasively fatty acid uptake, distribution, and tracer release as expressions of myocardial lipid metabolism. The uptake of the ^{11}C-palmitic acid into the human myocardium is rapid to a peak value reached at approximately 5 minutes after IV pulse injection. Thereafter, the tracer release has at least two components.[35,57] In the normal myocardium, these components relate to the rate of transfer of the labeled fatty acid from at least two different cellular pools into the mitochondria; one of these pools is in the complex lipids, and the other appears to be the protein-bound fatty acids, also referred to as the free fatty acid pool. In the mitochondria, rapid degradation physiologically by β-oxidation results in the generation of carbondioxide that is released practically instantaneously into the circulating blood and transported out of site of the observed ROI.

The uptake of the tracer into the myocardium depends, as stated above, on various factors, such as local perfusion, substrate diffusion, transport, and acceptance in the cytosol by binding to CoA.[19] Of these factors, local perfusion and binding to CoA are dominant in modifying the initial tracer accumulation in an observed myocardial segment.

$$CH_3-(CH_2)_{14}-COOH$$
Palmitic Acid (PA)

Figure 4.

The two principally observable quantities, namely, tracer uptake into and rate of release from the myocardium by dynamic imaging, have been interpreted diagnostically in various heart diseases.[10] However, the biochemical complexity of myocardial lipid metabolism asks for caution in an attempt to interpret the kinetic data diagnostically. Thus, it is prudent to set limits to what extent dynamic imaging of labeled palmitic acid may be used clinically. Also, adding imaging of local MBF to metabolic imaging usually enhances the diagnostic potential of labeled palmitic acid.

An obvious approach to using labeled palmitic acid diagnostically as with other labeled long-chain fatty acids or their applicable analogs is the observation of uptake and turnover in various myocardial regions. This may be done preferably at rest and at exercise or before and after changing myocardial metabolism, for example, by glucose loading. An alternative to physical stress testing is the pharmacologic stress testing, for example, with dobutamine.[58-60] This agent activates adrenoreceptors of the β_1, β_2, and α_1-types and thus has a potent inotropic effect. It increases myocardial oxygen demand but does not readily induce arrhythmias.

Early studies on dogs[35] with pulse-injected ^{11}C-labeled palmitic acid had revealed an extraction fraction of 65% ± 10% from the coronary blood circulation into the normal myocardium, with little influence on this value from physiological changes in blood flow, oxygen consumption, arterial concentrations, and myocardial consumptions of glucose and fatty acid and from the pH. The half-time of the initial portion of the turnover curve correlated with the myocardial oxygen consumption and with the release of labeled CO_2. The late portion of the turnover curve was interpreted to arise from complex lipids, mainly triglycerides. The turnover of this pool appeared to be independent of myocardial oxygen consumption. But the fraction of tracer incorporated into this pool was inversely proportional to that found in the pool that turned over rapidly. A considerable scatter of individual data in the turnover curves was noted. This set of data has been principally observed also in the human myocardium.

Ischemic Myocardium

In acutely ischemic myocardium of the dog the locally reduced uptake of ^{11}C-palmitic acid was concordant with the reduced local blood flow.[48,61,62] In addition, the extraction fraction was below that in normal myocardium. Also, in myocardial portions peripheral to the ischemic region, regional blood flow may be higher than in the control myocardium of normal heart; this was accompanied by a decrease of fatty acid extraction in the hyperperfused myocardium; it obscured the differences in fatty acid uptake between the various myocardial regions of the ischemic heart. The uptake of ^{11}C-palmitic acid in ischemic myocardium was reduced in the lipid fraction with fast turnover; it did not change in the fraction with a slow turnover. Accordingly, the rate of tracer releases from the myocardium was reduced relative to control. Again, the interindividual data scattered significantly more than the intraindividual data.

Also observed in the ischemic heart was an increased myocardial consumption of glucose in correlation with a release of lactate. This led to the dual tracer analysis using PET with a labeled glucose analog, ^{18}F-2-deoxyglucose (FDG), and a coronary blood flow agent such as ^{13}N-labeled ammonia.[48,61,63] This dual tracer approach has become clinically important for the determination of myocardial viability in hypoperfused myocardial regions.[46]

The sequential measurements of coronary blood flow and then of fatty acid uptake and turnover in the myocardium allowed the description of metabolic recovery after coronary thrombolysis. In a corresponding clinical simulation study in dogs,[64] the initial reduction in flow when expressed in percent of controls was restored to approximately 80% within 1 hour after thrombolysis with streptokinase or plasminogen activator. The initially reduced fatty acid uptake was restored by then to 65%–70%; then both fell again within 1 day to approximately 35% to return a week later to approximately 65%. Thereafter, flow remained at this reduced value, whereas on average, fatty acid uptake again decreased to 45% over a period of 3 weeks. This pattern of data corresponds to hibernating myocardium. Despite the relatively large scatter of interindividual data, the analysis of intraindividual data showed a strong correlation of the fatty acid uptake at 1 hour and at 4 weeks after thrombolysis. This led to the conclusion that measurement of ^{11}C-palmitic acid with PET 1 hour after thrombolysis may predict the ultimate salvage or degree of stunning or hibernation of the reperfused myocardium.

The metabolism of ^{11}C-palmitic acid was shown in normal dog myocardium to depend also on substrate availability.[38,57] Thus, after IV glucose-insulin infusion the plasma concentration of free fatty acids fell as that of glucose and lactate rose. With a near-normal myocardial oxygen consumption being maintained, the utilization of labeled palmitic acid for β-oxidation decreased to a higher degree than seen for the extraction fraction. This was related to a comparatively larger fraction of the tracer being incorporated into the slow-turnover lipid pool. The initial portion of the turnover curves also was prolonged under glucose load. In these experiments, again, the scatter of interindividual data surpassed that of the intraindividual data. Obviously, myocardial metabolism is regulated sensitively according to substrate availability in addition to other factors that are seemingly difficult to control.

This principal response of the kinetics of ^{11}C-palmitic acid was confirmed in normal human myocardium.[57,65] Tracer uptake into the normal and ischemic myocardium reached a maximum at approximately 5 minutes after pulse injection. The half-times of tracer release from the labeled fast and slowly renewing lipid pool again indicated relatively larger interindividual than intraindividual scatter in individuals with normal myocardium and in patients with various diseases. All patients had diminished cardiac pump function that was measured by the ejection fraction. Without glucose load, the average normal half-times of the rapid component of tracer release after overnight fasting was 19 ± 7 minutes [standard deviation (SD)] and in patients it was 20 ± 5 minutes. A similar scatter of data was seen when the tracer was injected following an oral glucose load; in fact, in the group of patients the oral glucose load provoked a prolonged half-time of the pool with rapid turnover in some individuals and a shortened half-time in others. The reason for these different patterns of response to glucose in the patient group remained unclear. One of the reasons for interindividual scatter of measured half-times of tracer release especially in the lipid fraction with fast turnover may be varying losses of fatty acid from the myocardial cells by retrograde diffusion or transport into the circulating blood.[66]

The measurements by dynamic external imaging of tracer kinetics following IV pulse injection of ^{11}C-palmitic acid do not a priori allow a differentiation between losses of tracer by metabolism and retrograde diffusion or transport, in short back-diffusion. However, the two pathways may be separated by imaging under metabolic intervention. Thus, back-diffusion may be induced by ketone bodies such as 3-hydroxybutyrate. Dogs were treated with this compound and were IV pulse injected with ^{11}C-palmitic acid. By examining the arteriovenous difference in the coronary circulation between ^{11}C bound to CO_2 and non-CO_2 compounds clearly revealed the decrease of β-oxidation during 3-hydroxybutyrate infusion in the presence of an enhanced tracer release. This indicates fatty acid back-diffusion under conditions of decreased transfer of fatty acid into β-oxidation. Ketone bodies may perhaps compete with fatty acids for carnitine acyltransferase in the carnitine shuttle and also for transport in the circulating blood.[67]

An appropriate, yet relatively simple, multicompartment model with few assumptions appeared appropriate to biokinetics data that had been obtained in dog hearts by external imaging with PET after pulse injection of ^{11}C-palmitic acid into the left atrium.[31]

The model allowed close fitting to the observed time-activity curves. This confirmed the data from parallel measurements of coronary blood flow, of fatty acid utilization and esterification into lipids, and of the fraction of tracer that underwent β-oxidation. The resulting rate constants demonstrated an increased back-diffusion on pharmacologic blockage of β-oxidation either through inhibition of the carnitine shuttle or through glucose load. Under both regimen, the fraction of incorporated tracer that was utilized for β-oxidation fell to approximately 15%–30% from approximately 80% in controls or under myocardial workload. The interindividual data scattered rather widely. However, the application of the compartment model in these various experimental dog studies under different metabolic conditions accurately conformed to the directly measured fatty acid transfers from the capillary blood into the myocardial lipid pools and from there into β-oxidation.

The above-mentioned experiments promise, indeed, the noninvasive description of fatty acid metabolism in individual patients if additional data are obtained. In a given patient, after a metabolic intervention these may describe the response of biokinetics that is measured by dynamic imaging following a repeated injection of the tracer. In this case, the patient is his or her own control or the biokinetics measurement is accompanied by an additional parallel analysis of the arterial blood; this may yield information on the rate of tracer disappearance and on the generation of labeled catabolites from β-oxidation; in this instance only a single injection of tracer is needed.

The former approach is less demanding in clinical practice and may be significant diagnostically. Thus, in patients with ischemic heart disease, dobutamine, as already referred to above, appears to be a safe and potent inotropic agent that increases the cardiac workload by activating adrenoreceptors of the β_1-, β_2-, and α_1-type with a low probability of causing arrhythmias. Measuring the uptake and release of the labeled fatty acid before and under the pharmacologic effect of dobutamine[58–60] allows the recognition of ischemia-induced changes in tracer turnover in the rapidly renewing pool in the affected regions of the myocardium. In normal myocardium, dobutamine was reported to shorten the mean half-times of tracer release to the range from 7.9 to 17.9 minutes, compared with the mean control range from 9.9 to 24.7 minutes. In patients with ischemic heart disease, the normally perfused myocardium had a mean tracer half-time in the rapidly renewing pool of 14.2 ± 4.4 minutes during dobutamine infusion and of 19.1 ± 4.4 minutes for control; yet in the myocardium at risk, dobutamine did not change the half-time that was prolonged prior to dobutamine infusion, from 26.3 ± 14.5 minutes to 26.5 ± 14.8 minutes. Regarding peak uptake of the tracer, only the myocardium at risk showed a significant decrease when the differences for each patient were tested. The deviation of response from control to dobutamine indicated reduced metabolic reserve; it was linked to abnormal regional wall motion, severity of coronary angiograms, and to the presence of Q-waves in the electrocardiograms (ECGs). The dobutamine-induced alterations of half-times were more sensitive than the ECG findings or the subjective symptoms.

For the above dobutamine test, the IV infusion of dobutamine started at a dose of 5 μg/kg per minute with an increase of 3–5 μg/kg per minute every 5 minutes while monitoring heart rate, blood pressure, and a 12-lead ECG until the systolic blood pressure reached 180 mm Hg and the heart rate was 120 beats/min or when the patient complained of chest discomfort. Then, with continued dobutamine infusion, the second tracer injection was given for renewed biokinetics analysis in the myocardium.

Nonischemic Cardiomyopathy

In nonischemic cardiomyopathy, the patterns of tracer uptake and turnover in different myocardial regions after IV pulse injection of the labeled fatty acid appear to differ from those seen in ischemic heart disease. In the latter, accumulation of defects usually are seen to conform to the region of supply of a coronary artery;[68] they also are relatively more homogeneous in the affected region. On the other hand, nonischemic cardiomyopathy causes multiple smaller, usually spotty accumulation defects resulting in marked heterogeneity of tracer uptake throughout the myocardium.[69] The distinct pattern of tracer distribution did not correlate with clinical findings nor the cause of this disease.

These findings were confirmed by a quantitative study.[70] Areas of homogeneously severely depressed accumulation of ^{11}C-palmitic acid were sized in reconstructed adjacent cross sections of the left ventricle. Defect regions representing 15% or more of the expected cross-sectional area were observed in 8 of 10 patients with ischemia but in none of the 10 patients with nonischemic cardiomyopathy, again irrespective of the cause of the disease. All normal individuals showed homogeneous tracer distribution in the LV wall.

The quite similar result with a long-chain fatty acid labeled with radioiodine such as ω-I-HDA is discussed later;[71] this and the wide availability of the γ-camera in the planar or SPECT mode encourages practical clinical application of fatty acid imaging for the noninvasive differential diagnosis between ischemic and nonischemic heart disease.

Some forms of cardiomyopathy appear to be determined genetically. One is caused by a deficiency of long-chain acyl-CoA-dehydrogenase that catalyzes the initial rate-limiting reaction in β-oxidation of fatty acids in the mitochondria. So far, at least three different types of this enzyme have been identified. They are specific for short-, medium- and long-chain fatty acids. Failure of any one of these enzymes may have no symptoms at all or it may cause grave clinical symptoms differing in childhood and adolescence. The type and degree of involvement of the myocardium is a diagnostic challenge.

One answer to that challenge is the observation of the biokinetics of labeled fatty acids of different chain lengths in a dual tracer approach with labeled acetate as an internal standard in myocardial metabolism; indeed, it yielded highly significant data of diagnostic relevance.[72] In a study with six patients suffering from long-chain acyl-CoA-dehydrogenase deficiency, the half-time of tracer release from the myocardium after pulse injection of ^{11}C-palmitic acid was prolonged. To correct for interindividual differences, ^{11}C-acetate was injected in each patient either shortly before or after the fatty acid injection for dynamic PET lasting an additional 20–30 minutes. The generated time-activity curve of labeled acetate represents the rate of tricarboxylic acid degradation as the final step in mitochondrial fatty acid degradation with release of [11]CO_2; that is, it validly estimates oxidative metabolism in the myocardium.[73–77]

If the time activity curves for labeled fatty acid and for acetate superimpose, the fatty acid is degraded fully. The degree of difference between slopes of these two curves then indicates the severity of inhibition of fatty acid β-oxidation caused by the lack of the particular acyl-CoA-dehydrogenase. The limitation of this method lies in the need to restrict the observation to all situations in which myocardial metabolism is at a steady state, that is, not influenced during the study by effects from substrate concentration in the circulating blood, hormones, workload, ischemia, and tracer back-diffusion. Nevertheless, such particular interventions if given under controlled conditions may have additional assets in designing a clinical study protocol.

In this manner, the localized effect of a genetic disorder can be determined noninvasively. This promises future clinical and research applications and may lead to a better understanding of metabolic consequences of genetic disorders. This applies especially in view of the evolution of the human genome program.

ω-^{123}I-heptadecanoic Acid and ω-^{123}I-hexadecanoic Acid

Principal Biokinetics

The demonstration of the potential of radioiodine-labeled fatty acid for myocardial scintigraphy in 1965 by Evans et al[4] initiated further work in the early 1970s. Thus, hexadecanoic acid was iodinated with ^{123}I at the terminal methyl group to 16-iodohexadecanoic acid.[7] After IV pulse injection of this labeled substrate in humans, myocardial images revealed reduced tracer uptake in the region of ischemia, and repetitive images indicated the possibility of measuring the clearance of the tracer from various myocardial segments. A normal half-time of the "degradation process" of the labeled fatty acid in the cells was seen to be <25 minutes.[6] In nine patients undergoing cardiac catheterization, widely varying clearance rates were stated but not documented.[7]

In a parallel investigation, HDA was iodinated at the terminal methyl group with ^{123}I to ω-I-HDA and thus became an analog of stearic acid (Fig. 5). The terminal iodination was chosen because the atomic radius of iodine and the molecular radius of the methyl group are both close to 0.2 nm.[9] Comparing labeling of different long-chain fatty acids with different radionuclides in different positions, the ω-I-HDA was found to be superior and to behave in the mouse myocardium kinetically like palmitic acid.[9]

Further experimental studies in animals indicated that the rate of binding of ω-I-HDA to CoA was practically indistinguishable from the binding measured with palmitic acid.[18] Also, the distribution of this fatty acid analog between the various lipid fractions within the rat myocardium was again indistinguishable from the distribution of stearic acid, the natural substrate; however, the distribution of palmitic acid within the various lipid fractions differed from that of stearic acid and its iodinated analog.[33] This particular difference between distributions of the various fatty acids and various analogs again was observed in the lipids of dog myocardium.[78]

A total of approximately 60% of the tracer at peak uptake in the rat myocardium, that is, within a few minutes after pulse injection of ω-I-HDA, was recovered as water-soluble free iodine.[33,79] A similar large fraction of free iodine was recovered soon after the tracer injection in the dog myocardium.[80,81] The large fraction of free ^{123}I in the rat and dog myocardium within minutes after pulse injection of the tracer led to the question of the meaning and validity of the clearance measurements obtained by external scintigraphy.[42,80-82] Another argument pertained to the possibility that the release of free iodine from the myocardium after fatty acid catabolism of ω-I-HDA was determined by the integrity of the mitochondrial membrane.[83]

Two investigations clarified these uncertainties. One group of studies proved the free ^{123}I that appeared in the rat myocardium soon after pulse injection of ω-^{123}I-HDA to derive, indeed, from β-oxidation.[34,79,83] The other study unequivocally showed the simultaneous release of both CO_2 and free iodine into the coronary sinus in humans

I-(CH$_2$)$_{16}$—COOH
ω-Iodo-heptadecanoic Acid (ω-I-HDA)

Figure 5.

following injection into the coronary artery of double-labeled ω-I-HDA; ^{14}C was in the carboxyl group and ^{123}I was on the ω-position of the carbon chain. Because the generation and release of ^{14}C-CO_2 in this study could only have come from fatty acid metabolism, the simultaneous generation and release of ^{123}I and ^{14}C not only confirmed the completion of β-oxidation of the labeled tracer but also precluded preferential trapping of free iodine over CO_2 in the myocardium over the observed time period of 15 minutes. On the other hand, ^{123}I-labeled NaI when injected into the coronary artery as a tracer of recirculating iodide had a longer residence time in the myocardium than the free iodine released together with CO_2 from catabolism into the venous side of the capillaries.[34] The latter indicates different exchange rates for substrates between the extravascular space and the arterial and venous sites of the capillary system.

The clinical application of ω-^{123}I-HDA yielded excellent images with the γ-camera, but the image was found to be contaminated by signals from free ^{123}I. Beyond 15 minutes after pulse injection of the tracer, the residual activity in the peripheral blood had fallen to 10%–15% of the initial value and by then 55%–75% of this was inorganic ^{123}I.[43,84] The circulating iodine pool is only 20%–30% of the total iodine pool in the body. The various amounts of ^{123}I in the total iodine pool at various times prevented the quantification of myocardial tracer clearance. Therefore, the contribution of free ^{123}I to the total images at various times was rather simply determined by the dual tracer technique and subtracted from the total image. In this manner, the biokinetics of lipid-bound ^{123}I in the human myocardium were obtained and evaluated.[11,43,85] The peak uptake was between 5 and 10 minutes after the tracer injection. In a normal control group, the average half-time of the first component of the turnover curve without correction for the second component was 24.4 ± 4.7 minutes (SD) for the entire LV wall.

Subsequent studies verified that the results with ω-I-HDA were comparable with the myocardial uptake and turnover of ^{11}C-palmitic acid that was measured with dynamic PET imaging in patients without heart disease.[41] The two sets of data were comparable, even superimposed, when the two curves were normalized to their peak values. Also, in the mouse myocardium, the labeled palmitic acid and the labeled ω-I-HDA were kinetically alike with their relatively rapid turnover rates.[9]

The concordance of data obtained with the two labeled fatty acids in mice and humans showing fast and relatively slow rates of tracer release must be viewed against the respective myocardial structures and functions. Thus, myocardial microstructures regarding the topographical relations between cells and capillaries are similar in both species, as are the mitochondrial masses per cell and functions of lipid membranes. However, the heart rates differ by a factor of 3–4, and the tracer release times are similarly different in the myocardium of mice and humans. This comparison of data thus supports the notion that the relatively low rates of release of tracer measured with ^{11}C-palmitic acid and the ω-^{123}I-labeled fatty acids in the human myocardium are indeed related to lipid turnover.[32]

The various experimental results show that ^{123}I-labeled ω-I-HDA is a metabolic indicator of natural fatty acid in the human myocardium provided the primary images are corrected for recirculating free ^{123}I.

Ischemic Myocardium

With regard to coronary artery disease (CAD), ω-I-HDA, like ^{11}C-palmitic acid, showed a reduced peak uptake in the ischemic region conforming to the supply zone of the stenosed coronary artery.[84] In these regions the rates of release were reduced more often than enhanced with both tracers.[43,49,86,87] In regions of myocardial infarction, enhanced rather than prolonged rates of tracer release were seen.[43,49,67] Also, the infusion of insulin and glucose or glucose alone reduced the tracer release after peak uptake similar to ^{11}C-palmitic acid.[57,87] Yet, the half-times of tracer release scattered much between the individual patients. In patients with myocardial ischemia (MI), the mean half-time of tracer release was 31.8 ± 19.6 minutes (SD) in the ischemic regions, with significant differences between myocardial regions of a given patient.[43] In general, the scatter of tracer turnover in normal and diseased myocardium was larger interindividually than intraindividually for both ω-I-HDA and ^{11}C-palmitic acid.[34,41,88]

The kinetics of ^{123}I-labeled ω-I-hexadecanoic acid was similar to ω-I-HDA.[49,89] The accumulation defects with ω-I-hexadecanoic acid correlated with perfusion defects, measured with [201]Tl.[89] Using the image substraction technique for background correction,[43,85] the average normal first-component half-time was 27.5 ± 3.0 minutes, and in infarcted zones it was 18.5 ± 2.5 minutes; yet, remote regions within the infarcted myocardium had half-times of 34.0 ± 8.4 minutes and were similar to those obtained with ^{123}I-labeled ω-I-HDA.[49]

Moreover, ^{123}I-labeled ω-I-hexadecanoic acid in these studies was analyzed kinetically in dog myocardium with implanted radiation detectors. After pulse injection of the tracer into the right atrium, time activity curves were obtained over a period of 3 hours from normal and ischemic myocardium without correction for catabolically released [123]I. The initial uptake of tracer was flow related and the half-times were not changed by a decrease in local perfusion; yet considerable recirculation of ^{123}I had occurred throughout the experiments.

Nonischemic Cardiomyopathy

In patients with different forms of nonischemic cardiomyopathy the pattern of tracer distribution at peak uptake was found for both tracers to be rather heterogeneously spotty, usually throughout the LV myocardium; moreover, large variations in the release rates in various myocardial regions did not correlate with the pattern of tracer distribution. This is in contrast to the situation with CAD where significant deviations of rates of tracer release were confined to the regions of significantly altered uptake.[69,70,71,90] One investigation of the myocardial uptake of ω-^{123}I-hexadecanoic acid in patients with nonischemic cardiomyopathy failed to correct for free ^{123}I and, probably for this reason, did not observe the distinct pattern of tracer uptake or reveal the typical time-activity curve with the tracer inflow to a peak prior to tracer release.[91] All data thus far promise imaging of myocardial kinetics of labeled natural fatty acids or their metabolically compatible analogs, either with the γ-camera or PET, to be particularly helpful in the differential diagnosis between CAD and nonischemic cardiomyopathy.

The advantage of these tracers is their easy applicability. The radiopharmaceutical preparation is relatively simple. Conventional planar γ-camera imaging is used widely, and SPECT in the fast dynamic mode is increasingly available. The images are excellent and reveal the pattern of tracer distribution in various myocardial regions. Disadvantages are the need for image correction for free ^{123}I and, compared with PET, currently lack the quantification of tracer uptake; yet, the rates of tracer releases are as quantitative as they are with ^{11}C-labeled fatty acid and PET.

The nearly equal results obtainable with ω-I-HDA, ω-^{123}I-hexadecanoic acid, and ^{11}C-palmitic acid also share the limitations of applying a single tracer to the diagnosis of myocardial metabolism. Of course, the single tracer technique does not permit the distinction between the routes by which the tracer is lost from the myocardium, be it by metabolic degradation or by back-diffusion/transport. The metabolic pathways that exist between fatty acid uptake into and release of catabolites or of the nondegraded fatty acid from the myocardium into the blood circulation is most complex. This makes the choice of an appropriate model to the analysis of time-activity curves most difficult. Still, some principal metabolic features obviously can be described, as discussed in the following section.

ω-(p-^{123}I-phenyl)pentadecanoic Acid

Principal Biokinetics

Phenylated long-chain fatty acids are metabolized similarly to straight-chain fatty acids.[92,93] The stability of iodine binding to the phenyl ring thus promised to label this fatty acid analog with ^{123}I for myocardial metabolic studies.[94] The metabolite of this tracer following β-oxidation is probably p-I-phenyl-propenoic acid rather than p-I-benzoic acid; both do not enter the iodine pool in the body but are lost rapidly by renal excretion.[95–97] Thus, the correction of images for ^{123}I in the free-iodine pool in the body is not required, a great advantage in the clinical setting.

By labeling ω-phenylpentadecanoic acid with radioiodine two isomers are obtained, the para- and orthoiodinated ω-phenyl-pentadecanoic acid, in short p-PPA and o-PPA (for p-PPA see Fig. 6). Testing the two isomers for kinetic behavior in the myocardium of the mouse, rat, and rabbit revealed that p-PPA behaves kinetically and biochemically similarly to palmitic acid.[33,98–101] Yet, in the rat myocardium, the rate of binding of p-PPA to CoA and that of early tracer release after peak uptake was significantly reduced compared with palmitic acid.[102] Uptake of p-PPA into the myocardium depended linearly on flow; this spanned in dog myocardium from 0.05 to 7 mL/min per gram tissue at rest and during exercise.[25] However, the uptake was only approximately 25% of the p-PPA that was delivered by the flow. This value is distinctly lower than with palmitic acid. In ischemic zones, the ratio between flow and uptake did not alter significantly.[28] Also, in these studies, the individual data scattered widely among the animals without clear explanation.

Again, in rodent myocardium, the incorporated p-PPA was esterified into various lipid fractions similarly to palmitic acid.[33,100,103,104] The rate of release of the tracer was exclusively caused by β-oxidation; back-diffusion or transport was not seen.[33,102,105] The slightly prolonged retention of p-PPA compared with palmitic acid probably is a steric hindrance by the terminal phenyl group in the enzyme-catalyzed reactions in comparison with normal long-chain fatty acids.[106]

The similar biochemical behavior of incorporated p-PPA and palmitic acid without the need of correcting for recirculating labeled catabolites made p-PPA the preferred substrate over ω-I-HDA for applying the γ-camera scintigraphy in the planar mode or as SPECT to the diagnostic evaluation of fatty acid metabolism in patients with various heart diseases.[107]

The distribution of peak uptake of the tracer in the LV myocardium was diagnostically revealing. On the other hand, as was stated above, the measured rates of tracer release in humans scattered interindividually so much more than intraindividually[108] that the

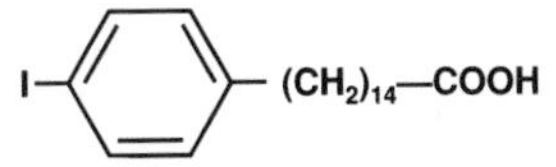

ω-(p-Iodo-phenyl)pentadecanoic Acid (p-PPA)

Figure 6.

diagnostic evaluation of an individual washout measurement became nearly invalid. To repeat, the metabolic pathways between fatty acid uptake into and release of catabolites or of nondegraded fatty acid from the myocardium is most complex. It makes the choice of an appropriate model to the analysis of single time-activity curves very difficult.

A relatively large number of reports on clinical applications of p-PPA principally confirmed the findings that were observed with labeled palmitic acid and ω-I-HDA.[107] Especially noteworthy is the influence of physical exercise on tracer uptake on the one hand and on the kinetics of tracer release on the other, following IV pulse injection of p-PPA.

Ischemic Myocardium

Myocardial p-PPA uptakes in patients with stable ischemic heart disease were, in a multicenter trial, very similar regarding presence, location, and severity of defects in 65% of the patients under fasting and nonfasting conditions and superior in 25% of the cases under the nonfasting condition.[109] The authors concluded that dietary restrictions are not necessary for optimal p-PPA imaging and, in fact, may lead to a reduced image quality in turnover studies.

In a dual tracer study with p-PPA and ^{201}Tl, patients with CAD and normal control individuals were IV pulse injected at and not after a maximal workload; all received a second injection of the two tracers at rest. Imaging began immediately after injection. Myocardial uptake of p-PPA varied with the degree of local blood supply at rest and at exercise and with the plasma concentration of free fatty acid. The gross myocardial images had been corrected using a modified interpolative background subtraction algorithm.[42,81,110] In normal individuals, the rate constant of fatty acid uptake fell from approximately 0.8 to 0.3 with an increased rate of fatty acid supply by a factor of 10; the latter value is given by the product of local perfusion and concentration of free fatty acid in the circulating blood. At a constant fatty acid concentration in the circulating blood, an increase of myocardial perfusion by a factor of approximately 3 caused the rate of tracer uptake to fall by a factor of approximately 2. In patients with one-vessel disease, the average rate constant of fatty acid uptake in the supply area of the affected coronary artery was reduced significantly compared with the control in normal myocardial segments. This indicates the need for analyzing local perfusion if the rate of fatty acid uptake is to be assayed quantitatively. No significant changes were seen in response to changes in plasma lactate concentration that ranged during exercise from approximately 5 to 60 mg/dL.

When imaging began 4 minutes after termination of maximal exercise and 5 minutes after pulse injection of p-PPA in patients with >70% stenosis of at least one coronary artery, the uptake in the ischemic region was increased in 63% of the patients, decreased in 11%, and no change from normal value was seen in 26%.[111] In normals, LV uptake was relatively uniform yet with considerable scatter between individuals. The mean maximal difference in four regional values of normal myocardium varied by 18% ± 7% at rest and 13% ± 5% after exercise; in the patients, these differences amounted to 36 ± 14 at rest and 30 ± 13 after exercise. The reason for the increased uptake in ischemic regions may be the short duration of the exercise-induced ischemia, the delayed start of the imaging, or a relatively reduced uptake in the normal myocardium under exercise. The release of the tracer was measured from 4 to 20 minutes after injection. It was, in normal individuals, 21.1 ± 10 minutes at rest and 12.6 ± 8.4 minutes after exercise. In the patient group these values varied considerably. In 74% of the noninfarcted segments in patients the release rates were reduced; in 96% of the regions some abnormality regarding uptake and release rates was registered. The data obviously indicate the need for a most careful design of study protocols with p-PPA for diagnostically valid information on MI.

Significant differences were seen between uptakes in three segments per myocardium of normal individuals and patients with CAD that was diagnosed by coronary angiography. The images had been corrected for background. The segmental data were expressed quantitatively in terms of the activity ratio myocardium to blood pool, the latter being taken as background. Both were measured 7 minutes after IV pulse injection of p-PPA at rest and immediately after exercise. Of the various modes of uptake analysis, this ratio was found to be depressed and the best parameter for differentiating between CAD and normal myocardium; the data obtained at exercise had the highest significance.[108]

The myocardial uptake of p-PPA may be a sign of myocardial viability. In attempts at assessing myocardial viability in patients with previous myocardial infarction, 39% of persistent myocardial perfusion defects that were seen with ^{99m}Tc-hexakis-2-methyl-isobutyl isonitrile (MIBI) at rest still showed p-PPA uptake following exercise, and in 25% p-PPA uptake was normal.[112] In another study using ^{201}Tl imaging following maximal exercise and again after reinjection at rest, p-PPA uptake at rest was a more frequent sign of viability than seen by uptake of reinjected ^{201}Tl.[113] This appears to support the p-PPA uptake to be a more sensitive indicator of viability than the ^{201}Tl reinjection technique at rest following an exercise scan.

The release rate of the tracer immediately after the peak uptake of p-PPA has only limited diagnostic power[108] and, moreover, was shown to vary with study protocols in patients with CAD. But repeat studies at rest and after exercise in the same individual may be revealing. Thus, in normal myocardium, maximal exercise increased the rate of the tracer release from the myocardium.[111] After submaximal exercise in another group of patients with CAD, the release rate was more increased than after maximal exercise.[114] Indeed, in patients with CAD, maximal exercise caused hardly any change or rather a decrease and rarely (15%) an increase in the rate of the tracer release.[111,115,116]

Despite the difficulty in judging singularly the meaning of the rate of the tracer release from the myocardium immediately after peak uptake in maximally exercised patients, the combined analysis with tracer distribution at peak uptake appeared to improve the diagnostic relevance. Thus, in patients with CAD, 63% of noninfarcted myocardial regions with ischemia had an increased uptake and 44% had a reduced rate of tracer release compared with normal individuals. Both parameters combined gave an 89% sensitivity and a 67% specificity when 1 SD difference from the mean values was used. The respective data were 72% and 100% when the differences were taken to be at least 2 SD from the mean values.[111] Similarly, high sensitivities and specificities were reported for other dynamic imaging studies in the planar mode with p-PPA.[117,118]

In all investigations and clinical applications of the diagnosis of CAD, first, the data scattered widely between different normal individuals and patients; this holds especially for the early release rate. Second, the generation and analysis of data for tracer uptake and release rate combined was labor-intensive and time-consuming. Third, the exercise-induced alterations of tracer uptake and release rate in patient sensitively depended on the study protocols including control of various substrate concentrations in the circulating blood. These various circumstances have led to only a limited diagnostic application of p-PPA scintigraphy in patients with CAD.

Nonischemic Cardiomyopathy

Imaging of labeled fatty acids at peak uptake has been helpful in differentiating between CAD and nonischemic cardiomyopathy. As was seen with ^{11}C-palmitic acid and ω-I-HDA, also p-PPA tracer distributes in the LV myocardium relatively heterogeneously spotty, "moth-eaten," irrespective of the cause of the disease, be it idiopathic, alcoholic, diabetic, viral, postpartum, or hypertensive cardiomyopathy.[119] In these studies, the tomographic images were taken over a period of 20 minutes beginning at 8 minutes and again at 40 minutes after IV pulse injection in fasting subjects at rest. Myocardial apical and basal short-axis sections were semiquantitatively analyzed through the construction of radial circumferential profile activity curves. These yielded the maximal percent variation of uptake in a given myocardium. The mean maximal percent variation in the control group was 18% ± 4%. It was 27% ± 12% for the patient group. The percent release of the tracer between 8 and 40 minutes amounted to 17 to 18 ± 6 in normal individuals and 24 to 26 ± 8 in patients. No significant correlation existed between the severity of altered tracer distribution in the myocardium and LV ejection fraction (LVEF). However, there was a positive correlation between heterogeneity of tracer uptake and the patient's New York Heart Association functional class.

In hypertensive cardiomyopathy with normal coronary arteries, the ^{201}Tl scans were normal, but the uptake of p-PPA was significantly heterogeneous in all patients, and this heterogeneity was increased in patients who were injected 1 minute prior to termination of maximal exercise. No significant correlation existed between the rates of tracer release in patients and normal volunteers; these rates showed again a wide scatter of individual data. Nevertheless, segments with accumulation defects tended to have a delayed rate of tracer release after exercise.[120] The concordance of the two parameters speaks in favor of spotty MI in spite of the negative thallium scans, as also was reported from animal studies.[121] This is in contrast to data from other forms of cardiomyopathy, where the local distribution of tracer uptake did not correlate with changes in the rate of tracer release, as seen with ω-I-HDA.[71,90] Also, in cardiomyopathies caused by congenital defects of specific enzymes, p-PPA imaging may be useful diagnostically.[72,122–124] However, significantly revealing data probably depend on using multiple tracer techniques with dynamic imaging that allow the recognition of defined metabolic steps.

Labeled Fatty Acids for Metabolic Trapping

Insertion of a Non-Carbon Nuclide Into the Carbon Chain

Soon after the introduction of labeled fatty acids for studying myocardial metabolism, efforts began to tailor their molecular structures in such a way that the labeled fatty acid or its labeled catabolites would become trapped at the site of β-oxidation. The initial attempts placed a foreign atom into the long carbon chain so that β-oxidation would be blocked at that molecular site. Tellurium showed promise in oleic acids, and the radioactive ^{123m}Te was selected to serve as label and blocker at the same time.[125–127] Also, in HDA, ^{123m}Te in the 9 position of the carbon chain lead to retention of the tracer in the myocardium. The release rate was about an order of magnitude below that of physiological long-chain fatty acids and allowed prolonged data collection for γ-camera imaging.[128] Excellent myocardial images in rats and dogs demonstrated a linear correlation of uptake with blood flow; infarcted myocardial regions were well delineated. In rat experiments, 3.7% ± 0.28% of the injected amount was taken up per gram of myocardial tissue.[128]

Interestingly, the degree of retention of the ^{123m}Te-labeled HDA declined with the distance of the position of the ^{123m}Te from the carboxyl group. Tellurium in the 5 position of the carbon chain caused full myocardial retention in dogs, while tellurium in the 11 position permitted about a 40% release of maximal uptake over 3 hours after pulse injection, without difference between normal and ischemic myocardium.[129]

The principle of tellurium placement into the carbon chain was further tested. Thus, p-PPA labeled with ^{123}I and carrying nonradioactive tellurium in the 6 position (Fig. 7) was incorporated rapidly into rat myocardium to approximately 5.6% (4.97%–6.29%) of the pulse-injected amount per gram of tissue with hardly any loss of tracer over a period

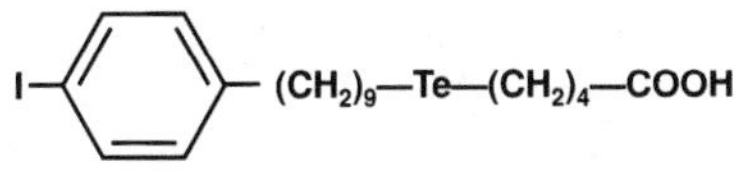

I—⟨benzene ring⟩—(CH$_2$)$_9$—Te—(CH$_2$)$_4$—COOH

ω-(p-Iodo-phenyl)-6-tellura-pentadecanoic
Acid (TPDA)

Figure 7.

of 2 hours.[130] The tracer rapidly cleared from the peripheral blood. Only minimal amounts of ^{123}I were set free to enter the iodine pool. Also, redistribution of this substrate was not seen.[131]

Other attempts at developing metabolically blocked fatty acids used triple fluorination of hexadecanoic acid with suboptimal results.[132] More recently, sulfur was chosen to replace tellurium in the carbon chain.[133–135] Placed in position 3 of the carbon chain, sulfur blocked completion of β-oxidation.[135] This led to the synthesis of 14-[^{18}F]-6-thia-HDA (FTHA) (Fig. 8) for use with PET in clinical cardiology.[133] Mouse studies indicated the near exclusive trapping of FTHA in mitochondria of the myocardium; activity was released with a half-time of approximately 2 hours. Excellent myocardial images were obtained by PET following pulse injection in cardiologically healthy patients in the fasting state.[136] The substrate was incorporated rapidly within <5 minutes after injection and was retained without recognizable loss over at least 40 minutes. The uptake increased significantly during exercise and slightly but not significantly after dipyridamole injection. The rate constant of uptake was significantly linearly related to the heart-rate–pressure product as an expression of myocardial oxygen consumption, with a correlation coefficient of 0.85.

Two dynamic PET studies in seven patients with CAD, one study under fasting conditions and the second one during euglycemic hypereinsulinemia, showed the suppressive effect of insulin on myocardial uptake of FTHA. The myocardial uptake in hyperinsulinemic patients was reduced to approximately 20% of the value in the fasting state, indicative of preferred glucose utilization in hyperinsulinemia.[137]

When myocardial retention of FTHA and BMIPP (see below) were compared in experimental MI in swine using extracorporeal perfusion, a 50% reduction of β-oxidation was measured in the ischemic group and an 80% reduction in the hypoxia group. Both labeled fatty acids showed a decreased retention in the ischemic group, while BMIPP had an increased uptake in the hypoxic group with FTHA uptake having the same mean value as the controls.[138] Thus, despite a significant reduction in β-oxidation during ischemia, BMIPP uptake was increased with no change of FTHA uptake compared with controls. The different kinetics between the two tracers in hypoxia indicate a specific dissociation between fatty acid transport into the myocardial cells expressed by both FTHA and BMIPP, esterification into lipids expressed by BMIPP, and β-oxidation that was measured independently in hypoxia; the failure of FTHA to respond to hypoxia might indicate some retention mechanism in the myocardial cell prior to β-oxidation, perhaps some

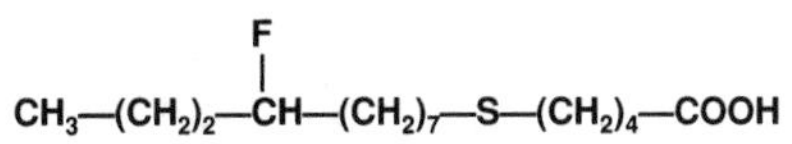

$$CH_3—(CH_2)_2—\overset{\overset{\text{F}}{|}}{CH}—(CH_2)_7—S—(CH_2)_4—COOH$$

14-R,S-Fluoro-6-thia-heptadecanoic Acid (FTHA)

Figure 8.

degree of esterification into complex lipids, or binding to fatty acid binding proteins, or some feedback control that enhances differentially the uptake of FTHA compared with normal fatty acid into mitochondria to enter β-oxidation.

The data promise the usefulness of FTHA for measuring in vivo by PET not only myocardial fatty acid metabolism, in general, but specifically the rate of substrate transfer into β-oxidation also under ischemic but not necessarily under hypoxic conditions. In this context, the multitracer method with o-PPA and p-PPA, as discussed later, may be particularly attractive.

Methylation of the Carbon Chain

A second principal approach toward trapping of fatty acid in myocardial metabolism used linking a methyl group onto the third carbon atom, the β-position, in the carbon chain of ω-I-HDA [β-methyl-heptadecanoic acid (BMHDA)].[139] In this way, β-oxidation of this fatty acid analog was expected to be inhibited. When BMHDA was labeled with ^{11}C in the carboxyl group, the tracer indeed was trapped and resulted in excellent PET images of dog myocardium; at 5 minutes after pulse injection, 2.3% of the injected amount was found per gram of myocardial tissue; the uptake was 2.7% approximately 1 hour later. The blood activity fell rapidly to <10% of the value found at 1 minute after injection. Infarcted myocardium was well delineated.[139]

In a subsequent study in perfused rat hearts, 66% of the [1-^{14}C]BMHDA in the myocardium was described to be β-oxidized slowly and 33% was esterified into complex lipids, while in the liver 53% was α-oxidized, 27% β-oxidized, and 20% esterified. No toxic effects were seen in perfused rat hearts when the substrate concentration was 1000 greater than that used for myocardial imaging.[140]

A quantitative measurement of the net extraction fraction of 1-[^{11}C]BMHDA in dog myocardium in vivo was made by PET.[141] This assumed steady-state metabolism of natural fatty acids at the time of examination. Normal fasting dogs and those after glucose and insulin infusion were measured. The myocardial uptake of BMHDA reached a plateau at approximately 15 minutes after pulse injection and remained unaltered for at least 60 minutes. The net extraction fractions were calculated from the time-activity curves in the peripheral arterial and venous blood and those obtained from myocardial imaging. The net extraction fraction was 0.22 in normal fasted dogs and fell to 0.10 during glucose and insulin infusion. The corresponding values for physiological fatty acids were 0.335 and 0.195, respectively. The rate of metabolism was defined as the product of the net extraction fraction, local blood flow, and arterial substrate concentration. This approach indicated that the rate of fatty acid utilization presumably by β-oxidation in the myocardium may be quantified with BMHDA and PET. This promises the recognition of viable tissue in CAD, where approximately 20% of so-called fixed ^{201}Tl defects are not infarcts but representative of ischemic tissue.

The search for optimization of myocardial imaging also led to dimethylation of ω-I-HDA, at the β-position of the carbon chain [β-dimethyl-HDA (DMHDA)].[142] The result was a reduced retention of tracer in the myocardium and a relatively high uptake in the lung, in contrast to the findings with dimethylated p-PPA as will be discussed later. The reason for these functional differences between the two dimethylated fatty acids is unknown; it again shows the potentially severe metabolic consequences of subtle structural changes of the substrate. The particular difference between dimethylated HDA and p-PPA seems to confirm a functional involvement of the ω-position of long-chain fatty acids in an early step of fatty acid metabolism, as also was seen in the different metabolic fates of p-PPA and o-IPPA, which will be discussed later.

Various long-chain fatty acids with ^{123}I labeling in the ω-position and dimethylation in the β-position were synthesized and tested in the rat myocardium. The ω-^{123}I-3,3-

dimethyl-nonadecanoic acid was well incorporated into the myocardium, 4.56% of the pulse-injected amount per gram of tissue at 2 minutes, with a retention similar to that of the DMHDA.[143]

The early success with BMHDA also prompted the synthesis and pharmacologic testing of p-PPA labeled with ^{123}I on the phenyl ring and carrying a methyl group in the 3 or β-position of the carbon chain (BMIPP).[144-146] Today this is the most widely used tracer of myocardial lipid metabolism in clinical cardiology.

β-Methyl-ω-(p-^{123}I-phenyl)pentadecanoic Acid

Principal Biokinetics

Myocardial uptake of BMIPP (Fig. 9) was seen to depend both on flow and on local myocardial fatty acid metabolism, as studied in dogs,[147] hamsters with cardiomyopathy,[148-150] and rabbits.[151] Also, the degree of uptake into the myocardial cells was found to correlate with intracellular ATP concentrations.[20,152] The distribution of activity between myocardial lipids 5 and 30 minutes following pulse injection of BMIPP in rats showed a relatively increased fraction of total activity in the triglycerides and a lesser fraction in phospholipids than seen with p-PPA. The fraction of activity of incorporated BMIPP in the mitochondria exceeded that from p-PPA.[153] In other in vivo and in vitro perfusion studies in rats, more BMIPP was found in the free-fatty acid pool than in complex lipids.[154,155]

Retention of the tracer was prolonged in rat myocardium compared with p-PPA; yet some release occurred contrary to BMHDA.[145] This indicated either back-diffusion or transport or some degree of metabolism. In normal human subjects, the average release rate in percent of maximal uptake was 6.2% per hour.[156] Thus, the initial expectation of predominant trapping of the tracer from BMIPP in the course of β-oxidation gave way to the realization that in addition to mitochondrial trapping BMIPP also was esterified quite effectively and probably kept in complex lipids. The reduced rate of tracer release from the normal myocardium may be attributed to a reduced rate of transfer of substrate from the lipid pool into β-oxidation and to a delay in the enzyme-catalyzed catabolism. A glucose load preceding a meal enriched in carbohydrates and proteins led in healthy volunteers to an only slightly increased myocardial BMIPP uptake compared with the fasting state; however, the washout rate increased from 13.1% $\pm$ 8.8% to 24.0% $\pm$ 3.7% as measured between 0.5 and 3.5 hours after tracer injection.[157] This indicates that for measuring BMIPP uptake fasting is not mandatory for getting adequate images.

In the dog myocardium, blocking the carnitine shuttle for fatty acids led to a significantly increased release rate of BMIPP. This was accompanied by a significant decrease of appearance of BMIPP catabolite from β-oxidation in the coronary sinus with concomitantly increased back-diffusion/transport of the BMIPP.[158] On the other hand, blocking the carnitine shuttle in the baboon myocardium caused a reduction in β-oxidation of

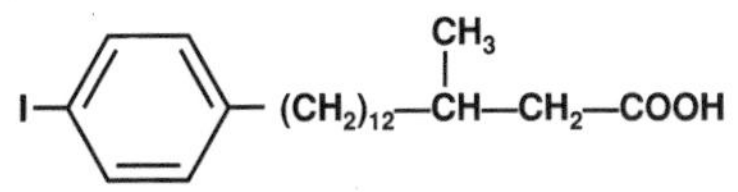

ω-(p-Iodo-phenyl)-3-R,S-methyl-pentadecanoic
Acid (BMIPP)

Figure 9.

BMIPP with a concomitant reduction of the release rate that would indicate no enhancement of back-diffusion/transport.[159] Similar reductions in release rates of the tracer from the baboon myocardium appeared following blocking of the carnitine shuttle in experiments with p-PPA and its orthoisomer o-PPA that will be discussed further later.[160] Interesting for clinical applications of BMIPP is the fact that in these studies image correction for background activity hardly improved image quality while background correction improved the images from p-PPA and o-PPA.

In the perfused rat heart, the catabolism of BMIPP appeared to begin with α-oxidation and then to continue with β-oxidation. The metabolic end-product was p-iodophenyl-acetic acid (PIPA) and not p-iodobenzoic acid (PIBA) as was previously assumed. Both α- and β-oxidation were stimulated by oleate and inhibited by glucose and insulin infusion. Acetate alone increased only α-oxidation.[106] Again, the reduced rate of catabolism of the phenylated fatty acid residues after α-oxidation was attributed to the terminal phenyl group; this is considered a hindrance in the enzymatic reaction in comparison with normal long-chain fatty acids.[97]

Also, two methyl groups were placed on the third carbon atom in the carbon chain of p-PPA [β-dimethyl-(ω-[p-^{123}I-phenyl])pentadecanoic acid (DMIPP)] as shown in Figure 10. This then was compared with BMIPP.[161] A similarly high myocardial uptake as with BMIPP was achieved in fasted rats; especially, the release rate from the myocardium was significantly lower with a half-time of approximately 8 hours, similar to the slow release rate of DMHDA.[161] The prolonged retention was confirmed in the dog myocardium in vivo[162] and in isolated perfused swine heart.[163]

Comparing the rates of incorporation of BMIPP, DMIPP, and p-PPA into various myocardial lipids in the rat, all three showed a ready uptake into triglycerides and phospholipids in various cellular fractions such as microsomes, mitochondria, and cytoplasm. However, the rates of uptake were different in that DMIPP lagged behind BMIPP. The accumulation of total activity in the mitochondrial fraction at 30 minutes after substrate injection was somewhat higher for DMIPP than for BMIPP, and both showed a higher fraction of total uptake in the mitochondria than did p-PPA; this may be related to the extent of trapping in the course of β-oxidation.[152] Indeed, the extent of trapping of DMIPP in fed rats was lower than seen at 24 hours after fasting, concomitant with a relative decrease in total uptake and an unaltered long retention time in the myocardium of fed animals.[164] In these studies, fasting caused the BMIPP uptake to be reduced in the mitochondrial and microsomal fraction and enhanced in the cytoplasmic fraction, while uptake of p-PPA was reduced, and uptake of DMIPP was enhanced in all three fractions. This different response of the fatty acid analogs to fasting is potentially important in clinical investigations and emphasizes the different involvements of the analogs in the various enzyme-catalyzed reactions in lipid metabolism in a given myocardium.

The findings with DMIPP in rat myocardium were somewhat different from those in the dog myocardium; uptake into various lipids and release rates of DMIPP, HDA, and p-PPA were compared. In dog myocardium, DMIPP showed the highest tissue-to-blood ratio because of its retention mainly in the triglycerides without recognizable fraction for oxidation. The highest uptake and fraction for oxidation had HDA with phospholipids

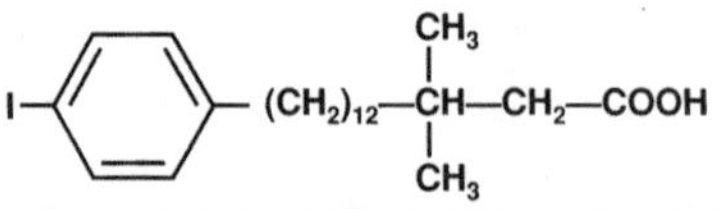

ω-(p-Iodo-phenyl)-3,3-dimethyl-pentadecanoic Acid (DMIPP)

Figure 10.

being the lipid fraction mainly labeled; p-PPA had a slightly lower uptake and fraction for oxidation with triglycerides being the main labeled lipid fraction.[162]

These sets of data with the various methylated fatty acid analogs again indicate the profound effects of relatively small changes in molecular structures on metabolic behavior. This was obvious in several steps of myocardial lipid metabolism involving esterification and catabolism; significant differences in these steps for the various fatty acid analogs appeared to be species specific.

Despite the particular properties of the dimethylated fatty acids compared with p-PPA and BMIPP, they have found less clinical attention than BMIPP. The latter is now commercially available as Cardioline (Japan) for routine use in nuclear cardiology. Recent reviews on BMIPP[107,165] state that, in Japan alone over 50 000 patient studies have been completed through December 1994. Also, many institutions in Europe currently use BMIPP. The reason for this broad acceptance of BMIPP mainly is the demonstrated stability of iodine on the phenyl ring and the usefulness of BMIPP for the time-demanding dynamic imaging of tracer uptake and release by SPECT that suits the practice of clinical cardiology.

The application of BMIPP in clinical cardiology has helped in identifying type and degree of myocardial pathology, be it caused by CAD or by cardiomyopathy without arteriosclerosis. In nearly all clinical applications of BMIPP, the dual tracer technique together with a flow tracer was revealing and crucial. Moreover, static imaging of myocardial uptake of BMIPP compared with that of a flow tracer, without reference to lipid turnover, often was diagnostically sufficient.

A more recent review entitled "Iodine-123–labeled fatty acids for myocardial single-photon emission tomography: Current status and future perspectives"[107] also discusses extensively clinical studies with BMIPP mainly regarding CAD and hypertrophic cardiomyopathy.

Ischemic Myocardium

Regarding ischemic heart disease in the dog heart model, the extraction fraction of BMIPP in acutely ischemic myocardium 30 minutes after coronary artery occlusion fell to 87% ± 5.6% of normal myocardium and was 75% ± 20.1% of control at 2 hours after reperfusion. At that time local blood flow was reduced to 64% ± 9% of control in the ischemic region, compared with 20% ± 5% in the infarcted region; yet, wall motion abnormalities were comparable in the reperfused and the infarcted regions.[166] As already stated, the uptake of BMIPP in the various myocardial regions was significantly parallel to the local ATP content.[152]

In patients with CAD, mismatches of uptake between BMIPP and a suitable flow tracer have diagnostic significance. Between 1.6 and 4.8 days after acute myocardial infarction, 37 patients were treated by early coronary reperfusion. The degrees of accumulation defects were evaluated after pulse injection of BMIPP and 3 days later with ^{201}Tl and classified to range from mild defect to complete defect. Four weeks later, the wall motion abnormalities were determined in these patients. A highly significant relative reduction in uptake of BMIPP compared with that of ^{201}Tl was found in correlation with the extent of improvement of the wall motion disturbance.[167] This study confirms the positive prognostic value of mismatch between uptake of BMIPP and a flow tracer in the myocardium.[168,169] The lower the ratio of uptakes of BMIPP and the flow tracer the higher appears to be the probability of myocardial viability in the observed region after acute infarction. On the other hand, microscopic and scintigraphic studies with BMIPP in dogs after 1 hour ischemia followed by reperfusion showed at 3 hours an increased fatty acid uptake per unit uptake of ^{201}Tl, in the border zone of the infarcted regions with only partial recovery of systolic function; this indicates local stunned but viable myocardium in the ischemic tissue surrounding the infarcts.[147] In a parallel study without reperfusion in dog myocardium, fatty acid uptake that was measured in the myocardial regions close to the infarct with ^{123}I-labeled ω-(p-iodophenyl)tetradecanoic acid again was relatively higher than that of [201]Tl.[170]

A recent systematic study on the mismatch between uptakes of BMIPP and a flow tracer (^{99m}Tc-Sestamibi) in 26 patients with myocardial infarction and after thrombolysis and revascularization showed three patterns: uptake of BMIPP more decreased than that of Sestamibi; uptake of BMIPP less reduced than that of Sestamibi; uptakes of both tracers equally reduced.[171] Myocardial wall segments with abnormal tracer uptakes were found in 24 patients. Only 6% of the segments with abnormal tracer uptake had no correlation with coronary artery stenosis; 75% were related to infarction and 19% to significant coronary artery stenosis of which one-fourth were in previously infarcted regions. When BMIPP uptake was more reduced than Sestamibi, about two-thirds of the segments belonged to reperfused myocardium. When BMIPP uptake was less reduced than Sestamibi uptake, nearly always a wall motion disturbance was found and more than two-thirds of these segments belonged to infarcted regions. Nearly half of the abnormal segments, 47.4%, showed both tracers equally reduced. The mismatch with relatively reduced BMIPP uptake appears again to indicate a good prognosis with a probability of 0.69 in this study. The reverse pattern with Sestamibi uptake being more reduced than BMIPP uptake may indicate increased fatty acid metabolism in stretched myocardial regions with wall motion abnormalities.

In 22 patients with subacute myocardial infarction and after coronary thrombolysis, the use of BMIPP and Sestamibi resulted again in a higher sensitivity of detection of ischemia than either Sestamibi or wall motion alone.[172] The high coincidence of wall motion abnormality with equally reduced uptake of BMIPP and Sestamibi also was related to a lack of inotropic reserve as tested with low-dose dobutamine and echocardiography.[173] On the other hand, segments with relatively lower BMIPP than Sestamibi uptake showed not only normal wall motion but also an inotropic reserve. Indeed, a normal perfusion study with Sestamibi together with reduced BMIPP uptake in patients with severe LV dysfunction after myocardial infarction correlated well with the positive response of wall motion to dobutamine during stress echocardiography indicative of viable versus scarred myocardium.[174] The combined perfusion-BMIPP study was more predictive of myocardial viability than was the perfusion study alone.

The observations of correlation between mismatches of relatively lower BMIPP than near normal flow tracer uptake on the one hand and successful reperfusion after acute MI on the other points to myocardial viability with residual metabolic disturbance; this also was confirmed by a relatively increased uptake of FDG in such myocardial segments.[175] Indeed, wall motion and inotropic reserve appear to recover faster than fatty acid metabolism after acute ischemia with reperfusion, indicative of myocardial stunning. If uptakes of BMIPP and flow tracer are both reduced after ischemia for longer periods of time, myocardial hibernation may be considered. If this does not persist it may express a beneficial adaptive response. Persistent reduction of both tracers, of course, occurs within myocardial scar tissue. An adaptive myocardial response in terms of cardioprotective effect could, indeed, be seen in patients with preinfarction angina; there was an augmented perfusion-BMIPP uptake mismatch in terms of significantly reduced relative perfusion associated with functional improvement following successful reperfusion compared with the patients without preinfarct angina.[176] This appears to confirm the observation in cases of unstable angina in contrast to acute MI; with unstable angina the ratio of uptakes of BMIPP and ^{201}Tl was more frequently elevated than being reduced and was associated with normal or hypokinetic wall motion rather than with akinesia most frequently seen in acute ischemia.[149]

Another study on 36 patients with chronic CAD with and without previous myocardial infarction investigated myocardial viability with the ^{201}Tl reinjection technique, added BMIPP uptake at rest, and wall motion scoring with echocardiography.[177] In myocardial segments with reversible defects on ^{201}Tl reinjection, 50% had a more severely decreased uptake of BMIPP than of ^{201}Tl; in 39% both tracers were reduced equally and only 11% showed a relatively higher BMIPP uptake than [201]Tl. On the other hand, of myocardial segments with persistent perfusion defects, 79% had equally reduced uptake of BMIPP and ^{201}Tl, only 7% had a more severely reduced uptake of BMIPP, and 14% showed a relatively increased BMIPP uptake. Wall motion was disturbed more in segments with relatively decreased uptake of BMIPP than of reinjected [201]Tl. This data again emphasizes the correlation between myocardial viability in ischemic myocardium, a relatively reduced BMIPP uptake compared with that of flow tracer and wall motion disturbance.

Uptake of BMIPP was measured by SPECT after IV pulse injection at maximal workload and, for the purpose of measuring tracer release, again 3 hours later at rest. This was followed by a renewed uptake measurement after reinjection of BMIPP at rest in 19 patients with CAD that was confirmed by coronary angiography. Wall motion also was evaluated by echocardiography.[156] This particular protocol permitted the observation of 14 out of 15 infarcted regions. The overall sensitivity of this approach for the diagnosis of CAD with >50% stenosis was 86% when tracer release was included in the evaluation. The specificity on visual inspection alone was 94%. Again, of the 14 myocardial segments with akinesia of the LV wall, only 4 or 28% had either normal or moderately reduced BMIPP uptake, while 39 out of 57 segments or 68% with hypokinesia were seen with normal or moderately reduced BMIPP uptake.

In a patient with effort angina the uptakes of BMIPP and of ^{201}Tl were compared prior to and 4 months after treatment with percutaneous transluminal coronary angioplasty (PTCA).[178] Prior to PTCA, BMIPP uptake at rest was reduced in the region with [210]Tl redistribution; after PTCA, the uptakes of BMIPP and ^{201}Tl had recovered fully. In another study, 38 patients with CAD including 18 with old infarcts had BMIPP dynamic scans 1 week before and 3 months after successful PTCA. The patients without restenosis showed on average a decreased BMIPP washout rate before PTCA in the affected myocardial regions with normal values after PTCA, concomitant with nonsignificant differences in the uptake values. Yet, for the patients who developed restenosis, the pre-PTCA washout rates appeared not different from control and did not change after PTCA.[179] The authors stress the decreased post-PTCA washout rate in the nonrestenosed patients with chronic CAD as an indicator of improved fatty acid utilization.

A significant improvement in the diagnosis of CAD used BMIPP and SPECT before and after oral glucose loading to a blood glucose level of 184 ± 40 mg/dL (mean ± SD).[68] Images were taken at 20 minutes and 4 hours following pulse injection of BMIPP. Of the 29 patients who all underwent coronary arteriography 22 had no previous myocardial infarction and 7 had a proven history of prior myocardial infarction. The glucose loading significantly increased the rate of tracer release after peak uptake different from the kinetics of ^{11}C-palmitic acid.[38,57] Also, the accumulation defect in the affected myocardial region became more prominent after glucose loading. The total defect score was in terms of the sum of early and late accumulation defects in each patient. In this way, the sensitivity of the detection of CAD with BMIPP significantly increased from 55% in the fasting state to 75% after glucose loading; the specificity remained at 78%.

Nonischemic Cardiomyopathy

Regarding cardiomyopathy, autoradiographic studies with 1-[^{14}C]-BMHDA and ^{131}I-labeled BMIPP on normotensive and hypertensive rat myocardium revealed the very heterogeneous distribution of the tracers in the hypertensive cardiomyopathy with decreased uptake in the endocardial regions.[155] Both tracers behaved alike.[180] Also, in clinical diagnostic studies, the distribution of BMIPP within the LV wall in hypertrophic cardiomyopathy was more heterogeneous and independent of perfusion that was assayed with ^{201}Tl.[181-183] In addition, uncoupling between BMIPP and ^{201}Tl became even more evident when the data on tracer release from BMIPP in the various myocardial regions, particularly in hypertrophic regions, were added to those of local uptake and flow.[182] This principally confirms observations made with other labeled long-chain fatty acids. Mismatches between uptakes of BMIPP and ^{201}Tl in the LV wall affected especially thickened wall regions where uptake of BMIPP tended to be decreased with normal or increased uptake of ^{201}Tl.

Contrary to the biokinetics in CAD, in cases with cardiomyopathy, myocardial regions with decreased BMIPP uptake often also had increased rates of tracer release.[182,184] It is not known whether increased release rates in these patients came from increased β-oxidation or back-diffusion/transport. However, when BMIPP uptake at rest in fasted patients was compared with ^{201}Tl uptake after stress and at rest, 6 of the 17 patients also showed thallium redistribution in the areas of decreased uptake of BMIPP.[183] This appears to indicate the involvement of ischemia in these patients with hypertrophic cardiomyopathy. Fatty acid back-diffusion/transport is known to occur in ischemic myocardial regions.

During and shortly following treatment of rats with adriamycin, myocardial uptake of the flow tracer ^{99m}Tc-MIBI was normal; yet the uptake of BMIPP decreased in the advanced stages of myocardial disease; this was somewhat less pronounced than, but concomitant with, a decrease in uptake of FDG.[185] The reduction of uptake of both tracers preceded deterioration of myocardial function that was measured by the LVEF.

In the genetically determined cardiomyopathy of the hamster the uptake of BMIPP and ^{201}Tl into the myocardium and LVEF were examined serially throughout the evolution of the disease.[148] Concomitant with the histologically proven deterioration of the myocardial structure the ratio of uptakes of BMIPP and ^{201}Tl dropped significantly and was paralleled by a drop in the ejection fraction. Also, the uptake ratios for ^{201}Tl in lung and myocardium increased significantly. Yet, the distribution of BMIPP in this type of myocardial disease was not heterogeneous, as was seen in dilated and hypertrophic cardiomyopathy in man. Also, even if the BMIPP uptake compared with that of ^{201}Tl was reduced relatively early in the development of the disease, the degree of change may be too subtle for detection by external imaging in man, if it occurs there as well.

ω-(o-^{123}I-phenyl)pentadecanoic Acid

Principal Biokinetics

When ω-phenyl-pentadecanoic acid is labeled with radioiodine two-thirds of the product shows the radioiodine in the paraposition on the phenyl ring (p-PPA), and one-third has the radioiodine in the orthoposition (o-PPA; Fig. 11.[33,94] First trials with rat

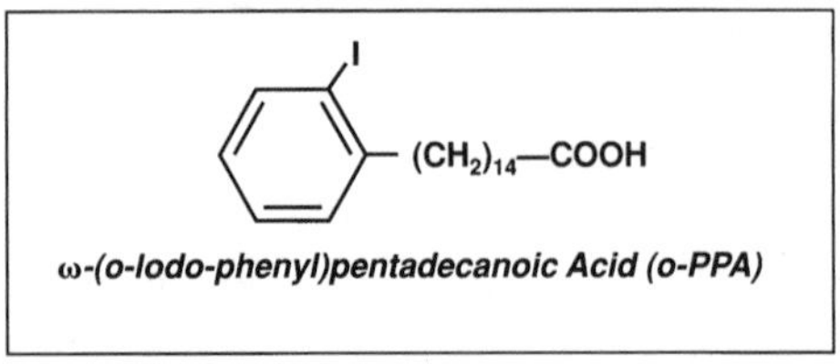

ω-(o-Iodo-phenyl)pentadecanoic Acid (o-PPA)

Figure 11.

myocardium showed these two isomers to behave quite different metabolically in that *o*-PPA was again rapidly lost after rapid uptake.[33,98] When applied to humans in an initial attempt to label the free-fatty acid pool as an internal standard in the measurement of myocardial lipid turnover, *o*-PPA was, contrary to expectation, observed to have a very low rate of tracer release.[186] This prompted follow-up investigations in rat myocardium in vivo and in vitro also using the isolated heart perfusion technique.[8,105,187]

The rapid uptake of *o*-PPA into the myocardium was similar to *p*-PPA. However, both isomers were significantly less readily bound in vitro to CoA by the enzyme acyl-CoA-sulfhydryl-thiolase than were palmitic acid and ω-I-HDA and HDA; after 30-minute incubation the binding was approximately 32% for *o*-PPA, approximately 48% for *p*-PPA, approximately 83% for HDA, and approximately 91% for palmitic acid.[102] A reason for the reduced rate of binding of *p*-PPA and *o*-PPA to CoA may be steric hindrance by way of the ω-position of the phenyl group on the long-chain fatty acid; also, the reaction demands ATP, so that the data may indicate an increased ATP dependence of *o*-PPA and *p*-PPA uptake into the myocardium compared with palmitic acid and ω-I-HDA.

The distribution of *o*-PPA and *p*-PPA within the lipid pool of rat myocardium differed greatly. In contrast to *p*-PPA, *o*-PPA was esterified hardly at all into complex lipids; it left the myocardium rapidly.[33] The rapid loss of tracer from the rat myocardium was identified not to be caused by β-oxidation. Blocking the carnitine shuttle and thus β-oxidation by injection of 2-[5-(4-chlorophenyl)-pentyl]-oxirane-2-carboxylate (POCA) did not alter the rate of tracer release following administration of *o*-PPA; yet, it led to a retention in the myocardium of *p*-PPA. Under this condition in vivo, *p*-PPA continued to be incorporated into triglycerides, while tracer in the free-fatty acid pool and in phospholipids diminished; also, *o*-PPA showed a tracer decline in the free-fatty acid pool with a slight rise in the triglyceride fraction to approximately 5% of the amount of tracer from *p*-PPA at 20 minutes after injection.[105,187] The results, thus, showed that in vivo *o*-PPA, in contrast to *p*-PPA, hardly crossed into the mitochondria for β-oxidation but remained largely nondegraded in the cytosol from where it rapidly was lost by back-diffusion or transport.

On the other hand and again surprisingly, in the baboon myocardium *o*-PPA entered β-oxidation similarly to *p*-PPA. This was demonstrated by measuring the release rates for both tracers from the myocardium without and with inhibiting palmitoyl transferase with ethylene 2-[6-(4-chlorophenoxy)hexyl]-oxirane-2-carboxylate (Etomoxir) for blocking the carnitine shuttle into mitochondria.[160] Also, in these studies the data scattered more interindividually than intraindividually.

The application of *o*-PPA to myocardial imaging in humans had shown that *o*-PPA after its rapid uptake into the myocardium at a rate similar to that of *p*-PPA was retained with prolonged half-times of several hours; catabolic end-products of *o*-PPA hardly appeared in the peripheral blood and urine.[186] The metabolic site of the myocardial trapping of *o*-PPA outside mitochondria in the cytosol of the human myocardial cells was confirmed essentially by diagnostic observations in patients.

In these studies, *o*-PPA was used double labeled with ^{123}I on the phenyl ring and with ^{14}C in the 2 position of the carbon chain. The rationale of this approach was the expectation of both tracers remaining together unless β-oxidation occurred. In case of ^{123}I trapping with ^{14}C appearing alone in the peripheral blood after IV pulse injection of the double-labeled *o*-PPA, β-oxidation would have occurred and the trapping would be localized in the mitochondria. If both labels would be retained in the myocardium, the site of the trapping would be in the cytosol outside the mitochondria.

After IV or, in another group of patients, intracoronary artery injection of ^{131}I and ^{14}C double-labeled *o*-PPA at the time of diagnostic coronary angiography, the two labels remained closely together in both sets of investigations.[102] After coronary artery injection of *o*-PPA, the ^{131}I-labeled catabolites and $^{14}CO_2$ appeared at a rate of approximately 0.2

the rate seen after p-PPA injection. In both instances, ^{131}I preceded ^{14}CO$_2$ by 5 to 10 minutes.

The conclusion of this work showed the usefulness of the dual tracer application of o-PPA together with p-PPA for probing the function of the carnitine shuttle in myocardial lipid metabolism. It also appeared justified in conjunction with the release rates from the total myocardium to assume either some reutilization of CO_2 and/or relatively rapid release of free iodine from the mitochondria for both phenylated fatty acids.

Ischemic Myocardium

The low rate of release of tracer from the myocardium after pulse injection of o-PPA prompted the clinical application of o-PPA for imaging with SPECT, for the purpose of detecting myocardial viability in hypoperfused areas. Thus, in 32 resting patients with a recent history of myocardial infarction the uptakes of o-PPA and of FDG were compared in myocardial regions with perfusion defects detected by ^{201}Tl.[188] All patients had, as usual, fasted overnight. Myocardial tissue with persistent perfusion defects following ^{201}Tl injection at stress and 3 hours later at rest are considered to contain viable myocardium when FDG was incorporated.[175,189] Of the segments with persistently decreased ^{201}Tl uptake, 50.5% had a decreased uptake of both o-PPA and FDG. Both tracers normally were accumulated in 21.8% of the ^{210}Tl defects. The uptake was normal for FDG but reduced for o-PPA in 17.4% and it was normal for o-PPA and reduced for FDG in 10.3% of the ^{201}Tl defects. The significant discrepancy between the incidences of uptake of o-PPA and FDG in myocardial regions with old infarcts may be caused by differences in metabolism in the observed regions with old infarcts; yet both tracers appear to signal the presence of viable tissue but with various degrees of metabolic derangements; some of the tissue may be more oriented to glycolysis indicative of persistent hypoxia in 17.4% of the ^{201}Tl defects, and the other, 10.3% of the ^{201}Tl defects, may be considered to have converted to normal utilization of fatty acids with reduced glycolysis perhaps also indicative of lipid storage in the affected regions. In all, within the 408 infarcted regions FDG uptake was normal in 39.2%, while o-PPA was normal in 32.1%. In 49.5% of the infarcted regions, one or the other tracer accumulated normally.

Following thrombolysis because of acute myocardial infarction wall motion abnormalities may persist or improve slowly or deteriorate within approximately 2 weeks. MBF imaging soon after reperfusion does not well predict the functional outcome of the therapy. Uptakes of o-PPA and of ^{99m}Tc-MIBI, as flow marker were compared by SPECT imaging in nine patients at rest and after overnight fasting within 5–12 days after thrombolytic therapy for acute myocardial infarction.[190] Of the total of 117 myocardial segments, 99 (85%) showed concordance for the two tracers. Less o-PPA uptake than MIBI was seen in 18 (15%) of the segments. No segment showed an excess of o-PPA over MIBI. Of the 23 segments with wall motion abnormalities on the day following thrombolytic therapy, 11 improved, and of these nine segments had less o-PPA than MIBI uptake and two segments had normal uptakes of both. All three segments with wall motion deterioration showed equal defects for o-PPA and MIBI. Of the nine segments without wall motion change, two had normal uptakes for both tracers, three had lower o-PPA than MIBI uptake, and in four segments uptakes of both were equally low. This set of data indicates the significant predictive value of comparatively low o-PPA versus flow tracer uptake in favor of wall motion improvement. It also confirms in humans that myocardial metabolism recovers with delay after reperfusion, and metabolic derangements may persist in regions with normal wall motion.[190]

Nonischemic Cardiomyopathy

The dual tracer technique with *o*-PPA and *p*-PPA was applied diagnostically in 15 patients with dilated cardiomyopathy. Data obtained from five patients without CAD or cardiomyopathy of any form served as controls.[191] The LVEF of the patients was 0.39 ± 0.11. The IV pulse injection of *o*-PPA preceded the injection of *p*-PPA by 50 minutes. PI in the dynamic mode with the camera head in the left anterior oblique 45° position began at the time of the first injection with a frame rate of 1 per minute for a total of 125 minutes. At 100 minutes of imaging, ^{123}I-NaI was IV given to correct, by image subtraction, for tracer outside myocardial lipids and in the circulating blood.[10,43] The images taken from 0–4 minutes after injection were scored parametrically for uptake. No significant differences in regional uptakes were found between patients and control subjects. After peak uptake the two tracers were analyzed quantitatively for their release rates in three defined myocardial regions per patient, with fitting by an iterative monoexponential method. The loss of tracer from *o*-PPA was taken to reflect mainly back-diffusion/transport into the circulating blood; the loss of tracer from *p*-PPA in the same patient was taken to be possibly caused by both β-oxidation and back-diffusion/transport; the difference between the two release rates of *o*-IPPA and *p*-PPA then would be related to the rate of β-oxidation in the observed myocardial regions of that given patient.

As was seen in other analyses with labeled fatty acids, in this dual tracer study the scatter of data was larger interindividually than intraindividually. However, significant alterations in lipid turnover were seen in at least 66% of the patients. They were identified by significant correlations within the nine findings per patient, three myocardial regions each with release rates of the two tracers and the difference between them. Three different patterns of lipid turnover indicated (1) predominantly increased β-oxidation; (2) predominantly decreased β-oxidation, in part with increased back-diffusion/transport; and (3) predominantly increased back-diffusion/transport. Interestingly, a highly significant increase in β-oxidation was seen in the posterolateral region of the myocardium compared with the anteroseptal and apical regions in both patients and control subjects.[191]

This study, contrary to the observations with ^{11}C-palmitic acid, ω-^{123}I-HDA, and *p*-PPA, did not show the spotty heterogeneity of tracer distribution in the LV wall at peak uptake first of *o*-PPA and then of *o*-PPA plus *p*-PPA. The reason for this may be the particular metabolic fate of *o*-PPA preceding the uptake of *p*-PPA. No significant correlation was seen between individual abnormal lipid turnover with the individually low ejection fraction.

Conclusions

Metabolically active substrates that are labeled with ^{123}I are increasingly available. This testifies to the increased applicability of the conventional γ-camera in the planar mode or in SPECT for the analysis of metabolism at defined tissue sites in the intact body. A decade ago, assaying metabolic reactions in vivo was widely believed to be restricted to PET and those substrates that could be labeled with positron emitting isotopes of nuclides occurring naturally in organic molecules such as ^{11}C, ^{13}N, ^{18}F, and [15]O. Radioiodine-labeled fatty acids indeed have played an important role in paving the way in the development of methods for measuring in vivo biochemical reactions, in general, and for the use with the conventional γ-camera in particular.

In principle, the following four aspects now may be addressed when lipid metabolism is to be studied in situ in diagnostic cardiology; these may be investigated with different fatty acids or their analogs (Fig. 1):

1. normal lipid metabolism, fatty acid uptake into and release from the myocardium, with ^{11}C-palmitic acid, ω-^{123}I-HDA, and p-PPA, also together with ^{11}C-acetate as interval standard;
2. preferential incorporation in complex lipids permitting partial β-oxidation, with BMIPP, without β-oxidation and back-diffusion/transport, with BMHDA, and with DMIPP;
3. preferential incorporation in free-fatty acid pool permitting back-diffusion/transport, with o-PPA;
4. preferential trapping in β-oxidation in mitochondria, with FTHA.

The single or combined use of these categories of fatty acids together with an appropriate flow tracer promises significant advances in the diagnosis and follow-up of myocardial disease. Yet, more work is expected before labeled fatty acids will be widely accepted as routine tools for noninvasively assessing myocardial metabolism in the practice of cardiology.

For clinical diagnostic use in answering the question of the degree and extension of and myocardial viability in ischemic heart disease, BMIPP in conjunction with an appropriate flow tracer such as ^{201}Tl or ^{99m}Tc-labeled isonitriles such as MIBI, presently appears to be an optimal tracer that has been evaluated most carefully.

For the diagnosis of cardiomyopathy, the labeled fatty acid should permit the observation of uptake into and release from the myocardium. The observation of tracer release either from β-oxidation or back-diffusion/transport adds to the analysis of the pattern of tracer uptake. Here, the most revealing appeared to be fatty acids of the above groups in 1 and 2. When the ^{123}I labeled analogs are used, especially HDA, the images need or improve on correction for tracer signals that originate from outside the myocardial lipid pool.

For the purpose of differentiating between various forms of cardiomyopathy and for clinical cardiological research in general, the dual fatty acid tracer analysis alone or in addition to imaging of flow seems promising, as was discussed above for the combination of p-PPA and o-PPA, the former as an analog for tracing physiological kinetics of fatty acid and the latter tracing nearly exclusively the free-fatty acid back-diffusion/transport. An example of a triple tracer technique alone or in addition to imaging flow may be the combination of HDA or p-PPA, with o-PPA and FTHA for additionally assessing nearly exclusively β-oxidation. In this manner, fatty acid uptake into the myocardium, its rate of being fed into β-oxidation, and its rate of back-diffusion/transport out of the myocardial cells into the circulating blood can be observed separately in a given patient. The dual use of ^{11}C-acetate and a labeled physiological fatty acid promises detailed information on mitochondrial function.

Multiple tracer techniques combined with the noninvasive assessment of myocardial flow yield relevant information for the differential and early diagnosis of cardiomyopathy and myocardial viability in ischemic heart disease. In this context, also the labeled methylated fatty acids in the above group 2 such as DMIPP and BMHDA are promising tracers for nearly exclusively observing the synthesis of complex lipids.

It is foreseen that metabolic imaging of myocardial lipids with ^{123}I-labeled fatty acid analogs may become an important component of the spectrum of diagnostic tools for the noninvasive and local analysis of myocardial cell integrity and metabolism.

Acknowledgments: The author appreciates the most useful provision of some original literature by D.R. Elmaleh and F.F. Knapp Jr. and the expert editorial help from Mrs. Joyce Rochek.

References

1. Bing RJ. Metabolic activity of the intact heart. *Am J Med* 1961;30:679–691.
2. Carlsten A, Hallgren B, Jagenburg R, et al. Myocardial metabolism of glucose, lactic acid, amino acids and fatty acids in healthy human individuals at rest and at different work loads. *Scand J Clin Lab Invest* 1961;13:418–428.

3. Gordon RS Jr, Cherkes A. Unesterified fatty acid in human blood plasma. *J Clin Invest* 1956;35:206–212.

4. Evans JR, Gunton RW, Baker RG, et al. Use of radioiodinated fatty acid for photoscans of the heart. *Circ Res* 1965;16:1–10.

5. Poe ND, Eber LM, Graham LS, et al. A critical evaluation of potassium-43 and cesium-129 for quantitative myocardial scanning. In: *Medical Radioisotope Scintigraphy*. Vol II. Vienna: International Atomic Energy Agency; 1972:365–378.

6. Poe ND, Robinson GD. Jr, MacDonald NS. Myocardial extraction of labeled long-chain fatty acid analogs. *Proc Soc Exper Biol Med* 1975;148:215–218 .

7. Poe ND, Robinson GD. Jr, Zielinski FW, et al. Myocardial imaging with 123-I-hexadecanoic acid. *Radiology* 1977;124:419–424 .

8. Weiss ES, Hoffman EJ, Phelps ME, et al. External detection and visualization of myocardial ischemia with 11-C-substrates in vitro and in vivo. *Circ Res* 1976;39:24–32.

9. Machulla H-J, Stoecklin G, Kupfernagel CH, et al. Comparative evaluation of fatty acids labeled with C-11, Cl-34m, Br-77, and I-123 for metabolic studies of the myocardium: Concise communication. *J Nucl Med* 1978;19:298–302.

10. Feinendegen LE, Vyska K, Freundlieb C, et al. Non-invasive analysis of metabolic reactions in body tissues, the case of myocardial fatty acids. *Eur J Nucl Med* 1981;6:191–200.

11. Freundlieb C, Hoeck A, Vyska K, et al. Use of ω-123-I-labeled heptadecanoic acid for non-invasively measuring myocardial metabolism. Proceedings, 15th International Meeting of the Society of Nuclear Medicine, Groningen 1977. Woldring M, Schmidt HAE, eds. New York: F.K. Schattauer, Stuttgart; 1978:216–219.

12. Jones GS Jr, Elmaleh DR, Strauss HW, et al. Synthesis and biodistribution of a new 99m-technetium fatty acid. *Nucl Med Biol* 1994;21:117–123.

13. Zaret BL, Beller GA, eds. *Nuclear Cardiology. State of the Art and Future Directions*. St Louis, Baltimore, Boston, Chicago, London, Philadelphia, Sydney, Toronto: Mosby; 1993.

14. Feinendegen LE. The dual parameter analysis for in vivo measuring metabolic reactions. In: Hoefer R., Bergmann H., eds. *Radioaktive Isotope in Klinik und Forschung*. Vienna: Egermann; 1984:465–486.

15. Logan J, Fowler JS, Volkow ND, et al. Graphical analysis of reversible radioligand binding from time-activity measurements applied to [N-11C-methyl]-(−)-cocaine PET studies in human subjects. *J Cereb Blood Flow Metab* 1990;10:740–747.

16. Patlak CS, Blasberg RG, Fenstermacher JD. Graphical evaluation of blood-to-brain transfer constants from multiple-time uptake data. *J Cereb Blood Flow Metab* 1983;3:1–7.

17. Myers DK, Feinendegen LE. Double labeling with 3-H-thymidine and 125-I-iododeoxyuridine as a method for determining the fate of injected DNA and cells in vivo. *J Cell Biol* 1975;67:484–488.

18. Ritzl F, Feinendegen LE. In vivo determination of site and rate of insulin catabolism using the double tracer technique with 51-Cr and 131-I. In: *Dynamic Studies with Radioisotopes in Medicine*. Vienna: International Atomic Energy Agency; 1971:57–68.

19. Lehninger AL, Nelson DL, Cox MM. Principles of Biochemistry. New York: Worth; 1993.

20. Neeley JR, Rovetto MJ, Oram JF. Myocardial utilization of carbohydrate and lipids. *Progr Cardiovasc Dis* 1972;15:289–329.

21. Opie LH. Metabolism of the heart in health and disease. *Am Heart J* 1969;77:383–410.

22. Stremmel W, Strohmeyer G, Berk PD. Hepatocellular uptake of oleate is energy dependent, sodium linked, and inhibited by an antibody to a hepatocyte plasma membrane fatty acid binding protein. *Proc Natl Acad Sci U S A* 1986;83:3584–3588.

23. Stremmel W. Fatty acid uptake by isolated rat heart myocytes represents a carrier mediated transport process. *J Clin Invest* 1988;81:844–852.

24. Wisneski JA, Gertz EW, Neese RA, et al. Myocardial metabolism of free fatty acids. *J Clin Invest* 1987;79:359–366.

25. Caldwell HJ, Martin GV, Link JM, et al. Iodophenylpentadecanoic acid-myocardial blood flow relationship during maximal exercise with coronary occlusion. *J Nucl Med* 1990;31:99–105.

26. Okada RD, Elmaleh D, Werre GS, et al. Myocardial kinetics of 123I-labeled-16-hexadecanoic acid. *Eur J Nucl Med* 1983;8:211–217.

27. Rothlin ME, Bing RJ. Extraction and release of individual free fatty acids by the heart and fat depots. *J Clin Invest* 1961;40:1380–1386.

28. Vyska K, Machulla HJ, Stremmel W, et al. Regional myocardial free fatty acid extraction in normal and ischemic myocardium. *Circulation* 1988;78:1218–1233.

29. Vyska K, Meyer W, Stremmel W, et al. Fatty acid uptake in normal human myocardium. *Circ Res* 1991;69:857–870.

30. Braunwald E, ed. *Heart Disease: A Textbook of Cardiovascular Medicine*. Philadelphia, Pa: Saunders; 1996.

31. Bergmann SR, Weinheimer CJ, Markham J, et al. Quantitation of myocardial fatty acid metabolism using PET. *J Nucl Med* 1996;37:1723–1730.

32. Feinendegen LE, Shreeve WW. On behalf of I-123 fatty acids for myocardial metabolic imaging. *J Nucl Med* 1987;28:545–546.

33. Beckurts TE, Shreeve WW, Schieren R, et al. Kinetics of different 123-I and 14-C-labeled fatty acids in normal and diabetic rat myocardium in vivo. *Nucl Med Commun* 1985;6:415–424.

34. Henrich MM, Grossmann K, Motz W, et al. Beta-oxidation of 1-[14-C]-17-[131-I]-iodoheptadecanoic acid following intracoronary injection in humans results in similar release of both tracers. *Eur J Nucl Med* 1993;20:225–230.

35. Schoen HR, Schelbert HR, Robinson G, et al. C-11 labeled palmitic acid for the noninvasive evaluation of regional myocardial fatty acid metabolism with positron-computed tomography, I: Kinetics of C-11 palmitic acid in normal myocardium. *Am Heart J* 1982;103:532–547.

36. Duwel CMB, Visser FC, Eenige van MJ, et al. The fate of 131-I-17-iodoheptadecanoic acid during lactate loading: Its oxidation is strongly inhibited in favor of its esterification. *Nucl Med* 1990; 29:24–27.

37. Oliver MF, Opie LH. Effects of glucose and fatty acids on myocardial ischemia and arrhythmias. *Lancet* 1994;343:155–158.

38. Schelbert HR, Henze E, Schon HR, et al. C-11 palmitate for the noninvasive evaluation of regional myocardial fatty acid metabolism with positron computed tomography, III: In vivo demonstration of the effects of substrate availability on myocardial metabolism. *Am Heart J* 1983;105:492–504.

39. Taegtmeyer H. Essential Fuels for the Heart and Mechanical Restitution. Chapter in: Dilsizian V, ed. *Myocardial Viability: A Clinical and Scientific Treatise*. Futura Publishing Company, Armonk, NY 2000.

40. Liedtke AJ, DeMaison L, Eggleston AM, et al. Changes in substrate metabolism and effects of excess fatty acids in reperfused myocardium. *Circ Res* 1988;62:535–542.

41. Notohamiprodjo G, Schmid A, Spohr G, et al. Comparison of myocardial metabolism of 11-C-palmitic acid (11-CPA) and 123-I-heptadecanoic acid (123-IHA) in man. In: Schmidt HAE , Vauramo DE, eds. *Nuklearmedizin-Nuklearmedizin in Forschung und Praxis*. New York: F.K. Schattauer, Stuttgart; 1984:233–236.

42. Eenige van MJ, Visser FC, Duwel CMB, et al. Analysis of myocardial time activity curves of I-123-heptadecanoic acid, I: Curve fitting. *Nucl Med* 1987;26:241–247.

43. Freundlieb C, Hoeck A, Vyska K, et al. Myocardial imaging and metabolic studies with [17–123-I]-iodoheptadecanoic acid. *J Nucl Med* 1980;21:1043–1050.

44. Gould KL, ed. *Coronary Artery Stenosis*. New York: Elsevier; 1991.

45. Marshall RC, Nash WH, Shine KI, et al. Glucose metabolism during ischemia due to excessive oxygen demand of altered coronary flow in the isolated arterially perfused rabbit septum. *Circ Res* 1981;49:64–68.

46. Tillisch J, Brunken R, Marshall R, et al. Reversibility of cardiac wall-motion abnormalities predicted by positron tomography. *N Engl J Med* 1986;314:884–888.

47. Bolukoglu H, Goodwin GW, Guthrie PH, et al. Metabolic fate of glucose in reversible low-flow ischemia of the isolated working rat heart. *Am J Physiol* 1996;270:H817–H826.

48. Schelbert HR, Henze E, Keen R, et al. C-11 palmitate for the noninvasive evaluation of regional myocardial fatty acid metabolism with positron-computed tomography, IV: In vivo evaluation of acute demand-induced ischemia in dogs. *Am Heart J* 1983;106:736–750.

49. van der Wall EE, den Hollander W, Heidendal GAK, et al. Dynamic myocardial scintigraphy with 123-I-labeled free fatty acids in patients with myocardial infarction. *Eur J Nucl Med* 1981;6:383–389.

50. Taegtmeyer H. Energy metabolism of the heart: From basic concepts to clinical applications. *Curr Probl Cardiol* 1994;14:62–113.

51. Taegtmeyer H. Metabolic support for the postischemic heart (Grand round). *Lancet* 1995; 345:1552–1555.
52. Downey JM, Cohen MV. Preconditioning. Chapter in: Dilsizian V, ed. *Myocardial Viability: A Clinical and Scientific Treatise*. Futura Publishing Company, Armonk, NY 2000.
53. Klocke FJ, Sherman AJ, Jain A. Reversible Myocardial Dysfunction: Stunning, Hibernation, or What? Chapter in: Dilsizian V, ed. *Myocardial Viability: A Clinical and Scientific Treatise*. Futura Publishing Company, Armonk, NY 2000.
54. Goodwin GW, Taegtmeyer H. Metabolic recovery of isolated working rat heart after brief global ischemia. *Am J Physiol* 1994;267:H462–H470.
55. Taegtmeyer H. Modulation of Responses to Myocardial Ischemia: Metabolic Features of Myocardial Stunning, Hibernation, and Ischemic Preconditioning. Chapter in: Dilsizian V, ed. *Myocardial Viability: A Clinical and Scientific Treatise*. Futura Publishing Company, Armonk, NY 2000.
56. Edwards WD. Cardiomyopathies. *Hum Pathol* 1987;18:625–635.
57. Schelbert HR, Henze E, Sochor H, et al. Effects of substrate availability on myocardial C-11 palmitate kinetics by positron emission tomography in normal subjects and patients with ventricular dysfunction. *Am Heart J* 1986;111:1055–1064.
58. Mason JR, Palac RT, Freeman ML, et al. Thallium-201 scintigraphy during dobutamine infusion: Nonexercise-dependent screening test for coronary disease. *Am Heart J* 1984;107: 481–485.
59. Meyer SL, Curry GC, Donsky MS, et al. Influence of dobutamine on hemodynamics and coronary blood flow in patients with and without coronary artery disease. *Am J Cardiol* 1976;38:103–108.
60. Tamaki N, Kawamoto M, Takahashi N, et al. Assessment of myocardial fatty acid metabolism with positron emission tomography at rest and during dobutamine infusion in patients with coronary artery disease. *Am Heart J* 1993;125:702–710.
61. Schelbert HR, Phelps ME, Huang SC, et al. N-13 ammonia as in indicator of myocardial blood flow. *Circulation* 1981;63:1259–1272.
62. Schelbert HR, Henze E, Phelps ME, et al. Assessment of regional myocardial ischemia by positron emission computed tomography. *Am Heart J* 1982;103:588–597.
63. Yoshida K, Mullani N, Gould KL. Coronary flow and flow reserve by PET simplified for clinical applications using rubidium-82 or nitrogen-13-ammonia. *J Nucl Med* 1996;37:1701–1712.
64. Knabb RM, Bergmann SR, Fox KAA, et al. The temporal pattern of recovery of myocardial perfusion and metabolism delineated by positron emission tomography after coronary thrombolysis. *J Nucl Med* 1987;28:1563–1570.
65. Schelbert HR, Czernin J. PET studies of myocardial blood flow and metabolism in patients with acute myocardial infarction. In: Zaret BL, Beller GA, eds. *Nuclear Cardiology. State of the Art and Future Directions*. St.Louis, Baltimore, Boston, Chicago, London, Philadelphia, Sydney, Toronto: Mosby; 1993:294–302.
66. Fox KAA, Abendschein DR, Ambos HD, et al. Efflux of metabolized and nonmetabolized fatty acid from canine myocardium: Implications for quantifying myocardial metabolism tomographically. *Circ Res* 1985;57:232–243.
67. Vanoverschelde JLJ, Wijns W, Kolanowski J, et al. Competition between palmitate and ketone bodies as fuels for the heart: Study with positron emission tomography. *Am J Physiol* 1993; 264:H701–H707.
68. Fujiwara S, Takeishi Y, Atsumi H, et al. Fatty acid metabolic imaging with iodine-123-BMIPP for the diagnosis of coronary artery disease. *J Nucl Med* 1997;38:175–180.
69. Geltman EM, Smith JL, Beecher D, et al. Altered regional myocardial metabolism in congestive cardiomyopathy detected by positron tomography. *Am J Med* 1983;74:773–785.
70. Eisenberg JD, Sobel BE, Geltman EM. Differentiation of ischemic from nonischemic cardiomyopathy with positron emission tomography. *Am J Cardiol* 1987;59:1410–1414.
71. Hoeck A, Freundlieb C, Vyska K, et al. Myocardial imaging and metabolic studies with [17-123-I]-iodoheptadecanoic acid in patients with idiopathic congestive cardiomyopathy. *J Nucl Med* 1983;24:22–28.
72. Kelly DP, Mendelsohn NJ, Sobel BE, et al. Detection and assessment by positron emission tomography of a genetically determined defect in myocardial fatty acid utilization (long-chain acyl-Co-A dehydrogenase deficiency). *Am J Cardiol* 1993;71:738–744.

73. Armbrecht JJ, Buxton DB, Schelbert HR. Validation of [1–11-C]acetate as a tracer for noninvasive assessment of oxidative metabolism with positron emission tomography in normal, ischemic, postischemic, and hyperemic canine myocardium. *Circulation* 1990;81:1594–1605.
74. Brown MA, Marshall DR, Sobel BE, et al. Delineation of myocardial oxygen utilization with carbon-11 labeled acetate. *Circulation* 1987;76:687–696.
75. Brown MA, Myears DW, Bergmann SR. Nonivasive assessment of canine myocardial oxidative metabolism with carbon-11 acetate and positron emission tomography. *J Am Coll Cardiol* 1988;12:1054–1063.
76. Brown MA, Myears DW, Bergmann SR. Validity of estimates of myocardial oxidative metabolism with carbon-11 acetate and positron tomography despite altered patterns of substrate utilization. *J Nucl Med* 1993;30:187–193.
77. Fischman AJ, Saito T, Dilsizian V, et al. Myocardial fatty acid imaging: Rationale, comparison of 11-C- and 123-I-labeled fatty acids, and potential clinical utility. *Am J Card Imaging* 1989;3:288–296.
78. Sloof GW, Visser FC, Teerlink T, et al. Incorporation of radioiodinated fatty acids into cardiac phospholipids of normoxic canine myocardium. *Mol Cell Biochem* 1992;116:79–87.
79. Luethy P, Chatelain P, Papageorgiou I, et al. Assessment of myocardial metabolism with iodine-123 heptadecanoic acid: Effect of decreased fatty acid oxidation on deiodination. *J Nucl Med* 1988;29:1088–1095.
80. Eenige van MJ, Visser FC, Duwel CMB, et al. Comparison of 17-iodine-131-heptadecanoic acid kinetics from externally measured time-activity curves and from serial myocardial biopsies in an open-chest canine model. *J Nucl Med* 1988;29:1934–1942.
81. Visser FC, Eenige van MJ, Westera G, et al. Metabolic fate of radioiodinated heptadecanoic acid in the normal canine heart. *Circulation* 1985;72:565–571.
82. Visser FC, Eenige van MJ, Duwel CMB, et al. Radioiodinated free fatty acids: Can we measure myocardial metabolism? *Eur J Nucl Med* 1986;12:S20–S23.
83. Kloster G, Stoecklin G, Smith EF, et al. Omega-halofatty acids: A probe for mitochondrial membrane integrity. *Eur J Nucl Med* 1984;9:305–311.
84. Eenige van MJ, Visser FC, Duwel CMB, et al. Clinical value of studies with radioiodinated heptadecanoic acid in patients with coronary artery disease. *Eur Heart J* 1990;11:258–268.
85. Freundlieb C, Hoeck A, Vyska K, et al. Nuklearmedizinische Analyse des Fettsaeureumsatzes im Myokard. In: Oeff K, Schmidt HAE, eds. *Nuklearmedizin-Nuklearmedizin und Biokybernetik*. Vol 1. Berlin: Medico-Informationsdienste; 1978:415–419.
86. Dudczak R. Myokardszintigraphie mit Jod-123 markierten Fettsaeuren. *Wien Klin Wochenschr* 1983;95:1–38.
87. Dudczak R, Kletter K, Frischauf H, et al. The use of 123-I-labeled heptadecanoic acid (HDA) as metabolic tracer: Preliminary report. *Eur J.Nucl Med* 1984;9:81–85.
88. Feinendegen LE. Single photon metabolic imaging in cardiology. In: Zaret BL, Beller GA, eds. *Nuclear Cardiology, State of the Art and Future Directions*. St.Louis, Baltimore, Boston, Chicago, London, Philadelphia, Sydney, Toronto: Mosby; 1993:260–274.
89. van der Wall EE, Heidendal GAK, den Hollander W, et al. I-123 labeled hexadecanoic acid in comparison with thallium-201 for myocardial imaging in coronary heart disease. *Eur J Nucl Med* 1980;5:401–405.
90. Hoeck A, Notohamiprodjo G, Spohr G, et al. Myocardial fatty acid metabolism after acute ethanol consumption. *Nucl Med Commun* 1986;7:671–682.
91. Rabinovitch MA, Kalff V, Allen R, et al. 123-I-hexadecanoic acid metabolic probe of cardiomyopathy. *Eur J Nucl Med* 1985;10:222–227.
92. Knoop F. Der Abbau aromatischer Fettsaeuren im Tierkoerper. *Beitr Chem Physiol Pathol* 1905;6:150–156.
93. Kulkarni PV, Corbett JR. Radioiodinated tracers for myocardial imaging. *Semin Nucl Med* 1990;20:119–129.
94. Machulla HJ, Marsmann M, Dutschka K. Biochemical concept and synthesis of a radioiodinated phenylfatty acid for in vivo metabolic studies of the myocardium. *Eur J Nucl Med* 1980;5:171–173.
95. Eisenhut M, Lehmann WD, Suetterle A. Metabolism of 15-(4'-123I-iodophenyl)pentadecanoic acid ([123I]IPPA) in the rat heart: Identification of new metabolites by high pressure

liquid chromatography and fast atom bombardment-mass spectrometry. *Nucl Med Biol* 1993; 6:747–754.

96. Reske SN, Sauer W, Machulla HJ, et al. Metabolism of 15(*p*-[123-I]iodophenyl)penta-decanoic acid in heart muscle and noncardiac tissues. *Eur J Nucl Med* 1985;10:228–234.

97. Schmitz B, Reske SN, Machulla HJ, et al. Cardiac metabolism of 15-(*p*-iodo-phenyl)-penta-decanoic acid: A gas-liquid chromatographic-mass spectrometric analysis. *J Lipid Res* 1984; 25:1102–1108.

98. Daus HJ, Reske SN, Machulla HJ, et al. Omega-*p*-131-I-phenylpentadecanoic acid, a highly promising radioiodinated fatty acid for myocardial imaging studies, II: Biodistribution in mice and rabbits. In: Hoefer R, Bergmann H, Verlag H, eds. *Radioaktive Isotope in Klinik und Forschung*. Wien; 369–376; 1980.

99. Daus HJ, Reske SN, Vyska K, et al. Pharmakokinetics of 15-(*p*-123-I-phenyl)-pentadecanoic acid in heart. In: *Nuklearmedizin-Nuklearmedizin im interdisziplinaeren Bezug*. Schmidt HAE, Wolf F, Mahlstedt J, Schattauer FK, New York: Stuttgart; 1981:108–111.

100. Reske SN, Sauer W, Machulla HJ, et al. 15(*p*-[123I]iodophenyl)pentadecanoic acid as tracer of lipid metabolism: Comparison with [1–14-C-]palmitic acid in murine tissues. *J Nucl Med* 1984;25:1335–1342.

101. Reske SN, Schoen S, Schmitt W, et al. Effect of myocardial perfusion and metabolic inter-ventions on cardiac kinetics of phenylpentadecanoic acid (IPPA)I123. *Eur J Nucl Med* 1986; 12:S27–S31.

102. Kaiser KP, Geuting B, Grossmann K, et al. Tracer kinetics of 15-(ortho-123/131-I-phenyl)-pentadecanoic acid (oPPA) and 15-(para-123/131-I-phenyl)-pentadecanoic acid (*p*PPA) in animals and man. *J Nucl Med* 1990;31:1608–1616.

103. Chien KR, Han A, White J, et al. In vivo esterification of a synthetic 125-I-labeled fatty acid into cardiac glycerolipids. *Am J Physiol* 1983;245:H693–H697.

104. Kropp J, Ambrose KR, Knapp FF Jr, et al. Incorporation of radioiodinated IPPA and BMIPP fatty acid analogues into complex lipids from isolated rat hearts. *Nucl Med Biol* 1992;19:283–288.

105. Grossmann K, Geuting B, Kaiser KP, et al. Metabolism of ortho- and para-131-I-phenyl-pentadecanoic acid (oPPA and pPPA) in normal and POCA (phenylalkyl-oxirane carboxylic acid) treated rat hearts in vivo. *Nucl Compact* 1990;21:223–225.

106. Yamamichi Y, Kusuoka H, Morishita K, et al. Metabolism of iodine-123-BMIPP in perfused rat hearts. *J Nucl Med* 1995;36:1043–1050.

107. Knapp FF (Russ) Jr, Kropp J. Iodine-123-labeled fatty acids for myocardial single photon emission tomography: Current status and future perspectives. *Eur J Nucl Med*. 1995;22:361–381.

108. Wieler H, Kaiser KP, Kuikka JT, et al. Standardized noninvasive assessment of myocardial free fatty acid kinetics by means of 15-(*p*-iodo-phenyl)pentadecanoic acid (123I-pPPA) scintig-raphy: Clinical results. *Nucl Med Commun* 1992;13:168–185.

109. Heller GV, Iskandrian AE, Orlandi C, et al. Fasting and nonfasting iodine-123-iodophe-nylpentadecanoic acid myocardial SPECT imaging in coronary artery disease. *J Nucl Med* 1998; 39:2019–2022.

110. Goris ML, Daspit SG, McLaughlin P, et al. Interpolative background substraction. *J Nucl Med* 1976;17:744–747.

111. Kennedy PL, Corbett JR, Kulkarni PV, et al. Iodine 123-phenylpentadecanoic acid myocar-dial scintigraphy: Usefulness in the identification of myocardial ischemia. *Circulation* 1986; 74:1007–1015.

112. Kuikka JT, Musalo H, Hietakorpi S, et al. Evaluation of myocardial viability with technetium-99m hexakis-2-methoxyisobutyl isonitrile and iodine-123 phenylpentadecanoic acid and sin-gle photon emission tomography. *Eur J Nucl Med* 1992;19:882–889.

113. Murray GL, Schad N, Magill HL. Dynamic low dose I-123-iodophenylpentadecanoic acid metabolic cardiac imaging: Comparison to myocardial biopsy and reinjection SPECT thal-lium in ischemic cardiomyopathy and cardiac transplantation. *Ann Nucl Med* 1993;7:SII79–SII85.

114. Pippin JJ, Jansen DE, Henderson EB, et al. Myocardial fatty acid utilization at various workloads in normal volunteers: Iodine-123 phenylpentadecanoic acid and single photon emission computed tomography to investigate myocardial metabolism. *Am J Cardiol Imag-ing* 1992;6:99–108.

115. Hansen CL, Corbett JR, Pippin JJ, et al. Iodine-123 phenylpentadecanoic acid and single photon emission computed tomography in identifying left ventricular metabolic abnormalities in patients with coronary heart disease: Comparison with thallium-201 myocardial tomography. *J Am Coll Cardiol* 1988;12:78–87.

116. Zimmermann R, Rauch B, Kapp M, et al. Myocardial scintigraphy with iodine-123 phenylpentadecanoic acid and thallium-201 in patients with coronary artery disease: A comparative dual-isotope study. *Eur J Nucl Med* 1992;19:946–954.

117. Schad N, Daus HJ, Ciavolella M, et al. Noninvasive functional imaging of regional rate of myocardial fatty acids metabolism. *Cardiologia* 1987;32:239–247.

118. Schad N. Dynamic IPPA studies: Techniques and applications. *Ann Nucl Med* 1993;7: SII57–SII58.

119. Ugolini V, Hansen CL, Kulkarni PV, et al. Abnormal myocardial fatty acid metabolism in dilated cardiomyopathy detected by iodine-123 phenylpentadecanoic acid and tomographic imaging. *Am J Cardiol* 1988;62:923–928.

120. Wolfe CL, Kennedy PL, Kulkarni PV, et al. Iodine-123 phenylpentadecanoic acid myocardial scintigraphy in patients with left ventricular hypertrophy: Alterations in left ventricular distribution and utilization. *Am Heart J* 1990;119:1338–1347.

121. Yonekura Y, Brill AB, Som P, et al. Regional myocardial substrate uptake in hypertensive rats: A quantitative autoradiographic measurement. *Science* 1985;227:1494–1496.

122. Dimauro S, Bonilla E, Zeviani M. Mitochondrial myopathies. *Ann Neurol* 1985;17:521–526.

123. Kropp J, Knapp FF Jr, Biersack HJ. Clinical use of fatty acids. In: Limouris GS, Shukla SK, Biersack KJ, eds. *Radionuclides for Cardiology*. Athens: Mediterra; 1994:159–204.

124. Turnbull DM, Sherratt HSA, Mitochondrial myopathies: Defects in β-oxidation. *Biochem Soc Trans.* 1985;13:645–648.

125. Knapp FF Jr, Ambrose KR, Callahan AP, et al. Tellurium-123m-labeled isosteres of palmitoleic and oleic acids show high myocardial uptake. In: Radiopharmaceuticals, II: Proceedings 2nd International Symposium Radiopharmaceuticals. New York: Society of Nuclear Medicine; 1979:101–108.

126. Knapp FF Jr. Selenium and tellurium as acron substitutes. In: Spencer PP, ed. *Radiopharmaceuticals: Structure-Activity Relationships*. New York: Grune and Stratton, Inc.; 1981:345–391.

127. Okada RD, Knapp FF Jr, Elmaleh DR, et al. Tellurium 123m-labeled-9-telluraheptadecanoic acid: A possible cardiac imaging agent. *Circulation* 1982;65:305–310.

128. Elmaleh DR, Knapp FF Jr, Yasuda T, et al. Myocardial imaging with 9-[Te-123m]telluraheptadecanoic acid. *J Nucl Med* 1981;22:994–999.

129. Okada RD, Knapp FF Jr, Goodman MM, et al. Tellurium labeled fatty acid analogs: Relationship of heteroatom position to myocardial kinetics. *Eur J Nucl Med* 1985;11:156–161.

130. Goodman MM, Knapp FF Jr, Callahan AP, et al. A new, well retained myocardial imaging agent: Radioiodinated 15-(*p*-iodophenyl)-6-tellurapentadecanoic acid. *J Nucl Med* 1982;23:904–908.

131. Bianco JA, Pape LA, Alpert JS, et al. Accumulation of radioiodinated 15-(*p*-iodophenyl)-6-tellurapentadecanoic acid in ischemic myocardium during acute coronary occlusion and reperfusion. *J Am Coll Cardiol* 1984;4:80–87.

132. Pochapsky SS, VanBrocklin HF, Welch MJ, et al. Synthesis and tissue distribution of fluorine-18 labeled trifluorhexadecanoic acids. Consideration in the development of metabolically blocked myocardial imaging agents. *Bioconjug Chem* 1990;1:231–244.

133. DeGrado TR, Coenen HH, Stoecklin G. 14(R,S,)-[18-F]fluoro-6-thia-heptadecanoic acid (FTHA): Evaluation in mouse of a new probe of myocardial utilization of long chain fatty acids. *J Nucl Med* 1991;32:1888–1896.

134. Hovik R, Osmundsen H, Berge R, et al. Effect of thia-substituted fatty acids on mitochondrial and peroxisomal beta oxidation. Studies in vivo and in vitro. *Biochem Biophys Acta* 1990;270:167–173.

135. Skrede S, Narce M, Bergseth S, et al. The effects of alkylthioacetic acids (3-thia fatty acids) on fatty acid metabolism in isolated hepatocytes. *Biochim Biophys Acta* 1989;268:296–302.

136. Ebert A, Herzog H, Stoecklin GL, et al. Kinetics of 14(R,S)-fluorine-18-fluoro-6-thia-heptadecanoic acid in normal human hearts at rest, during exercise and after dipyridamole injection. *J Nucl Med* 1994;35:51–56.

137. Mäki M, Haaparanta M, Nuutila P, et al. Free fatty acid uptake in the myocardium and sceletal muscle using fluorine-18-fluoro-6-thia-heptadecanoic acid. J Nucl Med. 1998;39:3120–1327.
138. Renstrom B, Rommelfanger S, Stone CK, et al. Comparison of fatty acid tracers FTHA and BMIPP during myocardial ischemia and hypoxia. *J Nucl Med* 1998;39:1684–1689.
139. Livni E, Elmaleh DR, Levy S, et al. Beta-methyl[1–11-C]heptadecanoic acid: A new myocardial metabolic tracer for positron emission tomography. *J Nucl Med* 1982;23:169–175.
140. Fink GD, Montgomery JA, David F, et al. Metabolism of β-methyl-heptadecanoic acid in the perfused rat heart and liver. *J Nucl Med* 1990;31:1823–1830.
141. Elmaleh DR, Livni E, Alpert NM, et al. Myocardial extraction of 1-[11-C]betamethylheptadecanoic acid. *J Nucl Med* 1994;35:496–503.
142. Jones GS, Livni E, Strauss HW, et al. Synthesis and biologic evaluation of 1-[11-C]-3,3-dimethylheptadecanoic acid. *J Nucl Med* 1988;29:68–72.
143. Goodman MM, Neff KN, Ambrose KR, et al. Effect of 3-methyl-branching on the myocardial retention of radioiodinated 19-iodo-18-nonadecenoic acid analogues. *Nucl Med Biol* 1989; 16:813–819.
144. Goodman MM, Kirsch G, Knapp FF Jr. Synthesis of radioiodinated ω-p-(iodophenyl)-substituted methyl-branched long chain fatty acids. *J Lab Cpd Radiopharm* 1982;19:1316–1318.
145. Goodman MM, Kirsch G, Knapp FF Jr. Synthesis and evaluation of radioiodinated terminal p-iodo-phenyl-substituted α- and β-methyl-branched fatty acids. *J Med Chem* 1984;27:390–397.
146. Knapp FF, Kropp J, Goodman MM, et al. The development of iodine-123-methyl-branched fatty acids and their application in nuclear cardiology. *Ann Nucl Med* 1993;7:SII1–SII14.
147. Miller DD, Gill JB, Livni E, et al. Fatty acid analogue accumulation: A marker of myocyte viability in ischemic-reperfused myocardium. *Circulation Res* 1988;63:681–692.
148. Nakai K, Ahmad M, Nakaki M, et al. Serial course of left ventricular function, perfusion and fatty acid uptake in the cardiomyopathic hamster. *J Nucl Med* 1993;34:1309–1315.
149. Saito T, Yasuda T, Gold HK, et al. Differentiation of regional perfusion and fatty acid uptake in zones of myocardial injury. *Nucl Med Commun* 1991;12:663–675.
150. Whitmer JT. Energy metabolism and mechanical function in perfused hearts of Syrian hamsters with dilated or hypertrophic cardiomyopathy. *J Mol Cell Cardiol* 1986;18:307–317.
151. Reinhardt CP, Weinstein H, Marcel R, et al. Comparison of iodine-123-BMIPP and thallium-201 in myocardial hypoperfusion. *J Nucl Med* 1995;36:1645–1653.
152. Fujibayashi Y, Yonekura Y, Tamaki N, et al. Myocardial accumulation of BMIPP in relation to ATP concentration. *Ann Nucl Med* 1993;7:15–18.
153. Ambrose KR, Owen BA, Goodman MM, et al. Evaluation of the metabolism in rat hearts of two new radioiodinated 3-methyl-branched fatty acid myocardial imaging agents. *Eur J Nucl Med* 1987;12:486–491.
154. Humbert T, Keriel C, Batelle DM, et al. Influence of the presence of a methyl group on the myocardial metabolism of 15-(para-iodophenyl)-3-methyl pentadecanoic acid (IMPPA). *Nucl Med Biol* 1990;17:745–749.
155. Humbert T, Luu-Doc C, Comet M, et al. Evaluation of cellular viability by quantitative autoradiographic study of myocardial uptake of a fatty acid analogue in isoproterenol-induced focal rat heart necrosis. *Eur J Nucl Med* 1991;18:870–878.
156. Kropp J, Joergens M, Glaenzer KP, et al. Evaluation of ischemia and myocardial viability in patients with coronary artery disease (CAD) with iodine-123 labeled 15-(p-iodophenyl)-3-R,S-methylpentadecanoic acid (BMIPP). *Ann Nucl Med* 1993;7:SII3–SII100.
157. De Geeter F, Caveliers V, Pansar I, et al. Effects of oral glucose loading on the biodistribution of BMIPP in normal volunteers. *J Nucl Med* 1998;39:1850–1856.
158. Hosokawa R, Nohara R, Fujibayashi Y, et al. Metabolic fate of iodine-123-BMIPP in canine myocardium after administration of Etomoxir. *J Nucl Med* 1996;37:1836–1840.
159. Dormehl IC, Hugo N, Rossouw D, et al. Planar myocardial imaging in the baboon model with iodine-123–15-(iodophenyl)pentadecanoic acid (IPPA) and iodine-123–15-(p-iodophenyl)-3-R,S-methylpentadecanoic acid (BMIPP), using time activity curves for evaluation of metabolism. *Nucl Med Biol* 1995;22:837–847.

160. Dormehl I, Feinendegen L, Hugo N, et al. Comparative myocardial imaging in the baboon with 123-I-labeled ortho and para isomers of 15-(iodophenyl)pentadecanoic acid (IPPA). *Nucl Med Commun* 1993;14:998–1004.

161. Knapp FF Jr, Goodman MM, Callahan AP, et al. Radioiodinated 15-(*p*-iodophenyl)-3,3-dimethylpentadecanoic acid: A useful new agent to evaluate myocardial fatty acid uptake. *J Nucl Med* 1986;27:521–531.

162. Sloof GW, Visser FC, Eenige van MJ, et al. Comparison of uptake, oxidation and lipid distribution of 17-iodoheptadecanoic acid, 15-(*p*-iodophenyl)pentadecanoic acid and 15-(*p*-iodophenyl)-3,3-dimethylpentadecanoic acid in normal canine myocardium. *J Nucl Med* 1993;34:649–657.

163. Reske SN, Knapp FF, Nitsch J, et al. 3,3-dimethyl-(*p*-I-123-phenyl)-pentadecanoic acid (DMIPP) uptake is excess to rMBF in reperfused myocardium. *Eur J Nucl Med* 1989;15:399.

164. Ambrose KR, Owen BA, Callahan AP, et al. Effects of fasting on the myocardial subcellular distribution and lipid distribution of terminal *p*-iodophenyl-substituted fatty acids in rats. *Nucl Med Biol* 1988;15:695–700.

165. Knapp FF Jr. Myocardial metabolism of radioiodinated BMIPP. *J Nucl Med* 1995;36:1051–1054.

166. Nohara R, Okuda K, Ogino M, et al. Evaluation of myocardial viability with iodine-123 BMIPP in a canine model. *J Nucl Med* 1996;37:1403–1407.

167. Ito T, Tanouchi J, Kato J, et al. Recovery of impaired left ventricular function in patients with acute myocardial infarction is predicted by the discordance in defect size on 123-I-BMIPP and 201-Tl SPECT images. *Eur J Nucl Med* 1996;23:917–923.

168. Tamaki N, Yonekura Y, Yamashita K, et al. Relation of left ventricular perfusion and wall motion with metabolic activity in persistent defects on thallium-201 tomography in healed myocardial infarction. *Am J Cardiol* 1988;62:202–208.

169. Tamaki N, Kawamoto M, Yonekura Y, et al. Regional metabolic abnormality in relation to perfusion and wall motion in patients with myocardial infarction: Assessment with emission tomography using an iodinated branched fatty acid analog. *J Nucl Med* 1992;33:659–667.

170. Kairento AL, Livni E, Mattila S, et al. Comparative evaluation of [123-I]4-*p*-iodophenyl-beta-methyltetradecanoic acid and thallium-201 in the detection of infarcted areas in the dog heart using SPECT. *Nucl Med Biol* 1988;15:333–338.

171. De Geeter F, Franken PR, Knapp FF Jr, et al. Relationship between blood flow and fatty acid metabolism in subacute myocardial infarction: A study by means of 99m-Tc-Sestamibi and 123-β-methyl-iodo-phenyl pentadecanoic acid. *Eur J Nucl Med* 1994;21:283–291.

172. Franken PR, De Geeter F, Dendale P, et al. Abnormal free fatty acid uptake in subacute myocardial infarction after coronary thrombolysis: Correlation with wall motion and inotropic reserve. *J Nucl Med* 1994;35:1758–1765.

173. Berthe C, Pierard LA, Hiernaux M, et al. Predicting the extent and location of coronary artery disease in acute myocardial infarction by echocardiography during dobutamine infusion. *Am J Cardiol* 1986;58:1167–1172.

174. Hambÿe A-SE, Vaerenberg MM, Dobbeleir AA, et al. Abnormal BMIPP uptake in chronically dysfunctional myocardial segments: Correlation with contractile response to low-dose dobutamine *J Nucl Med* 1998;39:1845–1850.

175. Tamaki N, Kawamoto M, Yonekura Y. Decreased uptake of I-123 BMIPP as a sign of enhanced glucose utilization assessed by FDG-PET. *J Nucl Med* 1991;32:1034.

176. Nakata T, Hashimoto A, Kobayashi H, et al. Outcome significance of thallium-201 and iodine-123-BMIPP perfusion-metabolism mismatch in preinfarction angina. *J Nucl Med* 1998;39:1492–1499.

177. Taki J, Nakajama K, Matsunari I, et al. Impairment of regional fatty acid uptake in relation to wall motion and thallium-201 uptake in ischemic but viable myocardium: Assessment with iodine-123 labeled beta-methyl-branched fatty acid. *Eur J Nucl Med* 1995;22:1385–1392.

178. Matsunari I, Saga T, Taki J, et al. Improved myocardial fatty acid utilization after PTCA. *J Nucl Med* 1995;36:1605–1607.

179. Yoshida S, Ito M, Mitsunami K, et al. Improved myocardial fatty acid metabolism after coronary angioplasty in chronic coronary artery disease. *J Nucl Med* 1998;39:933–938.

180. Yamamoto K, Som P, Brill AB, et al. Dual tracer autoradiographic study of β-methyl-(1–14-C)-heptadecanoic acid and 15-*p*-(131-I)-iodophenyl-β-methylpentadecanoic acid in normotensive and hypertensive rats. *J Nucl Med* 1986;27:1178–1183.

181. Kurata C, Tawarahara K, Taguchi T, et al. Myocardial emission computed tomography with iodine-123-labeled beta-methyl-branched fatty acid in patients with hypertrophic cardiomyopathy. *J Nucl Med* 1992;33:6–13.

182. Ohtsuki K, Sugihara H, Umamoto I, et al. Clinical evaluation of hypertrophic cardiomyopathy by myocardial scintigraphy using 123-I-labeled 15-(*p*-iodophenyl)-3,-*R*,*S*-methylpentadecanoic acid (123I-BMIPP). *Nucl Med Commun* 1994;15:441–447.

183. Taki J, Nakajima K, Bunko H, et al. 123-I-labeled BMIPP fatty acid myocardial scintigraphy in patients with hypertrophic cardiomyopathy: SPECT comparison with stress 201-Tl. *Nucl Med Commun* 1993;14:181–188.

184. Takeishi Y, Chiba J, Abne S, et al. Heterogeneous myocardial distribution of iodine-123 15-(*p*-iodophenyl)-3-*R*,*S*-methylpentadecanoic acid (BMIPP) in patients with hypertrophic cardiomyopathy. *Eur J Nucl Med* 1992;19:775–782.

185. Wakasugi S, Fischman AJ, Babich JW, et al. Myocardial substrate utilization and left ventricular function in adriamycin cardiomyopathy. *J Nucl Med* 1993;34:1529–1535.

186. Antar MA, Spohr G, Herzog HH, et al. 15-(ortho-123-I-phenyl)-pentadecanoic acid, a new myocardial imaging agent for clinical use. *Nucl Med Commun* 1986;7:683–696.

187. Geuting B, Grossmann K, Kaiser KP, et al. The different metabolic behavior of continuously infused 15-(ortho-131-I-phenyl)-pentadecanoic acid (oPPA) and 15-(para-131-I-phenyl)-pentadecanoic acid (pPPA) in the isolated perfused rat heart. *Nucl Compact* 1990;21:232–235.

188. Henrich MM, Vester E, von der Lohe E, et al. The comparison of 2–18-F-2-deoxyglucose and 15-(ortho-123-I-phenyl)-pentadecanoic acid uptake in persisting defects on thallium-201 tomography in myocardial infarction. *J Nucl Med* 1991;32:1353–1357.

189. Brunken R, Schwaiger M, Grover-McKay ME, et al. Positron emission tomography detects tissue metabolic activity in myocardial segments with persistent thallium perfusion defects. *J Am Coll Cardiol* 1987;10:557–567.

190. Franken PR, De Geeter F, Dendale P, et al. Regional distribution of 123-I-(ortho-iodophenyl)-pentadecanoic acid and 99m-Tc-MIBI in relation to wall motion after thrombolysis for acute myocardial infarction. *Nucl Med Commun* 1993;14:310–317.

191. Feinendegen LE, Henrich MM, Kuikka JT, et al. Myocardial lipid turnover in dilated cardiomyopathy: A dual in vivo tracer approach. *J Nucl Cardiol* 1995;2:42–52.

Positron Emission Tomography for the Assessment of Myocardial Viability:

Noninvasive Approach to Cardiac Pathophysiology

Heiko Schöder, MD and
Heinrich R. Schelbert, MD, PhD

Introduction

Positron emission tomography (PET) affords the noninvasive and quantitative assessment of myocardial blood flow (MBF) and metabolism. In clinical cardiology it is used most often for the analysis of extent and severity of coronary artery disease (CAD) and the assessment of "myocardial viability." Because leading cardiologists differ in their definition of the term ischemia,[1] the same appears to be true for the term viability. For practical purposes, we define it as regional left ventricular (LV) dysfunction which is reversible following coronary revascularization. Therefore, the term does not include normally contracting myocardium that only shows wall motion abnormalities during stress. Rather, this entity will be discussed separately in this chapter.

Reversible Left Ventricular Dysfunction—Implications for Positron Emission Tomography Imaging

The term viable myocardium does not necessarily preclude the presence of patchy areas of necrotic tissue. In a landmark study, Reimer and Jennings[2] described the so-called transmural wave front phenomenon of evolving myocardial infarction; that is, subendocardial myocardium is the first area that becomes functionally compromised when myocardial perfusion ceases. Likewise, one also would expect that cellular necrosis is not an all-or-non phenomenon in a given myocardial region. Therefore, tissue vulnerability may

From Dilsizian V (ed). *Myocardial Viability: A Clinical and Scientific Treatise.* Armonk, NY: Futura Publishing Co., Inc.; © 2000.

be related to inhomogeneities in residual blood flow and the occurrence of transient ischemic episodes. Depending on their frequency and severity, such transient ischemic episodes might cause patchy myocardial necrosis, morphological changes only at the microscopic level, or even exert a protective effect referred to as preconditioning. This concept is supported by recent morphological studies demonstrating a mixture of normal and abnormal myocytes and fibrotic tissue in dysfunctional myocardium which was classified as "viable" by PET.[3-5]

Clinical Findings—Myocardial Hibernation and Stunning

Functional abnormalities and impairment in MBF are associated with one another but do not necessarily occur in a parallel fashion. Examples are myocardial stunning and hibernation.[6-10] Both conditions characteristically exhibit an impairment in resting contractile function; in stunned myocardium as a response to preceding transient ischemic episodes, and in hibernating myocardium as a response to chronic hypoperfusion.

The classic concept of myocardial hibernation is derived from the clinical observations that patients with CAD may exhibit an improvement in regional contractile function in previously akinetic segments following revascularization.[10] The concept entails a concordant reduction in MBF and contractile function (perfusion contraction match), representing a new steady state between flow and function, though on a lower level. However, under experimental conditions, a proportional down-regulation of both myocardial perfusion and contractile function can be maintained only for short time periods.[11-13] Therefore, it remains uncertain whether these animal experimental findings can be extrapolated to the more complex situation in patients with chronic CAD and resting LV dysfunction. Consequently, the concept of myocardial hibernation has been challenged,[14] especially because quantitative PET measurements frequently revealed normal or nearly normal resting blood flow in chronically yet reversibly dysfunctional myocardium.[15-18] For instance, Vanoverschelde et al[18] studied patients with chronic CAD without prior myocardial infarction, yet with a completely occluded left anterior descending coronary artery. Regardless of presence or absence of wall motion abnormalities, the collateral dependent myocardium revealed normal or nearly normal resting flow and oxygen consumption. The only difference was a significantly reduced flow reserve in segments with impaired wall motion. Thus, these findings argue against the postulated perfusion–contraction match. In view of the normal resting blood flow, contractile dysfunction was attributed to repeated episodes of ischemia causing chronic stunning rather than to chronic hypoperfusion.

Further criticism to the concept of myocardial hibernation as a new steady state of supply and demand comes from histomorphological studies in patients with chronic LV dysfunction. The reported mixture of abnormal myocytes and fibrotic (scar) tissue suggest that the down-regulation of contractile function in response to decreased blood flow may be inadequate to maintain cellular integrity.[4,5,19] Myocytes in so-called hibernating myocardium may not survive indefinitely but rather undergo degeneration or apoptosis as a form of programmed cell death.[20] Long-term persistence of a balance between reduced flow and reduced contractile function (true hibernation) in patients with chronic CAD appears therefore uncertain. More likely, in the clinical setting there is a wide overlap of hibernation and stunning.[21] This scenario might even represent the majority of clinical cases with ischemic cardiomyopathy in which myocardial perfusion is reduced chronically but may fluctuate because of loss of autoregulatory compensating mechanisms. Reversibly dysfunctional myocardium responds to acute inotropic stimulation; however, the improvement in contractile function is accompanied by increased glucose utilization and a decrease in lactate extraction or lactate production.[2,22-24] Thus, intermittent increases in oxygen demand may not be accompanied by proportional increases in perfusion because of the impaired flow reserve. The resulting myocardial ischemia causes contractile dysfunction, which may persist even when oxygen demand and supply reach a balance again ("repetitive stunning"). Metabolic alterations in glucose utilization and oxidative metabolism in previously ischemic segments also may persist for some time after restoration of normal perfusion.[25–27]

Metabolic Alterations in Ischemic Myocardium

Myocardial ischemia entails an absolute or relative reduction in MBF leading to (1) inadequate supply of oxygen and nutrients and (2) limited washout of metabolites. Both factors alter myocardial substrate metabolism. Ischemia triggers a switch from predominantly free fatty acid metabolism to predominantly glucose metabolism as the main source of adenosine triphosphate (ATP) production.[28] Similarly, in chronically ischemic myocardium, glucose uptake is higher than in normal tissue and relatively independent from plasma substrate and insulin concentrations. Nevertheless, insulin may increase glucose utilization in both normal and dysfunctional myocardium, suggesting that glucose uptake in dysfunctional myocardium is not regulated only by local factors.[29]

During mild to moderate ischemia, increased glucose uptake and glycolysis may represent an important source of ATP which is primarily used for maintaining balanced plasma membrane ion fluxes.[35] However, more severe and chronic ischemia may limit myocardial glucose uptake by decreasing delivery. In addition, chronic ischemia causes an inhibition of oxidative metabolism, that is, the tricarboxylic acid (TCA) cycle and its regulatory enzymes. Cardiac metabolism relies then increasingly on anaerobic glycolysis. Yet, when tissue perfusion declines and no longer removes accumulating metabolites, acidosis and lactate accumulation inhibit further glycolysis.[36–38] In response, decreased ATP production and/or impaired energy utilization[39] lead to an impairment in cardiac function.

Under normal conditions the myocardial glucose uptake largely depends on the glucose transporter GLUT-4, which is regulated by insulin (Fig. 1). Ischemia and hypoxia[30] as well as increased levels of circulating catecholamines[31] may cause increased translocation of GLUT-4 from the cytoplasm to the sarcolemma. A similar translocation also has been described for GLUT-1,[32] the insulin-independent glucose transporter. In animal experiments, 6 hours of regional ischemia caused an increase in mRNA and polypeptide expression of GLUT-1. However, such increase was observed in both ischemic and nonischemic myocardium,[33] suggesting that (1) increased GLUT-1 expression is not responsible for increased glucose uptake in ischemic myocardium and (2) ischemia influences GLUT-1 expression only indirectly, for example, via release of mediator substances, which, in turn, cause GLUT-1 expression in the entire myocardium. In another study,[34] 60–90 minutes of moderate flow reduction caused an increased translocation of GLUT-4 and, to a lesser extent, also GLUT-1 from their intracellular storage pool to the sarcolemma. This was associated with increased glucose uptake in ischemic myocardium. Unfortunately, these findings during transient ischemia do not elucidate mechanisms involved in altered glucose metabolism [and hence potential mechanisms for increased ^{18}F-2-deoxyglucose (FDG) uptake] in chronically ischemic myocardium.

Reversibly dysfunctional *human* myocardium also shows increased gene expression of GLUT-1.[40] This augmented expression of glucose transporters was thought to explain the increased FDG uptake and glycogen content in abnormal myocytes found frequently in chronic dysfunctional myocardium.[3,5,19] However, such increased glycogen storage can be found in segments with preserved as well as reduced FDG uptake and at least one study observed a wide overlap in the degree of glycogen storage between segments with normal and abnormal wall motion.[3]

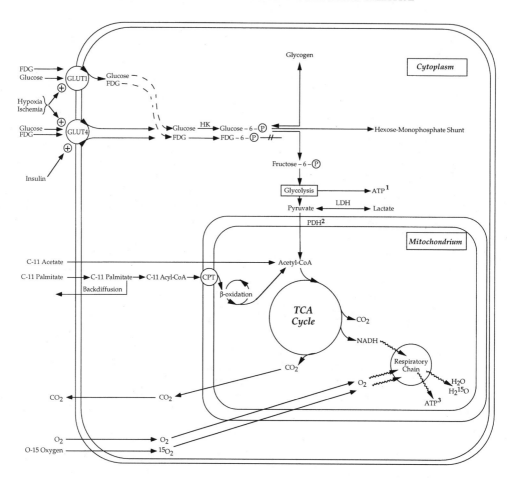

Figure 1. Scheme of cardiac metabolism and metabolic positron emission tomography (PET) tracers. The insulin-sensitive glucose transporter GLUT-4 accounts for the majority of glucose taken up by the myocardium in the postprandial state. GLUT-4 and another glucose transporter GLUT-1 may be stimulated by ischemia and hypoxia. (1) Adenosine triphosphate (ATP) produced by glycolysis is used predominantly for control of sarcolemmal ion flux and membrane potential. (2) Pyruvate dehydrogenase (PDH) is a key enzyme regulating substrate flux into the tricarboxylic acid cycle. (3) ATP derived from oxidative phosphorylation is used predominantly for contractile function. Stimulation of glucose metabolism can be achieved by glucose loading or pharmacologically by inhibition of lipolysis (eg, nicotinic acid derivatives) or inhibition of carnitine palmitoyl transferase (CPT1). Abbreviations: HK, hexokinase; LDH, lactate dehydrogenase; PDH, pyruvate dehydrogenase; CPT, carnitine palmitoyl transferase.

Detection of Viable Myocardium by Positron Emission Tomography

Introduction

Features critical for myocardial viability include the following:

1. Preservation of transmembrane ion concentration fluxes that depend on:
2. Persistence of some metabolic activity for production of ATP, which in turn depends on:

3. Some residual blood flow for sufficient supply of substrates as well as for washout of inhibitory metabolites.

The above parameters can be examined with PET as follows:

1. Integrity of membrane function

- ^{82}Rb

2. Metabolic activity for ATP generation

- Oxidative metabolism
  i. ^{11}C-acetate
  ii. ^{15}O oxygen

- Glucose uptake and phosphorylation by hexokinase
  i. FDG

3. Residual MBF

- ^{13}N-ammonia
- ^{15}O-water
- ^{82}Rb

Myocardial Blood Flow and Membrane Integrity

Cell survival depends on persistence of some residual blood flow and metabolic activity. The degree of residual blood flow therefore may offer some information regarding myocardial viability. It has been suggested that autoregulatory mechanisms for MBF remain operational down to flows of 0.4–0.5 mL/min per gram so that intracoronary pressures are maintained for oxygen exchange from blood to tissue.[41] Indeed, in a pig model of short-term hibernation, no myocardial infarction developed when microsphere blood flow remained >0.34 mL/min per gram.[12] Others identified a residual blood flow of 20% of normal as the threshold below which tissue survival and hence functional recovery are unlikely to occur.[42–44] Likewise, regional FDG uptake, an indicator of tissue viability, decreases significantly when blood flow declines below 20% of preischemic levels.[45] As blood flow initially declines, reductions in oxygen delivery are partially compensated for by an increase in oxygen extraction. However, below this threshold oxygen utilization declines steeply and nonoxidative metabolism dominates. Under these conditions removal of metabolic end products, in particular lactic acid and hydrogen ions, becomes limited.[37]

Myocardial perfusion can be assessed with the positron tracers ^{82}Rb, ^{15}O-water, ^{13}N-ammonia, and ^{62}Cu PTSM (the latter still being in the stage of experimental validation). For quantification of absolute MBF in ml/min per gram of tissue, tracer compartment models have been developed for ^{82}Rb, ^{15}O-water, and ^{13}N-ammonia.[46–49] Measurements of resting MBF in normal subjects yield comparable data regardless of different methodological approaches.[46,48,50] Factors like personal preference and experience, availability of a given tracer, ease of synthesis, and proximity of a cyclotron frequently determine the choice of the flow tracer.

^{15}O-water is metabolically inert and its first-pass extraction fraction approximates unity, making it an ideal blood flow tracer. However, the tracer distributes equally in blood pool and myocardium. Therefore, subtraction of blood pool activity is necessary for better visualization of the myocardium and quantification of blood flow. This usually is performed by labeling the blood pool with inhaled carbon monoxide.

Compared with the freely diffusible ^{15}O-water, ^{13}N-ammonia and [82]Rb are extracted and retained by the myocardium. ^{13}N-ammonia has a physical half-life time of ~10 minutes and, after initial back-diffusion, becomes effectively trapped in the myocardium. This allows longer data acquisition, a prerequisite for high-count density images.

[82]Rb has a half-life time of only 75 seconds. This might be advantageous when repeated studies are to be performed. However, lower intrinsic resolution caused by higher positron energy (high-energy positrons travel a longer distance before colliding with an electron, thus producing two γ-photons) might degrade image quality. Nevertheless, images with quality comparable with those with ammonia can be achieved with larger doses of approximately 50 mCi.[51] This tracer also has been proposed as a marker of myocardial viability: The cation [82]Rb is a potassium analog and a leakage of potassium ions from myocytes is an early marker of impaired cell membrane integrity, which correlates well with creatine kinase release from ischemic myocardium.[52,53] Consequently, attempts have been undertaken to assess myocardial viability with the rubidium cation. The tracer reveals a first-pass extraction fraction that is similar in acutely ischemic, post-ischemic, and normal myocardium.[54] However, there is a lack of retention or rapid washout of rubidium from necrotic myocardium.[54–56] In animal experiments, myocardial washout of rubidium was increased markedly in the infarct zone and there was a strong correlation between tracer washout and the severity of myocardial injury.[57]

Cardiac Metabolism

Essential metabolic processes and currently available PET tracers for the study of myocardial metabolism are outlined in Figure 1.

Oxidative Metabolism

Most of the ATP expended into contractile work is derived from oxidative metabolism.[58] At reperfusion, following a transient period of ischemia, functional recovery is contingent on a return of oxidative metabolism.[26,59–61] For instance, in canine myocardium with short-term ischemia (3 hours), viable and nonviable myocardium differs in the magnitude of residual oxidative metabolism and the recovery of contractile function in viable myocardium parallels the recovery in oxidative metabolism.[26] Similar findings also were reported in a chronic animal model.[62]

All oxidative fuels are metabolized via conversion to acetyl-coenzyme A (CoA) and passage through the TCA cycle. Therefore, ^{11}C-acetate, which is converted directly to acetyl-CoA and not metabolized via other major pathways in the myocardium,[63,64] should be an ideal indicator of myocardial oxidative metabolism. Uptake of ^{11}C-acetate is homogenous throughout the myocardium[65–67] and the tracer kinetics are largely independent of changes in substrate availability.[68,69] TCA cycle flux is measured by the production of ^{11}C carbon dioxide, which correlates closely with tracer clearance from the myocardium.

The initial tracer uptake depends on blood flow and therefore yields an indirect estimate of regional myocardial perfusion.[70,71] For quantification of oxidative metabolism and oxygen consumption, tracer kinetic models have been developed and evaluated under experimental conditions.[67,68,72,73] Other tracer kinetic models allow measurement of MBF in absolute terms, which correlate closely with measurements by ^{13}N-ammonia.[74,75] Alternatively, myocardial oxygen consumption now can be measured directly with the positron tracer [15]O oxygen.[76,77] However, this approach has not been used yet for clinical studies.

Glucose Utilization

Myocardial glucose utilization can be evaluated with FDG. This glucose analog traces the initial metabolic steps of glucose, that is, transmembrane uptake and subsequent phosphorylation by hexokinase. The phosphorylated product, FDG-6-phosphate (FDG-6-P), is not metabolized further and dephosphorylation is slow. Therefore FDG remains essentially trapped in the cytosol.[78-81]

Uptake and utilization of exogenous glucose and FDG in the myocardium correlate linearly at steady state[82] but changing levels of insulin or competing substrates may alter the relation between glucose and FDG uptake.[82-85]

Based on data derived from dynamic imaging and a suitable tracer kinetic model, FDG utilization also can be quantified.[82,86] However, such a quantitative approach does not necessarily improve the accuracy of FDG imaging for the assessment of myocardial viability,[87] which mainly is related to interindividual as well as regional myocardial differences in glucose metabolism.

Cardiac Imaging with ^{18}F-2-deoxyglucose

Dietary State of the Patient

The dietary state of the patient profoundly influences myocardial glucose utilization. After an overnight fast, normal myocardium preferentially consumes fatty acids, so that glucose metabolism accounts for only 40% of the energy derived from oxidative metabolism. However, with increasing plasma glucose and insulin levels, glucose becomes the preferred fuel substrate.[28,88] Consequently, cardiac imaging with FDG can be performed after oral glucose administration (glucose-loaded state) or in the fasted state. Four to five hours of fasting are sufficient to suppress glucose utilization in normal myocardium.[28,88]

Theoretically, studies in fasted patients may be more sensitive in detecting viable tissue because a positive signal (tracer uptake) is better to detect against a negative background. However, detection of small and scattered islands of residual viable tissue is of little importance because revascularization usually will not result in an improvement in contractile function. Additionally, poor image quality caused by low-count statistics may preclude accurate alignment of myocardial segments because of a lack of anatomic landmarks. Therefore, the glucose-loaded state is preferable for identifying dysfunctional myocardium that will improve contractile function following revascularization.

For quantitative analysis, steady-state conditions of plasma glucose and insulin are required but may not be present after oral glucose loading. To minimize these limitations, the intravenous (IV) administration of FDG usually is delayed for 60 minutes after oral glucose administration. By then, glucose and insulin should have reached stable plasma levels and imaging after oral glucose loading or with euglycemic hyperinsulinemic clamp appears to be equally accurate.[89]

Patients With Diabetes Mellitus

Despite a general disturbance in glucose uptake and utilization in diabetic patients, ischemic myocardium appears to use preferentially glucose as a substrate but rates of uninterpretable studies as high as 28% have been reported.[90] However, with appropriate control of plasma glucose levels and, if necessary, IV injection of small amounts of regular short-acting insulin, good image quality can be achieved in the majority of diabetic patients[91,92] and the diagnostic accuracy of blood flow/FDG imaging remains high.[92] Alternatively, continuous infusion of insulin and intermittent supplementary infusion of glucose are used to achieve stable plasma glucose concentrations.[93] This technique stimulates myocardial glucose uptake in nondiabetic patients as well as those with insulin-dependent diabetes mellitus, which improves the myocardium to blood pool activity ratio and, hence, the image quality. On quantitative analysis, both groups show similar rates of glucose metabolism.[89,93]

Limitations of ^{18}F-2-deoxyglucose Imaging

Several potential limitations of FDG imaging should be mentioned briefly. Inhomogeneity of myocardial FDG uptake, in particular in the fasted state, may occur.[65,94] In the posterolateral wall of the left ventricle relatively increased FDG and decreased ammonia uptake have been described in healthy individuals. This pattern reflects a kind of "physiological mismatch" and is not related to myocardial ischemia.

Most studies employing blood flow/FDG PET imaging were performed in patients with chronic CAD and at this time it remains uncertain whether the technique has the same accuracy in the early postinfarction period. It has been suggested that augmented glucose metabolism in hypoperfused myocardial segments may not be followed necessarily by an improvement in regional function after coronary revascularization in patients with recent myocardial infarction.[95,96] However, these studies did not use the original methodological approach: Relative FDG uptake was not normalized to areas with normal flow but rather to segments with maximal FDG uptake, which might explain discrepant results.

Last, FDG uptake has been reported in areas of acute myocardial infarction.[88,97] This probably reflects phagocytosis of FDG by monocytes and macrophages that accumulate in infarcted tissue. The phenomenon appears to be insignificant because leukocytes mainly are entrapped in necrotic regions where glucose uptake is decreased.[98]

Combined Blood Flow/Metabolism Imaging

Over the last decade data from clinical studies have substantiated the use of PET imaging for the assessment of myocardial viability. Most often used and today considered the "gold standard" is the combined analysis of myocardial perfusion and glucose utilization (by FDG) in corresponding myocardial segments. Three regional patterns of blood flow and glucose uptake have been identified[99,100] in dysfunctional myocardium of patients with chronic CAD, acute myocardial infarction, or stress-induced ischemia.[61,101–107]

These patterns include the following (Fig. 2):

- Normal—normal blood flow and glucose utilization
- Match—concordant reduction in regional blood flow and glucose utilization
- Mismatch—regional decrease in MBF with maintained or augmented glucose utilization.

The mismatch pattern has been associated with reversible myocardial dysfunction. However, the term "mismatch" does not necessarily imply the potential for full recovery of contractile function because scar and viable tissue frequently coexist in a given myocardial segment. For example, a subendocardial infarction may be associated with viable myocardium in the mid- and subepicardial layers of the myocardium,

NORMAL

NH₃

FDG

MATCH

NH₃

FDG

MISMATCH

NH₃

FDG

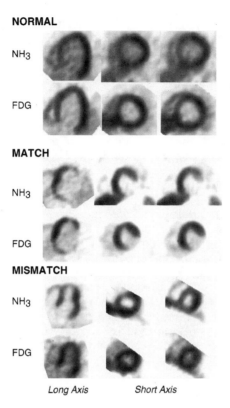

Long Axis   Short Axis

Figure 2. Patterns of myocardial blood flow (MBF)/glucose metabolism in horizontal long-axis and short-axis cuts of the left ventricle.

which precludes recovery of segmental contraction. Conversely, the term "match," although frequently used as a synonym for scar tissue, only implies that contractile function is unlikely to improve after revascularization.[100]

Alternative Imaging Protocols

For the combined perfusion/metabolism approach, institutions without a nearby cyclotron may prefer the combined single photon emission computer tomography (SPECT) perfusion and FDG PET approach (satellite PET concept). From a theoretical point of view the lack of attenuation correction for SPECT data may become a problem. Data based on analysis of myocardial perfusion using SPECT followed by FDG PET show nevertheless good agreement with those from PET imaging.[108–112]

In the past, thallium rest-redistribution has been thought to be an effective alternative for the detection of viable myocardium if FDG imaging is not available.[113,114] With special high-energy collimation it is now possible to perform FDG SPECT imaging.[115–120] In addition, new γ-cameras, which afford coincidence detection as well as attenuation correction algorithms, are currently being tested and should provide further improvement in FDG SPECT image quality.

Assessment of Viable Myocardium in Patients With Coronary Artery Disease

Clinical Relevance

PET for the assessment of myocardial viability is used most often in patients with ischemic cardiomyopathy. Therapeutic choices range from pharmacologic treatment to revascularization and cardiac transplantation. In three recent studies[121–123] the mortality for patients with ischemic cardiomyopathy and LV ejection fraction (LVEF) of ≤40% undergoing medical treatment ranged from 11% to 26% at 1 year and from 40% to 70% for 5 years.

Heart transplantation, a therapeutic alternative for patients with ischemic cardiomyopathy, suffers from rising costs and the limited number of donor hearts. This has led to a reexamination of coronary revascularization as a treatment. In unselected patients with end-stage CAD the long-term benefit of coronary revascularization exceeds that of medical therapy.[124] However, the main problem that remains is how to identify those patients who are likely to benefit most from bypass surgery. Despite recent advances in anesthesia, myocardial protection, and completeness of revascularization, the perioperative mortality in this patient population remains as high as 10%.[125–128] Therefore, from an ethical as well as economic aspect a risk-benefit analysis is necessary to decide which therapeutic approach should be chosen in an individual patient with ischemic cardiomyopathy.

Myocardial Blood Flow

Determination of Absolute Blood Flow Values

As expected, myocardial segments with reversible dysfunction demonstrate higher absolute blood flows than those with irreversible dysfunction. Consequently, attempts have been undertaken to utilize measurements of absolute MBF to distinguish reversibly from irreversibly dysfunctional myocardium and to define a certain threshold below which functional recovery is unlikely to occur.

In one study[129] viable myocardium was rarely present when blood flow fell below 0.25 mL/min per gram or 35% of normal flow, while blood flows >0.39 mL/min per gram were considered to indicate presence of viable myocardium based on preserved FDG uptake. In another study[130] the mean MBF in necrotic segments as judged by the FDG uptake was 0.45 mL/min per gram.

None of these above studies reported outcome data to assure the accuracy or limitations of this approach and only recently several studies that include patient follow-up have been reported. For instance, in a recent study by Wolpers et al,[74] MBF was the only independent predictor for functional recovery after revascularization in patients with acute myocardial infarction. Absolute blood flow was lower in segments with unchanged impairment of wall motion after revascularization (0.43 ± 0.18 mL/min per gram) compared with those that improved (0.73 ± 0.18 mL/min per gram) or normalized completely (0.85 ± 0.18 mL/min per gram).

Others found a significant negative correlation between the extent of fibrotic tissue, known to be a strong predictor for a postrevascularization improvement in ventricular function,[5,19] and the degree of residual MBF. However, even in this study, multiple regression analysis revealed absolute MBF as one, but not the strongest independent parameter for a functional improvement following revascularization.[5] In other studies,

Table 1

Table 1

Absolute Measurements of Myocardial Blood Flow in Normal, Reversibly, and Irreversibly Dysfunctional Myocardium

Author	Number Patients	Gold Standard	Tracer of Myocardial Blood Flow (MBF)	MBF in Normal Segments	MBF in Reversibly Dysfunctional Segments	MBF in Irreversibly Dysfunctional Segments
Gewirtz[129]	26	^{18}F-2-deoxyglucose (FDG) uptake	Ammonia	0.81 ± 0.23	>0.40	<0.25
Beanlands[130]	16	FDG uptake	Ammonia			<0.45
Grandin[132]	25	Recovery	Ammonia	0.93 ± 0.17	0.57 ± 0.19	0.77 ± 0.20
Deprè[5]	24	Recovery	Ammonia	N/A*	0.61 ± 0.12	0.88 ± 0.23
Wolpers[74]	30	Recovery	Acetate	1.04 ± 0.27	0.75 ± 0.18	0.43 ± 0.18
De Silva[136]	12	Recovery	Water	0.97 ± 0.22	0.73 ± 0.18	0.45 ± 0.11
Sun[24]	19	Mismatch	Ammonia	0.73 ± 0.23	0.53 ± 0.33	0.28 ± 0.09
Gerber[16]	39	Recovery	Ammonia	0.82 ± 0.18	0.96 ± 0.27	0.63 ± 0.26

Units are milliliters per minute per gram myocardial tissue.
* N/A, not applicable.

which also correlated histological alterations with PET findings, the postsurgical functional improvement was not predicted by preoperative flow values.[3]

Evidence for the contrary comes from a study by Czernin et al[61] who studied 22 patients with recent myocardial infarction using PET imaging with ^{13}N-ammonia, FDG, and ^{11}C-acetate. Myocardial blood flow in areas with concordant reduction in blood flow and glucose metabolism (match) averaged 0.32 ± 0.12 mL/min per gram. Oxidative metabolism was reduced severely in proportion to blood flow in these regions. However, despite statistical significance there was considerable overlap in flow values between segments with match, mismatch, and remote myocardium, indicating that measurement of blood flow alone is an unreliable method to assess tissue viability. Similar findings also were reported by Brunken et al.[131]

Grandin et al[132] studied patients with chronic CAD and preserved LV function. Reversibly dysfunctional myocardium exhibited higher absolute blood flows. However, a closer examination of these data reveals a considerable overlap in flow values between myocardial segments with reversible and irreversible dysfunction (0.77 ± 0.20 versus 0.57 ± 0.09 mL/min per gram), indicating that individual flow values discriminate poorly between viable and nonviable myocardium.

Finally, Tamaki et al[133] found resting flow studies to have the lowest accuracy for an improvement in regional LV function after revascularization: The positive and negative predictive accuracy of resting flow defects was 46% and 87%, as compared with 69% and 87% for stress-induced flow defects and 76% and 92% for the blood flow/glucose metabolism approach.

Semiquantitative methods to assess viable myocardium with flow tracers using either SPECT or PET and relative tracer activity distribution[134,135] also have been explored and found to be of limited value. In fact, one of these studies failed to demonstrate any correlation between the relative severity of flow defects and the presence of myocardial viability.[134]

Table 1 summarizes several recent studies and demonstrates the considerable variance in blood flow values in myocardial segments considered viable versus nonviable.

The Water Perfusable Tissue Index

Because restoration of blood flow can improve regional wall motion only in the absence of significant amounts of subendocardial scar tissue, it has been proposed that blood flow should be analyzed separately in the residual noninfarcted tissue in any given myocardial segment. This is the concept of the water perfusable tissue index (PTI), which is based on measurements of MBF with ^{15}O-water.[136,137] The index describes the myocardial tissue fraction that is able to rapidly exchange water, assuming that only viable myocardium exchanges water rapidly.

Yamamoto et al[137] studied a group of 26 patients with acute or chronic myocardial infarction. Regional glucose metabolism was considered the gold standard to indicate myocardial viability. In a control population, the PTI was 1.08 ± 0.07. The PTI in areas considered viable by blood flow/metabolism imaging, measured 0.75 ± 0.14 compared with 0.53 ± 0.12 $(p < 0.01)$ in nonviable segments. In a subgroup of early postinfarct patients who underwent successful thrombolysis, myocardial segments with functional recovery of wall motion had a PTI of 0.84 ± 0.10 as compared with 0.53 ± 0.11 in segments without recovery. Absolute MBFs were not different. In another study in 12 patients,[136] the same group reported that contractile function recovered only if the PTI was in excess of 0.7, that is, if at least 70% of the myocardial mass exchanged water rapidly. For example, the PTI averaged 0.99 ± 0.15 and thus was essentially normal, in segments with recovery of wall motion following revascularization. In contrast, if the PTI was <0.7 function did not improve (average 0.62 ± 0.06). Although these observations are intriguing, further validation of this method is needed.

In summary, quantitation of MBF alone appears to be of limited value for the detection of myocardial viability. Although severe reductions in blood flow may indicate irreversible LV dysfunction (ie, scar tissue), intermediate flow reductions are more difficult to interpret but do occur in the majority of patients in whom the assessment of myocardial viability is of clinical relevance. Therefore, additional methods are needed to better define these patients who are likely to benefit from coronary revascularization. Such methods might be based on the evaluation of membrane integrity (^{82}Rb kinetics), myocardial metabolism (^{11}C-acetate or palmitate and FDG), or contractile reserve (dobutamine echocardiography).

Assessment of Membrane Integrity

^{82}Rb also has been used for the assessment of myocardial viability. In patients with acute myocardial infarction, the uptake and rate of regional washout of ^{82}Rb were analyzed and compared with FDG uptake.[97,138] Uptake and retention of ^{82}Rb denoted viable myocardium as accurate as FDG. On follow-up in a subset of these patients, myocardial infarct size by ^{82}Rb (no tracer uptake or immediate washout) was related inversely to the cumulative 3-year mortality.[138] In patients with a reduced LV function (LVEF $\leq$ 43%) the absence of viable myocardium was an independent predictor of outcome; the mortality was 63% in patients without compared with 13% in those with viable myocardium.

Care must be taken when interpreting these data because 70% of the patients (in particular the vast majority of those with viable myocardium) underwent coronary revascularization during follow-up, regardless of their PET findings. The mortality rate in patients with viable myocardium was 8%; in those with nonviable myocardium it was 50%. In contrast to the authors own conclusion these findings therefore suggest that those patients with viable myocardium, who undergo coronary bypass surgery, have a good prognosis. This is in concordance with other reports that found presence and extent (and not the absence) of viable myocardium to be indicators of poor prognosis if no revascularization is performed.[139-141]

Others[142] analyzed regional Rb kinetics in patients with previous myocardial infarction and compared them with FDG uptake, which served as the gold standard for myocardial viability. Although the average Rb tissue clearance time was significantly different between normal, ischemic, and scar tissue, the data revealed a considerable scatter and overlap between the two latter groups, thereby compromising the clinical value of this approach.

Metabolic Activity as Parameter for Reversibly Dysfunctional Myocardium

First studies using metabolic PET imaging as a marker of myocardial viability date back to the 1980s and explored myocardial perfusion and glucose metabolism in dysfunctional myocardium of patients with CAD.[99,100,106] In their initial study, Tillisch et al[100] included 17 patients with 73 dysfunctional myocardial regions. Sixty-seven of these regions were revascularized adequately. At follow-up after 3 months, wall motion had improved significantly in 85% of segments with normal blood flow and glucose metabolism or blood flow/metabolism mismatches. In contrast, only 8% of segments with blood flow/metabolism match showed functional improvement. In these initial studies,[100,106] positive predictive values were 85% and 78% and negative predictive values 92% and 78%, respectively.

As expected, improvements in segmental function are associated with improved global LV function.[5,100,109,143] In the study by Tillisch et al,[100] for instance, the LVEF remained unchanged if a mismatch existed in only one of several myocardial segments, while it increased significantly from 30% ± 11% to 45% ± 14% ($p < 0.05$) in patients with two or more myocardial segments with mismatches.[100,106] More recently, it was reported that the magnitude of functional improvement after coronary revascularization is related inversely to, among other factors, the severity of preoperative wall motion abnormalities.[3,144] This might explain why one recent study found the predictive accuracy of PET imaging to be lower in myocardial segments with only preoperative mild hypokinesis as opposed to segments with severe hypo- or akinesis (positive predictive values 37% and 86%, respectively[42]).

Table 2 summarizes the predictive accuracy of PET FDG imaging for the recovery of regional LV function after revascularization.

The blood flow/glucose metabolism approach has been challenged by several investigators for various reasons.[74,94,137,138,145,146] For instance, persistence of residual oxidative metabolism assessed with ^{11}C-acetate has been advocated as a "better gold standard"

Table 2

Diagnostic Accuracy of Positron Emission Tomography Blood Flow/^{18}F-2-deoxyglucose Studies for Recovery of Regional Left Ventricular Dysfunction

Author	Number of Patients	Number Segments	Number Segments With WMA — Improved	Number Segments With WMA — Not Improved	Sensitivity	Specificity	PPV	NPV	Accuracy
Tillisch[100]	17	67	41	26	95	80	85	93	88
Tamaki[106]	22	46	23	23	78	78	78	78	78
Tamaki[105]	11	56	50	6	100	38	80	100	82
Marwick[27]	16	85	35	50	71	76	68	79	74
Lucignani[109]	14	54	39	15	92	86	95	80	91
Carrel[143]	21	23	19	4	95	50	84	75	83
Gropler[145–146]	34	116	73	43	83	50	52	81	63
Knuuti[101]	48	90	87	13	88	79	84	84	84
Tamaki[133]	43	130	59	71	88	82	76	92	85
Maes[3]	20	20	12	8	80	60	67	75	70
Gerber[16]	39	39	24	15	75	67	78	67	71

WMA, wall motion abnormalities prior to coronary revascularization; PPV, positive predictive value; NPV, negative predictive value.

for viable myocardium.[95,145,146] Thus, oxidative metabolism was reduced to 75% in reversibly but to 45% in irreversibly dysfunctional myocardium.[95] Reductions in blood flow were less severe (down to 74% and 63% of normal), implicating ^{11}C-acetate clearance rates as the better discriminator between viable and nonviable myocardium. The same authors also studied patients with chronic CAD before and after revascularization. Oxidative metabolism in dysfunctional but viable segments was comparable with that in normal myocardium. By contrast, in irreversibly dysfunctional segments, oxidative metabolism was reduced to 66% compared with normal myocardium.[145] In a subsequent study in a larger patient population these authors reported a higher predictive accuracy for ^{11}C-acetate than for FDG imaging.[146] Of note, the accuracy of FDG imaging in this particular study was remarkably low.

However, the use of ^{11}C-acetate for the detection of viable myocardium also has been challenged.[60,147] In patients with recent acute myocardial infarction, for instance, oxidative metabolism was found to correlate linearly with MBF and was reduced equally in segments with and without mismatch pattern.[60] Although follow-up data were not reported, these data suggest that in the early postinfarction period ^{11}C-acetate kinetics do not provide additional or independent information compared with the blood flow/glucose metabolism approach. Another, more recent study in patients with chronic CAD concludes that the assessment of oxidative metabolism does not provide any additional data when compared with measurements of absolute MBF alone.[74] Others are more optimistic and propose inotropic stimulation with low-dose dobutamine as a challenge for dysfunctional myocardium.[148] Using this approach, ^{11}C clearance rates uniformly increased in reversibly but remained unchanged or even declined in irreversibly dysfunctional myocardium.

In summary, the combined blood flow/glucose metabolism approach currently is used as the standard technique for the assessment of viable myocardium. Nevertheless, from a pragmatic point of view different institutions may prefer the technique(s) they are most familiar with. For fair comparison of different approaches, a large and prospective trial in a well-defined patient population would be necessary. Image readers should be blinded to clinical data and use prospectively defined criteria for study analysis.

Morphological Correlates of Chronic Left Ventricular Dysfunction and Their Relation to PET Findings

Significantly less fibrotic tissue is found in areas showing a mismatch of blood flow and glucose metabolism on PET imaging as compared with those exhibiting a match.[3,5,19,144] This is in concordance with and provides the rationale for the clinical observation that segments exhibiting a blood flow/metabolism mismatch are more likely to recover following coronary revascularization: at 3 months of follow-up after coronary bypass surgery, ventricular function improved in areas with mismatch but not with match.[3] Evidence suggests that an amount of 35% necrotic tissue is a threshold for postoperative functional recovery in a given segment.[3,5] Indeed, in one study stepwise regression analysis revealed the extent of fibrotic tissue as the most significant parameter predicting postrevascularization improvement in regional function.[5,19] Others[144] found the severity of preoperative wall motion abnormalities and a preserved glucose metabolism in these areas to be the strongest predictor for a postrevascularization improvement.

Abnormal myocytes in chronically dysfunctional myocardium were characterized by a loss of contractile material and an increase in glycogen deposits, reflecting what may be considered a "dedifferentiation" of mature cardiomyocytes.[3,5] Segments that showed functional recovery following coronary revascularization exhibited more cardiomyocytes, including a larger portion of cells with excessive glycogen storage.[3,5,19] Other studies demonstrated a reexpression of early proteins[149] and changes in the structure of titin, a sarcomer protein that is part of the actomyosin complex.[150] Under experimental conditions, this process of dedifferentiation appears to be reversible.[151]

Others have questioned the concept of de-differentiation: Schwarz et al analyzed biopsies from chronic ischemic myocardium exhibiting a mismatch of perfusion and glucose metabolism.[152] In their study morphological criteria such as number and structural alteration of the residual contractile material, structural alteration of mitochondria, extent of glycogen storage, and extent of fibrotic tissue did not distinguish between segments with and without functional recovery at 6 months after coronary bypass surgery. Although one might rightfully argue that the search for linear correlations between two arbitrarily chosen parameters (in particular if the biopsy material is limited) constitutes an overly simplistic approach to the complex phenomenon of myocardial ischemia, it is nevertheless reasonable to expect at least some differences in morphological changes between areas with and without functional recovery. However, these authors used a combined SPECT/PET approach for the evaluation of myocardial perfusion (sestamibi) and glucose metabolism (FDG). Differences in the definition of the term mismatch, including a potential misalignment between SPECT and PET image sets but also incomplete reperfusion, might have affected their data.

Nevertheless, the findings in all studies are in keeping with the notion that normal tissue and fibrosis/scar frequently coexist in a given myocardial segment. Reasonable interpretation of these data also shows that overly simplistic and mechanistic approaches are insufficient to understand complex biological phenomena such as myocardial ischemia. Thus, it cannot be expected that all myocardial segments showing the mismatch pattern will recover contractile function and those with matched reduction in perfusion and metabolism will never improve. Rather, match and mismatch indicate a certain likelihood with which functional improvement after revascularization can be expected. Depending on degree of morphological injury, myocytes may require a very long time to rebuild the contractile apparatus. In keeping with this concept, recent data show that the category of match, that is, segments with concordant reduction in MBF and glucose metabolism, is in itself inhomogenous; a higher amount of scar tissue was found in segments with the most severe match patterns.[3] Thus, some patients with a match pattern may in fact show a functional improvement after revascularization. The degree of loss of contractile material as well as increased myocyte glycogen accumulation appears to determine cell survival and, thus, the likelihood for functional recovery.[144] Moreover, fibrotic (scar) tissue and normal myocardium frequently coexist in a given myocardial segment and may involve the entire wall thickness in a patchy pattern or occur as predominant subendocardial scar with preserved normal myocardial tissue in the mid- and subepicardial wall. Restoration of MBF may promote functional recovery in the first scenario but not in the latter.

Prognostic Value of Positron Emission Tomography Viability Studies

From the above discussion it is obvious that a substantial amount of reversibly dysfunctional myocardium is a conditio sine qua non for any improvement in contractile function following revascularization. However, an improvement in segmental wall motion and contraction is of little clinical relevance as long as it does not lead to an improvement in global LV function because impaired LV function and survival are correlated strongly in patients with CAD.[153–155] Moreover, an increase in LVEF after revascularization is associated with an improvement in prognosis.[124] Other factors to be addressed include an improvement in life quality and amelioration in heart failure symptoms.

Consequently, studies have been undertaken to determine whether PET viability imaging might help to define patient groups who are most likely to benefit from coronary revascularization in terms of functional outcome and survival. For instance, Tamaki et al reported on a 2-year follow-up of 84 patients with stable CAD and prior myocardial infarction who had undergone FDG PET.[156] Increased FDG uptake was the single-most, independent prognostic parameter for subsequent cardiac events including sudden cardiac death, myocardial infarction, unstable angina, or need for revascularization. Stepwise multivariate analysis revealed increased FDG uptake to be a better prognostic indicator than the number of diseased coronary arteries or number and severity of thallium perfusion defects. Although encouraging, these data provided only first insights that PET viability imaging also might have prognostic implications. Thus, blood flow/metabolism imaging might be helpful in distinguishing regions with completed infarction from viable but ischemically compromised tissue and thereby possibly influence treatment decisions.

However, the search for viable myocardium is of more clinical relevance in patients with impaired LV function, that is,

1. Patients with undetermined leading cause for congestive heart failure (ischemic versus nonischemic cardiomyopathy)
2. Patients with known CAD and poor LVEF whose therapeutic alternatives include pharmacologic treatment, coronary bypass surgery, or heart transplantation.

Subsequent studies therefore have focused on these patient groups. Table 3 summarizes studies that indicate that coronary revascularization can substantially improve the prognosis of patients with ischemic cardiomyopathy if viable myocardium was shown by PET.[139–141] All three studies prove that patients benefit from revascularization in terms of nonfatal cardiac events. In addition, two of these studies found the presence of a mismatch pattern per se to be an independent indicator for cardiac death.[139,140] For instance, in the initial study by Eitzman et al[140] the 1-year mortality rate in patients with mismatch and medical therapy was 33% but was reduced to 3.8% in those who underwent bypass surgery. In comparison, patients with match had a 1-year mortality rate of 6%. Similar results were reported subsequently by Di Carli et al (Fig. 3).[139]

A quantitative relation between preoperative amount of PET viable myocardium and a postsurgical improvement in heart failure symptoms has been documented as well. Di Carli et al[157] studied 36 patients with CAD and an average LVEF of 28% ± 6% before and after coronary revascularization. The greatest improvement in heart failure symptoms occurred in patients with the largest mismatches (Fig. 4). A blood flow/metabolism mismatch involving ~20% of the left ventricle was the best predictor for an improvement in functional status following bypass surgery with a sensitivity of 76% and a specificity of 78%. At least in part, this might be related to an improvement in global left ventricular function; as shown recently, postrevascularization changes in LVEF correlate linearly with the amount of myocardium with flow/metabolism mismatch prior to bypass surgery.[157a]

It needs to emphasized that the above studies were performed retrospectively. A large prospective study is still missing. Such study should analyze quantitatively PET viability patterns and their relation to an improvement in regional and global LV function, in heart failure symptoms and survival. It also should consider the actual time between the PET study and bypass surgery because this time interval may critically affect functional improvement and patient survival.[158] This is of particular importance in patients with poor LV function and large amounts of viable myocardium, that is, those who would benefit most from coronary revascularization.

It cannot be emphasized enough that the issue of myocardial viability must not be isolated from the specific clinical context! Thus, any viability imaging should be part of a clinical algorithm that may include clinical evaluation, coronary angiography, and evaluation of regional and global LV function. Other factors that affect a patient's eligibility to undergo coronary bypass surgery also need to be considered: presence of suitable target vessels, LV diameter and volume, accompanying diseases, and biological age. All too often PET viability imaging is not part of such rigorous diagnostic algorithm. A large retro-

Table 3

Cardiac Event Rates in Studies Addressing Prognostic Value of PET Blood Flow/Metabolism Imaging

Author	Number of Patients	Age (y)	LVEF	Follow-up (months)	PET Viable		PET Nonviable	
					Revascularized	Medical Treatment	Revascularized	Medical Treatment
Di Carli[139]	93	65 ± 4	25 ± 6%	13 ± 6	3/26 (11.5%)	7/17 (41.2%)	1/17 (5.9%)	3/33 (9.1%)
Eitzman[140]	82	59 ± 10	35 ± 14%	12	3/26 (11.5%)	9/18 (50%)	1/14 (7%)	3/24 (12.5%)
Lee[141]	129	68 ± 12	35 ± 15%	17 ± 9	8/49 (16.3%)	13/21 (61%)	2/19 (10.5%)	7/40 (17.5%)
Total	304				14/101 (10.1%)	29/56 (52%)	4/50 (8%)	13/97 (13.4%)
					$p = 0.014$	$p = 0.042$		

PET, Positron Emission Tomography; LVEF, Left Ventricular Ejection Fraction.

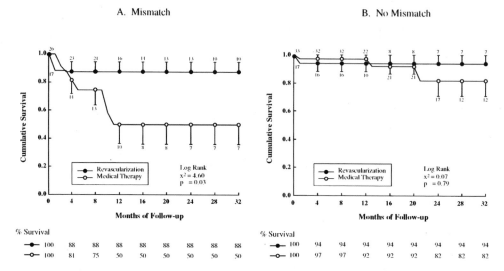

Figure 3. Cumulative survival of patients according to presence or absence of PET blood flow/metabolism mismatch and mode of treatment. Coronary revascularization in patients with mismatch significantly improves survival. Reproduced with permission from Reference 139.

spective study from our institution showed that a significant amount of viable myocardium (expected to result in improvement in LV function) was found in 50% of all patients referred for PET blood flow/glucose metabolism imaging over the last 10 years. However, in only 50% of them this actually was followed by coronary revascularization.[159]

In addition, a meta-analysis of the currently available data demonstrates that revascularization does not only improve the prognosis in patients with ischemic cardiomyop-

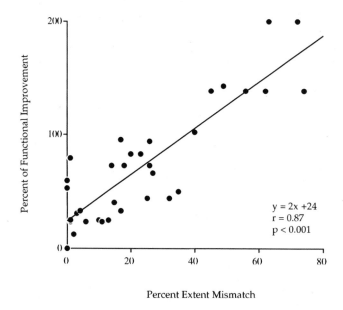

Figure 4. Relation between the anatomic extent of blood flow/metabolism mismatches [as percent of the left ventricular (LV) myocardium] and change in functional capacity after bypass surgery (as percent improvement from baseline). Reproduced with permission from Reference 157.

athy and mismatch, but the number of cardiac events also is reduced in patients with a match pattern undergoing bypass surgery (Table 3). There are two possible explanations for this finding. (1) It just reaffirms earlier data from the Coronary Artery Surgery Study (CASS)[124] that patients with multivessel disease and low LVEF benefit from revascularization regardless of other factors; and (2) even after subclassifying patients according to blood flow/metabolism patterns, none of these three groups (normal, mismatch, and match) is in itself homogenous. Other factors, such as clinical parameters indicative of ischemia (e.g., presence and severity of angina pectoris) and extent and severity of mismatch or match (complete or incomplete match) need to be considered. For instance, in a recent study with 4-year follow-up of patients with a mean ejection fraction of 25% ± 6%, coronary revascularization tended to improve survival in patients without mismatch who had severe angina pectoris.[160] Regardless, in many patients the combined stress and rest perfusion imaging, followed by the assessment of glucose metabolism might be the protocol of choice because the detection of stress-induced ischemia per se might influence the therapeutic decision (e.g. coronary revascularization or conservative management).

Second, the necessity and usefulness of myocardial viability studies in patients with acute myocardial infarction is debatable. This is because mounting evidence suggests that in these patients restoration of normal antegrade perfusion may always be beneficial, most likely because it prevents ventricular remodeling (open artery hypothesis[161–166]). "

Third, dysfunctional myocardium with normal resting perfusion also deserves further attention. Following revascularization its contractile function may or may not improve, depending on the underlying pathological mechanism. If abnormal wall motion is caused by (repeated) stunning, restoration of normal perfusion will help to prevent further ischemic episodes and therefore promote functional recovery. In contrast, dysfunctional segments with normal resting perfusion—in particular in patients with low ejection fraction—also may represent remodeled myocardium[167–170], (Table 4). Ventricular remodeling can develop progressively in patients with CAD, usually after a large acute

Table 4

Positron Emission Tomography Blood Flow/Glucose Metabolism Patterns and Their Clinical Correlates

Pattern	Clinical Finding	Blood Flow At Rest	Blood Flow During Inotropic Stimulation	Blood Flow Flow Reserve	FDG	Wall Motion At Rest	Wall Motion During Inotropic Stimulation
Normal							
	Normal myocardium	n	↑↑	n	n	n	↑↑
	Stunning	n	↑	↓	n*	↓	↑
	Remodeling	n or ↘	= or ↗	↓	n	↓	= or ↗
Match Incomplete							
	Nontransmural MI	↓	↗	↓	↓	↓	=
Complete							
	Transmural MI	↓↓	=	↓	↓↓	↓	=
Mismatch							
	Hibernation	↘ or ↓	↑	↓	↑	↓	↑

MI, myocardial infarction; n, normal; =, unchanged compared to rest.
* ^{18}F-2-deoxyglucose (FDG) uptake in stunned myocardium may vary.
Time course described in Reference 25.

myocardial infarction.[167,171] As shown recently, such remodeled myocardium often is not associated with increased interstitial fibrosis,[172] which is why resting absolute flow is frequently within normal limits. Even if fibrosis occurs, the expected decrease in resting flow may be offset by an increase in wall stress (and blood flow) in the residual myocardium. Because regions for measurement of MBF usually include the entire LV wall, flow per unit of tissue remains normal.[173] Depending on extent and severity of ventricular remodeling, the concerned segments may need a very long time to regain their functional capacity or not recover at all. Nevertheless, restoration of normal antegrade perfusion may help to prevent further remodeling so that the improvement of resting contractile function after revascularization may be a battered gold standard. Even in viable segments without functional recovery, revascularization can prevent further remodeling and thereby improve prognosis. In addition, resting contractile function can only improve if most of the subendocardium is still viable. Yet, stress- or exercise-induced increases in catecholamines still could increase thickening in the outer layer of the LV wall and so contribute to enhanced global systolic LV performance during these periods.

Summary

The assessment of myocardial viability, that is, the detection of LV dysfunction that is reversible after coronary revascularization, is of importance in a small, yet important subset of patients with CAD. PET provides a high predictive accuracy for an improvement in LV function following coronary revascularization. PET viability studies also provide prognostic information; they may help to select these patients with end-stage CAD who are most likely to benefit from coronary revascularization in terms of functional outcome and survival. Last, if applied in a reasonably selected population, this imaging approach may be cost-effective and, in fact, help to redirect considerable financial resources to other important sectors of health care.

References

1. Hearse D. Myocardial ischaemia: Can we agree on a definition for the 21st century? *Cardiovacs Res* 1994;28:1737–1744.
2. Reimer KA, Lowe JE, Rasmussen MM, et al. The wavefront phenomenon of ischemic cell death, I: Myocardial infarct size vs duration of coronary occlusion in dogs. *Circulation* 1977;56:786–794.
3. Maes A, Flameng W, Nuyts J, et al. Histological alterations in chronically hypoperfused myocardium. *Circulation* 1994;90:735–745.
4. Schwarz ER, Schaper J, vom Dahl J, et al. Myocyte degeneration and cell death in hibernating myocardium. *J Am Coll Cardiol* 1996;27:1577–1585
5. Deprè C, Vanoverschelde JL, Melin JA, et al. Structural and metabolic correlates of the reversibility of chronic left ventricular ischemic dysfunction in humans. *Am J Physiol* 1995; 268:H1265–H1275.
6. Braunwald E, Kloner RA. The stunned myocardium: Prolonged, postischemic ventricular dysfunction. *Circulation* 1982;66:1146–1149.
7. Braunwald E, Rutherford JD. Reversible ischemic left ventricular dysfunction: Evidence for "hibernating myocardium." *J Am Coll Cardiol* 1986;8:1467–1470.
8. Kloner RA, DeBoer LW, Darsee JR, et al. Prolonged abnormalities of myocardium salvaged by reperfusion. *Am J Physiol* 1981;241:H591–H599.
9. Kloner RA, Allen J, Cox TA, et al. Stunned left ventricular myocardium after exercise treadmill testing in coronary artery disease. *Am J Cardiol* 1991;68:329–334.
10. Rahimtoola SH. The hibernating myocardium. *Am Heart J* 1989;117:211–221.

11. Liedtke AJ, Renstrom B, Nellis SH, et al. Mechanical and metabolic functions in pig hearts after 4 days on chronic coronary stenosis. *J Am Coll Cardiol* 1995;26:815–825.

12. Schulz R, Rose J, Martin C, et al. Development of short-term myocardial hibernation: Its limitation by the severity of ischemia and inotropic stimulation. *Circulation* 1993;88:684–695.

13. Shen YT, Vatner SF. Mechanism of impaired myocardial function during progressive coronary stenosis in conscious pigs: Hibernation versus stunning? *Circ Res* 1995;76:479–488.

14. Vanoverschelde JL, Wijns W, Borgers M, et al. Chronic myocardial hibernation in humans. From bedside to bench. *Circulation* 1997;95:1961–1971.

15. Conversano A, Walsh JF, Geltman EM, et al. Delineation of myocardial stunning and hibernation by positron emission tomography in advanced coronary artery disease. *Am Heart J* 1996;131:440–450.

16. Gerber BL, Vanoverschelde JL, et al. Myocardial blood flow, glucose uptake, and recruitment of inotropic reserve in chronic left ventricular ischemic dysfunction. Implications for the pathophysiology of chronic myocardial hibernation. *Circulation* 1996;94:651–659.

17. Marinho NV, Keogh BE, Costa DC, et al. Pathophysiology of chronic left ventricular dysfunction. New insights from the measurement of absolute myocardial blood flow and glucose utilization. *Circulation* 1996;93:737–744.

18. Vanoverschelde JL, Wijns W, Depré C, et al. Mechanisms of chronic regional postischemic dysfunction in humans. New insights from the study of noninfarcted collateral-dependent myocardium. *Circulation* 1993;87:1513–1523.

19. Depré C, Vanoverschelde JL, Gerber B, et al. Correlation of functional recovery with myocardial blood flow, glucose uptake, and morphologic features in patients with chronic left ventricular ischemic dysfunction undergoing coronary artery bypass grafting. *J Thorac Cardiovasc Surg* 1997;113:371–378.

20. Chen C, Ma L, Linfert DR, et al. Myocardial cell death and apoptosis in hibernating myocardium. *J Am Coll Cardiol* 1997;30:1407–1412.

21. Bolli R. Myocardial stunning in man. *Circulation* 1992;86:1671–1691.

22. Indolfi C, Piscione F, Perrone-Filardi P, et al. Inotropic stimulation by dobutamine increases left ventricular regional function at the expense of metabolism in hibernating myocardium. *Am Heart J* 1996;132:542–549.

23. Schulz R, Guth B, Pieper K, et al. Recruitment of an inotropic reserve in moderately ischemic myocardium at the expense of metabolic recovery: A model of short term hibernation. *Circ Res* 1992;70:1282–1295.

24. Sun KT, Czernin J, Krivokapich J, et al. Effects of dobutamine stimulation on myocardial blood flow, glucose metabolism, and wall motion in normal and dysfucntional myocardium. *Circulation* 1996;94:3146–3154.

25. Buxton DB, Schelbert HR. Measurement of regional glucose metabolic rates in reperfused myocardium. *Am J Physiol* 1991;261:H2058–H2068.

26. Buxton DB, Vaghaiwalla-Mody F, Krivokapich J, et al. Quantitative assessment of prolonged metabolic abnormalities in reperfused canine myocardium. *Circulation* 1992;85:1842–1856.

27. Marwick T, MacIntyre W, Lafont A, et al. Metabolic responses of hibernating and infarcted myocardium to revascularization: A follow-up study of regional perfusion, function, and metabolism. *Circulation* 1992;85:1347–1353.

28. Opie LH. *The Heart: Physiology and Metabolism.* New York: Raven Press; 1991.

29. Mäki M, Luotolahti M, Nuutila P, et al. Glucose uptake in the chronically dysfunctional but viable myocardium. *Circulation* 1996;93:1658–1666.

30. Sun D, Nguyen N, DeGrado T, et al. Ischemia induces translocation of the insulin-responsive glucose transporter GLUT4 to the plasma membrane of cardiac myocytes. *Circulation* 1994; 89:793–798.

31. Rattigan S, Appleby GJ, Clark MG. Insulin-like action of catecholamines and Ca2+ to stimulate glucose transport and GLUT-4 translocation in perfused rat heart. *Biochim Biophys Acta.* 1991;1094:217–223.

32. Wheeler TJ, Fell RD, Hauck MA. Translocation of two glucose transporters in heart: Effects of rotenone, uncouplers, workload, palmitate, insulin and anoxia. *Biochim Biophys Acta* 1994; 1196:191–200.

33. Brosius, FC III, Liu Y, Nguyen N, et al. Persistent myocardial ischemia increases GLUT1 glucose transporter expression in both ischemic and non-ischemic heart regions. *J Mol Cell Cardiol* 1997;29:1675–1685.

34. Young LH, Renfu Y, Russell R, et al. Low-flow ischemia leads to translocation of canine heart GLUT-4 and GLUT-1 glucose transporters to the sarcolemma in vivo [see comments]. *Circulation* 1997;95:415–422.

35. Weiss JN, Lamp ST. Glycolysis preferentially inhibits ATP-sensitive K+ channels in isolated guinea pig cardiac myocytes. *Science* 1987;238:67–69.

36. Neely JR, Grotyohann LW. Role of glycolytic products in damage to ischemic myocardium. Dissociation of adenosine triphosphate levels and recovery of function of reperfused ischemic hearts. *Circ Res* 1984;55:816–824.

37. Cross HR, Clarke K, Opie LH, et al. Is lactate-induced myocardial ischemic injury mediated by decreased pH or increased intracellular lactate? *J Mol Cell Cardiol* 1995;27:1369–1381.

38. Owen P, Dennis S, Opie LH. Glucose flux rate regulates onset of ischemic contracture in globally underperfused rat hearts. *Circ Res* 1990;66:344–354.

39. Flameng W, Vanhaecke J, VanBelle H. Relation between coronary artery stenosis and myocardial purine metabolism, histology and regional function in humans. *J Am Coll Cardiol* 1987;9:1235–1242.

40. Schwaiger M, Sun D, Deeb M, et al. Expression of myocardial glucose transporter (GLUT) mRNA in patients with advanced coronary artery disease. *Circulation* 1994;90:I113. Abstract.

41. Feigl E, Neat G, Huang A. Interrelations between coronary artery pressure, myocardial metabolism and coronary blood flow. *J Mol Cell Cardiol* 1990;22:375–390.

42. vom Dahl J, Eitzman D, Al-Aouar A, et al. Relation of regional function, perfusion, and metabolism in patients with advanced coronary artery disease undergoing surgical revascularization. *Circulation* 1994;90:2356–2366.

43. Hearse D, Crome R, Yellon D, et al. Metabolic and flow correlates of myocardial ischemia. *Circ Res* 1983;38(suppl I):I52–I74.

44. Rivas F, Cobb F, Bache R, et al. Relationship between blood flow to ischemic regions and extent of myocardial infarction. *Circ Res* 1976;38:439–447.

45. Kalff V, Schwaiger M, Nguyen N, et al. The relationship between myocardial blood flow and glucose uptake in ischemic canine myocardium determined with fluorine-18-deoxyglucose. *J Nucl Med* 1992;33:1346–1353.

46. Hutchins G, Schwaiger M, Rosenspire K, et al. Noninvasive quantification of regional blood flow in the human heart using N-13 ammonia and dynamic positron emission tomographic imaging. *J Am Coll Cardiol* 1990;15:1032–1042.

47. Kuhle WG, Porenta G, Huang SC, et al. Quantification of regional myocardial blood flow using ^{13}N-ammonia and reoriented dynamic positron emission tomographic imaging. *Circulation* 1992;86:1004–1017.

48. Bergmann SR, Herrero P, Markham J, et al. Noninvasive quantitation of myocardial blood flow in human subjects with oxygen-15-labeled water and positron emission tomography. *J Am Coll Cardiol* 1989;14:639–652.

49. Herrero P, Markham J, Shelton M, et al. Implementation and evaluation of a two-compartment model for quantification of myocardial perfusion with rubidium-82 and positron emission tomography. *Circ Res* 1992;70:496–507.

50. Araujo L, Lammertsma A, Rhodes C, et al. Noninvasive quantification of regional myocardial blood flow in coronary artery disease with oxygen-15-labeled carbon dioxide inhalation and positron emission tomography. *Circulation* 1991;83:875–885.

51. Gould K. PET Perfusion Imaging and Nuclear Cardiology. *J Nucl Med*.1991;32:579–606.

52. Hill J, Gettes L. Effect of coronary artery occlusion on local myocardial extracellular potassium activity in swine. *Circulation* 1980;61:768–777.

53. Johnson R, Sammel N, Norris R. Depletion of myocardial creatine kinase, lactate dehydrogenase, myoglobin and potassium after coronary artery ligation in dogs. *Cardiovasc Res* 1981;15:529–537.

54. Goldstein RA. Kinetics of rubidium-82 after coronary occlusion and reperfusion. Assessment of patency and viability in open-chested dogs. *J Clin Invest* 1985;75:1131–1137.

55. Goldstein RA, Mullani NA, Wong WH, et al. Positron imaging of myocardial infarction with Rubidium-82. *J Nucl Med* 1986;27:1824–1829.

56. Goldstein RA. Rubidium-82 kinetics after coronary occlusion: Temporal relation of net myocardial accumulation and viability in open-chested dogs. *J Nucl Med* 1986;27:1456–1461.

57. Masazumi A, Links J, Takatsu H, et al. Regional Rb-82 washout assessed by PET reflects the severity and time course of myocardial ischemia-reperfusion injury. *J Am Coll Cardiol* 1993; 21:460A. Abstract.

58. Weiss J, Hiltbrand B. Functional compartmentation of glycolytic versus oxidative metabolism in isolated rabbit heart. *J Clin Invest* 1985;75:436–447.

59. Taegtmeyer H, Roberts A, Raine A. Energy metabolism in reperfused heart muscle: Metabolic correlates to return of function. *J Am Coll Cardiol* 1985;6:864–870.

60. Vanoverschelde J-LJ, Melin JA, Bol A, et al. Regional oxidative metabolism in patients after recovery from reperfused anterior myocardial infarction. *Circulation* 1992;85:9–21.

61. Czernin J, Porenta G, Brunken R, et al. Regional blood flow, oxidative metabolism, and glucose utilization in patients with recent myocardial infarction. *Circulation* 1993;88:885–895.

62. Weinheimer C, Brown M, Nohara R, et al. Functional recovery after reperfusion is predicated on recovery of myocardial oxidative metabolism. *Am Heart J* 1993;125:939–949.

63. Brown M, Marshall DR, Burton BS, et al. Delineation of myocardial oxygen utilization with carbon-11-labeled acetate. *Circulation* 1987;76:687–696.

64. Buxton DB, Schwaiger M, Nguyen A, et al. Radiolabeled acetate as a tracer of myocardial tricarboxylic acid cycle flux. *Circ Res* 1988;63:628–634.

65. Hicks RJ, Herman WH, Kalff V, et al. Quantitative evaluation of regional substrate metabolism in the human heart by positron emission tomography. *J Am Coll Cardiol* 1991;18:101–111.

66. Armbrecht JJ, Buxton DB, Brunken RC, et al. Regional myocardial oxygen consumption determined noninvasively in humans with [1-^{11}C] acetate and dynamic positron tomography. *Circulation* 1989;80:863–872.

67. Ng CK, Huang SC, Schelbert HR, et al. Validation of a model for [1-11C] acetate as a tracer of cardiac oxidative metabolism. *Am J of Physiol* 1994;266:H1304–H1315.

68. Armbrecht JJ, Buxton DB, Schelbert HR. Validation of [1-^{11}C] acetate as a tracer for noninvasive assessment of oxidative metabolism with positron emission tomography in normal, ischemic, post-ischemic and hyperemic canine myocardium. *Circulation* 1990;81:1594–1605.

69. Brown MA, Myears DW, Bergmann SR. Validity of estimates of myocardial oxidative metabolism with carbon-11 acetate and positron emission tomography despite altered patterns of substrate utilization. *J Nucl Med* 1989;30:187–193.

70. Chan SY, Brunken RC, Phelps ME, et al. Use of the metabolic tracer ^{11}C acetate for evaluation of regional myocardial perfusion. *J Nucl Med* 1991;32:665–672.

71. Gropler RJ, Siegel BA, Geltman EM. Myocardial uptake of carbon-11-acetate as an indirect estimate of regional myocardial blood flow. *J Nucl Med* 1991;32:245–251.

72. Buck A, Wolpers HG, Hutchins GD, et al. Effect of C-11 acetate recirculation on estimates of myocardial oxygen consumption by PET. *J Nucl Med* 1991;32:1950–1957.

73. Sun KT, Chen K, Huang S-C, et al. Compartment model for measuring myocardial oxygen consumption using [1-C-11] acetate. *J Nucl Med* 1997;38:459–466.

74. Wolpers HG, Burchert W, van den Hoff J, et al. Assessment of myocardial viability by use of 11C-acetate and positron emission tomography. Threshold criteria of reversible dysfunction. *Circulation* 1997;95:1417–1424.

75. van den Hoff J, Burchert W, Wolpers HG, et al. A kinetic model for PET with [1-carbon-11] acetate. *J Nucl Med* 1996;37:521–529.

76. Iida H, Rhodes CG, Araujo LI, et al. Noninvasive quantification of regional myocardial metabolic rate for oxygen by use of ^{15}O$_2$ inhalation and positron emission tomography. Theory, error analysis, and application in humans. *Circulation* 1996;94:792–807.

77. Yamamoto Y, de Silva R, Rhodes CG, et al. Noninvasive quantification of regional myocardial metabolic rate of oxygen by ^{15}O$_2$ inhalation and positron emission tomography. Experimental validation. *Circulation* 1996;94:808–816.

78. Gallagher BM, Ansari A, Atkins H, et al. Radiopharmaceuticals XXVII. ^{18}F-labeled 2-deoxy-2-fluoro-D-glucose as a radiopharmaceutical for measuring regional myocardial glucose me-

tabolism in vivo: Tissue distribution and imaging studies in animals. *J Nucl Med* 1977;18: 990–996.

79. Phelps ME, Huang SC, Hoffman EJ, et al. Tomographic measurement of local cerebral glucose metabolic rate in humans with (F-18) 2-fluoro-2-deoxy-D-glucose: Validation of method. *Ann Neurol* 1979;6:371–388.

80. Halama JR, Gatley SJ, DeGrado TR, et al. Validation of 3-deoxy-3-fluoro-D-glucose as a glucose transport analogue in rat heart. *Am J Physiol* 1984;16:H754–H759.

81. Krivokapich J, Huang SC, Selin CE, et al. Fluorodeoxyglucose rate constants, lumped constant, and glucose metabolic rate in rabbit heart. *Am J Physiol* 1987;252:H777–H787.

82. Ratib O, Phelps ME, Huang SC, et al. Positron tomography with deoxyglucose for estimating local myocardial glucose metabolism. *J Nucl Med* 1982;23:577–586.

83. Hariharan R, Bray M, Ganim R, et al. Fundamental limitations of F-18–2-deoxy-2-fluoro-D-glucose for assessing myocardial glucose uptake. *Circulation* 1995;91:2435–2444.

84. Ng CK, Holden JE, DeGrado TR, et al. Sensitivity of myocardial fluorodeoxyglucose lumped constant to glucose and insulin. *Am J Physiol* 1991;260:H593–H603.

85. Schneider CA, Nguyen VT, Taegtmeyer H. Feeding and fasting determine postischemic glucose utilization in isolated working rat hearts. *Am J Physiol* 1991;260:H542–H548.

86. Gambhir SS, Schwaiger M, Huang SC, et al. Simple noninvasive quantification method for measuring myocardial glucose utilization in humans employing positron emission tomography and fluorine-18 deoxyglucose. *J Nucl Med* 1989;30:359–366.

87. Knuuti MJ, Nuutila P, Ruotsalainen U, et al. The value of quantitative analysis of glucose utilization in detection of myocardial viability by PET. *J Nucl Med* 1993;34:2068–2075.

88. Choi Y, Brunken RC, Hawkins RA, et al. Factors affecting myocardial 2-[F-18]fluoro-2-deoxy-D-glucose uptake in positron emission tomography studies of normal humans. *Eur J Nucl Med* 1993;20:308–318.

89. Knuuti MJ, Nuutila P, Ruotsalainen U, et al. Euglycemic hyperinsulinemic clamp and oral glucose load in stimulating myocardial glucose utilization during positron emission tomography. *J Nucl Med* 1992;33:1255–1262.

90. vom Dahl J, Hicks RJ, Lee KS, et al. Positron emission tomography myocardial viability studies in patients with diabetes mellitus. *J Am Coll Cardiol* 1991;17:121A. Abstract.

91. Besozzi MC, Brown MD, Hubner KF, et al. Retrospective post therapy evaluation of cardiac function in 208 coronary artery disease patients evaluated by positron emission tomography. *J Nucl Med* 1992;33:885. Abstract.

92. Schöder H, Campisi R, Ohtake T, et al. Blood flow-metabolism imaging with positron emission tomography in patients with diabetes mellitus for the assessment of reversible left ventricular contractile dysfunction. *J Am Coll Cardiol* 1999;33:1328–1337

93. Hicks R, von Dahl J, Lee K, et al. Insulin-glucose clamp for standardization of metabolic conditions during F-18 fluoro-deoxyglucose PET imaging. *J Am Coll Cardiol* 1991;17: 381A.

94. Gropler RJ, Siegel BA, Lee KJ, et al. Nonuniformity in myocardial accumulation of fluorine-18-fluorodeoxyglucose in normal fasted humans [see comments]. *J Nucl Med* 1990;31: 1749–1756.

95. Gropler RJ, Siegel BA, Sampathkumaran K, et al. Dependence of recovery of contractile function on maintenance of oxidative metabolism after myocardial infarction. *J Am Coll Cardiol* 1992;19:989–997.

96. Pierard L, De Landsheere C, Berthe C, et al. Identification of viable myocardium by echocardiography during dobutamine infusion in patients with myocardial infarction after thrombolytic therapy: Comparison with positron emission tomography. *J Am Coll Cardiol* 1990; 15:1021–1031.

97. Gould LK, Yoshida K, Hess MJ, et al. Myocardial metabolism of fluorodeoxyglucose compared to cell membrane integrity for the potassium analogue Rubidium-82 for assessing infarct size in man by PET. *J Nucl Med* 1991;32:1–9.

98. Wijns W, Melin JA, Leners N, et al. Accumulation of polymorphonuclear leukocytes in reperfused canine myocardium: Relation with tissue viability assessed by fluorine-18–2-deoxy-glucose uptake. *J Nucl Med* 1988;29:1826–1832.

99. Marshall RC, Tillisch JH, Phelps ME, et al. Identification and differentiation of resting myocardial ischemia and infarction in man with positron computed tomography 18F-labeled fluorodeoxyglucose and N-13 ammonia. *Circulation* 1983;67:766–778.

100. Tillisch J, Brunken R, Marshall R, et al. Reversibility of cardiac wall motion abnormalities predicted by positron tomography. *New Engl J Med* 1986;314:884–888.
101. Knuuti MJ, Saraste M, Nuutila P, et al. Myocardial viability: Fluorine-18-deoxyglucose positron emission tomography in prediction of wall motion recovery after revascularization. *Am Heart J* 1994;127:785–796.
102. Camici P, Araujo LI, Spinks T, et al. Increased uptake of 18F-fluorodeoxyglucose in post-ischemic myocardium of patients with exercise-induced angina. *Circulation* 1986;74:81–88.
103. Marwick T, Nemec J, Lafont A, et al. Prediction by postexercise fluoro-18 deoxyglucose positron emission tomography of improvement in exercise capacity after revascularization. *Am J Cardiol* 1992;69:854–859.
104. Schwaiger M, Brunken R, Grover-McKay M, et al. Regional myocardial metabolism in patients with acute myocardial infarction assessed by positron emission tomography. *J Am Coll Cardiol* 1986;8:800–808.
105. Tamaki N, Ohtani H, Yonekura Y, et al. Significance of fill-in after thallium-201 reinjection following delayed imaging: Comparison with regional wall motion and angiographic findings. *J Nucl Med* 1990;31:1617–1623.
106. Tamaki N, Yonekura Y, Yamashita K, et al. Positron emission tomography using fluorine-18 deoxyglucose in evaluation of coronary artery bypass grafting. *Am J Cardiol* 1989;64:860–865.
107. Tamaki N, Yonekura Y, Yamashita K, et al. Value of rest-stress myocardial positron tomography using nitrogen-13 ammonia for the preoperative prediction of reversible asynergy. *J Nucl Med* 1989;30:1302–1310.
108. Altehoefer C, Kaiser H-J, Dörr R, et al. Fluorine-18 deoxyglucose PET for assessment of viable myocardium in perfusion defects in ^{99m}Tc-MIBI SPET: A comparative study in patients with coronary artery disease. *Eur J Nucl Med*. 1992;19:334–342.
109. Lucignani G, Paolini G, Landoni C, et al. Presurgical identification of hibernating myocardium by combined use of technetium-99m hexakis 2-methoxyisobutylisonitrile single photon emission tomography and fluorine-18 fluoro-2-deoxy-D-glucose positron emission tomography in patients with coronary artery disease. *Eur J Nucl Med* 1992;19:874–881.
110. Paolini G, Lucignani G, Zuccari M, et al. Identification and revascularization of hibernating myocardium in angina-free patients with left ventricular dysfunction. *Eur J Cardiothor Surg* 1994;8:139–144.
111. Schneider C, Voth E, Theissen P, et al. Vitalitätsbeurteilung chronischer Myokardinfarkte durch 18-F-fluorodeoxyglucokose-positronenemissionstomographie und durch ^{99m}Tc-MIBI-SPECT. (Assessment of viability in chronic myocardial infarction using F-18 fluoro-deoxyglucose and 99m Tc sestamibi SPECT). *Z Kardiol* 1994;83:124–131.
112. vom Dahl J, Altehoefer C, Sheehan FH, et al. Myocardial viability assessed by combined nuclear imaging using myocardial scintigraphy and positron emission tomography: Impact on treatment and functional outcome following revascularization. *J Am Coll Cardiol* 1994;23:117A. Abstract.
113. Dilsizian V, Bonow R. Current diagnostic techniques of assessing myocardial viability in patients with hibernating and stunned myocardium. *Circulation* 1993;87:1–20.
114. Schöder H, Friedrich M, Topp H. Myocardial viability: What do we need? *Eur J Nucl Med* 1993;20:792–803.
115. Bax JJ, Cornel JH, Visser FC, et al. Prediction of recovery of myocardial dysfunction after revascularization. Comparison of fluorine-18 fluorodeoxyglucose/thallium-201 SPECT, thallium-201 stress-reinjection SPECT and dobutamine echocardiography. *Eur J Nucl Med* 1997;24:558–564.
116. Bax J, Visser F, Van Lingen A, et al. Feasibility of assessing myocardial uptake of 18F-fluorodeoxyglucose using single photon emission computed tomography. *Eur Heart J* 1993;14:1675–1682.
117. Cornel JH, Bax JJ, Fioretti PM, et al. Prediction of improvement of ventricular function after revascularization. ^{18}F-fluorodeoxyglucose single-photon emission computed tomography vs low-dose dobutamine echocardiography. *Eur Heart J* 1997;18:941–948.
118. Martin W, Debelke D, Patton J, et al. FDG SPECT: Correlation with FDG PET. *J Nucl Med* 1995;36:988–995.

119. Delbeke D, Videlefsky S, Patton J, et al. Rest myocardial perfusion/metabolism imaging using simultaneous dual-isotope acquisition SPECT with technetium-99m-MIBI/fluorine-18-FDG. *J Nucl Med* 1995;36:2110–2119.

120. Sandler MP, Patton JA. Fluorine-18 labeled fluorodeoxyglucose myocardial single-photon emission computed tomography: An alternative for determining myocardial viability. *J Nucl Cardiol* 1996;3:342–349.

121. Bounous EP, Mark DB, Pollock BG, et al. Surgical survival benefits for coronary disease patients with left ventricular dysfunction. *Circulation* 1988;78:I151–I157.

122. Califf R, Harrell F, Lee K, et al. The evolution of medical and surgical therapy for coronary artery disease. *JAMA* 1989;261:2077–2086.

123. Luciani GB, Faggian G, Razzolini R. Severe ischemic left ventricular failure: Coronary operation or heart transplantation? *Ann Thorac Surg* 1993;55:719–723.

124. Alderman EL, Fisher LD, Litwin P, et al. Results of coronary artery surgery in patients with poor left ventricular function (CASS). *Circulation* 1983;68:785–795.

125. Elefteriades J, Tolis G Jr, Levi E, et al. Coronary artery bypass grafting in severe left ventricular dysfunction: Excellent survival with improved ejection fraction and functional state. *J Am Coll Cardiol* 1993;22:1411–1417.

126. Christakis G, Wesiel R, Fremes S, et al. Coronary artery bypass grafting in patients with poor ventricular function. *J Thorac Cardiovasc Surg* 1992;103:1083–1092.

127. Freeman A, Walshhi W, Giles R. Early and long-term results of coronary artery bypass grafting with severely depressed left ventricular performance. *Am J Cardiol* 1984;54:749–754.

128. Dreyfus GD, Duboc D, Blasco A, et al. Myocardial viability assessment in ischemic cardiomyopathy: Benefits of coronary revascularization. *Ann Thorac Surg* 1994;57:1402–1408.

129. Gewirtz H, Fischman AJ, Abraham S, et al. Positron emission tomographic measurements of absolute regional myocardial blood flow permits identification of nonviable myocardium in patients with chronic infarction. *J Am Coll Cardiol* 1994;23:851–859.

130. Beanlands RS, deKemp R, Scheffel A, et al. Myocardial viability determination using N-13 ammonia kinetics and PET. *Circulation* 1993;88:I199. Abstract.

131. Brunken R, Schwaiger M, Tillisch J, et al. Severity of segmental myocardial blood flow reduction and persistence of metabolic activity in patients with chronic ischemic heart disease. *J Nucl Med* 1986;27:891.

132. Grandin C, Wijns W, Melin JA, et al. Delineation of myocardial viability with PET. *Circulation* 1995;92:1911–1918.

133. Tamaki N, Kawamoto M, Tadamura E, et al. Prediction of reversible ischemia after revascularization: Perfusion and metabolic studies using positron emission tomography. *Circulation* 1995;91:1697–1705.

134. Go R, MacIntyre W, Saha G, et al. Hibernating myocardium versus scar: Severity of irreversible decreased myocardial perfusion in prediction of tissue viability. *Radiology* 1995;194:151–155.

135. Altehoefer C, vom Dah J, Buell U, et al. The accuracy of thallium-201 SPECT at rest for evaluation of myocardial viability in comparison to fluorine-18 FDG PET differs for the vascular supply territories. J Nucl Med 1993;34(Suppl):148P. Abstract.

136. de Silva R, Yamamoto Y, Rhodes CG, et al. Preoperative prediction of the outcome of coronary revascularization using positron emission tomography. *Circulation* 1992;86:1738–1742.

137. Yamamoto Y, de Silva R, Rhodes C, et al. A new strategy for the assessment of viable myocardium and regional myocardial blood flow using ^{15}O-water and dynamic positron emission tomography. *Circulation* 1992;86:167–178.

138. Yoshida K, Gould KL. Quantitative relation of myocardial infarct size and myocardial viability by positron emission tomography to left ventricular ejection fraction and 3-year mortality with and without revascularization. *J Am Coll Cardiol* 1993;22:984–997.

139. Di Carli MF, Davidson M, Little R, et al. Value of metabolic imaging with positron emission tomography for evaluating prognosis in patients with coronary artery disease and left ventricular dysfunction. *Am J Cardiol* 1994;73:527–533.

140. Eitzman D, Al-Aouar Z, Kanter HL, et al. Clinical outcome of patients with advanced coronary artery disease after viability studies with positron emission tomography. *J Am Coll Cardiol* 1992;20:559–565.

141. Lee KS, Marwick TH, Cook SA, et al. Prognosis of patients with left ventricular dysfunction, with and without viable myocardium after myocardial infarction. Relative efficacy of medical therapy and revascularization. *Circulation* 1994;90:2687–2694.

142. vom Dahl J, Muzik O, Wolfe ER, et al. Myocardial Rubidium-82 tissue kinetics assessed by dynamic positron emission tomography as a marker of myocardial cell membrane integrity and viability. *Circulation* 1996;93:238–245.

143. Carrel T, Jenni R, Haubold-Reuter S, et al. Improvement of severely reduced left ventricular function after surgical revascularization in patients with preoperative myocardial infarction. *Eur J Cardiothorac Surg* 1992;6:479–484.

144. Shivalkar B, Maes A, Borgers M, et al. Only hibernating myocardium invariably shows early recovery after coronary revascularization. *Circulation* 1996;94:308–315.

145. Gropler RJ, Geltman EM, Sampathkumaran K, et al. Functional recovery after coronary revascularization for chronic coronary artery disease is dependent on maintenance of oxidative metabolism. *J Am Coll Cardiol* 1992;20:569–577.

146. Gropler RJ, Geltman EM, Sampathkumaran K, et al. Comparison of carbon-11-acetate with fluorine-18-fluorodeoxyglucose for delineating viable myocardium by positron emission tomography. *J Am Coll Cardiol* 1993;22:1587–1597.

147. Hicks RJ, Melon P, Kalff V, et al. Metabolic imaging by positron emission tomography early after myocardial infarction as a predictor of recovery of myocardial function after reperfusion. *J Nucl Cardiol* 1994;1:124–137.

148. Hata T, Nohara R, Fujita M, et al. Noninvasive assessment of myocardial viability by positron emission tomography with ^{11}C acetate in patients with old myocardial infarction. Usefulness of low-dose dobutamine infusion. *Circulation* 1996;94:1834–1841.

149. Ausma J, Schaart G, Thone F, et al. Chronic ischemic viable myocardium in man: aspects of dedifferentiation. *Cardiovasc Pathol* 1995;4:29–37.

150. Ausma J, Furst D, Thone F, et al. Molecular changes of titin in left ventricular dysfunction as a result of chronic hibernation. *J Mol Cell Cardiol* 1995;27:1203–1212.

151. Borisov AB. Myofibrillogenesis and reversible disassembly of myofibrils as adaptive reactions of cardiac muscle cells. *Acta Physiol Scand* 1991;S599:71–80.

152. Schwarz ER, Schaper J, vom Dahl J, et al. Myocyte degeneration and cell death in hibernating human myocardium. *J Am Coll Cardiol* 1996;27:1577–1585.

153. Mock M, Ringqvist I, Fisher L, et al. Survival of medically treated patients in the coronary artery surgery study (CASS) registry. *Circulation* 1982;66:562–568.

154. Hammermeister K, Derouen T, Dodge H. Variables predictive of survival in patients with coronary artery disease: Selection by univariate and multivariate analysis from the clinical, elctrocardiographic, exercise, arteriographic and quantitative angiographic evaluations. *Circulation* 1979;59:412–427.

155. The Multicenter Post-infarction Research Group. Risk stratification and survival after myocardial infarction. *N Engl J Med* 1983;309:331–336.

156. Tamaki N, Kawamoto M, Takahashi N, et al. Prognostic value of an increase in fluorine-18 deoxyglucose uptake in patients with myocardial infarction: Comparison with stress thallium imaging. *J Am Coll Cardiol* 1993;22:1621–1627.

157. Di Carli M, Asgarzadie F, Schelbert HR, et al. Quantitative relation between myocardial viability and improvement in heart failure symptoms after revascularization in patients with ischemic cardiomyopathy. *Circulation* 1995;92:3436–3444.

157a. Schöder H, Campisi R, Auerbach M, et al. Extent of PET blood flow/metabolism mismatches can predict the magnitude of post-revascularization improvement in global left ventricular function. *J Nucl Med* 1998;39:162P.

158. Beanlands RS, Hendry P, Masters R, et al. Delay in revascularization is associated with increased mortality in patients with severe left ventricular dysfunction and viable myocardium on FDG PET imaging. *Circulation* 1997;96:I434. Abstract.

159. Allen-Auerbach M, Schöder H, Hoh C, et al. Prevalence of myocardial viability as detected by positron emission tomography in patients with ischemic cardiomyopathy. Circulation 1999;99: 2921–2926

160. Di Carli MF, Maddahi J, Rokhsar S, et al. Long-term survival of patients with coronary artery disease and left ventricular dysfunction: Implications for the role of myocardial viability assessment in management decisions. *Circulation* 1997;96:I434. Abstract.

161. Brodie BR, Stuckey TD, Kissling G, et al. Importance of infarct-related artery patency for recovery of left ventricular function and late survival after primary angioplasty for acute myocardial infarction. *J Am Coll Cardiol* 1996;28:319–325.
162. Welty F, Mittleman M, Lewis S, et al. A patent infarct-related artery is associated with reduced long-term mortality after percutaneous transluminal coronary angioplasty for postinfarction ischemia and an ejection fraction <50%. *Circulation* 1996;93:1496–1501.
163. Fortin DF, Califf RM. Long term survival from acute myocardial infarction: Salutary effect of an open coronary vessel. *Am J Med* 1990;88:9–15N.
164. White HD, Cross DB, Elliot DM, et al. Long term prognostic importance of patency of the infarct-related coronary artery after thrombolytic therapy for acute myocardial infarction. *Circulation* 1994;89:61–67.
165. Hochman JS. Has the time come to seek and open all occluded infarct-related arteries after myocardial infarction? *J Am Coll Cardiol* 1996;28:846–848.
166. Kim CB, Braunwald E. Potential benefits of late reperfusion of infarcted myocardium. The open artery hypothesis. *Circulation* 1993;88:2426–2436.
167. Pfeffer MA, Braunwald E. Ventricular remodeling after myocardial infarction. *Circulation* 1990;81:1161–1172.
168. Pfeffer MA, Braunwald E, Moyé LA, et al. Effect of captopril on mortality and morbidity in patients with left ventricular dysfunction after myocardial infarction. Results of the survival and ventricular enlargement trial. The SAVE Investigators [see comments]. *N Engl J Med* 1992;327:669–677.
169. Klug D, Robert V, Swynghedauw B. Role of mechanical and hormonal factors in cardiac remodeling and the biologic limits of myocardial adaptation. *Am J Cardiol* 1993;71:46A–54A.
170. Tsutsui H, Ishihara K, Cooper G. Cytoskeletal role in the contractile dysfunction of hypertrophied myocardium. *Science* 1993;260:682–687.
171. Pfeffer MA, Pfeffer JM, Lamas GA. Development and prevention of congestive heart failure following myocardial infarction. *Circulation* 1993;87:IV120–IV125.
172. Marijanowski MM, Teeling P, Becker AE. Remodeling after myocardial infarction in humans is not associated with interstitial fibrosis of noninfarcted myocardium. *J Am Coll Cardiol* 1997;30:76–82.
173. Neglia D, Parodi O, Gallopin M, et al. Myocardial blood flow response to pacing tachycardia and dipyridamole infusion in patients with dilated cardiomyopathy without overt heart failure. *Circulation* 1995;92:796–804.

Chapter 18

Nuclear Magnetic Resonance and Myocardial Viability

William J. Thoma, PhD, Mark A. Lawson, MD,
William T. Evanochko, PhD, and
Gerald M. Pohost, MD

Introduction

Nuclear magnetic resonance (NMR) provides a versatile tool to evaluate the myocardium. The scope of NMR applications range from high-resolution structural and functional imaging [magnetic resonance imaging (MRI)] to probes of the metabolic status of myocardial regions [magnetic resonance spectroscopy (MRS)]. This text reviews the ways NMR can be applied to the assessment of myocardial viability.[1]

Clinical Magnetic Resonance Imaging

MRI has excellent spatial and temporal resolution and is suited ideally for visualization of cardiac morphology and function. Substantial data are available on the application of MRI to patients with coronary artery disease to evaluate cardiac function and geometry. Current investigations are directed toward the use of NMR to image myocardial perfusion and the coronary arteries. Thus, MRI may offer the most comprehensive ability to assess the genesis and the effects of myocardial ischemia and infarction.

Magnetic Resonance Approaches to Assess Ischemic Heart Disease

Evaluation of Morphology and Function

MRI has the ability to image the heart in any selected tomographic plane without interference from surrounding soft tissue, lungs, or bones. Cardiac images are obtained using spin-echo or "dark blood" acquisitions yielding static, high-resolution depictions of

[1]Readers unfamiliar with the physical principles and terminology of NMR or MRI are encouraged to consult a general text such as *NMR in Physiology and Biomedicine*, Robert Gillies ed. Academic Press, San Diego, Calif,

1994. From Dilsizian V (ed). *Myocardial Viability: A Clinical and Scientific Treatise*. Armonk, NY: Futura Publishing Co., Inc.; © 2000.

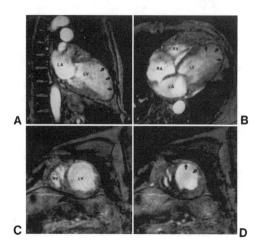

Figure 1. Gradient-echo images of the heart in a patient with prior anterior myocardial infarction. (**A**) End-systolic vertical long-axis image. (**B**) End-systolic horizontal long-axis image. (**C**) End-systolic short-axis image. (**D**) End-diastolic short-axis image. RA, right atrium; RV, right ventricle; LA, left atrium; LV, left ventricle.

cardiac anatomy, while gradient-echo or "bright blood" acquisitions producing images that, when viewed as a continuous loop movie, show ventricular contraction and relaxation, so called cine-MRI. The most common orientations used in cardiac imaging include the vertical long axis, the horizontal long axis, and the short axis (Fig. 1).

Typically, the intrinsic contrast between the endocardium and intracavitary blood eliminates the need to use contrast material, making cardiac MRI a truly noninvasive imaging modality. The use of multiple imaging planes allows visualization of the precise extent of regional wall motion abnormalities. Global ventricular function can be determined tomographically from end-systolic and end-diastolic images. Left ventricular (LV) volumes and ejection fraction are derived accurately either by applying the area-length method to long-axis images or Simpson's rule to serial short-axis images.[2] Right ventricular (RV) function can be assessed more accurately using MRI with, for example, serial short-axis imaging than with any other imaging modality.

MRI allows assessment of the complications of myocardial infarction. Location, extent, and functional significance of LV aneurysms are assessed easily [Fig. 2(A)]. Mural thrombus formation is noted as a poorly defined intracavitary structure adherent to thinned myocardial wall and projecting into the LV chamber [Fig. 2(B)]. However, thrombus is more difficult to detect when mobile such as with marked dyskinesis. Peri-

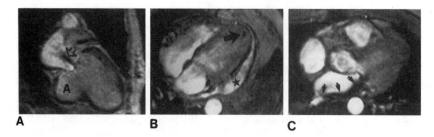

Figure 2. Complications of prior myocardial infarction. (**A**) Inferoposterior aneurysm (A) and mild mitral regurgitation (open arrow). (**B**) Apical thrombus (arrow) and pericardial effusion (*). (**C**) Severe eccentric jet of mitral regurgitation.

cardial effusion associated with postinfarction pericarditis can be imaged, even if small, using either spin-echo or gradient-echo techniques. The presence of mitral regurgitation resulting from papillary muscle dysfunction or ventricular dilatation is confirmed by a dark jet (signal void) of turbulent blood flow appearing in the left atrium during ventricular systole [Fig. 2(C)]. The mitral regurgitation can be quantitated by a technique known as phase velocity mapping. Likewise, ventricular septal rupture can be detected and quantitated. Of course, in this case the signal void emanates from the interventricular septum as blood flows from the left into the right ventricle. Phase velocity mapping can be used to quantitate the size of the shunt.

Acutely infarcted myocardium appears as brighter than normal tissue on T_2-weighted images.[3–7] This image contrast is related to differing proton relaxation characteristics. Thus, the observed signal characteristics are different in normal and acutely infarcted myocardium. Although changes in acutely infarcted myocardium are complex following coronary occlusion, this increase in signal is caused by, in large part, the increased proton (H^+) content of edematous tissue.[5,8] The area of signal enhancement generally corresponds to the size of the myocardial ischemia. Reperfusion enhances regional edema and may lead to an overestimate of the size of infarction.[9] Such enhancement in signal intensity of acutely infarcted myocardium can persist for weeks. On the other hand, infarcted myocardium does not consistently produce alterations in relaxation times over the long term, and therefore infarct sizing may be less precise.[10] However, regional myocardial wall thinning at the site of prior infarction can be demonstrated (Fig. 1). The presence of myocardium with enhanced signal after acute myocardial ischemia is consistent with irreversible damage.

Magnetic Resonance Coronary Angiography

Perhaps the most intriguing application of MRI for evaluating ischemic heart disease is coronary magnetic resonance angiography (MRA). Although not a direct indicator of myocardial viability, the ability to visualize coronary anatomy when viability is in question would be quite helpful. Using MRA, the coronary arteries may be visualized in-plane as in Figure 3, viewed using computer-aided projection techniques, or as three-dimensional (3-D) reconstructions. Currently, coronary MRA is limited to the larger and less tortuous arteries. Artifacts and alignment errors resulting from cardiac and respiratory motion confound the final product. Further, the high-signal epicardial fat that usually surrounds the coronaries can reduce the contrast between the coronary artery and epicardial fat

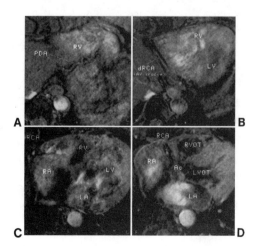

Figure 3. Coronary magnetic resonance angiogram (MRA) of the right coronary artery viewed in multiple transaxial planes (inferior to superior). (**A**) Inferior plane with posterior descending artery (PDA) (**B**) Distal right coronary artery (dRCA) in the atrioventricular (AV) groove. (**C**) Midcardiac plane with RCA in AV groove. (**D**) RCA near the origin from the aorta.

making visualization of the arteries even more difficult. Imaging of the arteries can be improved by using methodologies, such as "saturation pulses," to remove fat signals. The proximal two-thirds of the coronary arteries have been imaged successfully in-plane using breath-hold, respiratory gating, or respiratory feedback monitoring techniques to minimize respiratory artifacts.[11–15] Patent saphenous vein grafts can be visualized using gradient-echo techniques as a bright visible intraluminal signal. However, there must be sufficient flow to generate contrast between the lumen and the wall. Graft MRA can be limited by signal dropout associated with the ferromagnetic properties of sternal wires and hemostatic clips used in internal mammary grafts. Phase velocity imaging can be applied to the evaluation of coronary blood flow and has been used to visualize grafts.[16]

Detection of the Presence and Extent of Myocardial Ischemia

Dynamic exercise within the magnetic resonance scanner is difficult. Furthermore, motion and respiratory artifacts increase with the level of exercise. Thus, pharmacologic agents such as dobutamine have been used to induce stress. An alternate pharmacologic approach to dobutamine is dipyridamole.

Dobutamine

As with dobutamine stress echocardiography, ischemic wall motion changes can be detected by cine-MRI during an infusion of dobutamine. In one series the sensitivity of this approach, compared with coronary angiography, to detect single-vessel disease was 88%, while sensitivity for multivessel disease was 100%.[17] In another series there was 90%–95% agreement reported between magnetic resonance–detected wall motion abnormalities and the site and extent of perfusion defects on ^{201}Tl imaging.[18]

Recently, Dendale et al addressed the issue of viable myocardium after acute myocardial infarction.[19] They hypothesized that viable tissue could be characterized either by demonstration of recovery of wall motion under dobutamine stress or by perfusion patterns after paramagnetic contrast agent administration. Using a gradient-echo magnetic resonance technique at rest and with low-dose dobutamine administration, they examined 28 patients within the first 2 weeks after acute myocardial infarction. They also performed contrast enhanced spin-echo MRI using gadolinium (Gd)-tetraazacyclo-dodecane-tetraacetic acid (DOTA) and classified the enhancement patterns as either subendocardial, transmural, or a doughnut pattern. Finally, they scored wall motion at rest and with stress to assess the contractile reserve of the infarct regions. They reported that in 31 of 37 patients, subendocardial or absent enhancement was related to functional recovery with stress. Absence of functional recovery in 10 of 17 transmural infarct segments indicated nonviability. Finally, the doughnut pattern was associated exclusively with the absence of viability. They concluded that the contrast enhancement patterns were related to residual myocardial viability.

Dendale et al also studied the relationship between abnormalities in myocardial wall thickening (WT) during dobutamine infusion and relation to changes in both myocardial perfusion and fatty acid metabolism.[20] Utilizing low-dose dobutamine MRI, 15 patients with a myocardial infarction underwent (1) MRI to assess their WT and contractile reserve; (2) technetium-99m (^{99m}Tc) sestamibi (MIBI) to assess myocardial perfusion; and (3) β-methyl-iodophenyl-pentadecanoic acid (BMIPP) single photon emission computed tomography (SPECT) to assess fatty acid uptake. They reported that the WT at rest was significantly related to the uptake of MIBI ($p < 0.001$) but not to abnormalities in the uptake of BMIPP. An abnormal uptake of MIBI was seen in all of the akinetic segments. Some of the hypokinetic segments had a normal uptake while others had a mildly to moderately reduced uptake. Of significance was the relation between abnormalities of fatty acid metabolism and the contractile reserve. They concluded that there was a close relation between WT and residual perfusion. In contrast, abnormal contractile reserve was associated with abnormalities of fatty acid metabolism. Also, by using cine-MRI in combination with low-dose dobutamine stimulation Dendale,et al predicted viability after infarction with an accuracy of 80%. They also noted that ability to assess viability was underestimated in akinetic segments.[21]

Dipyridamole

Although dipyridamole is not truly a stress-inducing agent, reversible wall motion abnormalities can be detected following the administration of dipyridamole and have been observed. Such abnormalities were present in 67% of patients with reversible defects on ^{201}Tl tomography using standard dipyridamole infusions (0.56 mg/kg).[22] However, an increase to 78% in sensitivity was observed when the dose was increased (0.75 mg/kg).[23] Dipyridamole leads to such abnormal wall motion by coronary flow reduction rather than induction of increased stress. Flow reductions sufficient to induce wall motion abnormalities usually require higher doses of dipyridamole that may not be well tolerated by patients. We do not recommend dipyridamole to induce wall motion abnormalities because the sensitivity of this approach is limited compared with that of a stress test.

Contrast Agents

Stress-induced reduction in segmental wall motion can be used to assess the extent of jeopardized myocardium. Changes in myocardial blood flow (MBF) might, in theory, be visualized by standard gradient-echo imaging techniques. Such changes have not been visualized using standard magnetic field strengths. Therefore, magnetic resonance contrast agents are necessary to visualize heterogeneity of MBF. There are two classes of currently available magnetic resonance contrast agents: paramagnetic and magnetic-susceptibility agents. Paramagnetic agents (eg, Gd-based agents) shorten T_1 relaxation. Thus, myocardium perfused by the agent will appear brighter than jeopardized myocardium. These magnetic resonance contrast agents behave like plasma; when a first-pass imaging approach is used a bolus of intravenously (IV) injected contrast agent can be tracked through the central circulation and into the myocardium (Fig. 4). After administration of the contrast agent, myocardial regions supplied by stenotic coronary arteries show decreased signal intensity that correspond to ^{201}Tl perfusion defects (Fig. 5).[24] A

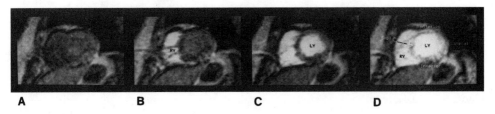

Figure 4. Serial images demonstrating the first pass of contrast during myocardial perfusion imaging. (**A**) Prior to contrast injection. (**B**) Contrast appearing first in the right ventricle. (**C**) Contrast next appearing in the left ventricle. (**D**) Contrast finally appearing in the myocardium.

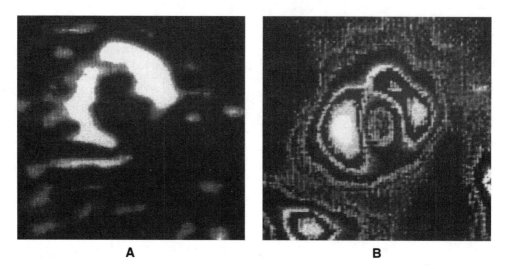

Figure 5. (**A**) Magnetic resonance imaging (MRI) and (**B**) nuclear short-axis perfusion images in a patient with a defect involving the inferolateral and inferior segments.

homogenous distribution of contrast has been observed in healthy subjects. When contrast-enhanced magnetic resonance perfusion imaging was repeated after revascularization, there was normalization of signal intensity in the revascularized territory when compared with the previous MRI study. Inhomogeneity in myocardial perfusion is generally induced with an infusion of dipyridamole. When compared with ^{201}Tl tomography, contrast-enhanced MRI correlated well with thallium images.[25] Changes in signal intensity during the first-pass data can be displayed as an intensity-time curve for separate myocardial segments. Jeopardized myocardium demonstrates diminished wash-in of contrast (decreased up slope) and lower peak signal intensity (Fig. 6).[24]

Early studies were limited by acquiring images in a single tomographic plane. To reliably determine the extent of coronary artery disease, multiple tomographic planes are necessary. Validation of acquisition techniques that can obtain multiple tomographic

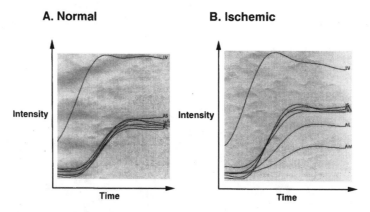

Figure 6. Signal intensity-time curves. The uppermost curve represents the left ventricle (LV). The lower curves represent the six short-axis myocardial segments. (**A**) Normal patient with homogeneous wash-in to all segments. (**B**) Patient with ischemic heart disease with a perfusion defect of the anterior and anterolateral segments. Ant, anterior; AL, anterolateral; IL, inferolateral; Inf, inferior; IS, inferoseptal; AS, anteroseptal.

planes while maintaining temporal resolution adequate to evaluate contrast agent kinetics during a first-pass study have been reported.[26–28] Magnetic susceptibility agents (eg, dysprosium) cause signal reduction in normal myocardium, while hypoperfused myocardium appears bright ("hot spot"). Image acquisition techniques are being optimized.[29] A goal of magnetic resonance perfusion imaging is to establish a relationship between alterations of relaxation time, contrast agent concentration, and MBF. A better understanding of these variables would provide improved quantitative estimation of MBF (milliliters per second per gram).[30] An MRI approach known as magnetization transfer, which exhibits sensitivity to tissue perfusion that obviates the need for contrast agents, is under investigation.[31]

Kim et al also examined myocardial Gd-diethylenetriamine penta-acetic acid (DTPA) contrast enhancement on proton MRIs and found that this approach demonstrated the extent and severity of injury in acutely reperfused myocardium.[32] Based on prior knowledge, it has been shown that contrast medium-enhanced MRI of acute, reperfused infarcts have both hypoenhanced and hyperenhanced regions in areas of injured myocardium. Because the mechanisms that lead to these altered enhancement patterns are unknown, an isolated rabbit heart model was used to evaluate altered enhancement patterns to myocardial perfusion and viability. Using T_1-weighted spin-echo images and stepwise changes in perfusate Gd-DTPA concentration, the Gd clearance time constants indicated the severity of microvascular damage. Using spatial maps of such washout time constants, the size of regions with abnormal time constants correlated with histologically determined infarct size. These authors concluded that the differential image intensities of Gd-DTPA primarily were caused by regional differences in contrast agent wash-in and washout time constants in the contrast-enhanced MRI. The extent and severity of myocardial injury can be deduced by these regional differences in time constants.

Assessment of Myocardial Viability

Magnetic Resonance Imaging

The role of standard MRI to differentiate viable from nonviable myocardium, like echocardiography, relies on the imaging of regional thinning and of reduced regional systolic WT. Nonviable myocardial regions having <50% peak ^{201}Tl counts or <50% uptake of ^{18}F-2-deoxyglucose (FDG) have a significantly lower end-diastolic wall thickness and percent systolic WT in the involved myocardial segments when compared with the normal myocardial segments [Fig. 1(C) and 1(D)].[33,34] However, the presence of severe regional wall motion abnormalities alone does not reliably indicate nonviable myocardium because such regions may be "hibernating" or "stunned." It has been shown that asynergic regions that are metabolically active by FDG positron emission tomography (PET) maintain a greater end-diastolic wall thickness than those without metabolic activity. By using a threshold value for end-diastolic wall thickness of 8 mm for akinetic or dyskinetic segments, the sensitivity and specificity for predicting metabolic activity is 74% and 79%, respectively. Dobutamine infusion has been used in conjunction with echocardiography to assess the viability in asynergic segments. Similarly, but with the advantage of true 3-D information and no interference from bone or lung, MRI has been used to assess functional changes during dobutamine infusion. Low-dose dobutamine infusion generally will lead to wall motion improvement in viable asynergic myocardial segments but no such improvement in nonviable segments. Larger infusions of dobutamine can lead to worsening of ischemic asynergic segments and reduction in specificity. Wall thickness and WT are indirect indicators of viability. However, a unique aspect of magnetic resonance methods is the ability to assess metabolism providing a more direct means to evaluate viability using spectroscopy.

Hsu et al used the isolated perfused rabbit heart model to study the delayed reduction of tissue water diffusion after myocardial ischemia using MRI techniques.[35] The apparent diffusion coefficient of normally perfused myocardium remained constant while the nonperfused region showed a gradual decrease. Myocyte swelling, which is known to occur during the onset of myocardial infarction, appears to be linked to the observed decrease in diffusion coefficient. Because of this relation, the strategy might provide another approach to noninvasive determination of viability of ischemic myocardium.

Lawson et al have looked at the correlation of thallium uptake with LV wall thickness by cine-MRI in patients with acute and healed myocardial infarcts.[36] This study used a three-pronged approach: first, the relation between both end-diastolic and end-systolic wall thickness and normalized thallium-201 uptake was examined in a group of patients with myocardial ischemia; second, the relation between regional WT and normalized thallium uptake was determined; and finally, the relation between thallium uptake and wall thickness both early and late after infarction was evaluated. A total of 24 myocardial ischemia patients underwent both routine SPECT imaging and cine-MRI soon after infarct ($n = 7$) and late after infarct ($n = 17$). MRI wall thickness at end-diastole and end-systole were correlated to normalized thallium activity in 18 segments. End-systolic wall thickness correlated significantly with normalized thallium uptake in the vast majority of segments (14 of 18); in contrast, end-diastolic wall thickness correlated with only 4 of 18 segments; likewise WT correlated with only 3 of 18 segments. These authors concluded that end-systolic wall thickness was an excellent parameter for diagnosing severely reduced myocardial scar.

Magnetic Resonance Spectroscopy

In addition to the proton many other nuclei exist for evaluating normal and abnormal myocardium using NMR spectroscopy (NMRS). Table 1 lists several important nuclei that can and have been used to study myocardium and their natural abundance in tissue. One can see that the quantities of other nuclei are dramatically less than those of protons, resulting in substantially less signal. Under most circumstances, there is not enough signal to produce even low-resolution images in vivo utilizing these nuclei. Despite these limitations, NMRS utilizing these nuclei provides unique information unavailable from other noninvasive methods.

Table 1

Physical Properties of Magnetic Nuclei

Nucleus	Percent Natural Abundance	Spin	Frequency at 1.5 T (MHz)
$^{23}Na^1H$	99.98	1/2	64
^{13}C	1.11	1/2	16
^{19}F	100	1/2	60
^{23}Na	100	3/2	16.8
^{31}P	100	1/2	25.6

Phosphorus-31 Nuclear Magnetic Resonance

Phosphorus-31 (^{31}P) is a nuclear species that can be detected noninvasively from myocardium. NMRS using ^{31}P can provide information on the metabolic status of the cardiac myocyte. Adenosine triphosphate (ATP) is the source of chemical energy for myocardial contraction. The concentration of ATP is maintained within the cell by transfer of the high-energy phosphate of phosphocreatine (PCr) to adenosine diphosphate (ADP) via the creatine kinase reaction. The phosphorus resonance of PCr, as well as the three peaks from ATP, can be identified readily in the ^{31}P spectrum (Fig. 7). The concentration of ATP is maintained at the expense of PCr under conditions where cellular respiration is impaired (such as ischemia). This buffering of ATP by PCr allows the ratio of PCr to ATP to be used as an indicator of the metabolic status of the myocardium.

Under ischemic conditions, the hydrolysis of ATP produces significant quantities of inorganic phosphate (P_i). The P_i resonance often is obscured by overlapping peaks from phosphodiesters such as diphosphoglycerate (2,3-DPG) from red blood cells that have a similar spectral position. Observation of the P_i peak can be improved by the use of proton decoupling.[37] In this technique, the nuclear interactions between protons and neighboring phosphorus nuclei are changed by radio frequency irradiation of the protons while observing the phosphorus. One of the major interactions decoupling removes normally causes broadening of the ^{31}P resonances. Therefore, proton decoupling increases the frequency resolution by narrowing the ^{31}P resonances. When the P_i peak can be resolved, the ratio of PCr/P_i would provide an even more sensitive marker of myocardial insult as

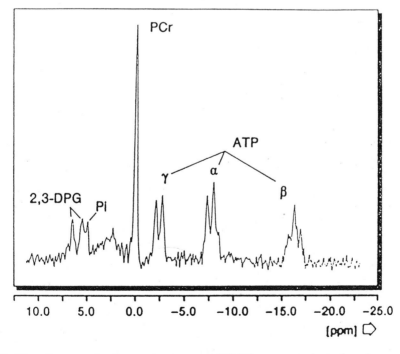

Figure 7. Phosphorus nuclear magnetic resonance (NMR) spectrum obtain from human myocardium at 1.5 T. The prominent peaks from left to right are phosphocreatine (PCr), third phosphate of adenosine triphosphate (γ-ATP), first phosphate of adenosine triphosphate (α-ATP), and second phosphate of adenosine triphosphate (β-ATP). This spectrum is from one slice from a 32-slice chemical shift imaging (CSI) set. Total acquisition time was approximately 35 minutes.

has been seen in a rat model of cardiac allograft rejection.[38] In addition, the chemical shift (spectral position) of the P_i peak is related to the intracellular pH and provides a noninvasive means to assess intracellular pH.

To utilize the metabolic information derived from ^{31}P NMR, it is important to understand the metabolic derangements that occur under different ischemic conditions. Metabolic and histological studies by Jennings and Reimer have shown that the two major hallmarks of irreversible cell injury are an inability to maintain transmembrane potential and near total depletion of ATP.[39] Under conditions of ischemia, the myocardium attempts to maintain ATP concentrations through the creatine kinase reaction, but eventually ATP is lost. The amount of ATP depletion depends on the duration and severity of the ischemia.[40] With moderate ischemia, myocardial function is depressed rapidly, and though PCr concentration can be depleted dramatically, ATP is decreased only mildly. If the ischemia is not severe, myocardial function may return rapidly on reperfusion, consistent with the concept of myocardial hibernation.[41] If ischemia is more severe, reperfusion may not lead to the rapid normalization of myocardial function, although the tissue may still be viable, consistent with the concept of stunning.[42] In these circumstances, ATP is not depleted severely and recovers slowly to preischemic levels. This slow return of nucleotide levels may be caused by the depletion of adenine nucleotides during the period of reduced flow. ATP concentration in regions subjected to severe and prolonged ischemia decreases significantly and does not recover on reperfusion. Histologically, these regions show myocardial necrosis, particularly in the subendocardial region.

Three studies using NMRS have attempted to identify metabolic factors that may be related to contractile function. Schwartz et al[43] found a close relationship between segment shortening and phosphorus metabolites during early ischemia. Korestune et al[44] found that metabolite changes occur too slowly to account for function decline. Instead, they offered evidence that mechanical factors related to perfusion pressure may be regulatory. Clarke et al[45] found that only phosphorylation potential (the ratio $[ATP]/[ADP][P_i]$) changed at a rate greater than contractile function. The control of contractile function remains an area for future investigation.

Rehr et al have applied ^{31}P NMR spectroscopic methods to the identification of viable myocardium in a canine model. They studied the myocardium after coronary occlusions of up to 6 hours with NMR examinations performed up to 72 hours after reperfusion.[46,47] They found that their ^{31}P NMR measurements accurately predicted myocardial viability.

These data suggest that ^{31}P might be a useful means to identify viable myocardium. Such ^{31}P NMR spectra were obtained rapidly from a surface coil sewn directly into the canine myocardium, but obtaining data specific to the myocardium from a coil placed outside of the chest wall requires the use of a localization spectroscopic technique. Several localization techniques have been developed and applied with some success to the study of myocardial viability. In clinical work, when the surface coil cannot be placed directly on the tissue to be studied, several localizing techniques can be applied.

Localization

The signal density obtained in ^{31}P NMR spectroscopic imaging of the myocardium is not sufficient to allow spatial mapping with the resolution of conventional proton MRI. Therefore, techniques that localize the signal to the area of interest must be implemented. Surface coils often are used for excitation and reception of the radiofrequency (rf) signal. This, in itself, provides a degree of localization based on the size of the coil and its limited volume of sensitivity. The volume of tissue observed, in general, is confined to a region under the coil a distance of one coil radius below the surface of the sample. Very small coils can localize specific vascular territories in animal models with sufficiently large hearts and clinically. In smaller hearts, such as those of rat or ferret, measurements generally are made of the entire myocardium.

Several techniques have been used to localize spectroscopic signals to the myocardium. Signal can be acquired from a localized area using magnetic field gradients for selective excitation in 1-D, 2-D, or 3-D.[48] This can be combined with phase encoding to obtain signals from multiple regions or planes within a sample[49] and, if enough signal or time is available for acquisition, a 3D map of the distribution of a specific nucleus can be obtained.[50]

With the exception of a surface coil sewn directly onto the myocardium in a high-field system, multiple signal averages must be taken to obtain spectra of reasonable signal-to-noise (S/N). In addition, because the relaxation time (T_1) of PCr exceeds that of the α-, β-, or γ-phosphorus in ATP, the acquisition approach can artificially decrease the measured ratio between PCr and ATP. Finally, discomfort and tolerance limits patient studies to under 2 hours in the magnet and, practically speaking, only studies of 1 hour or less are likely to be successful.

The ability of NMR to determine metabolic differences across the myocardial wall has been tested in two animal models. A porcine model was used at the Oxford University[51] to generate a map of transmural distribution of phosphorus metabolites using a rotating frame approach. Unfortunately, this approach suffers from off-resonance effects, which cause a nonuniform excitation profile across the spectral width. A form of the Fourier series window approach was applied to the porcine model by Gober et al.[52] They observed a heterogeneous response of the tissue to a period of regional ischemia. The largest body of work in this area has come from the group at the University of Minnesota using a canine model. They have used a Fourier series windows approach together with adiabatic pulses[53,54] to observe transmural metabolite levels associated with graded reductions in flow,[55] in hypertrophy,[56] and in the uptake of 2-deoxyglucose.[57]

Detection of Myocardial Ischemia

Building on the knowledge obtained from the animal studies cited above, localized ^{31}P NMR spectra have been used to identify the effects of ischemia in human subjects. Weiss et al[58] performed spectroscopic imaging studies in 16 patients with known coronary artery disease. Each of these patients had significant stenosis of the left anterior descending (LAD) or left main coronary artery as seen by coronary angiography. The subjects were positioned prone within the magnet and an isometric hand grip exercise. ^{31}P NMR spectra were collected before, during, and after exercise using a surface coil and 1-D phase encoding for localization of the myocardial signal. In patients with significant angiographic coronary artery disease, the PCr/ATP ratio dropped significantly with exercise and returned to normal during recovery. Normal subjects with nonischemic heart disease showed no change in PCr/ATP. When five of the nine patients with coronary artery disease were restudied after revascularization, they had normal PCr/ATP during exercise.

A similar exercise protocol was used by Yabe et al[59] to compare ^{31}P NMR spectroscopic images with redistribution on thallium imaging. They studied 27 patients with known LAD stenosis with either fixed or reversible thallium defects in the anterior wall. In this series the patients were studied supine, which is better tolerated. Patients with transient thallium defects had a lower resting PCr/ATP than controls and patients with fixed defects had a lower PCr/ATP than those with transient defects. Only those patients with reversible thallium defects showed a significant decrease in PCr/ATP with isometric exercise. Normal subjects with fixed defects showed no change in their PCr/ATP with exercise. The observation of lower resting PCr/ATP with fixed thallium defects has been confirmed in our laboratory.[60]

To demonstrate the usefulness of in vivo ^{31}P NMRS in the evaluation of patients with ischemic heart disease, Mitsunami et al reported major findings from three clinical cardiac MRS investigations.[61] The first study evaluated the relation between ^{31}P MRS with handgrip exercise and detection of myocardial ischemia as defined by exercise ^{201}Tl redistribution. Contrary to findings in normal subjects or patients with fixed thallium defects, the ratio of PCr to ATP decreased significantly during exercise in patients with reversible thallium defects. In the second study, PCr and ATP content was measured by ^{31}P MRS and compared in human myocardium with ischemia or scar diagnosed by exercise thallium imaging. Although the PCr content decreased in patients with either reversible or fixed thallium defects, the ATP content decreased only in the latter group. In the third study, postischemic myocardium with chronic mechanical dysfunction that exhibits recovery after revascularization (hibernating myocardium) was characterized metabolically using quantitative cardiac ^{31}P MRS. Postischemic myocardium with reversible mechanical dysfunction demonstrated reduced PCr but normal ATP content. These results suggest that ^{31}P MRS is a clinically useful approach both for the detection of myocardial ischemia and for the evaluation of myocardial viability.

Such studies demonstrate that PCr/ATP changes with exercise can be used to identify ischemic myocardium. Unfortunately, there are two drawbacks to this approach. First, it is only possible to interrogate the anterior myocardium, that is, that myocardium in closest proximity to the chest wall and thus the surface coil. Second, exercise studies limit the amount of time available for acquisition to steady-state exercise and could cause patient movement. To date, no one has applied pharmacologic stress to this population with, for example, dobutamine. Pharmacologic stress should reduce patient movement. If the stress can be maintained at constant levels for prolonged time intervals, signal averaging will allow improvement in data quality through an increased S/N ratio.

The animal and cell culture data of Jennings and Reimer predict that scarred and nonviable myocardium could be identified by quantifying the [ATP] in a given myocardial region. The volume of myocardial tissue could be estimated from high-resolution proton images. If a reference sample containing a phosphorus standard is placed within the area of the surface coil (after correction for relative position of the coil) the concentration of high-energy phosphates can be calculated. When this was done by Mitsunami et al[62] they found that patients with both Q-wave and non-Q-wave myocardial ischemias had reduced absolute concentrations of ATP and PCr. They also found a correlation between the concentration of ATP and a viability score derived from thallium uptake.

The limitation of localized ^{31}P spectroscopy, that is, S/N, can be improved by specialized excitation pulse.[63] Such pulsing approaches improve data quality by providing more uniform excitation, but the most effective way to improve S/N is to increase the strength of the magnetic field.

Two different approaches have been applied to take advantage of the increased signal higher field strength provides. Menon et al[64] have used a Fourier series window technique to obtain multiple thin slices across the myocardium at a field strength of 4 T. They were able to obtain good S/N spectra from voxels with volumes of 8 cc that were entirely contained within the myocardium. This substantially eliminates contamination from blood pool and allows metabolic information from the endocardium to be separated from that from the epicardium. Again, acquisition was limited to the anterior wall of the left ventricle.

Hetherington et al[65] have taken a different approach. They applied a 3D chemical shift imaging (CSI) approach first described at lower field strength of 2 T by Twieg et al[66] to a whole body 4.1-T system. Also, they have been able to acquire good S/N spectra from voxels with a nominal volume of 8 cc. Instead of using the increased S/N to slice through the anterior wall, they have obtained data from as much of the left ventricle as can been seen from a surface coil. Individual spectra from the anterior wall, interventricular septum, and even a portion of the lateral wall could be identified. Images of the distribution of ATP and PCr can be generated from the area under the respective ^{31}P peaks.

With refinement in methodologies, it may be possible to interrogate virtually the entire myocardium allowing evaluation of different regions of the left ventricle or different layers of the myocardial wall.

Chemical Shift and Shift Reagents

The NMR signal contains much more information than the simple proton maps that are used for imaging. Small changes in the local magnetic field are brought about by the electron environment. These small interactions with the magnetic field produce a small shift in the resonance frequency, termed the chemical shift. This allows the identification of chemical species. Using the ^{31}P spectrum as an example, one can identify resonances corresponding to each of the three phosphates of ATP as well as PCr. In addition, there are peaks corresponding to 2,3-DPG from the red blood cells within the blood pool, which in most cases obscure the myocardial inorganic phosphate peak.

In addition to identification of individual nuclear species the chemical shift can provide information about the local molecular environment. The chemical shift of the P_i peak, for instance, is dependent on the pH of the surrounding milieu. Accordingly, myocardial pH can be assessed noninvasively using the position of the inorganic myocardial peak. Shift reagents can be added to shift the peak of extracellular versus intracellular components, such as in the case of ^{23}Na.

Other Nuclei

To date there have been no in vivo human spectroscopy studies published using nuclei other than phosphorus. ^{1}H, ^{23}Na, and ^{19}F spectra have characteristics that have allowed unique metabolic information to be obtained in animal models.

Though the vast majority of the ^{1}H NMR signal used for imaging is derived from in-water molecules, a small and variable portion is derived from other molecules. Using techniques that suppress the water signal, the nonwater portion of the spectrum can be visualized. Peaks derived from portions of lipid molecules can be identified (Fig. 8). With

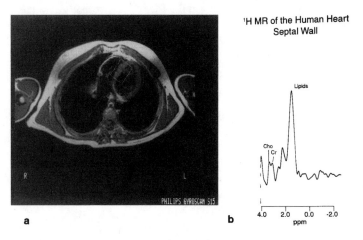

a   **b**

Figure 8. Proton NMR spectrum obtained from human myocardium at 1.5 T.

the use of this technique one can visualize the accumulation of lipids under ischemic conditions.[67]

The peaks derived from lipid protons have been studied extensively. Lipid droplets can be seen on gross histological specimens in the border zones of myocardial infarctions. This has been investigated in dog models of myocardial ischemia in our laboratory by Reeves et al.[68] We found increased intensity of NMR lipid signal in regions of moderate reduction in myocardial flow, but no significant change in the regions with severe flow reduction. It has been suggested that the prolonged recovery from an ischemic insult (stunning) is caused by, at least in part, such lipid accumulation in viable cells. Other mechanisms for myocardial stunning include calcium accumulation.[69] Myocardial calcium concentration has been measured using[19]F NMRS. The NMR visible Ca^{2+} chelator 5F-bis-(o-aminophenoxy)-N,N,N',N'-tetraacetic acid (5F-BAPTA) can be introduced into the myocardial cell by a perfusion technique. The chemical shift of the ^{19}F in the compound is dependent on the binding of Ca^{2+}. The relative proportion of an upfield to downfield signal reflects the concentrations of bound and free concentrations of BAPTA in the intracellular space and is proportional to the intracellular concentration of free Ca^{2+}.[69] Cardiac gating of signal acquisition can be added and measurements of intracellular Ca^{2+} can be made with temporal resolution of 50 ms.[70] Studies of ischemia and reperfusion using ^{19}F NMR have shown increasing intracellular Ca^{2+} in stunned myocardium as well as an increase in the size of Ca^{2+} transients during ischemia. This approach is a difficult one and the possibility of Ca^{2+} is not clinically likely.

Bottomley and Weiss recently presented an elegant approach for detecting nonviable infarcted myocardium.[71] They argue that because creatine kinase levels in the blood are used widely to diagnose cardiac necrosis, a noninvasive method to assess local creatine concentrations in the healthy and diseased human myocardium might prove clinically useful. Therefore, they measured total myocardial creatine by spatially localized ^1H MRS at 1.5 T in 10 healthy volunteers (controls) and 10 patients with a history of myocardial infarction. They report that total creatine was significantly lower in regions of infarction than in regions of noninfarcted myocardium in patients. They conclude from their data that spatially localized ^1H MRS may provide a means to assess myocardial creatine noninvasively and the assessment of regional creatine (creatine depletion) may distinguish viable (no creatine depletion) from nonviable (creatine depletion) myocardium.

^{23}Na NMR has been used to measure intracellular sodium concentration, in vitro. This technique takes advantage of the paramagnetic effect to produce a chemical shift. A specific paramagnetic shift reagent [based on dysprosium (Dy)] is added to the extracellular fluid of an isolated perfused heart preparation. This leads to a shifted signal from extracellular Na^+ up/downfield from the (non-Dy labeled) intracellular Na^+ signal such that concentration of Na_i^+ can be measured from the area of this peak. Pike et al[72] have used this technique, interleaved with ^{31}P NMR, to measure the effects of ischemia on isolated perfused rat hearts. They found that though high-energy phosphates and LV function decline rapidly at the onset of ischemia, $[Na^+]_i$ rises more gradually. Recently, they have observed that some hearts experience a rapid rise in $[Na^+]_i$, and that this often is associated with the onset of ventricular fibrillation.[73] Return of the $[Na^+]_i$ to normal levels appears to be associated with a return to normal contractile function in these hearts.

Kim et al recently used fast ^{23}Na MRI of acutely reperfused myocardial infarction as a means to assess myocardial viability.[74] This strategy is based on the theory that the ability of the myocyte to maintain an ionic sodium concentration gradient is an excellent indicator of myocardial viability. Using both rabbit and canine models, the relation of ^{23}Na intensity on MRIs to viability was assessed. Acutely infarcted, myocardium was identified by absence of triphenyltetrazolium chloride (TTC) staining. Regions of infarcted myocardium by TTC showed a significant elevation in ^{23}Na as determined by increase in MRI intensity compared with viable regions. These authors concluded that following acute infarction and reperfusion, nonviable myocardium is associated with a regional increase in ^{23}Na MRI intensity. A reduction in ^{23}Na imaging times using fast gradient-echo imaging techniques can be achieved to just a few minutes. Finally, it was suggested that ^{23}Na MRI may be a useful experimental and, in the future, clinical tool for assessing viable myocardium.

Conclusions

Cardiac NMRS and MRI are versatile tools for the evaluation of myocardium under normal and ischemic conditions. Imaging techniques presently in clinical use are helpful in visualizing the structural and functional integrity of specific cardiac regions after an ischemic insult. Augmenting standard MRI with more specialized imaging sequences and physical or pharmacologic stress to highlight compromised regions will increase the clinical value of this technique. Finally, NMR is a valuable research tool and provides a nondestructive measurement of many intracellular metabolic functions. Translation of spectroscopic techniques into clinically relevant procedures should help to determine reversibility after an ischemic or other myocardial insult including cardiomyopathy, allograft rejection, and cardiotoxcity. Coupled with the other insights that NMR can provide, spectroscopic procedures should be of great clinical value early in the 21st century.

References

1. Guilles R, ed. *NMR in Physiology and Biomedicine*. San Diego, Calif: Academic Press; 1994.
2. Cranney GB, Lotan CS, Dean L, et al. Left ventricular volume measurement using cardiac axis nuclear magnetic resonance imaging. *Circulation* 1990;82:154–163.
3. McNamara MT, Higgins CB, Schechtmann N, et al. Detection and characterization of acute myocardial infarction in man with use of gated magnetic resonance. *Circulation* 1985;71:717–724.
4. Dilworth LR, Aisen AM, Mancini GBJ, et al. Serial nuclear magnetic resonance imaging in acute myocardial infarction. *Am J Cardiol* 1987;59:1203–1205.
5. Johnston DL, Mulvagh SL, Cashion RW, et al. Nuclear magnetic resonance imaging of acute myocardial infarction within 24 hours of chest pain onset. *Am J Cardiol* 1989;64:172–179.
6. Johns JA, Leavitt MB, Newell JB, et al. Quantitation of acute myocardial infarct size by nuclear magnetic resonance imaging. *J Am Coll Cardiol* 1990;15:143–149.
7. Johnston DL, Wendt RE, Mulvagh SL, et al. Characterization of acute myocardial infarction by magnetic resonance imaging. *Am J Cardiol* 1992;69:1291–1295.
8. Chatham JC, Ackerman S, Blackard SJ. High-resolution ^{1}H NMR imaging of regional ischemia in the isolated perfused rabbit heart at 4.7 T. *Magn Reson Med* 1991;21:144–150.
9. Ryan T, Tarver RD, Duerk JL, et al. Distinguishing viable from infarcted myocardium after experimental ischemia and reperfusion by nuclear magnetic resonance imaging. *J Am Coll Cardiol* 1990;15:1355–1364.
10. McNamara MT, Higgins CB. Magnetic resonance imaging of chronic myocardial infarcts in man. *AJR* 1986;146:315–320.
11. Manning WJ, Li W, Edelman RR. A preliminary report comparing magnetic resonance coronary angiography with conventional angiography. *N Engl J Med* 1993;328:828–832.
12. Pennell DJ, Keegan J, Firmin DN, et al. Magnetic resonance imaging of coronary arteries: Techniques and preliminary results. *Br Heart J* 1993;70:315–326.
13. Manning WJ, Li W, Boyle NG, et al. Fat-suppressed breath-hold magnetic resonance coronary angiography. *Circulation* 1993;87:94–104.
14. Edelman RR, Manning WJ, Pearlman J, et al. Human coronary arteries: Projection angiograms reconstructed from breath-hold two-dimensional MR images. *Radiology* 1993;187:719–722.
15. Wang Y, Christy PS, Korosec FR, et al. Coronary MRI with a respiratory feedback monitor: The 2D imaging case. *Magn Reson Med* 1995;33:116–121.

16. Hoogendoorn LI, Pattynama PMT, Buis B, et al. Noninvasive evaluation of aortocoronary bypass grafts with magnetic resonance flow mapping. *Am J Cardiol* 1995;75:845–848.

17. van Rugge FP, van der Wall EE, de Roos A, et al. Dobutamine stress magnetic resonance imaging for detection of coronary artery disease. *J Am Coll Cardiol* 1993;22:431–439.

18. Pennell DJ, Underwood SR, Manzara CC, et al. Magnetic resonance imaging during dobutamine stress in coronary artery disease. *Am J Cardiol* 1992;70:24–40.

19. Dendle P, Francine PR, Block P, et al. Contrast enhanced and functional magnetic resonance imaging for the detection of viable myocardium after infarction. *Am Heart J* 1998;135:875–880.

20. Dendale P, Franken PR, van der Wall EE, et al. Wall thickening at rest and contractile reserve early after myocardial infarction: Correlation with myocardial perfusion and metabolism. *Coron Artery Dis* 1997;8:259–264.

21. Dendale P, Franken PR, Holman E, et al. Validation of low-dose dobutamine magnetic resonance imaging for assessment of myocardial viability after infarction by serial imaging. *Am J Cardiol* 1998;82:375–377.

22. Pennell DJ, Underwood SR, Ell PJ, et al. Dipyridamole magnetic resonance imaging: A comparison with thallium-201 emission tomography. *Br Heart J* 1990;64:362–369.

23. Baer FM, Smolarz K, Jungehulsing M, et al. Feasibility of high-dose dipyridamole-magnetic resonance imaging for detection of coronary artery disease and comparison with coronary angiography. *Am J Cardiol* 1992;69:51–56.

24. Manning WJ, Atkinson DJ, Grossman W, et al. First-pass nuclear magnetic resonance imaging studies using gadolinium-DTPA in patients with coronary artery disease. *J Am Coll Cardiol* 1991;18:959–965.

25. Schaefer S, van Tyen R, Saloner D. Evaluation of myocardial perfusion abnormalities with gadolinium-enhanced snapshot MR imaging in humans. *Radiology* 1992;185:795–801.

26. Eichenberger AC, Schuiki E, Kochli VD, et al. Ischemic heart disease: Assessment with gadolinium-enhanced ultrafast MR imaging and dipyridamole stress. *JMRI* 1994;4:425–431.

27. Lawson MA, Walsh EG, Doyle M, et al. Multislice MRI in the assessment of myocardial perfusion: A comparison with radionuclide methods. *Circulation* 1994;90:I411.

28. Edelman RR, Li W. Contrast-enhanced echo-planar MR imaging of myocardial perfusion: Preliminary study in humans. *Radiology* 1994;190:771S–777S.

29. Sakuma H, O'Sullivan M, Lucas J, et al. Effect of magnetic susceptability contrast medium on myocardial signal intensity with fast gradient-recalled echo and spin-echo MR imaging: Initial experience in humans. *Radiology* 1994;190:161–166.

30. Wilke N, Simm C, Zhang J, et al. Contrast-enhanced first pass myocardial perfusion imaging: Correlation between myocardial blood flow in dogs at rest and during hyperemia. *Magn Reson Med* 1993;29:485–497.

31. Prasad PV, Burstein D, Edelman RR. MRI evaluation of myocardial perfusion without a contrast agent using magnetization transfer. *Magn Reson Med* 1993;30:267–270.

32. Kim RJ, Chen EL, Lima JA, et al. Myocardial Gd-DTPA kinetics determine MRI contrast enhancement and reflect the extent and severity of myocardial injury after acute reperfused infarction. *Circulation* 1996;94:3318–3326.

33. Perrone-Filardi P, Bacharach SL, Dilsizian V, et al. Metabolic evidence of viable myocardium in regions with reduced wall thickness and absent wall thickening in patients with chronic ischemic left ventricular dysfunction. *J Am Coll Cardiol* 1992;20:161–168.

34. Perrone-Filardi P, Bacharach SL, Dilsizian V, et al. Regional left ventricular wall thickening: Relation to regional uptake of [18]fluorodeoxyglucose and ^{201}Tl in patients with chronic coronary artery disease and left ventricular dysfunction. *Circulation* 1992;86:1125–1137.

35. Hsu EW, Xue R, Holmes A, et al. Delayed reduction of tissue water diffusion after myocardial ischemia. *Am J Physiol* 1998; 275:H697–H702.

36. Lawson MA, Johnson LL, Coghlan L, et al. Correlation of thallium uptake with left ventricular wall thickness by cine magnetic resonance imaging in patients with acute and healed myocardial infarcts. *Am J Cardiol* 1997;70:434–441.

37. Luyten PR, Bruntink G, Sloff FM, et al. Broadband proton decoupling in human ^{31}P NMR spectroscopy. *NMR Biomed* 1989;1:177–183.

38. Canby RC, Evanochko WT, Barrett LV, et al. Monitoring the bioenergetics of cardiac allograft rejection using in-vivo P-31 nuclear magnetic resonance spectroscopy. *JACC* 1987;9:1067–1074.

39. Jennings RB, Reimer KA. Lethal myocardial ischemic injury. *Am J Pathol* 1981;102:241–255.
40. Neill WA, Ingwall JS. Stabilization of a derangement in adenosine triphosphate metabolism during sustained, partial ischemia in the dog heart. *JACC* 1986;8:894–900.
41. Rahimtoola SH. The hibernating myocardium in ischaemia and congestive heart failure. *Eur Heart J* 1993;14(suppl A):22–26. Review.
42. Braunwald E, Kloner RA. The stunned myocardium: Prolonged postischemic ventricular dysfunction. *Circulation* 1982;60:1146–1149.
43. Schwartz GG, Schaefer S, Meyerhoff DJ, et al. Dynamic relation between myocardial contractility and energy metabolism during and following brief coronary occlusion in the pig. *Circ Res* 1990;67:490–500.
44. Koretsune Y, Corretti MC, Kusuoka H, et al. Mechanism of early ishemic contractile failure. Inexcitability, metabolite accumulation, or vascular collapse *Circ Res* 1991;68:255–262.
45. Clarke K, O'Conner AJ, Willis RJ. Temporal relation between energy metabolism and myocardial function during ischemia and reperfusion. *Amer J Physiol* 1987;253:H412–H421.
46. Rehr RB, Fuhs BE, Lee F, et al. Differentiation of reperfused-viable (stunned) from reperfused-infarcted myocardium at 1 to 3 days postreperfusion by in vivo phosphorus-31 nuclear magnetic resonance spectroscopy. *Am Heart J* 1991;122:1571–1582.
47. Rehr RB, Tatum JL, Hirsch JI, et al. Effective separation of normal, acutely ischemic, and reperfused myocardium with P-31 MR spectroscopy. *Radiology* 1988;168:81–89.
48. Aue W. Localization methods for in vivo nuclear magnetic resonance spectroscopy. *Rev Magn Reson Med* 1986;1:21–72.
49. Brown TR, Kincaid BM, Ugurbil K. NMR Chemical shift imaging in three dimensions. *Proc Natl Acad Sci U S A* 1982;79:3523–3536.
50. Maudsley AA, Hilal SK, Perman WH, et al. Spatially resolved high resolution spectroscopy by "four dimensional" NMR. *J Magn Reson* 1982;51:147–152.
51. Rajagopalan B, Bristow JD, Radda GK. Measurements of transmural distribution of phosphorus metabolites in the pig heart by magnetic resonance spectroscopy. *Cardiovasc Res* 1989; XXIII:1015–1026.
52 Gober JR, Schaefer S, Camacho SA, et al. Epicardial and endocardial localized 31P magnetic resonance spectroscopy: Evalutation of metabolitic heterogeneity during regional ischemia. *Magn Reson Med* 1990;13:204–215.
53. Robitaille PM, Merkle H, Sublett E, et al. Spectroscopic imaging and spatial localization using adiabatic pulses and application to detect transmural metabolite distribution in the canine heart. *Magn Reson Med* 1989;10:14–37.
54. Robitaille PM, Lew B, Merkle H, et al. Transmural metabolite distribution in regional myocardial ischemia as studied by 31-PNMR. *Magn Reson Med* 1989;10:108–118.
55. Path G, Robitaille PM, Tristani M, et al. The correlation between transmural high energy phosphate levels and myocardial blood flow in the presence of graded coronary stenosis. *Circ Res* 1990;67:660–673.
56. Zhang J, Duncker DJ, Xu Y, et al. Glucose uptake in the severely hypertrophied left ventricle. *Circulation* 1990;88(suppl 1):1–37.
57. Yoshiyama M, Merkle H, Garwood M, et al. Transmural distribution of 2-deoxyglucose uptake in normal and post-ischemic canine myocardium. *NMR Biomed* 1995;8:9–18.
58. Weiss RG, Bottomley PA, Hardy CJ, et al. Regional myocardial metabolism of high-energy phosphates during isometric exercise in patients with coronary artery disease. *N Engl J Med* 1990;323:1593–1600.
59. Yabe T, Mitsunami K, Okada M, et al. Detection of myocardial ischemia by ^{31}P magnetic resonance spectroscopy during handgrip exercise. *Circulation* 1994;89:1709–1716.
60. Luney DJE, den Hollander JA, Evanochko WT, et al. ^{31}P Nuclear magnetic resonance spectroscopy of human myocardial scar. Proceedings, Society of Magnetic Resonance in Med., 12th Annual Meeting, August 14–20, 1993 New York, NY; 1993:1091.
61. Mitsunami K, Yabe T, Kinoshita M. Diagnosis of myocardial ischemia and viability by 31P nuclear magnetic resonance spectroscopy. *Rinsho Byori* 1998;46:348–353.
62. Mitsunami K, Okada M, Inoue T, et al. In vivo ^{31}P nuclear magnetic resonance spectroscopy in patients with old myocardial infarction. *Jpn Circ J* 1992;56:614–619.
63. Ugurbil K, Garwood M, Bendall MR. Amplitude and frequency modulated pulses to achieve 90 degree plane rotations with inhomogeneous B1 fields. *J Magn Reson* 1987;72:177–185.

64. Menon RS, Hendrich K, Hu X, et al. ^{31}PNMR spectroscopy of the human heart at 4T: Detection of substantially uncontaminated cardiac spectra and differentiation of subepicardium and subendocardium. *Magn Reson Med* 1992;26:368–376.
65. Hetherington HP, Luney DJE, Vaughan JT, et al. 3D 31P spectroscopic imaging of the human heart at 4.1T. *Magn Reson Med* 1995;33:427–431.
66. Twieg DB, Myerhoff DJ, Hubesch B, et al. Phosphorus-31 magnetic resonance spectroscopy in humans by spectroscopic imaging: Localized spectroscopy and metabolite imaging. *Magn Reson Med* 1989;12:291–305.
67. Evanochko WT, Reeves RC, Canby RC, et al. Proton NMR spectroscopic studies of "stunned" myocardium. In: Cohen SM, ed. *Physiological NMR Spectroscopy: From Isolated Cells to Man. Ann New York Acad Sci* 1987;508:460–462.
68. Reeves RC, Evanockho WT, Canby RC, et al. Demonstration of increased myocardial lipid with postischemic dysfunction ("myocardial stunning") by proton magnetic resonance spectroscopy. *JACC* 1989;13:739–744.
69. Marban E, Kitakaze M, Kusuoka H, et al. Intracellular free calcium concentration measured with 19F NMR spectroscopy in intact ferret hearts. *Proc Natl Acad Sci U S A* 1987;84:6005–6009.
70. Kirschenlohr HL, Metcalf JC, Morris PG, et al. Ca^{2+} transient, Mg^{2+}, and pH measurements in the cardiac cycle by ^{19}F NMR. *Proc Natl Acad Sci U S A* 1988;85:9017–9021.
71. Bottomley PA, Weiss RG. Non-invasive magnetic-resonance detection of creatine depletion in non-viable infarcted myocardium. *Lancet* 1998;351:714–718.
72. Pike MM, Luo CS, Clark MD, et al. NMR measurements of Na^+ and cellular energy in ischemic rat heart: Role of Na^+-H^+ exchange. *Am J Physiol* 1993;265:H2017–H2026.
73. Pike MM, Luo CS, Yanagida S, et al. $^{23}Na^+$ and ^{31}P nuclear magnetic resonance studies of ischemia-induced ventricular fibrillation. Alterations of intracellular Na^+ and cellular energy. *Circ Res* 1995;77:773–783.
74. Kim RJ, Lima JA, Chen EL, et al. Fast 23Na magnetic resonance imaging of acute reperfused myocardial infarction. Potential to assess myocardial viability. *Circulation* 1997;95:1877–1885. Footnotes

INDEX

Page numbers in *italics* indicate figures. Page numbers followed by "t" indicate tables.

Acetoacetate
    CoASH, 2-oxoglutarate, NAD+, intramitochondrial concentrations of, mitochondria oxidizing, 96t
    mitochondria oxidizing, NAD+, 2-oxoglutarate, 96t
    pyruvate, CoASH, 2-oxoglutarate, NAD+, intramitochondrial concentrations of, mitochondria oxidizing, 96t
Acetyl-CoA, ketone bodies, metabolism of, regulatory sites in, 95
Adenosine triphosphate
    activated nonspecific cation channel, 145
Aerobic, *versus* anaerogic energy production, 28, 28–29
Amino acids, branched-chain, 97
Anaerogic, *versus* aerobic energy, 28, 28–29
Anaplerosis, 96–98, 97, 98
Anti-infarct effect of preconditioning, models, 56–57
Apoptosis, 5–7, 6
Arterial input function, measuring, tracer kinetics, 257–259, 258
Asynergic myocardium, diagnostic features, ischemic heart disease, 208t
Asynergy
    ischemic cardiomyopathy, 208t, 208–209
    segmental, left, ventricular, structural correlates, reversible, irreversible, 209–212
Attenuation correction, SPECT, 305

Beta-methyl-w-(p-^{123}I-phenyl)penta-decanoic acid, 371–376
Bloodpool tomography, gated, 164–171

Branched-chain amino acids, 97
    isoleucine, 97
    leucine, 97
    valine, 97

Cl-channels, sarcoplasmic reticulum, 128
    ^{11}C-palmitic acid, 357–362
Capillary density, nonmyocyte compartment, 212
Carbon chain, methylation of, 370–371
Carboxylation, decarboxylation pathways, pyruvate metabolism, in heart muscle, 98
Cardiomyopathy, ischemic
    asynergy, 208t, 208–209
    histomorphological changes, 7–8, 8
    structural changes, 7–8, 8
Cation channel, nonspecific, adenosine triphosphate-activated, 145
Cell death
    excitotoxic, 150–151
    myocardial, 5–7
        apoptosis, 5–7, 6
        necrosis, 5
Cell membrane integrity, 249–436
Cell survival, programmed, 26, 26–27, 27
Cellular physiology, 77–159
Channels, 117–150, 118
    adenosine triphosphate-activated nonspecific cation channel, 145
    Cl-channels, sarcoplasmic reticulum, 128
    chloride channels, 145–147, 146
    connexins, topology of, 148
    excitotoxic cell death, 150–151
    intercellular channels, 147–150, 148
    K+ channels, 132–142, 133, 134, 135, 136, 137, 138–139, 140–141
    L-type calcium channel, 128–131, 129, 130
    Na+ channel, 142–145, 143, 144

nonsarcolemmal channels, 118–128
P-type Ca^{2+} channel, 132
ryanodine receptor, *118*, 118–127, *119, 120, 121, 122, 123, 124, 124–125, 127*
sarcolemmal channels, 128–147
sarcoplasmic reticulum, 118–128
sodium channel structure, *143*
T-type Ca^{2+} channel, 132
Chemical shift, shift reagents, nuclear magnetic resonance, 431
Chloride channels, 145–147, *146*
Citric acid cycle, depletion of, *95*, 95–96, 96t
CoASH
    acetoacetate, 2-oxoglutarate, NAD+, intramitochondrial concentrations of, mitochondria oxidizing, 96t
Connexins, topology of, *148*
Contractile reserve, 181–206
    after myocardial infarction, prognosis, *186*, 186–188, *187*
    assessment, postextrasystolic potentiation, 222
    clinical markers, myocardial viability, 181–182
    dobutamine echocardiography
        after acute myocardial infarction, 183–185, *184*
        single photon emission computerized tomography, positron emission tomography, compared, 193–197, *194*
    hibernating myocardium, 188–189
    Kaplan-Meier survival curves, *186, 193*
    left ventricular dysfunction
        acute, reversible, 182–188
        chronic, 189
            dobutamine echocardiography in, *189*, 189–192, *190, 191, 192*
            persistent, 188–193
    stunned myocardium, 182–183, *183*
    stunning, *versus* acute hibernation, *185*, 185–186
Contraction, perfusion, mismatch, match, 4–5, *5*
Contraction-perfusion, mismatch, match, 4–5, *5*
Contrast agents, nuclear magnetic resonance, *423*, 423–425, *424*
Copper coil model, myocardial viability, *83*, 83–84

Coronary artery, transient occlusion, model, 86–87
Coronary artery disease
    chronic
        dobutamine stress echocardiogram, 221
        identifying, thallium-201 scintigraphy, protocol, 289–291, *290*
        thallium imaging patients with, 270–271
    positron emission tomography, 400–410

Decarboxylation pathways, pyruvate metabolism, in heart muscle, *98*
Depletion, citric acid cycle, *95*, 95–96, 96t
Diabetes mellitus, positron emission tomography with, 397–398
Diagnostic techniques, *13*, 13–16, *14, 15*
Dietary state of patient, positron emission tomography and, 397
Dihydropyridine receptor. *See* L-type calcium channel
Dipyridamole, nuclear magnetic resonance, 423
Dobutamine, nuclear magnetic resonance, 422–423
Dobutamine echocardiography, 212–216, *213*, 215t, 216–222
    after acute myocardial infarction, contractile reserve, 183–185, *184*
    chronic coronary artery disease, 221
    left ventricular dysfunction, contractile reserve, *189*, 189–192, *190, 191, 192*
    microvascular integrity, 218–221, *219, 220*
    myocyte membrane integrity, 218
    safety, with reduced left ventricular systolic function, 221–222
    single photon emission computerized tomography
        compared, contractile reserve, 193–197, *194*
        positron emission tomography, compared, 193–197, *194*
    technical limitations, 216–218, *218, 219*, 219t
Echocardiographic assessment, viable, nonviable myocardium, 212–222

Electrical injury model, myocardial
    viability, 79–82, *80, 81, 82*
End effector, preconditioning, 62–63
Energetics of heart, 105–113
    cellular targets, 108t, 108–109, *109*
    L-argine, chemical structure, *106*
    mitochondria, 109–110, *110*
    molecular targets, nitric oxide, 108t,
        108–109, *109*
    nitric oxide synthase, regulation of,
        107–108
    nitric oxide synthesis, 105–107, *106*
        localization of, 107
    oxygen consumption, whole animal,
        110–111
    pathophysiology, 111–112
    physiology, 109–111
    respiration, control of, 109–111
Energy production, anaerogic, aerobic
    versus, 28, *28*–29
Everted segment model, myocardial
    viability, 86
Excitotoxic cell death, 150–151
Experimental models, 79–90
    copper coil model, *83,* 83–84
    coronary artery, transient occlusion,
        86–87
    electrical injury model, 79–82, *80, 81,*
        82
    everted segment model, 86
    Folts' model, 84–86, *85*
    irreversibly injured myocardium,
        histological detection, 87
    myocardial viability, 79–90
    reversed electrical potentials, thrombus
        formation in aortas, model, *80*
    thrombin injection model, 86
    thrombosis
        coronary artery
            electrical injury model, *82*
            model, *81*
        coronary artery occlusion by, 87–88

^{18}F-2-deoxyglucose, positron emission
    tomography, 397–398
Fatty acids
    labeled, lipid metabolism, imaging,
        349–390
        dual parameter analysis, dynamic,
            noninvasively measuring
            metabolism, 351–352
        instruments, 352

living organism, constraints of
    measuring, 350–351
myocardial fatty acid metabolism,
    354, 354–357, *356*
    beta-methyl-w-(p-^{123}I-phenyl)-
        pentadecanoic acid, 371–376
    ^{11}C-palmitic acid, 357–362
    carbon chain, methylation of,
        370–371
    w^{123}I-heptadecanoic acid, 362–365
    metabolic trapping, labeled fatty
        acids for, 368–371
    nuclide, non-carbon, insertion into
        carbon chain, 368–370, *369*
    w-(o-^{123}I-phenyl)pentadecanoic
        acid, 376–379
    w-(p-^{123}I-phenyl)pentadecanoic
        acid, 365–368
    types of labeled fatty acids, 352–354,
        353
    w^{123}I-hexadecanoic acid, 362–365
    metabolism of, regulatory sites in, *95*
    oxidative metabolism pathways, *99*
FDG imaging. *See* ^{18}F-fluoro-
    deoxyglucose imaging thallium-
    201 scintigraphy, 294–300
Fibrinolytic therapy, myocardial salvage,
    timing, *236,* 236–237, *237*
Fibrous matrix, nonmyocyte
    compartment, 211–212
Folts' model, myocardial viability, 84–86,
    85
Free radicals, oxygen-derived, 30
Fuels, heart, mechanical restitution, 91–104
    acetoacetate, CoASH, 2-oxoglutarate,
        NAD+, intramitochondrial
        concentrations of, mitochondria
        oxidizing, 96t
    anaplerosis, 96–98, *97, 98*
    branched-chain amino acids, *97*
    cardiac metabolism, control, regulation
        of, 92t
    citric acid cycle, depletion of, *95,* 95–
        96, 96t
    CoASH, 2-oxoglutarate, NAD+,
        intramitochondrial
        concentrations of, mitochondria
        oxidizing, 96t
fatty acids
    metabolism of, regulatory sites in,
        95
    oxidative metabolism pathways, *99*

glucose
    metabolism of, regulatory sites in, *95*
    oxidative metabolism pathways, *99*
isoleucine, branched-chain amino acids, *97*
ketone bodies
    to acetyl-CoA, metabolism of, regulatory sites in, *95*
    oxidative metabolism pathways, *99*
leucine, branched-chain amino acids, *97*
moiety-conserved cycles, 98–99, *99*
    cardiovascular system, 94t
    ischemic heart muscle, depletion, replenishment of, *100*, 100–101
pyruvate metabolism, in heart muscle, carboxylation, decarboxylation pathways, *98*
pyruvate or acetoacetate, CoASH, 2-oxoglutarate, NAD+, intramitochondrial concentrations of, mitochondria oxidizing, 96t
respiration, control of, 98–99, *99*
valine, branched-chain amino acids, *97*
Furifosmin, technetium-99m, 340

Gated bloodpool single photon emission computer tomography, regional function, 169–171, *170*
Gated bloodpool tomography, 164–171
Gated perfusion
    metabolic imaging, 171–177
    metabolism imaging, regional function, 171–175, *172, 173*
Gated perfusion/metabolism scans, global function, 175–176
Gated single photon emission computer tomography
    perfusion/metabolism images, acquisition of, 176–177
Global function
    from gated perfusion/metabolism scans, 175–176
    from tomographic gated bloodpool, 167–169, *168, 169*
Glucose
    metabolism of, regulatory sites in, *95*
    oxidative metabolism pathways, *99*
Graded ischemia, 29–30
Graded metabolic responses, 29–30

Heart failure
    left ventricular dysfunction, 3–4, *4*
    treatment options, 9–13
        heart transplantation, 12–13
        medical therapy, 9–11, *10*
        revascularization, *11*, 11–12, *12*
Heart transplantation, 12–13
Hibernation, 25–36
    acute, *versus* stunning, contractile reserve, *185*, 185–186
    contractile reserve, 188–189
    histologic features of, 211t
Histomorphological changes, ischemic cardiomyopathy, 7–8, *8*
Histopathology, diagnostic features, asynergic myocardium, ischemic heart disease, 208t

Imaging, advances in, 161–248
Infarct size
    left ventricular function, myocardial salvage, timing, 238–240, *239*
    myocardial salvage, timing, relationship between, *239*
Infarction, myocardial, acute, thallium imaging after, 270
Input function, arterial, measuring, tracer kinetics, 257–259, *258*
Intercellular channels, 147–150, *148*
Ionic tracers, intravenously injected, *266*, 266–268, *267*
Irreversibly injured myocardium, histological detection, 87
Ischemia
    asynergy, 208t, 208–209
    graded, 29–30
    histomorphological changes, 7–8, *8*
    multiple mediators, preconditioning, *59*, 59–60
    nuclear magnetic resonance, 419–425
    structural changes, 7–8, *8*
    stunning, 116–117, 151–153
Ischemic preconditioning, 25–36
Isoleucine, branched-chain amino acids, *97*
W^{123}I-heptadecanoic acid, 362–365

K+ channels, 132–142, *133, 134, 135, 136, 137, 138–139, 140–141*
Kaplan-Meier survival curves, contractile reserve, *186, 193*

Ketone bodies
  to acetyl-CoA, metabolism of, regulatory sites in, *95*
  oxidative metabolism pathways, *99*
Kinase C, protein, signal transduction pathway for, 57–59, *58*
Kinetic models
  application to cardiac studies, 257
  tracer kinetics, application to cardiac studies, 257
Kinetics, tracer, 251–264
  arterial input function, measuring, 257–259, *258*
  complicated models, 262, *262*
  kinetic models, application to cardiac studies, 257
  myocardial uptake, quantitating, 263–264, *264*
  partial volume effects, correction for, *260*, 260–262
  simple model, 251–257, *252, 254, 255, 256*
  spillover, correction for, *260*, 260–262
  three-compartment model, *262*
  tissue time activity curve, measuring, *259*, 259–260

L-argine, chemical structure, *106*
L-type calcium channel, 128–131, *129, 130*
Labeled fatty acids, lipid metabolism, imaging, 349–390
  dual parameter analysis, dynamic, noninvasively measuring metabolism, 351–352
  instruments, 352
  living organism, constraints of measuring, 350–351
  myocardial fatty acid metabolism, *354,* 354–357, *356*
    beta-methyl-*w*-(p-^{123}I-phenyl)-pentadecanoic acid, 371–376
    ^{11}C-palmitic acid, 357–362
    carbon chain, methylation of, 370–371
    w^{123}I-heptadecanoic acid, 362–365
    metabolic trapping, labeled fatty acids for, 368–371
    nuclide, non-carbon, insertion into carbon chain, 368–370, *369*
    w-(o-^{123}I-phenyl)pentadecanoic acid, 376–379

    w-(p-^{123}I-phenyl)pentadecanoic acid, 365–368
  types of labeled fatty acids, 352–354, *353*
  w^{123}I-hexadecanoic acid, 362–365
Left ventricular dysfunction
  heart failure, 3–4, *4*
  reversible, positron emission tomography, 391–394
Left ventricular remodeling, 9
Leucine, branched-chain amino acids, *97*
Lipid metabolism, labeled fatty acids, imaging, 349–390
  dual parameter analysis, dynamic, noninvasively measuring metabolism, 351–352
  instruments, 352
  living organism, constraints of measuring, 350–351
  myocardial fatty acid metabolism, *354,* 354–357, *356*
    beta-methyl-*w*-(p-^{123}I-phenyl)-pentadecanoic acid, 371–376
    ^{11}C-palmitic acid, 357–362
    carbon chain, methylation of, 370–371
    w^{123}I-heptadecanoic acid, 362–365
    metabolic trapping, labeled fatty acids for, 368–371
    nuclide, non-carbon, insertion into carbon chain, 368–370, *369*
    w-(o-^{123}I-phenyl)pentadecanoic acid, 376–379
    w-(p-^{123}I-phenyl)pentadecanoic acid, 365–368
  types of labeled fatty acids, 352–354, *353*
  w^{123}I-hexadecanoic acid, 362–365
Long-axis slice, creation of, *166*

Magnetic resonance, nuclear, 419–436
  chemical shift, shift reagents, 431
  contrast agents, *423,* 423–425, *424*
  dipyridamole, 423
  dobutamine, 422–423
  ischemia, 422
  ischemic heart disease, 419–425
  magnetic resonance coronary angiography, *421,* 421–422
  magnetic resonance spectroscopy, 426, 426t
  phosphorus-31 nuclear magnetic resonance, *427,* 427–429
Magnetic resonance spectroscopy, 426, 426t

Match, mismatch, contraction-perfusion, 4–5, *5*
Mechanical restitution, fuels, 91–104
  acetoacetate, CoASH, 2-oxoglutarate, NAD+, intramitochondrial concentrations of, mitochondria oxidizing, 96t
  anaplerosis, 96–98, *97, 98*
  branched-chain amino acids, *97*
  cardiac metabolism, control, regulation of, 92t
  citric acid cycle, depletion of, *95,* 95–96, 96t
  CoASH, 2-oxoglutarate, NAD+, intramitochondrial concentrations of, mitochondria oxidizing, 96t
  fatty acids
    metabolism of, regulatory sites in, *95*
    oxidative metabolism pathways, *99*
  glucose
    metabolism of, regulatory sites in, *95*
    oxidative metabolism pathways, *99*
  isoleucine, branched-chain amino acids, *97*
  ketone bodies
    to acetyl-CoA, metabolism of, regulatory sites in, *95*
    oxidative metabolism pathways, *99*
  leucine, branched-chain amino acids, *97*
  moiety-conserved cycles, 98–99, *99*
    cardiovascular system, 94t
    ischemic heart muscle, depletion, replenishment of, *100,* 100–101
  pyruvate metabolism, in heart muscle, carboxylation, decarboxylation pathways, *98*
  pyruvate or acetoacetate, CoASH, 2-oxoglutarate, NAD+, intramitochondrial concentrations of, mitochondria oxidizing, 96t
  respiration, control of, 98–99, *99*
  valine, branched-chain amino acids, *97*
Medical therapy, heart failure, 9–11, *10*
Metabolic imaging, gated perfusion, 171–177
Metabolic trapping, labeled fatty acids for, 368–371
Metabolism, 249–436
  control, regulation of, 92t

Microvascular integrity, dobutamine stress echocardiogram, 218–221, *219, 220*
Mismatch, match, contraction-perfusion, 4–5, *5*
Mitochondria
  nitric oxide, 109–110, *110*
  oxidizing pyruvate, acetoacetate, NAD+, 2-oxoglutarate, 96t
Model
  experimental, 79–90
    copper coil model, *83,* 83–84
    coronary artery, transient occlusion, 86–87
    electrical injury model, 79–82, *80, 81, 82*
    everted segment model, 86
    Folts' model, 84–86, *85*
    irreversibly injured myocardium, histological detection, 87
    reversed electrical potentials, thrombus formation in aortas, model, 80
    thrombin injection model, 86
    thrombosis
      coronary artery
      coronary artery occlusion by, 87–88
  tracer kinetics
    application to cardiac studies, 257
    complicated, 262, *262*
    simple, 251–257, *252, 254, 255, 256*
    three-compartment, *262*
Moiety-conserved cycles, 94t, 98–99, *99*
  ischemic heart muscle, depletion, replenishment of, *100,* 100–101
Myocardial cell death, 5–7
  apoptosis, 5–7, *6*
  necrosis, 5
Myocardial fatty acid metabolism, *354,* 354–357, *356*
Myocardial infarction, acute, thallium imaging after, 270
Myocardial perfusion tracers, technetium-99m-labeled, 315–348
  acute coronary artery disease, 332–337
  chronic coronary artery disease, *326,* 326–332
  technetium-99m-bis nitrido technetium, 340–341
  technetium-99m-furifosmin, 340
  technetium-99m sestamibi, 317–326
  technetium-99m-teboroxime, 337–338

technetium-99m-tetrofosmin, *338,* 338–340, *339*
Myocardial salvage, timing, 233–248
    fibrinolytic therapy, *236,* 236–237, *237*
    infarct size
        left ventricular function, 238–240, *239*
        relationship between, *239*
    National Heart Attack Alert Program, 242t
    perfusion, 249–436
    recanalization, angiographic, patency, 237–238
    reperfusion strategies, patency profile, *243*
    revascularization multicenter trials, salvage, 233–248
    streptokinase
        intracoronary, 234
        for occluded coronary artery trials, 240–242, 241t, *242*
    thrombolytic agents, 235
    thrombolytic multicenter trials, salvage, 233–248
    thrombolytic therapy, mortality, 234–235, *237*
Myocardial stunning, 25–36
Myocardial uptake, quantitating, tracer kinetics, 263–264, *264*
Myocardium
    morphological, echocardiographic features, 207–232
    stunned
        contractile reserve, 182–183, *183*
        thallium-201 scintigraphy, protocol for identifying, 291–293, *292, 293*
Myocyte, with major metabolic pathways, regulatory steps, 14
Myocyte dysfunction, reversible, 210–211, 211t
Myocyte membrane integrity, dobutamine stress echocardiogram, 218

NAD+, 2-oxoglutarate, mitochondria oxidizing, pyruvate, acetoacetate, 96t
National Heart Attack Alert Program, 242t
Necrosis, cell, 5
Nitric oxide, 105–113
    cellular targets, 108t, 108–109, *109*
    L-argine, chemical structure, *106*

mitochondria, 109–110, *110*
molecular targets, 108t, 108–109, *109*
    nitric oxide, 108t, 108–109, *109*
oxygen consumption, whole animal, 110–111
pathophysiology, 111–112
physiology, 109–111
respiration, control of, 109–111
synthase, regulation of, 107–108
synthesis, 105–107, *106*
    localization of, 107
No-reflow phenomenon, thallium imaging, *293*
Nonmyocyte compartment, 211–212
Nonsarcolemmal channels, 118–128
Nuclear magnetic resonance, 419–436
    chemical shift, shift reagents, 431
    contrast agents, *423,* 423–425, *424*
    dipyridamole, 423
    dobutamine, 422–423
    ischemia, 422
    ischemic heart disease, 419–425
    magnetic resonance coronary angiography, *421,* 421–422
    magnetic resonance spectroscopy, 426, 426t
    phosphorus-31 nuclear magnetic resonance, *427,* 427–429
Nuclide, non-carbon, insertion into carbon chain, 368–370, *369*

Occluded coronary artery trials, streptokinase, myocardial salvage, timing, 240–242, 241t, *242*
Osmotic fragility curves, ischemia, 61
W-(o-^{123}I-phenyl)pentadecanoic acid, 376–379
W-(p-^{123}I-phenyl)pentadecanoic acid, 365–368
Oxidative metabolism pathways
    fatty acids, *99*
    glucose, *99*
2-oxoglutarate
    CoASH, acetoacetate, NAD+, intramitochondrial concentrations of, mitochondria oxidizing, 96t
    NAD+, mitochondria oxidizing, pyruvate, acetoacetate, 96t
Oxygen consumption, whole animal, nitric oxide and, 110–111

P-type Ca^{2+} channel, 132
P38 MAPK, tyrosine 182 of,
    phosphorylation, 60
Partial volume effects, correction for,
    tracer kinetics, *260*, 260–262
Patency profile, reperfusion strategies,
    myocardial salvage, timing, *243*
Perfusion
    contraction, mismatch, match, 4–5, *5*
    gated, metabolic imaging, 171–177
    myocardial salvage, timing, 249–436
Perfusion/metabolism scans, gated,
    global function, 175–176
Pharmacologic preconditioning, 63–64
Phosphorus-31 nuclear magnetic
    resonance, *427*, 427–429
Positron emission tomography, 391–418
    ^{18}F-2-deoxyglucose, 397–398
    with coronary artery disease, 400–410
    with diabetes mellitus, 397–398
    dietary state of patient, 397
    reversible left ventricular dysfunction,
        391–394
    single photon emission computerized
        tomography, dobutamine
        echocardiography, compared,
        contractile reserve, 193–197,
        194
Postextrasystolic potentiation, contractile
    reserve assessment, 222
Preconditioning, 55–75
    anti-infarct effect of, models, 56–57
    end effector, 62–63
    in humans, 64–66
    ischemia, multiple mediators, *59*, 59–60
    ischemic, 25–36
    natural history of, 55–56
    osmotic fragility curves, ischemia, 61
    pharmacologic, 63–64
    protection, second window, 66–67
    protein kinase C, signal transduction
        pathway for, 57–59, *58*
    receptors, 57
    signal transduction pathway, 59
    tyrosine 182 of p38 MAPK,
        phosphorylation, 60
    tyrosine kinases, *60*, 60–62, *61*
Programmed cell survival, *26*, 26–27, *27*
Protein kinase C, signal transduction
    pathway for, 57–59, *58*
Protocols, thallium, 271–283, *272*
    late redistribution imaging, 275–277,
        276

    stress-3- to-4-hour-redistribution
        imaging, 273–275
    thallium reinjection, *277*, 277–283
Pyruvate
    acetoacetate, CoASH, 2-oxoglutarate,
        NAD+, intramitochondrial
        concentrations of, mitochondria
        oxidizing, 96t
    mitochondria oxidizing, acetoacetate,
        NAD+, 2-oxoglutarate, 96t
Pyruvate metabolism, in heart muscle,
    carboxylation, decarboxylation
    pathways, *98*

Recanalization, angiographic, patency, myo-
    cardial salvage, timing, 237–238
Receptors, preconditioning, 57
Regional function
    from gated bloodpool single photon
        emission computer tomography,
        169–171, *170*
    from gated perfusion/metabolism
        images, 171–175, *172, 173*
Regulatory steps, myocyte, with major
    metabolic pathways, 14
Remodeling, ventricular, left, 9
Reperfusion injury, 30
Reperfusion strategies, patency profile,
    myocardial salvage, timing, *243*
Reserve, contractile, 181–206
    after myocardial infarction, prognosis,
        186, 186–188, *187*
    clinical markers, myocardial viability,
        181–182
    dobutamine echocardiography
        after acute myocardial infarction,
            183–185, *184*
        single photon emission computerized
            tomography, positron emission
            tomography, compared, 193–
            197, *194*
    hibernating myocardium, 188–189
    Kaplan-Meier survival curves, *186, 193*
    left ventricular dysfunction
        acute, reversible, 182–188
        chronic, 189
            dobutamine echocardiography in,
                189, 189–192, *190, 191, 192*
        persistent, 188–193
    stunned myocardium, 182–183, *183*
    stunning, *versus* acute hibernation, *185*,
        185–186

Reserve assessment, contractile, postextrasystolic potentiation, 222

Respiration, control of, 98–99, *99*
nitric oxide, 109–111

Restitution, mechanical, fuels, 91–104
2-oxoglutarate, NAD+, mitochondria oxidizing, pyruvate, acetoacetate, 96t
acetoacetate, CoASH, 2-oxoglutarate, NAD+, intramitochondrial concentrations of, mitochondria oxidizing, 96t
anaplerosis, 96–98, *97, 98*
branched-chain amino acids, *97*
cardiac metabolism, control, regulation of, 92t
citric acid cycle, depletion of, *95,* 95–96, 96t
CoASH, 2-oxoglutarate, NAD+, intramitochondrial concentrations of, mitochondria oxidizing, 96t
fatty acids
metabolism of, regulatory sites in, *95*
oxidative metabolism pathways, *99*
glucose
metabolism of, regulatory sites in, *95*
oxidative metabolism pathways, *99*
isoleucine, branched-chain amino acids, *97*
ketone bodies
to acetyl-CoA, metabolism of, regulatory sites in, *95*
oxidative metabolism pathways, *99*
leucine, branched-chain amino acids, *97*
moiety-conserved cycles, 98–99, *99*
cardiovascular system, 94t
ischemic heart muscle, depletion, replenishment of, *100,* 100–101
pyruvate metabolism, in heart muscle, carboxylation, decarboxylation pathways, *98*
pyruvate or acetoacetate, CoASH, 2-oxoglutarate, NAD+, intramitochondrial concentrations of, mitochondria oxidizing, 96t
respiration, control of, 98–99, *99*
valine, branched-chain amino acids, *97*

Reticulum, sarcoplasmic, 118–128

Revascularization, *11,* 11–12, *12*

Revascularization multicenter trials, myocardial salvage, timing, salvage, 233–248

Revascularization response, diagnostic features, asynergic myocardium, ischemic heart disease, 208t

Reversed electrical potentials, thrombus formation in aortas, model, 80

Reversible myocardial dysfunction, 37–54
coronary flow, in early postischemic period, 39–41, *40*
flow limitation, regional, global responses to, 47
flow reduction, hibernation, short-term, 42–44
hibernation, chronic, models of, 44–45
hypocontractile myocardium, resting flow in, 47–49, *49*
ischemia, hibernation, short-term, 42–44
myocardial oxygen consumption, in early postischemic period, 39–41, *40*
porportionate, disproportionate reductions in flow, function, distinguishing, 41–42, *42*
structural changes, mechanisms underlying, 46–47
stunning, *versus* hibernation, 37–38

Ryanodine receptor, *118,* 118–127, *119, 120, 121, 122, 123, 124, 124–125, 127*

Safety, dobutamine stress echocardiogram, with reduced left ventricular systolic function, 221–222

Salvage, myocardial, timing, 233–248
fibrinolytic therapy, *236,* 236–237, *237*
infarct size
left ventricular function, 238–240, *239*
relationship between, *239*
National Heart Attack Alert Program, 242t
perfusion, 249–436
recanalization, angiographic, patency, 237–238
reperfusion strategies, patency profile, *243*
revascularization multicenter trials, salvage, 233–248
streptokinase
intracoronary, 234

for occluded coronary artery trials, 240–242, 241t, *242*

thrombolytic agents, 235

thrombolytic multicenter trials, salvage, 233–248

thrombolytic therapy, mortality, 234–235, *237*

Sarcolemmal channels, 128–147

Sarcoplasmic reticulum, 118–128

Scintigraphy

  thallium, with reinjection, low-dose transesophageal echocardiography, concordance, 14

  thallium-201, 265–314

    clinical applications, 270–271

    ^{18}F-fluoro-deoxyglucose imaging, 294–300

    historical background, 265–270

    prognostic value of, 300–304

    protocol, 271–283, *272*

      identifying chronic coronary artery disease, 289–291, *290*

      for identifying stunned myocardium, 291–293, *292, 293*

      strengths, thallium reinjection, 283–289

      weaknesses

        recent advances, 304–305

        thallium reinjection, 283–289

Segmental asynergy, left, ventricular, structural correlates, reversible, irreversible, 209–212

Sestamibi, technetium-99m, 317–326

Shift reagents, chemical shift, nuclear magnetic resonance, 431

Signal transduction pathway, 59

Signal transduction pathway for protein kinase C, 57–59, *58*

Single photon emission computer tomography

  acquisition of, 176–177

  dobutamine echocardiography, compared, contractile reserve, 193–197, *194*

  gated, acquisition of, 176–177

  gated bloodpool acquisition, 165–167, *166*

  positron emission tomography, dobutamine echocardiography, compared, contractile reserve, 193–197, *194*

Single photon emission tomography imaging

  attenuation correction, 305

  gated thallium, 304–305, *305*

  instrumentation, advances, 304–305

  technology, advances, 304–305

Size, infarct, myocardial salvage, timing, relationship between, *239*

Sodium channel, 142–145, *143, 144*

Sodium channel structure, *143*

SPECT imaging. *See* Single photon emission tomography imaging

Spillover, correction for, tracer kinetics, *260*, 260–262

Streptokinase

  intracoronary, myocardial salvage, timing, 234

  for occluded coronary artery trials, myocardial salvage, timing, 240–242, 241t, *242*

Stress-redistribution-reinjection thallium SPECT, FDG, SPECT FDG PET, concordance between, 16

Structural changes, ischemic cardiomyopathy, 7–8, *8*

Stunning, 25–36

  contractile reserve, 182–183, *183*

  ischemia, 116–117, 151–153

  thallium-201 scintigraphy, protocol for identifying, 291–293, *292, 293*

  versus acute hibernation, contractile reserve, *185*, 185–186

Survival

  cell, programmed, *26*, 26–27, *27*

  for medically treated, surgically treated patients, 11

T-type Ca^{2+} channel, 132

Teboroxime, technetium-99m, 337–338

Technetium-99m-bis nitrido technetium, 340–341

Technetium-99m-furifosmin, 340

Technetium-99m-labeled myocardial perfusion tracers, 315–348

  acute coronary artery disease, 332–337

  chronic coronary artery disease, *326*, 326–332

  technetium-99m-bis nitrido technetium, 340–341

  technetium-99m-furifosmin, 340

  technetium-99m sestamibi, 317–326

  technetium-99m-teboroxime, 337–338

technetium-99m-tetrofosmin, *338,* *338*–340, *339*

Technetium-99m sestamibi, 317–326

Technetium-99m-teboroxime, 337–338

Technetium-99m-tetrofosmin, *338,* 338–340, *339*

Tetrofosmin, technetium-99m, *338,* 338–340, *339*

Thallium-201 scintigraphy, 265–314
  clinical applications, 270–271
  ^{18}F-fluoro-deoxyglucose imaging, 294–300
  historical background, 265–270
  prognostic value of, 300–304
  protocol, 271–283, *272*
    identifying chronic coronary artery disease, 289–291, *290*
    for identifying stunned myocardium, 291–293, *292, 293*
  strengths, thallium reinjection, 283–289
  weaknesses
    recent advances, 304–305
    thallium reinjection, 283–289

Thallium protocols, 271–283, *272*
  late redistribution imaging, 275–277, *276*
  stress-3- to-4-hour-redistribution imaging, 273–275
  thallium reinjection, *277,* 277–283

Thallium scintigraphy, with reinjection, low-dose transesophageal echocardiography, concordance, 14

Three-compartment model, tracer kinetics, *262*

Thrombin injection model, myocardial viability, 86

Thrombolytic agents, myocardial salvage, timing, 235

Thrombolytic multicenter trials, salvage, myocardial salvage, timing, 233–248

Thrombolytic therapy, myocardial salvage, timing, mortality, 234–235, *237*

Thrombosis
  coronary artery
    electrical injury model, 82
    model, 81
  coronary artery occlusion by, 87–88

Timing, myocardial salvage, 233–248
  fibrinolytic therapy, *236,* 236–237, *237*
  infarct size

left ventricular function, 238–240, *239*
  relationship between, *239*

National Heart Attack Alert Program, 242t

perfusion, 249–436

recanalization, angiographic, patency, 237–238

reperfusion strategies, patency profile, *243*

revascularization multicenter trials, salvage, 233–248

streptokinase
  intracoronary, 234
  for occluded coronary artery trials, 240–242, 241t, *242*

thrombolytic agents, 235

thrombolytic multicenter trials, salvage, 233–248

thrombolytic therapy, mortality, 234–235, *237*

Tissue time activity curve, measuring, *259,* 259–260

Tomographic gated bloodpool, global function, 167–169, *168, 169*

Tracer kinetics, 251–264
  arterial input function, measuring, 257–259, *258*
  complicated models, 262, *262*
  kinetic models, application to cardiac studies, 257
  myocardial uptake, quantitating, 263–264, *264*
  partial volume effects, correction for, *260,* 260–262
  simple model, 251–257, *252, 254, 255, 256*
  spillover, correction for, *260,* 260–262
  three-compartment model, *262*
  tissue time activity curve, measuring, *259,* 259–260

Transient occlusion, coronary artery, model, 86–87

Transplantation, heart, 12–13

Treatment options, heart failure, 9–13
  heart transplantation, 12–13
  medical therapy, 9–11, *10*
  revascularization, *11,* 11–12, *12*

Tyrosine 182, of p38 MAPK, phosphorylation, 60

Tyrosine kinases, preconditioning, *60,* 60–62, *61*

Uptake, myocardial, quantitating, tracer kinetics, 263–264, *264*

Valine, branched-chain amino acids, *97*
Vascular biology, 77–159
Ventricular dysfunction, left
    acute, reversible, contractile reserve, 182–188
    chronic, contractile reserve, 189
        dobutamine echocardiography in, *189,* 189–192, *190, 191, 192*
        persistent, 188–193
    heart failure, 3–4, *4*
    reversible, positron emission tomography, 391–394
Ventricular function, left, infarct size, myocardial salvage, timing, 238–240, *239*
Ventricular function measurement, 163–180
    gated bloodpool tomography, 164–171
    gated perfusion, metabolic imaging, 171–177
    gated single photon emission computer tomography
        perfusion/metabolism images, acquisition of, 176–177
    global function
        from gated perfusion/metabolism scans, 175–176
        from tomographic gated bloodpool, 167–169, *168, 169*
    long-axis slice, creation of, *166*
    regional function
        from gated bloodpool single photon emission computer tomography, 169–171, *170*
        from gated perfusion/metabolism images, 171–175, *172, 173*
    single photon emission computer tomography, gated bloodpool acquisition, 165–167, *166*
Ventricular remodeling, left, 9
Ventricular systolic function, left, reduced, safety, dobutamine stress echocardiogram, 221–222

Viability, myocardium, 3–22
    cardiomyopathy, ischemic
        histomorphological changes, 7–8, *8*
        structural changes, 7–8, *8*
    contraction-perfusion, mismatch, match, 4–5, *5*
    definition of, 16–18, *17*
    diagnostic techniques, *13,* 13–16, *14, 15*
    heart failure
        left ventricular dysfunction, 3–4, *4*
        treatment options, 9–13
    ischemic cardiomyopathy
        histomorphological changes, 7–8, *8*
        structural changes, 7–8, *8*
    left ventricular dysfunction, heart failure, 3–4, *4*
    left ventricular remodeling, 9
    myocardial cell death, 5–7
        apoptosis, 5–7, *6*
        necrosis, 5
    myocyte, with major metabolic pathways, regulatory steps, 14
    perfusion, contraction, mismatch, match, 4–5, *5*
    remodeling, ventricular, left, 9
    stress-redistribution-reinjection thallium SPECT, FDG SPECT, FDG PET, concordance between, 16
    survival, for medically treated, surgically treated patients, 11
    thallium scintigraphy, with reinjection, low-dose transesophageal echocardiography, concordance, 14
    treatment options, heart failure, 9–13
        heart transplantation, 12–13
        medical therapy, 9–11, *10*
        revascularization, *11,* 11–12, *12*
    ventricular dysfunction, left, heart failure, 3–4, *4*
    ventricular remodeling, left, 9